EVIDENCE-BASED PRACTICE
in Nursing & Healthcare
A GUIDE TO BEST PRACTICE

EVIDENCE-BASED PRACTICE
in Nursing & Healthcare
A GUIDE TO BEST PRACTICE

● **Bernadette Mazurek Melnyk, PhD, RN, CPNP/NPP, FAAN, FNAP**
Dean and Distinguished Foundation Professor in Nursing
Arizona State University
College of Nursing
Tempe, Arizona
Associate Editor, *Worldviews on Evidence-Based Nursing*
Founder and Director, the National Association of Pediatric Nurse Practitioners'
  (NAPNAP)
KySS (Keep your children/yourself Safe and Secure) Mental Health Promotion Campaign.

● **Ellen Fineout-Overholt, PhD, RN**
Clinical Associate Professor
Director, the Center for Advancement of Evidence-Based Practice
Arizona State University
College of Nursing
Tempe, Arizona

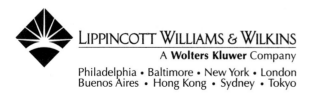

LIPPINCOTT WILLIAMS & WILKINS
A **Wolters Kluwer** Company
Philadelphia • Baltimore • New York • London
Buenos Aires • Hong Kong • Sydney • Tokyo

Acquisitions Editor: Elizabeth Nieginski
Managing Editor: Helen Kogut
Developmental Editor: Deedie McMahon
Editorial Assistant: Josh Levandowski
Production Editor: Diane Griffith
Director of Nursing Production: Helen Ewan
Managing Editor / Production: Erika Kors

Art Director: Carolyn O'Brien
Cover: BJ Crim
Senior Manufacturing Manager: William Alberti
Indexer: Alexandra Nickerson
Compositor: Lippincott Williams & Wilkins
Printer: R.R. Donnelley–Crawfordsville

9 8 7 6 5 4 3

Library of Congress Cataloging-in-Publication Data
Melnyk, Bernadette M.
   Evidence-based practice in nursing & healthcare : a guide to best practice / Bernadette M. Melnyk and Ellen Fineout-Overholt.
      p. ; cm.
   Includes bibliographical references and index.
   ISBN 0-7817-4477-6 (alk. paper)
   1. Evidence-based nursing. 2. Evidence-based medicine. I. Title: Evidence-based practice in nursing and healthcare. II. Fineout-Overholt, Ellen. III. Title.
   [DNLM: 1. Evidence-Based Medicine--methods. 2. Nursing--methods. 3. Nurse Clinicians. WY 100 M526e 2005]
   RT42.M44 2005
   610.73—dc22

                                                                        2004009913

Care has been taken to confirm the accuracy of the information presented and to describe generally accepted practices. However, the authors, editors, and publisher are not responsible for errors or omissions or for any consequences from application of the information in this book and make no warranty, express or implied, with respect to the content of the publication.

The authors, editors, and publisher have exerted every effort to ensure that drug selection and dosage set forth in this text are in accordance with the current recommendations and practice at the time of publication. However, in view of ongoing research, changes in government regulations, and the constant flow of information relating to drug therapy and drug reactions, the reader is urged to check the package insert for each drug for any change in indications and dosage and for added warnings and precautions. This is particularly important when the recommended agent is a new or infrequently employed drug.

   Some drugs and medical devices presented in this publication have Food and Drug Administration (FDA) clearance for limited use in restricted research settings. It is the responsibility of the health care provider to ascertain the FDA status of each drug or device planned for use in his or her clinical practice.

LWW.com

I dedicate this book to my loving and supportive family: my husband, John;
and my three daughters; Angela, Megan, and Kaylin; as well as to my father,
who always taught me that anything can be accomplished with
a spirit of enthusiasm and determination.

Bernadette Mazurek Melnyk

This book is dedicated in loving memory to my Dad, Arthur J. Fineout,
who taught me to think critically, apply what I learned, and never give up.

Ellen Fineout-Overholt

contributors

Chapter Contributors
(listed in alphabetical order)

Patricia E. Benner, RN, PhD, FAAN, FRCN
Professor & Thelma Shobe Endowed Chair in
    Ethical and Spiritual Dimensions of Nursing
    Care, Department of Social and Behavioral
    Sciences
University of California San Francisco
San Francisco, California
Chapter 7

Cecily Betz, PhD, RN, FAAN
Assistant Professor
University of Southern California
Department of Nursing
Los Angeles, California
Editor, *Journal of Pediatric Nursing*
Chapter 14

Donna Ciliska, RN, PhD
Professor, School of Nursing
McMaster University
Ontario, Canada
Chapter 8

Robert Cole, PhD, MS
Associate Professor of Clinical Nursing
Center for High-Risk Children and Youth
University of Rochester School of Nursing
Rochester, New York
Chapter 10

John F. Cox III, MD
Clinical Instructor in Medicine
University of Rochester
School of Medicine and Dentistry
Rochester, New York
Chapter 15

Alba DiCenso, BScN, MSc, PhD
Professor and Joint Member
School of Nursing and Clinical Epidemiology and
    Biostatistics
McMaster University
Faculty of Health Sciences
Health Sciences Centre
Ontario, Canada
Chapter 8

Y'Vonne Lane Gray, MS, RN
Visiting Assistant Professor
School of Nursing
Adelphi University
Garden City, New York
Chapter 15

Gail Ingersoll, EdD, RN, FAAN, FNAP
Professor of Nursing
Director of Clinical Nursing Research
Director, Office of Evaluation
University of Rochester Medical Center
Rochester, New York
Chapter 12

Linda Johnston, PhD, RN
Professor and Chair, Neonatal Nursing Research
The Royal Children's Hospital and
The University of Melbourne
Deputy Director
The Victorian Centre for Nursing Practice
    Research
Melbourne, Australia
Chapter 5

Victoria Wynn Leonard, RN, FNP, PhD
Assistant Professor
University of San Francisco School of Nursing
San Francisco, California
Chapter 7

Richard Nollan, MLS, MA, AHIP
Assistant Professor & Special Collections
    Librarian
The University of Tennessee Health Science
    Center Library
Memphis, Tennessee
Chapters 2 & 3

Bethel Ann Powers, RN, PhD
Associate Professor
Associate Director, Center for Clinical Research
    on Aging
University of Rochester School of Nursing
Rochester, New York
Chapters 6 & 11, Appendices B & F

Tom Rickey, BA
Manager of National Media Relations & Senior
    Science Editor
University of Rochester Medical Center
Rochester, New York
Chapter 14

Brett Robbins, MD
Assistant Professor of Internal Medicine and
    Pediatrics
School of Medicine and Dentistry
Residency Program Director, Medicine-Pediatrics
    Residency Program
University of Rochester Medical Center
Rochester, New York
Chapter 15

Jean Slutsky, PA, MSPH
Acting Director
Center for Outcomes and Evidence
Director, National Guidelines Clearinghouse
Agency for Healthcare Research
    and Quality
Washington, DC
Chapter 9

Kathryn Smith, RN, MN
California Medical Home Project
Los Angeles Medical Home Project
CCS Workgroup
Assistant Nursing Director
University Southern California University
    Affiliated Program
Children's Hospital Los Angeles
Los Angeles, California
Chapter 14

Julia F. Sollenberger, MLS
Director, Health Science Libraries and
    Technologies
Assistant Professor of Medical Informatics
University of Rochester Medical Center
Rochester, New York
Chapter 3

Priscilla L. Stephenson, MSLS, MSEd
Academy of Health Information Professionals
Assistant Professor, Coordinator, Reference
    Services
University of Tennessee Health Science Center,
    Health Sciences Library and
    Biocommunications Center
Memphis, Tennessee
Chapters 2 & 3

Cheryl Stetler, PhD, RN, FAAN
Specialist for Evidence-Based Practice
Amherst, Massachusetts
Chapter 8

Kathleen R. Stevens, RN, EdD, FAAN
Professor and Director
Academic Center for Evidence-Based Nursing
The University of Texas Health Science Center at
    San Antonio
San Antonio, Texas
Chapter 4

● **Appendices**

Rona F. Levin PhD, RN
Project Director, Joan M. Stout, RN
Evidence Based Practice Initiative
Lienhard School of Nursing
Pace University
Pleasantville, New York
Professor Emeritus
Felician College
Lodi, New Jersey
Appendix E

Joanne K. Singleton, PhD, RN, CS, FNP
Professor, Leinhard School of Nursing
Pace University
New York, New York
Appendix E

Harriet R. Feldman, PhD, RN
Dean and Professor in Nursing
Leinhard School of Nursing
Pace University at Pleasantville
New York, New York
Appendix E

Nancy Watson, PhD, RN
Director, Center for Clinical Research on Aging
University of Rochester School of Nursing
Rochester, New York
Appendix J

- ## Specialty Evidence Review Chapters on CD-ROM

Chapter 18 Acute and Critical Care

Editors

Anne W. Wojner, PhD, RN, CCRN
Assistant Professor of Neurology & Neuroscience
    Critical Care Medicine
University of Texas–Houston, Stroke Team
Medical School, Department of Neurology
Houston, Texas

and

Jill T. Jesurum, PhD, ARNP, ACNP
Clinical Scientist
Department of Cardiovascular Research
Swedish Medical Center
Seattle, Washington

Contributors
(*listed in alphabetical order*)

Patti L. Barkley, RN, BSN
Cardiovascular Outcomes Manager
St. Luke's Episcopal Hospital
Houston, Texas

Quana D. Bert, ARNP, MSN, RN-C
Clinical Effectiveness
Cardiac Outcomes Data Coordinator
Swedish Medical Center
Seattle, Washington

Jan Foster, PhD, RN, CNS, CCRN
Assistant Professor of Nursing
Texas Woman's University
Houston, Texas

Sandra K. Hanneman, PhD, RN, FAAN
Associate Dean for Research
Center for Nursing Research
University of Texas Health Science
    Center–Houston
Houston, Texas

Robin Hardwicke, RN, MSN, CCRN, FNP-C
Texas Woman's University
Doctoral Student
Houston, Texas

Janie Heath, RN, PhD(c), CCRN, ANP, ACNP
Assistant Professor and Director
Acute Care NP & Critical Care CNS Program
Georgetown University
School of Nursing and Health Studies
Washington, DC

Susan Houston, RN, PhD, CNAA, FAAN
Assistant Vice President
St. Luke's Episcopal Hospital
Houston, Texas

Dorothy M. Kite-Powell, MSN, RN, CCRN, CNS
Manager, Outcomes Management and Research
St. Luke's Episcopal Hospital
Houston, Texas

Srisuda Lecagoonporn, RN, MSN
Texas Woman's University
Doctoral Student
Houston, Texas

Carolyn C. Lewis, MN, RN
Texas Woman's University
Doctoral Student
Houston, Texas

Susan Parnell, RN, MSN, MPH, CIC
Texas Woman's University
Doctoral Student
Houston, Texas

Joya D. Pickett, RN, MSN, CCRN
Critical Care Clinical Nurse Specialist
Swedish Medical Center
Clinical Faculty, University of Washington
Seattle, Washington

Vicki M. Pruitt, RN, BSN, CIC
Infection Control Practitioner
St. Luke's Episcopal Hospital
Houston, Texas

Susan Reed, MN, ARNP, CCRN
Cardiology Nurse Practitioner
Department of Cardiovascular Research
Swedish Medical Center
Seattle, Washington

Lisa M Tedeschi, RN, MS
Faculty, Associate Degree Nursing Program
Bellevue Community College
Bellevue, Washington

Valerie P. Waldmeier, APRN, C-FNP
Texas Woman's University
Doctoral Student
Houston, Texas

Chapter 19 Adult Primary Care

Editors

Joanne K. Singleton, PhD, RN, CS, FNP
Professor, Leinhard School of Nursing
Pace University
New York, New York

Carol Green-Hernandez, PhD, ANP/FNP-BC
Associate Professor in the Primary Care Nurse
    Practitioner Program
University of Vermont
Burlington, Vermont

and

Edwin McMillan, MS, RN, FNP
Director, The Institute for Healthy Aging
Leinhard School of Nursing
Pace University
New York, New York

Contributors
(listed in alphabetical order)

Maria Claudia Escobar, RN, FNP, MPH
Sidney Hillman Family Practice
New York, New York

Joyce Knestrick, PhD, FNP
Associate Professor
Wheeling Jesuit University
Wheeling, West Virginia

Mary McCormack, APNC, MSN, MPH
The Medical Institute of New Jersey
Cedar Knolls, New Jersey

Randi Moskowitz, RN, MPH, MBA
Manager, Oncology Services
Saint Vincent Catholic Medical Centers
Brooklyn/Queens Service Division
Jamaica, New York

Mary B. Neiheisel, BSN, MSN, EdD, CNS,
  APRN-FNP
Professor of Nursing
Pfizer/Ardoin Endowed Professor
College of Nursing and Allied Health Professions
University of Louisiana at Lafayette and Faith
    House
Lafayette, Louisiana

Jill R. Quinn, PhD, RN, CS-ANP
Assistant Professor, Center for Clinical Research
    on Aging
University of Rochester School of Nursing
Rochester, New York

Agatha A. Quinn, PhD, APRN, FNP, CNS
Associate Professor
University of Colorado Health Sciences Center
Denver, Colorado

Chapter 20 Aging Adults

Editor

Margaret J. Bull, PhD, RN, FAAN
Professor
Marquette University
College of Nursing
Milwaukee, Wisconsin

Contributors
(listed in alphabetical order)

Fay L. Bower, DNSc, FAAN
Chair, Department of Nursing
Holy Names College
Oakland, California
Acquisitions Editor for Books
Sigma Theta Tau International

Merrie J. Kaas, DNSc, RN, CS
Associate Professor
University of Minnesota School of Nursing
Minneapolis, Minnesota

Hong Li, PhD, RN
Assistant Professor, Center for Research on Aging
University of Rochester School of Nursing
Rochester, New York

Cyndi S. McCullough, MSN
Senior Consultant
HDR, Inc.
Omaha, Nebraska

Ruth E. McShane, PhD, RN
Clinical Assistant Professor
RN-BSN-MSN Program Coordinator
Marquette University
College of Nursing
Milwaukee, Wisconsin

Mary H. Palmer, PhD, RNC, FAAN
Helen W. and Thomas L. Umphlet Distinguished
    Professor in Aging
Professor, University of North Carolina Chapel Hill
School of Nursing
Chapel Hill, North Carolina

Sarah A. Wilson, PhD, RN
Associate Professor
Marquette University
College of Nursing
Milwaukee, Wisconsin

Chapter 21 Emergency and Trauma Care

Editor

Lisa Marie Bernardo, RN, PhD, MPH
Associate Professor
University of Pittsburgh School of Nursing
Pittsburgh, Pennsylvania

Contributors
(listed in alphabetical order)

Bonnie J. Clemence, RN, MSN
Nurse Consultant
Mechanicsburg, Pennsylvania

Susan Hohenhaus, RN
Project Manager
EMSC Enhancing Pediatric Patient Safety
Duke University Medical Center
Columbia, South Carolina

Jessica Muto, SN
University of Pittsburgh School of Nursing
Pittsburgh, Pennsylvania

Ann M. Mitchell, PhD, RN
Assistant Professor of Nursing
University of Pittsburgh School of Nursing
Pittsburgh, Pennsylvania

Teresa J. Sakraida, DNSc, RN
Assistant Professor of Nursing
University of Pittsburgh School of Nursing
Pittsburgh, Pennsylvania

Renee Semonin-Holleran, RN, PhD, CEN, CCRN,
    CFRN
Chief Flight Nurse
Emergency Clinical Specialist
University Air Care
University of Cincinnati
Cincinnati, Ohio

Tener Goodwin Veenema, PhD, MPH, MS, CPNP
Associate Professor of Clinical Nursing
Center For High-Risk Children & Youth
University of Rochester School of Nursing
Department of Emergency Medicine
University of Rochester School of Medicine &
    Dentistry
Rochester, New York

Catherine Vladutui, MPH
Intern, CDC Emerging Leaders Program
Washington, D.C.

Kirstyn K. Zalice, CRNP
Instructor of Nursing
University of Pittsburgh School of Nursing
Pittsburgh, Pennsylvania

Chapter 22 High-risk Children and Youth

Editors

Marion E. Broome, PhD, RN, FAAN
Professor and Associate Dean
Center for Nursing Research
School of Nursing
University of Alabama at Birmingham
Birmingham, Alabama

and

Bernadette Mazurek Melnyk, PhD, RN,
    CPNP/NPP, FAAN
Associate Dean for Research and Professor
Director, Center for Research and Evidence-Based
    Practice and PNP and Dual PNP/Psychiatric
    Mental Health Programs
University of Rochester School of Nursing and
School of Medicine and Dentistry
Rochester, New York

Contributors

(listed in alphabetical order)

Marilyn J. Aten, PhD, RN
Associate Professor of Nursing
Center for High-Risk Children and Youth
University of Rochester School of Nursing
Rochester, New York

Michelle A. Beauchesne, DNSc, RN, CPNP
Associate Professor & Coordinator of Primary
    Care
School of Nursing
Bouve College of Health Sciences
Northeastern University
Boston, Massachusetts

Debra H. Brandon, PhD, RN
Duke University School of Nursing and
Duke University Medical Center
Durham, North Carolina

Margaret-Ann Carno, PhD, RNC, CCRN
Post Doctoral Fellow
Center for High Risk Children and Youth
University of Rochester School of Nursing
Rochester, New York

Mary Katharine Cornwell, MSN, RN, NNP
Memorial Hermann Children's Hospital
Houston, Texas

Michelle Czarnecki, MSN, RN, CPNP
Advanced Practice Nurse
Acute Pain Service
Jane B. Pettit Pain and Palliative Care Center
Children's Hospital of Wisconsin
Milwaukee, Wisconsin

Margaret Grey, DrPH, FAAN, CPNP
Independence Foundation Professor
Associate Dean for Research Affairs
Yale School of Nursing
New Haven, Connecticut

Donna Harris, MS, RN, PNP-CS
Clinical Nurse Specialist
Chronic Pain Service
Jane B. Pettit Pain and Palliative Care Center
Children's Hospital of Wisconsin
Milwaukee, Wisconsin

Myra Martz Huth, PhD, RN
Assistant Vice President
Center for Excellence
Cincinnati Children's Hospital Medical Center
Cincinnati, Ohio

Sheri Kanner, DNSc (c), CPNP
Doctoral Candidate
Yale School of Nursing
New Haven, Connecticut

Barbara Kelley, EdD, RN, MPH, CPNP
Associate Professor
Director of Graduate Program
School of Nursing
Bouve College of Health Sciences
Northeastern University
Boston, Massachusetts

Renee Ladwig, MSN, RN, CS
Clinical Nurse Specialist
Chronic Pain Service
Jane B. Pettit Pain and Palliative Care Center
Children's Hospital of Wisconsin
Milwaukee, Wisconsin

Dianne Morrison-Beedy, PhD, RN, WHNP
Brody Professor and Associate Professor of
    Nursing
Center for High-Risk Children and Youth
University of Rochester School of Nursing
Rochester, New York

Leigh Small, PhD, RN-CS, NP
Assistant Professor of Nursing and
Evidence-Based Practice Mentor
Center for High-Risk Children and Youth and
    Center for Research and Evidence-Based
    Practice
University of Rochester School of Nursing
Rochester, New York

Barbara S. Turner, RN, DNSc, FAAN
Associate Dean for Research
Duke University School of Nursing and
Duke University Medical Center
Durham, North Carolina

Barbara Velsor-Friedrich, PhD, RN
Associate Professor
Niehoff School of Nursing
Loyola University
Chicago, Illinois

Robin Whittemore, PhD, APRN
Associate Research Scientist and Lecturer
Yale School of Nursing
New Haven, Connecticut

Chapter 23 Psychiatric Mental Health

Editor

Patricia Wilke, MSN, RN
Clinical Instructor
Kent State University College of Nursing
Kent, Ohio

Contributors

(listed in alphabetical order)

Sarah P. Farrell, PhD, APRN, BC
Associate Professor
University of Virginia School of Nursing and
    Health Evaluation Sciences
School of Medicine
Charlottesville, Virginia

Alice R. Kempe, PhD, RN, CS
Associate Professor
Breen School of Nursing
Ursuline College
Pepperpike, Ohio

Rene Love, MSN, APRN, BC
Associate in Psychiatry
Community Mental Health Center
Vanderbilt University Medical Center
Nashville, Tennessee

Irma H. Mahone, MSN
Doctoral Student
University of Virginia
Charlottesville, Virginia

Wanda K. Mohr, PhD, RN, FAAN
Associate Professor
University of Medicine and Dentistry of New
    Jersey
Newark, New Jersey

Doris Noel Ugarriza, PhD
Associate Professor
University of Miami School of Nursing
Coral Gables, Florida

Jacqueline A. Zauszniewski, PhD, RNC
Associate Professor
Frances Payne Bolton School of Nursing
Case Western Reserve University
Cleveland, Ohio

reviewers

● Reviewers

Jane Barnsteiner, PhD, RN, FAAN
Professor of Pediatric Nursing
University of Pennsylvania
Philadelphia, Pennsylvania

Anne M. Berger, MS, MBA, RN
Doctoral Fellow
Connell School of Nursing
Boston College
Boston, Massachusetts

Jacqueline Byers, PhD, RN, CNAA
Associate Professor
School of Nursing
College of Health and Public Affairs
Orlando, Florida

Anita Carroll, EdD, MSN, RN
Director of the Associate Degree Nursing Program
Navarro College
Corsicana, Texas

Karla Dalley, RN, PhD
Assistant Professor of Nursing
School of Nursing
University of Nevada
Las Vegas, Nevada

Beulah E. Hall, RN EdD
Associate Professor of Nursing
Drexel University
College of Nursing and Health Professions
Philadelphia, Pennsylvania

Rita Hammer, PhD, RN, CS
Professor of Nursing
Quinnipiac University
Hamden, Connecticut

Carole Hanks, DrPH, MSPH, RN, FNP
Associate Professor
Louise Herrington School of Nursing
Baylor University
Waco, TX.

Lisa Hopp, PhD, RN
Associate Professor
School of Nursing
Purdue University Calumet
Hammond, Indiana

Roberta Kaplow, RN, PhD
Professor (Clinical)
Nell Hodgson Woodruff School of Nursing
Emory University
Atlanta, Georgia

Becky Keele-Smith, PhD, APRN, BC
Associate Professor of Nursing
Department of Nursing
New Mexico State University
Las Cruces, New Mexico

Peggy Leapley, PhD, RN, CNS, FNP-C
Professor and Director of Nurse Practitioner
    Program
California State University, Bakersfield
Bakersfield, California

Jane Lemke, RN, BHSc COHN MEd
Program Manager, Instructor
Occupational Health Nurse Certificate Program
Mohawk College
Hamilton Ontario, Canada.

Dorothy Lemmey, Ph.D., RN
Assistant Professor
Kent State University
Kent, Ohio

Eileen Lumb, MS RN FNP
Assistant Professor of Clinical Nursing
University of Rochester School Of Nursing
Rochester, New York

Marylou K. McHugh, RN, EdD
Adjunct Faculty
Drexel University and Temple University
Philadelphia, Pennsylvania

Margaret E. Miller, PhD, RN
Professor, MSN Faculty
Bellarmine University
Louisville, Kentucky

Diana M. L. Newman, EdD, RN
Associate Professor
The University of Massachusetts
Boston College of Nursing and Health Sciences
Boston, Massachusetts

Susan T. Pierce, EdD, MSN, RN
Associate Professor, College of Nursing
Northwestern State University
Shreveport, Louisiana

Margaret Prydun, PhD, RN
Assistant Professor
Texas Women's University
College of Nursing Houston Center
Houston, Texas

Nancy A. Sowan, PhD, RN
Associate Professor
College of Nursing and Health Sciences
University of Vermont
Burlington, Vermont

Kathleen O. Williams, PhD, RN
Assistant Professor
College of Nursing
Kent State University
Kent, Ohio

Michael Zito, MS
Associate Professor Physical Therapy
University of Connecticut
Storrs, Connecticut

foreword

Like many of you, I have appreciated healthcare through a range of experiences and perspectives. As someone who has delivered healthcare as a combat medic, paramedic, nurse, and trauma surgeon, the value of evidence-based practice is clear to me. Knowing what questions to ask, how to carefully evaluate the responses, maximize the knowledge and use of empirical evidence, and provide the most effective clinical assessments and interventions are important assets for every healthcare professional. The quality of U.S. and global healthcare depends upon clinicians being able to deliver on these and other best practices.

The Institute of Medicine calls for all healthcare professionals to be educated to deliver patient-centered care as members of an interdisciplinary team, emphasizing evidence-based practice, quality improvement approaches, and informatics. Although many practitioners support the use of evidence-based practice, and there are indications that our patients are better served when we apply evidence-based practice, there are challenges to successful implementation. One barrier is knowledge. Do we share a standard understanding of evidence-based practice and how such evidence can best be used? We need more textbooks and other references that clearly define and provide a standard approach to evidence-based practice.

Another significant challenge is the time between the publication of research findings and the translation of such information into practice. This challenge exists throughout public health. Determining the means of more rapidly moving from the brilliance that is our national medical research to applications that blend new science and compassionate care in our clinical systems is of interest to us all.

As healthcare professionals who currently use evidence-based practice, you recognize these challenges and others. Our patients benefit because we adopt, investigate, teach, and evaluate evidence-based practice. I encourage you to continue the excellent work to bring about greater understanding and a more generalizable approach to evidence-based practice.

Richard H. Carmona, MD, MPH, FACS
VADM, USPHS
United States Surgeon General

The 2001 IOM report, Crossing the Quality Chasm: A New Health System for the 21st Century, challenged health professionals to provide care based upon the best available scientific evidence. This is not an easy challenge to meet. That practice should be based upon high quality research is well accepted. The difficulty is in transferring such knowledge into the practice of clinicians, practice settings, and health policy. Melnyk and Fineout-Overholt's new book, *Evidence-Based Practice in Nursing and Healthcare*, is a significant addition to the field and will provide great impetus to the needed paradigm shift to evidence-based practice in nursing and related disciplines. The book offers the reader a clearly delineated and demystified pathway to the establishment of an evidence-based practice. The focus on both the individual—whether a clinician or a patient—and the systems in which care is provided is a particularly strong aspect of this book. Melnyk and Fineout-Overholt's book should be required reading in all master's programs. Their text has provided a blueprint for the future of nursing practice and a rigorously substantiated and clearly described means for nurse clinicians, educators, and administrators to participate in improving quality of care.

Janet D. Allan, PhD, RN, CS, FAAN
Dean and Professor
University of Maryland School of Nursing and
Vice-Chair, U.S. Preventive Services Task Force

preface

This book was written with our shared philosophy of "anything is possible if you have a big dream and believe in your ability to accomplish that dream." It was this vision and belief along with sheer persistence through many "character-building experiences" during the writing and editing of this book that have resulted in the culmination of a user-friendly guide that will assist advanced practice nurses, nurses, and other healthcare professionals in the delivery of the highest quality, evidence-based care in order to produce the best outcomes for their patients.

The decision to write this book was, in large part, stimulated by our desire to accelerate the rate at which research findings are translated into practice in order to improve clinical care. Although there are many interventions/treatments that have been found to result in positive outcomes in the literature, few of these interventions are being implemented in clinical practice. It is daunting for us to think that it takes an average of 17 years to move research findings into practice. Therefore, aggressive initiatives must be undertaken to reduce this very large research–practice gap.

We are hopeful that this book will cultivate a foundational understanding of the steps of evidence-based practice (EBP), clarify misperceptions about the implementation of EBP, and provide readers with practical action strategies for the implementation of evidence-based care so that widespread acceleration of EBP across the country becomes a reality. Because we also know that motivation is an important component of change, we have intertwined **inspirational quotes** throughout our book to encourage readers to build their beliefs and abilities to actively engage in EBP and accomplish any desired goals.

We believe this book contains *key, usable, relatable* content for all levels of practitioners and learners, with **many exemplars** that bring to life the concepts within the chapters. For those who want to build their knowledge and skills, this book contains the foundational steps of EBP. For those clinicians who desire to stimulate or lead a change to EBP in their practice sites, this book has information and practical strategies/models on how to introduce change, how to overcome barriers in implementing change, and how to conduct an outcomes assessment of that change. For those in advanced roles or educational programs, the chapters on generating quantitative and qualitative evidence as well as how to write a successful grant proposal should be of particular interest. For educators, we have included a special chapter on teaching EBP and hope that this book will facilitate a change in how research concepts and critical appraisal are being taught in professional programs throughout the country.

Key features of this book, not typically included in EBP books, include: **"real-life" examples** that assist the reader in actualizing important concepts and overcoming barriers in the implementation of evidence-based care; efficient critical appraisal of both quantitative and qualitative evidence; how to factor in a clinician's expertise and patient preferences/values when making decisions about patient care; chapters on outcomes management and how to create a vision to motivate a change to best practice; chapters on generating both qualitative and quantitative evidence when little evidence exists to guide clinical practice; how to write a successful grant proposal to fund a study or outcomes management project; as well as a chapter on how to disseminate evidence to other professionals, the media, and policy-makers.

We also have included **web alerts** that direct readers to helpful Internet resources and sites that can be used to further develop EBP knowledge and skills.

In addition, in an **accompanying CD-ROM**, we have included **40 evidence reviews** written by experts in the field that answer burning clinical questions across *six specialty areas; adults in critical/acute care; adults in primary care; aging; emergency and trauma care; high-risk children and youth; and psychiatric mental health.* These evidence reviews, along with the chapters in this book, all of which have been peer reviewed, will hopefully stimulate changes in clinical care that result in the best patient outcomes.

Finally, readers have the opportunity to obtain **continuing education contact hours** for reading chapters of our book. Since we believe in constructive feedback, we hope to hear from many readers of our book on what was most helpful for them and what can be done to improve a future edition.

It is important to remember that EBP is a problem-solving approach to practice, one that cultivates an excitement for implementing the highest quality of care as well as a spirit of inquiry and life-long learning. However, EBP also is a journey, one that takes time and becomes easier when the principles of this book are placed into action with enthusiasm on a consistent daily basis. As you embark on your EBP journey, whether it be to first learn the steps of EBP or to lead a successful EBP change effort, we leave you with the words of Les Brown: "Shoot for the moon. Even if you miss, you land among the stars."

Bernadette Mazurek Melnyk and Ellen Fineout-Overholt
Bernadette_Melnyk@urmc.rochester.edu
Ellen_Fineout@urmc.rochester.edu

acknowledgments

This book could not have been accomplished without the support, understanding, and assistance of many wonderful colleagues, staff, family, and friends. First, I would like to acknowledge the outstanding work of my co-editor, Ellen–thank you for all of your efforts, friendship, attention to detail, and ongoing support throughout this process–I could not have accomplished this without you. Second, a heartfelt thanks is extended to all of our contributing authors and reviewers as the final product reflects an outstanding team effort by everyone. Third, along with my wonderful husband and daughters, I am appreciative for the ongoing love and support that I receive from my mother, Anna May Mazurek, my brother and sister-in-law, Fred and Sue Mazurek, and my sister, Christine Warmuth, whose famous words to me "Just get out there and do it" have been a key to many of my successful endeavors. I also would like to thank my wonderful colleagues and staff at the University of Rochester School of Nursing, especially those in the Center for Research & Evidence-Based Practice and my COPE study team, for their support, understanding, and ongoing commitment to our projects and their roles throughout this process, especially Nancy Feinstein, Eileen Fairbanks, Nancy Watson, Leigh Small, Hong Li, Holly Brown, Zendi Moldenhauer, Lisa Spath, and Pamela Sawdey. In addition, I would like to thank each of my close friends, especially Ann Marie Lagonegro, for the much-needed encouragement and support that they provided me during the writing and editing of this book, especially during my "character-building times." Finally, I would like to acknowledge Elizabeth Nieginski at Lippincott Williams & Wilkins for her ongoing enthusiasm and adaptability throughout this process as well as Deedie McMahon and Helen Kogut for their assistance with and dedication to keeping this project "on-track."

Bernadette Mazurek Melnyk

Books are not written only by the people whose names are on the cover or the pages...there are many who support them and the credit for any success must be shared. I sincerely thank my dear husband, Wayne, and my precious 2-year-old daughter, Rachael, both of whom have missed Mommy while I worked many hours on this book. I would like to thank my dear family, the Texas Fineouts (especially Grandginny, John, Angela, Ashton, and Aubrey) and the many friends who have prayed for me throughout this journey. I could not have asked for a greater collaborating colleague than Bernadette Melnyk. She has been a true kindred spirit in this journey. Thanks Bern! As a novice to writing books, I am grateful for the support and sage advice provided by Deedie McMahon and Helen Kogut from Lippincott Williams & Wilkins. We had a great group of contributors, and I very much appreciate their investment throughout this process. In addition, I am so thankful for the support provided by many of my faculty and staff colleagues at the University of Rochester School of Nursing, Leigh Small in particular. Lastly, I give grateful thanks to my Jesus, who sustained me through many late nights, early mornings, long days, illnesses, and hardships to see this endeavor come to fruition.

Ellen Fineout-Overholt

contents

Appendices

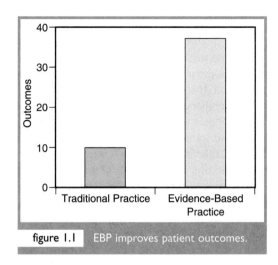

figure 1.1   EBP improves patient outcomes.

a result of this gap, initiatives such as the federal funding of EBP centers have been implemented. (AHRQ, 2002; Felch & Scanlon, 1997; Straus & Sackett, 1998). National leaders and professional organizations also continue to voice an urgent need for *speedier* mechanisms that translate research findings into clinical practice (Cronenwett, 2002; Hinshaw, 2000; Melnyk, 2002). Sponsored by the Johnson & Johnson Pediatric Institute and Sigma Theta Tau International, a hallmark "think tank" on maternal-child health was conducted that brought 17 national experts together to identify priorities and strategic initiatives to improve the care and outcomes for mothers and children for the next decade. The promotion of EBP was one of four high-priority areas identified by the experts (Johnson & Johnson Pediatric Institute and Sigma Theta Tau International, 2002).

There also is some evidence to indicate that healthcare providers who use an evidence-based approach to delivering patient care experience higher levels of satisfaction than those who deliver care that is steeped in tradition (Dawes, 1996). With recent reports of pervasive "burnout" among healthcare professionals and the pressure that many influential healthcare organizations exert on providers to deliver high-quality, safe care under increasingly heavy patient loads, the use and teaching of EBP may be key not only to providing outstanding care to patients and saving healthcare dollars (Titler, Cullen, & Ardery, 2002), but also to reducing the escalating turnover rate in certain healthcare professions.

Without current best evidence, practice is rapidly outdated, often to the detriment of patients. As an example, for years, pediatric primary care providers advised parents to place their infants in a prone position while sleeping, with the underlying reasoning that this is the best position to prevent aspiration in the event of vomiting. With evidence indicating that prone positioning increases the risk of sudden infant death syndrome, the American Academy of Pediatrics (AAP) released a clinical practice guideline recommending a supine position for infant sleep (AAP, 2000). As another example, despite strong evidence that use of beta blockers following an acute myocardial infarction reduces morbidity and mortality, these medications are considerably underused in older adults (Slutsky, 2003). Specifically, research has indicated that the risk of death doubles with the use of calcium channel blockers versus beta blockers

(Soumerai, McLaughlin, Spiegelman, Hertzmark, Thibault, & Goldman, 1997). Although this evidence is noteworthy, many practitioners choose to use calcium channel blockers as the medication of choice in treating acute myocardial infarction. Therefore, the critical question that all healthcare providers need to ask themselves is, Can we continue to implement practices that are not based on sound evidence and, if so, at what cost (e.g., physical, emotional, and financial) to our patients and their family members?

Even if health professionals answer this question negatively and remain resistant to implementing EBP, in the not-too-distant future, it can be expected that third-party payers will provide reimbursement only for healthcare practices whose effectiveness is supported by scientific evidence (Melnyk, 1999). In addition to pressure from third-party payers, a growing number of patients and family members are seeking out the latest evidence posted on Web sites about the most effective treatments for their health conditions. This is likely to exert even greater pressure on healthcare providers to provide the most up-to-date practices and health-related information. Therefore, despite resistance from some healthcare providers who are skeptical or who oppose EBP, it is likely that the EBP movement will continue with full force.

Another important reason that clinicians must include the latest evidence in their decision making is that evidence continually evolves. For example, as a result of findings from the Prempro arm of the Women's Health Initiative Study, sponsored by the National Institutes of Health, the clinical trial on hormone replacement therapy with Prempro was ceased early—after only 2.5 years—because the overall health risks (e.g., myocardial infarction, venous thromboembolism, and invasive breast cancer) of taking this combined estrogen/progestin hormone replacement therapy were found to be far greater than the benefits (e.g., prevention of osteoporosis and endometrial cancer). Compared with women taking a placebo, women who received Prempro had a 29% greater risk of coronary heart disease, a 41% higher rate of stroke, and a 26% increase in invasive breast cancer (Hendrix, 2002a). For years, practitioners prescribed long-term hormone therapy in the belief that it protected menopausal women from cardiovascular disease because many earlier studies supported this practice. However, there were studies that left some degree of uncertainty and prompted further investigation (i.e., the Prempro study) of what was best practice for these women. As a result of the Women's Health Initiative Study, practice recommendations have changed. The evolution of evidence in this case is a good example of the importance of basing practice on the latest, best evidence available and of engaging in a lifelong learning approach (i.e., EBP) about how to gather, generate, and apply evidence.

Definition and Evolution of Evidence-Based Practice

Evidence-based practice is the conscientious use of current best evidence in making decisions about patient care (Sackett, Straus, Richardson, Rosenberg, & Haynes, 2000). It is a problem-solving approach to clinical practice that integrates:

- A systematic search for and critical appraisal of the most relevant evidence to answer a burning clinical question
- One's own clinical expertise
- Patient preferences and values (Figure 1-2)

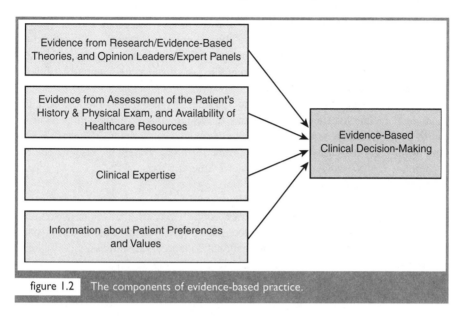

figure 1.2   The components of evidence-based practice.

Unlike **research utilization**, which is the use of knowledge typically based on a single study, EBP takes into consideration the expertise of the practitioner as well as patient preferences and values (Barnsteiner & Prevost, 2002).

Components of Evidence-Based Practice

Although evidence from **systematic reviews** of **randomized clinical trials** (RCTs) has been regarded as the strongest level of evidence on which to base practice decisions, evidence from **descriptive** and **qualitative studies** as well as from **opinion leaders** should be factored into clinical decisions when randomized trials are not available. **Evidence-based theories** also should be included as evidence. In addition, patient preferences, values, and concerns should be incorporated into the evidence-based approach to decision making along with the practitioner's assessment of the patient's condition through subjective history taking, objective physical examination findings, and laboratory reports, as well as healthcare resources available to implement the chosen treatment(s).

History of the Movement

The EBP movement was founded by Dr. Archie Cochrane, a British epidemiologist, who struggled with the efficacy of healthcare and challenged the public to pay only for care that had been empirically supported as effective (Enkin, 1992). In 1972, Cochrane published a landmark book that criticized the medical profession for not providing rigorous reviews of evidence so that policy makers and organizations could make decisions about healthcare. Cochrane was a strong proponent of using evidence from randomized clinical trials because he believed that this was the strongest evidence on which to base clinical practice decisions. He asserted that reviews of research evidence across all specialty areas need to be prepared systematically through a rigorous process and that they should be maintained to consider the generation of new evidence (Cochrane Collaboration, 2001).

In an exemplar case, Cochrane noted that thousands of low-birth-weight premature infants died needlessly. He emphasized that the results of several randomized clinical trials supporting the effectiveness of corticosteroid therapy to halt premature labor in high-risk women had never been analyzed and compiled in the form of a systematic review. The data from that systematic review showed that corticosteroid therapy reduced the odds of premature infant death from 50% to 30% (Cochrane Collaboration, 2001).

Dr. Archie Cochrane died in 1988. However, as a result of his influence and call for updates of systematic reviews of randomized controlled trials, the Cochrane Center was launched in Oxford, England in 1992, and the Cochrane Collaboration was founded a year later. The major purpose of the Center and international collaboration is to assist individuals in making well-informed decisions about healthcare by developing, maintaining, and updating systematic reviews of healthcare interventions and ensuring that these reviews are accessible to the public (Cochrane Collaboration, 2001).

Further information about the Cochrane Center and Collaboration can be accessed at **http://www.cochrane.org/cochrane/ cc-broch.htm#cc**.

Key Steps of Evidence-Based Practice

The five critical steps of EBP (summarized in Box 1-1) include:

1. Asking the burning clinical question in the format that will yield the most relevant and best evidence (i.e., PICO format, which is discussed later in this chapter)
2. Collecting the most relevant and best evidence to answer the clinical question, including searching for systematic reviews/meta-analyses or clinical practice guidelines first
3. Critically appraising the evidence that has been collected for its validity, relevance, and applicability
4. Integrating the evidence with one's clinical expertise, assessment of the patient's condition, and available healthcare resources along with the patient's preferences and values to implement a clinical decision
5. Evaluating the change resulting from implementing the evidence in practice

Step 1: Formulate the Burning Clinical Question

In step 1 of EBP, clinical questions should be asked in **PICO format** (i.e., patient population, intervention of interest, comparison intervention or status, and outcome) to yield the most relevant and best evidence. For example, a well-designed PICO question would be, In teenagers

---

box 1.1

Five Steps of Evidence-Based Practice

1. Ask the burning clinical question.
2. Collect the most relevant and best evidence.
3. Critically appraise the evidence.
4. Integrate all evidence with one's clinical expertise, patient preferences, and values in making a practice decision or change.
5. Evaluate the practice decision or change.

(the patient population), how effective is Depo-Provera (the intervention) versus oral contraceptives (the comparison intervention) in the prevention of pregnancy (the outcome). Asking questions in PICO format results in an effective search that yields the best, relevant information and saves an inordinate amount of time (Melnyk & Fineout-Overholt, 2002a). In contrast, an inappropriately formed question (e.g., What is the best type of birth control to use?) would probably lead to irrelevant information.

For other clinical questions that are not intervention focused, the meaning of the letter **I** can be "interest area" instead of "intervention." An example of a nonintervention question would be, What is the duration of breast feeding in new mothers who have breast-related complications in the first 3 months after the infants' birth versus those who do not have breast-related complications? In this question, the population is new breast-feeding mothers, the area of interest is breast-feeding complications, the comparison is those mothers who do not have complications, and the outcome is breast-feeding duration.

When a clinical problem generates multiple clinical questions, priority should be given to those questions with the most important consequences or those that occur most frequently (i.e., those clinical problems that occur in high volume and/or those that carry high risk for negative outcomes to the patient). For example, nurses and physicians on a surgical unit routinely encounter the question, In postoperative patients, how effective is morphine versus hydromorphone in relieving pain? Another question might be, What is the most effective intervention for preventing pressure sores in postoperative, middle-aged patients? The clinical priority would be answering the first question because pain is a daily occurrence, versus seeking an answer to the second question because pressure ulcers rarely occur in postoperative, middle-aged patients. Chapter 2 provides more in-depth information about formulating PICO questions.

Step 2: Search for Best Evidence

The search for best evidence, step 2 in EBP, should first begin with systematic reviews or **meta-analyses** and evidence-based **clinical practice guidelines**, which are regarded as the strongest level of evidence on which to base practice decisions (Guyatt & Rennie, 2002). Although there are many hierarchies of evidence available in the literature (e.g., Guyatt & Rennie, 2002; Harris et al., 2001), we have chosen to present a hierarchy that encompasses a broad range of evidence, including systematic reviews of qualitative evidence (see Box 1-2). A systematic review is a summary of evidence on a particular topic, typically by an expert or expert panel that uses a rigorous process for identifying, appraising, and synthesizing studies to answer a specific clinical question. Conclusions are then drawn about the data gathered through this process (e.g., How effective is massage versus pharmacologic agents in reducing pain in adult women with arthritis? What are the major factors that predict heart disease in women?). Using a rigorous process of well-defined, preset criteria to select studies for inclusion in the review, bias is overcome, and results are more credible.

Many systematic reviews incorporate quantitative methods to summarize the results from multiple studies. These reviews are called meta-analyses. A meta-analysis often yields an overall summary statistic that represents the effect of the intervention across multiple studies. Because a meta-analysis combines the samples of each study included in the review to create one larger study, the summary statistic is more precise than the individual findings from any one of the contributing studies alone (Ciliska, Cullum, & Marks, 2001). Thus, systematic reviews and meta-analyses yield the strongest level of evidence on which to base practice decisions.

In addition to the Cochrane Database of Systematic Reviews, *Worldviews on Evidence-Based Nursing* by Sigma Theta Tau International provides systematic reviews to guide nursing practice across many topic areas. More information can be found at **www.nursingsociety.org**.

box 1.2

Rating System for the Hierarchy of Evidence

Level I: Evidence from a systematic review or meta-analysis of all relevant randomized controlled trials (RCTs), or evidence-based clinical practice guidelines based on systematic reviews of RCTs

Level II: Evidence obtained from at least one well-designed RCT

Level III: Evidence obtained from well-designed controlled trials without randomization

Level IV: Evidence from well-designed case-control and cohort studies

Level V: Evidence from systematic reviews of descriptive and qualitative studies

Level VI: Evidence from a single descriptive or qualitative study

Level VII: Evidence from the opinion of authorities and/or reports of expert committees

Modified from Guyatt & Rennie, 2002; Harris et al., 2001.

Evidence-based clinical practice guidelines are specific practice recommendations that are based on a methodologically rigorous review of the best evidence on a specific topic. As such, they have tremendous potential to improve the quality of care, the process of care, and patient outcomes (Grimshaw & Russell, 1993; Grimshaw et al., 1995). More information about guideline development and implementation may be found in Chapter 9.

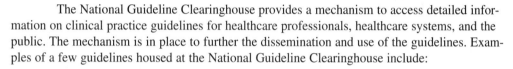

In addition, the Agency for Healthcare Research and Quality (AHRQ), in collaboration with the American Medical Association and the American Association of Health Plans, provides a public resource for clinical practice guidelines at **www.guideline.gov.**

The National Guideline Clearinghouse provides a mechanism to access detailed information on clinical practice guidelines for healthcare professionals, healthcare systems, and the public. The mechanism is in place to further the dissemination and use of the guidelines. Examples of a few guidelines housed at the National Guideline Clearinghouse include:

- "Elderly suicide: secondary prevention" by the University of Iowa Gerontological Nursing Interventions Research Center (June 2002)
- "2001 Consensus guidelines for the management of women with cervical cytological abnormalities" by the American Medical Association
- Anthrax as a biological weapon, 2002: Updated recommendations for management.

The Association of Women's Health, Obstetric and Neonatal Nurses (AWHONN) has been on the forefront of professional organizations that heavily advocate the use of evidence to guide practice. Consistent with this advocacy, AWHONN (www.awhonn.org) has developed a host of evidence-based clinical practice guidelines to inform practice that include such topics as neonatal skin care, breast-feeding support, and nursing management of the second stage of labor. A major advantage of the AWHONN guidelines is that they include the strength of evidence on which each recommendation is based.

Although clinical practice guidelines have tremendous potential to improve the quality of care and outcomes for patients, their success depends on a highly rigorous guideline development process and the incorporation of the best evidence available. In addition, guideline success depends on proper implementation (Graham, Harrison, Brouwers, Davies, & Dunn, 2002).

A toolkit to enhance the use of clinical practice guidelines was developed by the Registered Nurses Association of Ontario (RNAO; DiCenso et al., 2002) and can be downloaded from the RNAO Web site at **www.rnao.org.**

If systematic reviews or evidence-based guidelines are not available, the search process should proceed with an investigation for original randomized controlled trials in databases such as MEDLINE or CINAHL (Cumulative Index of Nursing and Allied Health Literature). If randomized trials are not available, the search should continue for other types of studies that generate evidence to guide clinical decision making (e.g., descriptive or qualitative studies). Chapter 3 contains more detailed information on searching for evidence.

Step 3: Critical Appraisal

The third step in the EBP process is vital in that it involves the critical appraisal of the evidence obtained from the search process. Although professionals typically view critical appraisal as an exhaustive, time-consuming process, it can be efficiently accomplished by answering three key questions (summarized in Box 1-3):

1. What were the results of the study? For example, in intervention trials, this includes how large are the treatment effects; in qualitative studies, this includes evaluating whether the research approach fits the purpose of the study.
2. Are the results valid? For example, in intervention trials, it would be important to determine whether the subjects were randomly assigned to treatment or control groups and whether they were equal on key characteristics prior to the treatment.
3. Will the results of the study facilitate the care of the practitioner's patients? This third critical appraisal question should include asking whether the subjects in the study were similar to the patients for whom care is being delivered and whether the benefits are greater than the risks of treatment.

The answers to these questions ensure relevance and transferability of the evidence from the search to the specific population for whom the practitioner provides care. For example, if a systematic review provided evidence to support the positive effects of using distraction to alleviate pain in postsurgical patients between the ages of 20 and 40 years, those same results may not be relevant for postsurgical patients who are 65 years or older. In addition, even if a randomized controlled trial supported the effectiveness of a specific intervention with a patient population, careful consideration of the risks and benefits of that intervention must be considered before its implementation. Unit Two contains in-depth information on the critical appraisal (step 3 in EBP) of all types of evidence, from expert opinion and qualitative studies to randomized controlled trials.

Step 4: Integrate the Evidence

The fourth key step in EBP is integrating the evidence found from the literature search with the healthcare provider's expertise, clinical assessment of the patient and available healthcare resources, as well as patient preferences and values to implement a decision. In addition to ethical considerations related to involving patients in treatment decisions, consumers of healthcare services want to participate in the clinical decision-making process (Kee, 1996). Even if the evidence found from a rigorous search and critical appraisal strongly supports that a certain treatment is beneficial (e.g., hormone replacement therapy [HRT] to prevent osteoporosis in a very high-risk woman), a discussion with the patient may reveal her intense fear of developing breast cancer while taking HRT or other reasons that the treatment is not acceptable. Moreover, as part of the history-taking process or physical examination, a comorbidity or contraindication may be found that increases the risks of HRT (e.g., prior history of stroke). Therefore, despite compelling evidence to support the benefits of HRT

box 1.3

Key General Critical Appraisal Questions

What were the results of the study?
Are the results valid?
Will the results help me in caring for my patients?

in preventing osteoporosis in high-risk women, a decision against its use may be made after a thorough assessment of the individual patient and a discussion of the risks and benefits of treatment.

Similarly, a clinician's assessment of healthcare resources that are available to implement a treatment decision is a critical part of the EBP decision-making process. For example, on follow-up evaluation, a clinician notes that the first-line treatment of acute otitis media in a 3-year-old patient was not effective. The latest evidence indicates that antibiotic A has slightly greater efficacy than antibiotic B in the second-line treatment of acute otitis media in young children. However, because antibiotic A is far more expensive than antibiotic B and the family of the child does not have prescription coverage, the practitioner and parents together may decide to use the less expensive antibiotic to treat the child's unresolved ear infection.

Step 5: Evaluate Effectiveness

The fifth key step in EBP is evaluating the evidence-based intervention in terms of how the treatment worked or how effective the clinical decision was with a particular patient or practice setting. This type of evaluation is essential in determining whether the change based on evidence resulted in the expected outcomes. If the treatment did not produce the expected effects, outcomes analysis should include the formulation of all possible alternative explanations for the findings (e.g., nonadherence to the treatment regimen by the patient, lack of appropriate dosage of medication, different demographic characteristics of the provider's patients versus those used in the studies reviewed). Chapter 12 contains information on how to evaluate outcomes of an intervention based on evidence.

Several excellent online Web sites with tutorials teach the five steps of EBP. Two excellent sites with these learning modules include Teaching/Learning Resources for Evidence Based Practice at Middlesex University in London at **http://www.mdx.ac.uk/www/rctsh/ebp/ main.htm** and the University of Rochester Medical Center at **http://www.urmc.rochester.edu/HSLT/miner/resources/ evidence_based/index.cfm**

Controversies Surrounding Evidence-Based Practice

One controversy surrounding EBP is that it is basically a new term for **research utilization**, which is the use of some portion of a single study in practice that is similar to the manner in which it was used in the original study. Although research utilization is a component, EBP requires a larger and more complex knowledge base and skill set.

A second controversy is that some individuals believe that EBP is "cookbook" care in which there is a disregard for the individualization of patient care. Although the temptation to use evidence as a "cookbook" may be present with EBP, decisions are made based on the evidence being considered and its relevance for a specific clinical situation or patient. The incorporation of research evidence into practice should consistently include the patient's unique clinical circumstances, his or her preferences and values, and available healthcare resources.

Third, some experts argue that EBP contains evidence only from RCTs. Although a synthesis of data from RCTs is regarded as the strongest evidence because bias and confounding variables are controlled through the use of random assignment to experimental and control groups, evidence from other types of studies is recognized as valuable. For example, data from qualitative and quantitative descriptive studies are especially useful in guiding practice when there are limited or no clinical trials that evaluate the effectiveness of clinical interventions and when the clinical question cannot be answered by an RCT. In addition, qualitative evidence is important in that it incorporates patients' voices into the process of EBP (Pearson, 2002).

Because it is being increasingly recognized that EBP and systematic reviews should consider evidence from both quantitative and qualitative studies, researchers are beginning to establish frameworks or systems for the critical appraisal of qualitative research for EBP (Pearson, 2002; Sandelowski, 2000). One such framework is the Qualitative Assessment and Review Instrument (QARI) or FAME Scale, which ranks qualitative evidence in terms of its Feasibility, Appropriateness, Meaningfulness, and Effectiveness (Pearson, 2002).

Fourth, there is controversy about the use of evidence-based clinical practice guidelines. A criticism of evidence-based guidelines and reports is that various experts can appraise the same data from studies and come to different conclusions about which practice should be based on the evidence reviewed (Cronenwett, 2002). In addition, Lohr, Eleazer, and Mouskopf (1998) propose that guidelines alone have little impact if they cannot be translated into tools that healthcare providers can use in everyday practice. Some individuals also question whether EBP guidelines can be produced and updated frequently enough to consider new evidence from the most recently completed studies.

Finally, some contend that EBP does not consider theory as well as the humanistic aspects of care. However, theories that have accumulated evidence to support their propositions should be incorporated into EBP. For example, self-regulation theory by Johnson and Leventhal (Johnson, Fieler, Jones, Wlasowicz, & Mitchell, 1997) contends that provision of concrete objective information to patients undergoing stressful medical events will enhance their understanding, predictability, and confidence. As a result, they will have better emotional and functional coping outcomes (e.g., less anxiety and higher activity level) than patients who do not receive this type of information. Numerous RCTs provide data to support this theory with adults and children undergoing intrusive or stressful procedures, cancer patients being treated with chemotherapy and radiation, as well as parents of hospitalized and critically ill children and low-birth-weight premature infants (Johnson, 1984; Johnson,

Kirchhoff, & Endress, 1975; Johnson, Rice, Fuller, & Endress, 1978; Melnyk, 1994; Melnyk, Alpert-Gillis, Hensel, Cable-Beiling, & Rubenstein, 1997; Melnyk et al., 2001). As a result, providers should consider this evidence-based theory as one that is useful in guiding their practices.

Regarding the humanistic components of care, recognized experts in EBP acknowledge that implementing EBP is necessary but not sufficient for delivering the highest quality of patient care (DiCenso, Cullum, Ciliska, & Guyatt, 2004).Without the ability to deliver EBP within a context of caring that embraces compassion, cultural sensitivity, and respect for patients and their families, healthcare would fall painfully short of its ultimate goal of providing safe, effective, and holistic care that meets the bio/psycho/social needs of its consumers (see Figure 1-3).

Frequently, this is where the expertise of a practitioner affects the clinical decision. For example, a seasoned nurse who has practiced on a surgical unit that has a high percentage of elderly Native American patients reviews the latest systematic review on a new treatment that may speed postoperative recovery time. Despite this strength of evidence for the new treatment, the nurse knows that it will be in direct conflict with the traditions and values of Native American elderly patients and, as a result, would precipitate much emotional anxiety in them. Therefore, as part of the EBP process, the nurse advocates for the unit to continue the standard versus newer treatment with this population of patients.

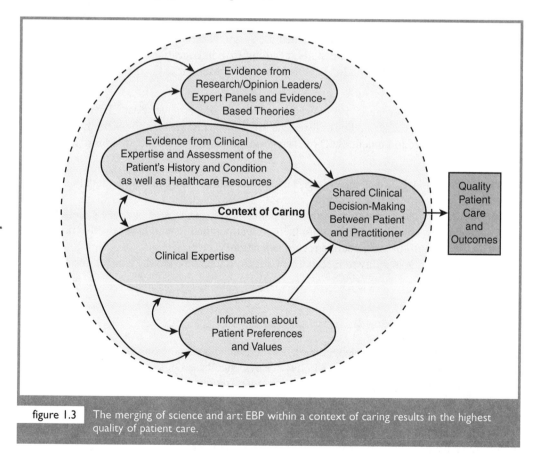

figure 1.3   The merging of science and art: EBP within a context of caring results in the highest quality of patient care.

Obstacles and Opportunities

Healthcare providers are struggling to deliver evidence-based care while managing demanding patient loads and attempting to keep pace with the volume of journal articles related to their clinical practices.

Barriers to Evidence-Based Practice

Nurses, physicians, and other health professionals cite a number of barriers to EBP that include:

- Lack of knowledge regarding EBP strategies
- Misperceptions or negative views about research and evidence-based care
- Lack of belief that EBP will result in more positive outcomes than traditional care
- Voluminous amounts of information in professional journals
- Lack of time and resources to search for and appraise evidence
- Overwhelming patient loads
- Organizational constraints, such as lack of administrative support or incentives
- Demands from patients for a certain type of treatment (e.g., patients who demand antibiotics for their viral upper respiratory infections when they are not indicated)
- Peer pressure to continue with practices that are steeped in tradition
- Inadequate content and behavioral skills regarding EBP in educational programs (Barnsteiner & Prevost, 2002; Cronenwett, 2002; McKibbon, 1999; Melnyk, 2002; Melnyk et al., 2000; Silagy & Haines, 1998).

Cabana and colleagues (1999) used a review of 5,658 articles about EBP guidelines from which they selected 76 studies to formulate their own framework of barriers that affect practitioner adherence to guidelines. Three categories of barriers were identified through this review, including:

- Knowledge and lack of awareness (e.g., lack of familiarity with guidelines, guideline accessibility)
- Attitudes (e.g., lack of confidence in the guideline developer, lack of outcome expectancy that the guideline will be effective with their patient population, and lack of self-efficacy or motivation to perform the guideline recommendations)
- Behaviors (e.g., the inability to incorporate patient preferences into the clinical decision-making process)

Facilitators of Evidence-Based Practice

To overcome the barriers in implementing EBP, there must be champions and mechanisms to support the cause as well as a variety of effective evidence-based models for advancing this type of care. With the downsizing of many healthcare organizations nationally, few providers can devote their time to the mission of facilitating EBP.

For healthcare professionals to advance the use of EBP, misconceptions about how to implement practice based on scientific evidence need to be corrected, and knowledge and skills in this area must be enhanced (Melnyk, 2002; Melnyk et al., 2000).

unit I

16

Facilitating conditions that have been found to enhance EBP include:

- Support and encouragement from administration
- Time to critically appraise studies and implement their findings
- Clearly written research reports (Omery & Williams, 1999)

In addition, findings from a recent survey with advanced practice nurses revealed that mentorship in EBP was a key factor for implementing evidence-based care (Melnyk & Fineout-Overholt, 2002b). Facilitating conditions believed to specifically affect the use of EBP guidelines include:

- Organizational capacity for change that includes strong support and interest at all levels of leadership
- Implementation infrastructure (e.g., adequate resources and time)
- Characteristics of the healthcare team (e.g., a shared vision and mission)
- Guideline characteristics (e.g., importance of the guideline to clinicians, credibility of the guideline) (Solberg et al., 2000)

In a recent study, Grimshaw and colleagues (2001) determined the effectiveness of various types of interventions to enhance the translation of research findings into practice by physicians. Interventions found to be effective from a review of 41 systematic reviews included educational outreach and multifaceted interventions based on the assessment of potential barriers. However, studies have yet to determine which components of these multifaceted interventions are most effective. Using only passive approaches, such as didactic lectures on EBP information, is not likely to be successful in producing a behavior change to evidence-based care.

In a systematic review to determine the effects of introducing clinical practice guidelines via multiple strategies (e.g., in-services, lectures, opinion leaders) to nurses, midwives, and other nonphysician health professionals, Thomas and colleagues (1999) concluded that there is some evidence to support that care based on evidence-based guidelines is effective and does lead to improved patient outcomes. However, the investigators noted that caution should be used in generalizing the findings from their review because only 18 studies and 467 health professionals were included. In addition, many of these studies had limited follow-up on the outcomes measures used.

A panel of international experts also rated organizational capability for change as well as infrastructure as key factors that facilitated the use of EBP guidelines by physicians (Solberg et al., 2000). The top five of a possible 25 identified strategies included:

1. System supports (e.g., reminders)
2. Emphasis on physician benefit (e.g., how the change would make practice easier)
3. Barrier reduction
4. Measurement of improvement
5. Information and training

Overcoming Barriers to Evidence-Based Practice

For evidence-based care to become the "gold standard" of practice, EBP barriers must be overcome. Federal agencies, healthcare organizations and systems, health insurers, policy makers, and regulatory bodies must advocate for and require its use. Funding agencies must establish translational research as a high priority.

Promoting Acceptance

Australia and the United Kingdom have been leaders on the forefront of widespread implementation of EBP. In the United States, a paradigm shift to EBP is occurring; however, U.S. healthcare systems will need to learn more from these leaders and rapidly accelerate the integration of strategies being used in Australia and the United Kingdom for providing evidence-based care. For example, Australia was able to establish EBP as an integral part of its healthcare system because EBP is subscribed to as the basis of the public health system by the federal government. In Australia, EBP is recognized as an essential ingredient of continuous quality improvement (CQI) by accreditation agencies and regarded as centrally important by health insurers. In addition, it is designated as a priority by the National Health & Medical Research Council and required by regulatory bodies as the basis for healthcare providers' undergraduate and graduate educational curricula (Pearson, 2002). Similarly, the Department of Health in the United Kingdom has stipulated that the practice of nursing, midwifery, and health visiting needs to be evidence-based (U.K. Department of Health, 1999).

As an initial step, barriers to EBP must be assessed within a particular system. Surveys or focus groups should first be conducted with healthcare providers to assess their baseline knowledge, attitudes/beliefs, and behaviors regarding EBP. An additional benefit of conducting surveys or focus groups at the outset of any new EBP initiative is that research shows that these strategies also are effective in raising awareness and stimulating a change to evidence-based care (Jolley, 2002).

As part of the survey or focus group, practitioners should be asked about their baseline knowledge of EBP as well as to what extent they believe that implementing EBP will result in improved care and better patient outcomes. This is a critical question in that providing information alone usually does not change behavior (Melnyk, 2002). Although practitioners must possess basic knowledge and skills about EBP, it is critical for them to believe that EBP will produce better outcomes in order for changes in their practices to occur.

> ❝*Belief at the beginning of any successful undertaking is the one ingredient that will ensure success.*❞
>
> *William James*

Healthcare providers who do not believe that EBP results in improved care and patient outcomes need to be exposed to real-case scenarios in which evidence-based care resulted in better outcomes than care that was steeped in traditional practices. For example, many primary care providers continue to prescribe antidepressants as the sole treatment for adolescents when systematic reviews of their effectiveness have indicated that medication alone is not beneficial in treating mild to moderate adolescent depression (Moldenhauer & Melnyk, 1999). In addition, although rigorous systematic reviews of the effectiveness of metered-dose inhalers (MDIs) versus nebulizers in administering bronchodilators to children have indicated that MDIs are just as effective with fewer side effects and less emergency room time, nebulizers continue to be the preferred route of administration in emergency rooms (Melnyk, 1999).

Correcting Misperceptions

Because misperceptions about EBP constitute another barrier to its implementation, clarifying these perceptions and teaching the basics of EBP are critical to advancing evidence-based care. For example, many practitioners believe that searching for and critically appraising research articles is an overwhelming, time-consuming process. However, practitioners who have this belief frequently have not had exposure to databases such as the *Cochrane Library* and the **National Guidelines Clearinghouse** that can provide them with quick, easily retrievable systematic reviews and evidence-based guidelines to inform their practices. In addition, because many educational curriculums continue to teach the in-depth critique of a single study versus time-efficient approaches to the gathering and critical appraisal of a body of empirical studies, clinicians may have the misperception that the EBP process is not feasible in the context of their current practice environments. Therefore, the basics of EBP (e.g., how to formulate a searchable question that will yield the best evidence and how to search for and critically appraise relevant studies) must first be taught in order to create baseline knowledge and skills.

The teaching of EBP can and should be accomplished with multiple strategies, including continuing education conferences, interactive workshops, and dissemination of educational materials, such as journal articles, textbooks, and informational handouts (Davies, 2002). The best learning method incorporates the teaching of didactic information with interactive behavioral skills. Therefore, creating opportunities for clinicians to practice the skills that they are learning about in didactic sessions is superior to didactic sessions alone.

More detailed information about teaching EBP can be found in Chapter 15. Moreover, three centers housed in nursing schools in the United States can serve as resources for the teaching and implementation of EBP.

1. The Academic Center for Evidence-Based Nursing (ACE) at the University of Texas Health Science Center at San Antonio
   http://www.acestar.uthscsa.edu/
2. The Center for Research & Evidence-Based Practice (CREP) at the University of Rochester School of Nursing in New York
   (**www.urmc.rochester.edu/son/ebp/**)
3. The Sara Cole Hirsch Institute for Best Nursing Practice Based on Evidence at Case Western Reserve School of Nursing at
   http://fpb.cwru.edu/HirshInstitute/

Both the ACE and CREP offer annual national EBP continuing education (CE) conferences for nurses and other healthcare professionals, with funding support from the Agency for Healthcare Research and Quality (AHRQ). The focus of the CREP's annual national/international conference is to highlight the best evidence to guide practice in four substantive areas: care of high-risk children and youth, acute/critical care, care of older adults, and psychiatric/mental healthcare.

Preconference interactive workshops also are held in conjunction with the CREP's annual conference and focus on such topics as the foundations of EBP, in-depth critical appraisal skills, teaching EBP, disseminating evidence, and developing and implementing EBP guidelines. In addition, the Sara Hirsch Institute also offers a certificate through a continuing education program in implementing best nursing practices.

Centers for EBP also have been established internationally in Australia, New Zealand, Hong Kong, Germany, the United Kingdom, and Canada. The mission of these centers is to educate clinicians through workshops or formal courses on EBP (Ciliska, DiCenso, & Cullum, 1999).

Abstraction journals, such as *Evidence-Based Medicine, Evidence-Based Nursing, Evidence-Based Mental Health,* and *Evidence-Based Health Policy & Management,* are another mechanism through which professionals can find evidence to guide their practice. These journals summarize high-quality studies that have important clinical implications and provide a commentary by an expert in the field. The commentary addresses strengths and limitations of the research reviewed. In addition, EBP columns to guide practice are now regularly appearing features in professional journals such as *Pediatric Nursing* and *Maternal-Child Nursing.*

Questioning Clinical Practices: Developing Guidelines

❝*Never stop questioning!***❞**

S u s a n   L .   H e n d r i x

After basic EBP knowledge and skills are attained, it is important for healthcare professionals to ask questions about their current clinical practices (e.g., Is the use of pacifiers effective in decreasing neonatal pain during intrusive procedures? Is heparin or anti-embolic stockings the best prophylaxis for prevention of deep vein thrombosis?). Efforts also should be made to prioritize practice problems within an organization or practice setting. One strategy for prioritizing practice problems is described by Rosenfeld and colleagues (2000), who conducted a survey and focus groups with nurses in a large academic health center. The purpose of the survey and focus groups was to develop specific action plans around particular patient problems. Once high-priority areas are recognized, it is helpful to identify colleagues who have an interest in the same clinical question so that a collaboration can be formed to search for and critically appraise the evidence found. The results of this search and appraisal can be shared with colleagues through a variety of mechanisms (e.g., journal clubs, EBP practice rounds, or informational handouts). If a current practice guideline does not exist, one can be developed and implemented. However, guideline development is a rigorous endeavor, and adequate time must be allotted for the individuals who will complete the work (Davies, 2002). Useful processes for developing and implementing clinical practice guidelines are described in Chapter 9. To complete the EBP process, evaluation of the outcome of guideline implementation is essential to determine its effects on the process and outcomes of care.

Change to EBP within an organization or practice requires a clear vision, a written strategic plan, a culture in which EBP is valued and expected, and persistence to make it happen.. In addition, the chance to succeed in making a change to EBP will be greater where there is administrative support, encouragement, and allocated resources. It is often best to start with a small change (Gennaro, Hodnett, & Kearney, 2001), especially when there is high skepticism about EBP and elevated levels of stress or complacency within a system, rather than to expect a complete change to EBP to happen within a short period of time. For example, finding a mechanism for routinely disseminating and discussing evidence-based literature, such as journal clubs or EBP rounds, that can spark interest and enhance "buy-in" from colleagues and administration may be a wonderful start to facilitating a change to EBP.

> ❝*I don't think there is any other quality so essential to success of any kind as the quality of perseverance. It overcomes almost everything, even nature.*❞
>
> *John D. Rockefeller*

Further information about how to infuse EBP into clinical settings is provided in Chapter 8, which reviews a variety of specific EBP strategies and implementation models. In addition, Chapter 16 outlines assessment strategies for determining an organization's stage of change. It also provides multiple suggestions for motivating a vision for change to best practice, based primarily on evidence-based organizational change principles. For two case examples on how evidence-based care can positively impact patient outcomes, see the Appendix "EBP in Action." These two case examples are success stories of how EBP can improve both the process and outcomes of patient care. Countless examples similar to these can be found in the literature. Evidence-based success stories stem from asking compelling clinical questions, which emphasizes the need to cultivate a never-ending spirit of inquiry within our colleagues, our students, and ourselves. These two case examples, along with the Women's Health Study, teach a valuable lesson: never stop questioning because providers need to take evidence-based responsibility for clinical decisions and stay up to date with data that can further support or dramatically change their practice standards (Hendrix, 2002b). Once that spirit of inquiry is promulgated within us and our clinical settings, the journey toward a change to EBP will begin.

We have come to a time when the credibility of health professions will be judged by practices based on the best and latest evidence from sound scientific studies in combination with clinical expertise, astute assessment, and respect for patient values and preferences. The chance to influence health policy also rests on the ability to provide policy makers with the best evidence on which to make important decisions. However, it is important to remember that high-quality healthcare also depends on the ability to deliver EBP within a context of caring, which is the merging of science and art.

For EBP to evolve more quickly, commitments to advancing evidence-based care must be made by both individuals and organizations. Basic and graduate professional programs must teach the value and processes of EBP, leveled appropriately. Doctoral programs must create researchers and leaders who advance EBP through the generation of new knowledge from research to support the most effective practices, as well as the testing of established and new models of EBP implementation so that it can be determined which models are most effective on both staff and patient outcomes. Researchers and practitioners across disciplines also must unite to produce evidence on the effectiveness of numerous practices and to answer high-priority, compelling clinical questions, as well as to determine how best those interventions can be translated into practice.

The time has come for practitioners from all healthcare professions to embrace EBP and quickly move from practices that are steeped in tradition to those that are supported by sound evidence from well-designed studies. In doing so, patients, healthcare professionals, and healthcare systems will be able to place more confidence in the care that is being delivered and know that the best outcomes for patients and their families are being achieved.

references

AAP (2000). Changing concepts of sudden infant death syndrome: Implications for infant sleeping environment and sleep position. Elk Grove Village, IL: American Academy of Pediatrics. Retrieved from http://www.guidelines.gov.

AHRQ (2002). Evidence-based practice centers. Overview. October, 2002. Rockville, MD: Agency for Healthcare Research and Quality (AHRQ). Retrieved from http://www.ahrq.gov/clinic/epc/.

Balas, E. A., & Boren, S. A. (2000). Managing clinical knowledge for healthcare improvements (pp. 65–70). Germany: Schattauer Publishing Company.

Barnsteiner, J., & Prevost, S. (2002). How to implement evidence-based practice. Some tried and true pointers. *Reflections on Nursing Leadership, 28* (2), 18–21.

Bostrom, J., & Suter, W. N. (1993). Research utilization: Making the link to practice. *Journal of Nursing Staff Development, 9*, 28–34.

Cabana, M. D., Rand, C. S., Powe, N. R., Wu, A. W., Willson, M. H., Abboud, P. A., & Rubin, H. R. (1999). Why don't physicians follow clinical practice guidelines? A framework for improvement. *JAMA, 282*, 1458–1465.

Camiah, S. (1997). Utilization of nursing research in practice and application strategies to raise awareness amongst nurse practitioners: a model for success. *Journal of Advanced Nursing, 26*, 1193–1202.

Ciliska, D., Cullum, N., & Marks, S. (2001). Evaluation of systematic reviews of treatment or prevention interventions. *Evidence-Based Nursing, 4*, 100–104.

Ciliska D, DiCenso A, Cullum N. (1999). Centres of evidence-based nursing: directions and challenges. *Evidence-Based Nursing, 2*, 102–104.

Cochrane, A. L. (1972). *Effectiveness and efficiency. Random reflections on health services.* London: Nuffield Provincial Hospitals Trust.

Cochrane Collaboration. (2001). Retrieved January 22, 2002 from http://www.cochrane.org/cochrane/cc-broch.htm#cc.

Committee on Quality of Health Care in America, Institute of Medicine (2001). *Crossing the quality chasm: A new health system for the 21st century.* Washington, DC: National Academy Press.

Cretin, S., Farley, D. O., Dolter, K. J., & Nicholas, W. (2001). Evaluating an integrated approach to clinical quality improvement. *Medical Care, 39* (Suppl. 2), 1170–1184.

Cronenwett, L. (2002). Research, practice and policy: Issues in evidence based care. *Online Journal of Issues in Nursing.* Retrieved from http://www.nursingworld.org/ojin/keynotes/speech_2.htm.

Davies, B. L. (2002). Sources and models for moving research evidence into clinical practice. *Journal of Obstetric, Gynecologic, and Neonatal Nursing, 31*, 558–562.

Dawes, M. (1996). On the need for evidence-based general and family practice. *Evidence-Based Medicine, 1*, 68–69.

DiCenso, A., Cullum, N., Ciliska, D., & Guyatt, G. (2004). Introduction to evidence-based nursing. In A. DiCenso, N. Cullum, D. Ciliska, & G. Guyatt (Eds.), *Evidence-based nursing: A guide to clinical practice.* Philadelphia: Elsevier.

DiCenso, A., Virani, T., Bajnok, I., Borycki, E., et al. (2002). A toolkit to facilitate the implementation of clinical practice guidelines in healthcare settings. *Hospital Quarterly, 5* (3), 55–60.

Enkin, M. (1992). Current overviews of research evidence from controlled trials in midwifery obstetrics. *Journal of the Society of Obstetricians and Gynecologists of Canada, 9*, 23–33.

Estabrooks, C. A. (1998). Will evidence-based nursing practice make practice perfect? *Canadian Journal of Nursing Research, 30*, 15–36.

Felch, W., & Scanlon, D. (1997). Bridging the gap between research and practice: The role of continuing medical education. *JAMA, 277,* 155–156.

Gennaro, S., Hodnett, E., & Kearney, M. (2001). Making evidence-based practice a reality in your institution. *American Journal of Maternal Child Nursing, 26,* 236–244.

Graham, I. D., Harrison, M. B., Brouwers, M., Davies, B. L., & Dunn, S. (2002). Facilitating the use of evidence in practice: Evaluating and adapting clinical practice guidelines for local use by health care organizations. *Journal of Obstetric, Gynecologic, and Neonatal Nursing, 31,* 599–611.

Grimshaw, J. M., & Russell I. (1993). Effect of clinical guidelines on medical practice: A systematic review of rigorous evaluations. *Lancet, 342* (8883), 1317–1322.

Grimshaw, J., Freemantle, N., Wallace, S., Russell, I., Hurwitz, B., Watt, I., Long, A., & Sheldon, T. (1995).Developing and implementing clinical practice guidelines. *Quality Health Care, 4* (1), 55–64.

Grimshaw, J. M., Shirran, L., Thomas, R., Mowatt, G., Fraser, C., Bero, L., et al. (2001). Changing provider behavior: An overview of systematic reviews of interventions. *Medical Care, 39* (Suppl. 2), II-2–II-45.

Guyatt, G., & Rennie, D. (2002). *Users' Guides to the Medical Literature.* American Medical Association: AMA Press.

Harris, R. P., Hefland, M., Woolf, S. H., et al. (2001). Current methods of the U.S. Preventive Services Task Force: A review of the process. *American Journal of Preventive Medicine, 20,* 21–35.

Heater, B., Becker, A., & Olson, R. (1988). Nursing interventions and patient outcomes: A meta-analysis of studies. *Nursing Research, 37,* 303–307.

Hendrix, S. L. (2002a). Implications of the women's health initiative. *A Supplement to the Female Patient,* November, 3–8.

Hendrix, S. L. (2002b). Summarizing the evidence. *A Supplement to the Female Patient,* November, 32–34.

Hinshaw, A. (2000). Nursing knowledge for the 21st century: Opportunities and challenges. *Journal of Nursing Scholarship, 32* (2), 117–123.

Kee, F. (1996). Patients' prerogatives and perceptions of benefit. *British Medical Journal, 312* (7138), 1151–1153.

Johnson, J. E. (1984). Coping with elective surgery. In H. H. Werley & J. J. Fitzpatrick (Eds.), *Annual Review of Nursing Research* (pp. 107–132). New York: Springer-Verlag.

Johnson, J. E., Fieler, V. K., Jones, L. S., Wlasowicz, G. S., & Mitchell, M. L. (1997). *Self-regulation theory: Applying theory to your practice.* Pittsburgh, PA: Oncology Nursing Press.

Johnson, J. E., Kirchhoff, K. T., & Endress, M. P. (1975). Altering children's distress behavior during orthopedic cast removal. *Nursing Research, 24* (6), 404–410.

Johnson, J. E., Rice, V. H., Fuller, S. S., & Endress, M. P. (1978). Sensory information, instruction in a coping strategy, and recovery from surgery. *Research in Nursing & Health, 1* (1), 4–17.

Johnson & Johnson Pediatric Institute, L. L. C., & Sigma Theta Tau International (2002). *Nurses Investing in Maternal-Child Health.* New Jersey: Johnson & Johnson Pediatric Institute, L. L. C.

Jolley, S. (2002). Raising research awareness: A strategy for nurses. *Nursing Standard, 16* (33), 33–39.

Lohr, K. N., Eleazer, K., & Mauskopf, J. (1998). Health policy issues and applications for evidence-based medicine and clinical practice guidelines. *Health Policy, 46,* 1–19.

McKibbon, A. (1999). *PDQ. Evidence-based principles and practice.* Hamilton: B.C. Decker

Melnyk, B. M. (1994). Coping with unplanned childhood Hospitalization: Effects of informational interventions on mothers and children. *Nursing Research, 43,* 50–55.

Melnyk, B. M. (1999). Building a case for evidence-based practice: Inhalers vs. nebulizers. *Pediatric Nursing, 25 ,* 101–103.

Melnyk, B. M. (2002). Strategies for overcoming barriers in implementing evidence-based practice. *Pediatric Nursing, 28 ,* 159–161.

Melnyk, B. M., Alpert-Gillis, L., Feinstein, N. F., Fairbanks, E., Schultz-Czarniak, J., Hust, D., et al. (2001). Improving cognitive development of LBW premature infants with the COPE program: A pilot study of the benefit of early NICU intervention with mothers. *Research in Nursing and Health, 24,* 373–389.

Melnyk, B. M., Alpert-Gillis, L., Hensel, P. B., Cable-Beiling, R. C., & Rubenstein, J. (1997). Helping mothers cope with a critically ill child: A pilot test of the COPE intervention. *Research in Nursing & Health, 20,* 3–14.

Melnyk, B. M., & Fineout-Overholt, E. (2002a). Key steps in evidence-based practice: Asking compelling clinical questions and searching for the best evidence. *Pediatric Nursing, 28 ,* 262–263, 266.

Melnyk, B. M., & Fineout-Overholt, E. (2002b). Putting research into practice. Rochester ARCC. *Reflections on Nursing Leadership, 28* (2), 22–25.

Melnyk, B. M., Fineout-Overholt, E., Stone, P., & Ackerman, M. (2000). Evidence-based practice: The past, the present, and recommendations for the millennium. *Pediatric Nursing, 26,* 77–80.

Moldenhauer, Z., & Melnyk, B. M. (1999). Use of antidepressants in the treatment of child and adolescent depression: Are they effective? *Pediatric Nursing, 25 ,* 643–645.

Omery, A., & Williams, R. P. (1999). An appraisal of research utilization across the United States. *Journal of Nursing Administration, 12,* 50–56.

Pearson, A. (2002). Nursing takes the lead. Redefining what counts as evidence in Australian health care. *Reflections on Nursing Leadership, 28* (4), 18–21, 37.

Rosenfeld, P., Duthie, E., Bier, J., Bowar-Ferres, S., Fulmer, T., Iervolino, L., et al. (2000). Engaging staff nurses in evidence-based research to identify nursing practice problems and solutions. *Applied Nursing Research, 13 ,* 197–203.

Sackett, D. L., Straus, S. E., Richardson, W. S., Rosenberg, W., & Haynes, R. B. (2000). *Evidence-based medicine: How to practice and teach EBM.* London: Churchill Livingstone.

Sandelowski, M. (2000). Combining qualitative and quantitative sampling, data collection, and analysis techniques in mixed-method studies. *Research in Nursing & Health, 23,* 246–255.

Silagy, C. & Haines, A. (1998). *Evidence based practice in primary care.* London: BMJ Books.

Shonkoff, J. P., & Phillips, D. A. (2000). *From neurons to neighborhoods: The science of early childhood development* [Electronic version]. Washington, DC: National Academy Press.

Shorten, A., & Wallace, M. (1997). Evidence-based practice. When quality counts. *Australian Nursing Journal, 4*(11), 26–27.

Slutsky, J. (2003). Clinical guidelines: Building blocks for effective chronic illness care. Slide presentation at Web-assisted audio conference, "Causes of and potential solutions to the high cost of healthcare." Rockville, MD: AHRQ. Retrieved August 25, 2003 from http://www.ahrq.gov/ news/ulp/hicosttele/

Soumerai S. B., McLaughlin T. J., Spiegelman D., Hertzmark E., Thibault G., & Goldman L. (1997). Adverse outcomes of underuse of beta-blockers in elderly survivors of acute myocardial infarction. *JAMA. 277,* 115–21.

Solberg, L. I., Brekke, M. L., Fazio, C. J., Fowles, J., Jacobsen, D. N., Kotke, T. E. et al. (2000). Lessons from experienced guideline implementers: Attend to many factors and use multiple strategies. *Joint Commission Journal on Quality Improvement, 26,* 171–188.

Straus, S. & Sackett, D. (1998). Getting research into practice: using research findings in clinical practice. *British Medical Journal, 317* (7154), 339–342.

Thomas, L. H., McColl, E., Cullum, N., Rousseau, N., & Souter, J. (1999). Clinical guidelines in nursing, midwifery and the therapies: A systematic review. *Journal of Advanced Nursing, 30,* 40–50.

Titler, M. G., Cullen, L., & Ardery, G. (2002). Evidence-based practice: An administrative perspective. *Reflections on Nursing Leadership, 28* (2), 26–29, 46.

U.K. Department of Health (1999). Making a difference: Strengthening the nursing, midwifery and health visiting contribution to health and healthcare. Retrieved from http://www.doh.gov.uk/nurstrat.htm

Asking Compelling Clinical Questions

Richard Nollan, Ellen Fineout-Overholt, and Priscilla Stephenson

chapter 2

> *"Nothing is a waste of time if you use the experience wisely."*
>
> Auguste Rodin

How healthcare professionals seek and use information has changed over the past several decades (Leggat, 2003). The proliferation of information and mechanisms that make it more readily available (e.g., the Internet) along with the increasing complexity of patient illness require that practitioners become proficient at getting to the information they need when they need it. This does not happen automatically (Novins & Armstrong, 1999). Resources (e.g., computers, databases, and libraries) have to be put into place to make sure that practitioners can retrieve needed information so they can do their jobs. Not all practice environments have these resources. For example, Rasch and Cogdill (1999) found that of 134 nurse practitioners, 86 of them reported having computer access in their practice settings. Of those, only 58% had access to the World Wide Web. Estabrooks and colleagues (2003) found that although nurses were increasing their use of the Internet and e-mail at home, their work use was not comparable. There are many variables that influence whether a practitioner has the capacity to gather information quickly (e.g., financial ability to purchase a computer, availability of Internet service providers); however, every clinician must be able to articulate the clinical issue in such a way that maximizes the information obtained with the least amount of time investment. Hence, the first step in getting to the right information is to determine the "real" clinical issue, that is, asking a searchable, answerable question. This chapter provides the practitioner with strategies to hone their skills in formulating the clinical question to minimize the time spent in searching for relevant, valid evidence to answer it.

A Needle in a Haystack: Finding the Right Information at the Right Time

The key to success for any healthcare professional involved in patient care is to stay informed and as up to date as possible. *External* pressure to be up to date increasingly comes from patients, employers, certifying organizations, and insurers (Melnyk, 1999). The clinician's personal desire to provide the best, most up-to-date care possible along with expectations from healthcare consumers that practice will be based on the latest and best evidence fosters evidence-based practice (EBP). However, desiring to gather the right information in the right way at the right time is not sufficient. Practical, lifelong learning skills (e.g., asking focused questions, learning to search efficiently) are required to negotiate the information rich environment that every clinician encounters. With the amount of information that clinicians have available to them today, finding the right information at the right time is much like weeding through the haystack to find the proverbial needle. If one has any hope of finding the needle, there must be some sense of the needle's characteristics. Formulating the clinical question is much like identifying the characteristics of the needle. Question components guide the searching strategies undertaken. Knowing how to sift through the haystack is also important (see Chapter 3 for searching strategies); however, without having a well-built question to guide the search for evidence, clinicians are likely to waste time and energy in finding what they need.

The Haystack: Too Much Information

Although there is plethora of information available, news of clinical advances diffuses slowly through the literature and can still fail to reach more than a small percentage of clinicians (Shorten & Wallace, 1997; Straus & Sackett, 1998). Healthcare practitioners are finding it increasingly more difficult to keep up with and be confident in innovation. For example, Anderson and colleagues (1991) wanted to know whether patients at high risk for venous thromboembolism at 16 short-stay hospitals in central Massachusetts were receiving adequate prophylaxis. The researchers performed an 18-month retrospective medical record review of an estimated 150,000 patients and identified 17% as being at high risk. Despite the extensive progress in the prevention of venous thromboembolism and the broad consensus by leading clinicians as to its importance, only 32% of those at high risk for venous thromboembolism received prophylaxis. Similarly, Agu, Hamilton, and Baker (1999) found that despite the known benefit of graduated compression stocking in prophylaxis of deep vein thrombosis (DVT), there is still a wide variation in their routine use for patients at high risk for DVT. These studies do not speculate on why these important clinical advances were not better utilized, but the results raise questions about the limitations of conventional formats for communicating healthcare information to practitioners.

Clinicians are challenged with the task of effectively, proactively, and rapidly sifting through the haystack of scientific information to find the right needle full of the best applicable information for a patient or practice. In a study about information-seeking behavior in nurse practitioners (NPs), Codgill (2003) found that NPs most frequently used colleagues, drug reference manuals, textbooks, and protocol manuals as information sources. In addition, Cogdill found that NPs were more likely to find answers to questions about drug therapy from a print resource and to discuss needs about diagnosis with a colleague. One of the aims of EBP is to emphasize first asking a well-built question, then searching the literature for an answer to the question. This will better prepare the clinician to discuss the literature with colleagues. The EBP process focuses on incorporating good information-seeking habits into a daily routine. However, in a busy clinical setting, there is seldom time to look for information. The purchase of a good medical text and regular perusal of the top journals in a specialty were once considered adequate for keeping up with new information, but scientific information is expanding faster than anyone could have foreseen. The result is that significant clinical advances occur so rapidly that they can easily be overlooked. Reading every issue of the top three or four journals in your field from cover to cover does not guarantee that your professional and clinical knowledge is current. With the increase of biomedical knowledge (especially information about clinical advances), it is clear that the traditional notion of "keeping up with the literature" is no longer practical. A clinician would have to read 17–19 journal articles a day, 365 days a year to remain current (Haynes, 1993). Instead, the emphasis must shift to more proactive information-seeking skills, starting with formulating an answerable, patient-specific question.

Digitization and the Internet have improved accessibility to information, regardless of space and time; however, these innovations have not resolved the issue of finding the right information at the right time. It is important to become friendly with and proficient at utilizing information technology, including the Internet and other electronic information resources, which means that clinicians must be skilled in using a computer. Learning to use computers comfortably is easily learned and essential to EBP and best practice. In addition, other barriers described by nurses and other health professionals to getting to the right information at the right time include a low comfort level with library and search techniques and a lack of time to search for the best evidence (Cook, Mulrow, & Haynes, 1997; Melnyk & Fineout-Overholt, 2002; Sackett, Straus, Richardson, Rosenberg, & Hayes, 2000). These barriers can be diminished by first learning how to ask a searchable, answerable question.

Asking Searchable, Answerable Questions

Finding the right information amidst an overwhelming amount of information in a timely way is imperative. The first step to accomplish this goal is to formulate the clinical issue into a searchable, answerable question. Smith, Ganschow, and colleagues (2000) conducted a clinical trial to evaluate the effectiveness of an education program on medical residents' EBP skills. They found that after the intervention, the residents were better at asking answerable questions, searching for relevant evidence, and understanding the results of quantitative studies. The importance of asking the "right" question cannot be overemphasized.

It is important to distinguish between the two types of questions that clinician might ask—background questions and foreground questions. **Background questions** are those that need to be answered as a foundation for asking the searchable, answerable foreground question. Sackett and colleagues (2000) describe background questions as those that ask for general information about a clinical issue. This type of question has two components: the starting place of the question (e.g., what, where, when, why and how) and the outcome of interest (e.g., the clinical diagnosis). For example, a background question could be, How does the drug acetaminophen work to affect fever? The answer to this question can be found in a drug pharmacokinetics text. Another example could be, How do hemodynamics differ with positioning? This answer can be found in textbooks, as well. Often, background questions cover the "full range of biologic, psychologic, and sociologic aspects of human illness" (Sackett et al., 2000, p. 16). If a clinician does not realize that the question at hand is a background question, time may be lost in searching for an answer in the wrong haystack (e.g., research databases versus a textbook).

Foreground questions are those that can be answered from scientific evidence about diagnosing, treating, or assisting patients with understanding their prognosis. These questions focus on specific knowledge. In the examples, the subsequent foreground questions could be, Which is more effective in reducing fevers in children, acetaminophen or ibuprofen? and Which is more effective in patients with acute respiratory distress syndrome (ARDS), prone or supine positioning? The first question builds on the background knowledge of how acetaminophen works but can be answered only by a study that compares the two listed medications. The second question requires knowledge of how positioning changes hemodynamics (i.e., the background question), but the two types of positioning must be compared in a specific population of patients in order to answer it. Recognizing the difference between the two types of questions is the challenge. Sackett and colleagues (2000) state that as a novice, one may need to ask primarily background questions. As one gains experience, the background knowledge has grown, and the focus becomes foreground questions. Although background questions are essential and must be answered, it is the foreground questions that are the searchable, answerable questions and the focus of this chapter.

Clinical Inquiry and Uncertainty in Generating Clinical Questions

Where clinical questions come from (i.e., their origin) is an important consideration. On a daily basis, most clinicians encounter situations for which they do not have all the information they need (i.e., uncertainty) to care for their patients as they would like (Counsell, 1997). The role of uncertainty is to spawn **clinical inquiry**. Horowitz and colleagues (1996) described clinical inquiry as a process in which clinicians gather data together using narrowly defined clinical parameters. This process allows for an appraisal of the available choices of treatment for the purpose of finding the most appropriate choice of action.

Clinical inquiry must be cultivated in the work environment. To foster clinical inquiry, a level of comfort must be had with uncertainty. Lindstrom and Rosyik (2003) state that uncertainty is a sequela of ambiguity. Clinicians live in a rather ambiguous world. What works for this patient may not work for that patient. The latest product on the market says it is the answer to all of the issues that come with wound healing, but is it? Formulating clinical questions in a structured, specific way, such as with PICO formatting (discussed later in this chapter), assists the clinician in finding the right evidence to answer those questions and decrease uncertainty. These successes then foster further clinical inquiry.

Questions often are considered in the areas of etiology, diagnosis, therapy, prevention, and prognosis. Qualitative questions are a part of clinical inquiry and are appropriate. These types of questions may be asked to determine meaning, to provide insight and scope to a phenomenon, to appreciate a patient's experience, or to help understand the influence of culture on healthcare. As well, interpreting patient assessment data (i.e., clinical findings), trying to determine the more likely cause of the patient's problem among the many it could be (i.e., differential diagnosis), or simply wanting to improve one's clinical skills in a specific area may prompt a question. Whatever the reason for the question, the components need to be considered and formulated carefully to facilitate efficiently finding relevant evidence to answer the questions.

Posing the Question Using PICO

Focused foreground questions are essential to judiciously finding the right evidence to answer them (Oxman et al., 1993). Foreground questions usually have four components, termed *PICO*. The acronym comes from the following:

Patient population of interest
Intervention of interest
Comparison of interest
Outcome of interest

Thoughtful consideration of each component can provide a clearly articulated question. Table 2-1 provides a quick overview of the PICO question components. Well-built, focused clinical questions drive the subsequent steps of the EBP process (*Cochrane Reviewer's Handbook*, online, accessed July 30, 2003).

The patient population (P) may seem easy to identify. However, without explicit description of who the population is, the clinician can get off on the wrong foot in searching. The *Cochrane Reviewer's Handbook* (2003) suggests careful consideration of the patient and the setting of interest. Limiting the population to those in a certain age group or other special subgroup is a good idea if there is a valid reason for doing so. Arbitrary designations for the patient population will not assist the clinician in retrieving the most relevant evidence.

The intervention of interest (I) may include but is not limited to any exposure, treatment, patient perception, diagnostic test, or prognostic factor. The more specifically the intervention of interest is defined, the more focused the search will be.

The comparison (C) needs special consideration. The comparison can be a true control, such as placebo. More commonly, the comparison is another treatment, sometimes the usual standard of care. For example, the clinician wants to ask the question, In caring for the disabled, does use of level-access showers improve patient hygiene more than bed bathing? The intervention of interest is level-access showers, and the comparison is the usual care of bed bathing.

The outcome (O) in the example is patient hygiene. Specifically identifying the outcome enables the searcher to find evidence that examined the same outcome variable, although the variable may be measured in various ways.

In some questions, there may be more than one outcome of interest found in a study, but all of these outcomes fall under one umbrella. For example, the question may be, In preschool-aged children, is an electrolyte, flavored drink more effective at reducing dry mouth,

table 2.1   PICO: Components of an answerable, searchable question

PICO	
Patient population/disease	The patient population or disease of interest, for example: ● age ● gender ● ethnicity ● with certain disorder (e.g., hepatitis)
Intervention	The intervention or range of interventions of interest, for example: ● Exposure to disease ● Prognostic factor A ● Risk behavior (e.g., smoking)
Comparison	What you want to compare the intervention against, for example: ● No disease ● Placebo or no intervention/therapy ● Prognostic factor B ● Absence of risk factor (e.g. non-smoking)
Outcome	Outcome of interest, for example: ● Risk of disease ● Accuracy of diagnosis ● Rate of occurrence of adverse outcome (e.g., death)

tachycardia, fever, and irritability than water alone? Instead of formulating the question this way, it would be better to use the umbrella term *dehydration* for all these symptoms that are listed. The question would then be, In preschool-aged children, is an electrolyte, flavored drink more effective at reducing dehydration (e.g., dry mouth, tachycardia, fever, irritability) than water alone? Specifying the outcome will assist the clinician in focusing the search for relevant evidence.

Three Ps of Proficient Questioning: Practice, Practice, Practice

The best way to become proficient in formulating searchable, answerable questions is to practice. This section of the chapter has six clinical scenarios from which you can formulate a clinical question. First, read the scenario and try to formulate the question using the template provided in Box 2-1, if needed. Then read the following paragraphs for help in determining the success of your question formulation.

Clinical Scenario 2-1 gives you practice in formulating a searchable, answerable question. Given the suggested format for a therapy question, fill in the blanks with information from the clinical scenario.

---

box 2.1

Question Templates for Asking PICO Questions

THERAPY

In _____, what is the effect of _____ on

_____ compared with _____?

ETIOLOGY

Are _____ who have _____ at _____ risk

for/of _____ compared with _____

with/without _____?

DIAGNOSIS OR DIAGNOSTIC TEST

Are (Is) _____ more accurate in diagnosing

_____ compared with _____?

PREVENTION

For _____ does the use of _____ reduce

the future risk of _____ compare with

_____?

PROGNOSIS

Does _____ influence _____ in patients who

have _____?

MEANING

How do _____ diagnosed with _____ perceive _____?

> ### Clinical Scenario 2.1
>
> ## Therapy Example
>
> A 17-year-old African-American woman is brought to the ER by her mother with a 3-day history of nausea, vomiting, and headache. Her medical and social histories are benign. The only drug she is taking is acetaminophen (Tylenol) 1 gram three times a day (t.i.d.) for her headache. Her physical exam is benign. The first laboratory results reveal nothing; however, the second reveal that she has a hepatitis B infection, for which she will receive appropriate treatment. The mother tells you she has heard that acetaminophen can cause liver problems, and she wonders whether her daughter should continue taking the drug for her headache, considering the diagnosis.

In _____, what is the effect of _____ on _____ _____compared with _____?

Remember that a well-formulated question is the key to a successful search. The question could be, In African-American female adolescents with hepatitis (P), what is the effect of <u>acetaminophen</u> (I) on <u>liver function</u> (O) compared with <u>ibuprofen</u>? (C)? A more general question might read, In people with hepatitis, what is the effect of acetaminophen on liver function compared with ibuprofen? Background knowledge would be necessary to know whether there were ethnic variations in how acetaminophen functioned or whether only the disease process was essential to the question.

In this example, the mother's concern has to do with diagnosis coupled with the knowledge that acetaminophen has a known hepatotoxic effect. Thus, the patient is an African-American adolescent female with hepatitis B, the intervention is acetaminophen (for the headache), the comparison might be another analgesic less toxic to the liver than acetaminophen, and the outcome is liver function. As is often the case, the answer to this clinical question can give rise to further questions. In this case, questions may be raised about the exact nature of acetaminophen's hepatotoxicity and prompt discussion about whether it should be used by any patient with hepatitis.

Clinical Scenario 2-2 contains an etiologic scenario. Given the format for etiology questions, fill in the blanks with information from the clinical scenario.

Are _____ who have _____ at _____ risk for/of _____ compared with _____ with/without _____?

Etiology questions help clinicians to address causality (Holloway et al., 2000). The question could read, Are <u>30- to 50-year-old women</u> (P) who have <u>high blood pressure</u> (I) at <u>in-</u>

Clinical Scenario 2.2

Etiology Example

A 40-year-old woman comes to the clinic for her regularly scheduled physical exam. Her blood pressure is 128/80. The rest of her history, physical assessment findings, and laboratory work are benign. When you discuss her findings with her, she asks you about her chance of having a heart attack, because her blood pressure is now considered hypertension. Given the discussions about hypertension parameters, you decide to search the literature to find the best evidence to answer her question.

---

creased risk for <u>an acute myocardial infarction</u> (O) compared with <u>women </u>without <u>high blood pressure</u>? (C)

Clinical Scenario 2-3 contains a scenario about diagnosis. Given the format for diagnosis questions, fill in the blanks with information from the clinical scenario.

Are _____ more accurate in diagnosing _____ compared with _____?

Diagnosis questions assist the clinician in determining which diagnostic tests will be best to confirm or exclude a diagnosis and with what degree of precision (Holloway et al., 2000). As well, cost, feasibility, and availability of the diagnostic test can be part of the ques-

---

Clinical Scenario 2.3

Diagnosis Example

A 50-year-old man comes to your clinic with complaints of mild indigestion for 3 days. His heart rate and blood pressure are within acceptable limits. His father had an acute myocardial infarction at 60 and coronary artery bypass surgery at 75. He died of unrelated causes at 85. The rest of the history, physical assessment findings, and laboratory test results are benign. You do an initial screening electrocardiogram (ECG). The patient asks whether it is beneficial to do more ECGs. You know what your clinic usually does for these types of patients, but you want to know what evidence is out there to support current practice.

> ## Clinical Scenario 2.4
>
> ## Prevention Example
>
> You are coordinator of the flu shot program at a retirement center. A group of participants at the center has asked you to come and talk with them about why it is important for people their age to get an annual flu shot. You want to be well prepared for this savvy group of elders, so you search the literature to find the best evidence to answer any question they may have. In the past 2 years, there have been two pneumonia-related deaths in the group, and you know that they will ask questions about whether there is a relationship between getting a flu shot and acquiring pneumonia.

tion. The question could read, Are <u>serial 12-lead ECGs</u> (I) more accurate in diagnosing (O) <u>an acute myocardial infarction</u> (P) compared with <u>one initial 12-lead ECG</u>? (C)

Clinical Scenario 2-4 contains a scenario about prevention. The following is the format for prevention questions. Fill in the blanks with information from the clinical scenario.

For _____, does the use of _____ reduce the future risk of _____ compared with _____?

Prevention questions assist the clinician in identifying risk factors that if adjusted can help to reduce the chance of developing the disease (Holloway et al., 2000). The question could read: For <u>patients 65 years and older</u> (P), does the use of <u>an influenza vaccine</u> (I) reduce the future risk of <u>pneumonia (O)</u> compared with <u>patients who have not received the vaccine</u>? (C)

Clinical Scenario 2-5 contains a scenario about prognosis. The following is the format for prognosis questions. Fill in the blanks with information from the clinical scenario.

Does _____ influence _____ in patients who have _____?

Prognosis questions assist the clinician in estimating a patient's clinical course across time (Holloway et al., 2000). The question could read, Does <u>smoking status (e.g., smoker [I] versus nonsmoker [C])</u> influence <u>death and infarction rate</u> (O) in patients who have <u>experienced an acute myocardial infarction</u>? (P)

Clinical Scenario 2-6 contains a scenario about meaning. The following is the format for meaning questions. Fill in the blanks with the information from the clinical scenario.

How do _____ with _____ perceive _____?

The question could read, How do <u>women</u> (P) diagnosed with <u>fibromyalgia</u> (I) perceive (O) <u>others' perceptions of their physical limitations</u>? (C)

Clinical Scenario 2.5

Prognosis Example

You are coordinator of the local support group for smokers who are trying to quit smoking or maintain their commitment to smoking abstinence. You are working on the program for the next quarter. An innovation you are trying out is to have clinicians and their patients come to a joint session on smoking cessation. You know that there have been three participants in the group who have not given up their cigarettes and who have had their second myocardial infarctions in the last 6 years. It is likely, you reason, that there will be questions and discussion about smoking and subsequent heart attacks. You want to provide the latest and best evidence to both of these key stakeholders to spur on their commitment to smoking cessation.

All of these examples and templates are for practicing. There may be various ways in which to ask a certain type of question. Do not get stuck in the mindset that there is only one way to ask a therapy or prevention question. Look at the your clinical scenario and try to put the PICO components into words. Then formulate the question. If the templates work and make sense for the scenario, by all means, use them. However, it is not wise action to try to form cookie-cutter questions, because some important component most assuredly will be missed.

Clinical Scenario 2.6

Meaning Example

You are caring for a 35-year-old woman admitted to the hospital after a motor vehicle accident (MVA). In talking with her, you find out that she was diagnosed with fibromyalgia 5 years ago. Until then, she had an active lifestyle. Since her diagnosis, she often feels fatigued and unable to perform to her own expectations. She is having difficulty with the physical therapy and tells you that she gets tired quickly. The healthcare team suspects that she may be anemic and wants to do blood tests. You think that her fatigue may be from her fibromyalgia and the subsequent stress of the MVA. When you discuss the team's plans, the patient becomes concerned. She wants to make sure that her diagnosis of fibromyalgia is being taken seriously. As a patient advocate, you want to provide the team with the best and latest evidence on what it feels like to have fibromyalgia and how the disorder manifests itself.

Why Work Hard at Formulating the Question?

Without a well-formulated question, the clinician is apt to search for wrong, too much, or irrelevant information. Honing one's skills in formulating a well-built question can provide confidence that the search will be more successful and timely. From their vast experience, Sackett and his colleagues (2000) suggested several other benefits to putting together good questions, including clearly communicating patient information with colleagues, helping learners more clearly understand content taught, and furthering the initiative to become better clinicians through the positive experience of asking a good question, finding the best evidence, and making a difference. Various Web-based resources can assist you in understanding how to formulate a searchable, answerable question.

Find Web-based information on formulating searchable, answerable questions at the following sites:
University of Illinois College of Medicine at Peoria:
http://www.uicomp.uic.edu/IntMedRes/teach/question.htm
Studentbmj.com: International Medical Student's Journal:
http://www.studentbmj.com/back_issues/0902/education/313.html

Formulating a well-built question is worth the time and effort it takes. A well-formulated question facilitates a focused search (Stone, 2002), decreasing searching time and improving search results. Formulating a well-built question is the first—and some have said the most challenging—step toward providing evidence-based care to your patients (Sackett et al., 2000).

> **"***My basic principle is that you don't make decisions because they are easy; you don't make them because they are cheap; you don't make them because they're popular; you make them because they're right.***"**
>
> *Fr. Theodore Hesburgh*

references

Agu, O., Hamilton, G., Baker, D. Graduated compression stockings in the prevention of venous thromboembolism. *British Journal of Surgery, 86*(8), 992–1004.

Anderson F., Wheeler H., Goldberg R., Hosmer D., Forcier A., & Patwardhan, N. (1991). Physician practices in the prevention of venous thromboembolism. *Annals of Internal Medicine, 115*, 591–595.

Cochrane Reviewer's Handbook (2003). Section 4: Formulating the problem. Found at http://www.cochrane.dk/cochrane/handbook/hbook.htm. Accessed July 30, 2003.

Cogdill, K. W. (2003). Information needs and information seeking in primary care: study of nurse practitioners. *Journal of the Medical Library Association, 91*(2), 203–215.

Cook, D. J., Mulrow, C. D., & Haynes, R. B.

(1997). Systematic reviews: Synthesis of best evidence for clinical decisions. *Annals of Internal Medicine, 126*(5), 376–380.

Counsell, C. (1997). Formulating questions and locating primary studies for inclusion in systematic reviews. *Annals of Internal Medicine, 127,* 380–387.

Estabrooks, C., O'Leary, K., Ricker, K., & Humphrey, C. (2003). The Internet and access to evidence: How are nurses positioned? *Journal of Advanced Nursing, 42,* 73–81.

Haynes, R. (1993). Where's the meat in clinical journals? *ACP Journal Club, 119,* A23–24.

Holloway, R., Benesch, C., Berg, M., Hinchey, J., Kieburtz, K., Marshall, F., Plotkin, K., Richard, I., & Schwid, S. (2000). *Journal club: Evidence-based medicine for the neurology residents. Syllabus and supporting materials.* Rochester, NY: University of Rochester Medical Center.

Horowitz, R., Singer, B., Makuch, R., & Viscoli, C. (1996). Can treatment that is helpful on average be harmful to some patients? A study of the conflicting information needs of clinical inquiry and drug regulation. *Journal of Clinical Epidemiology, 49,* 395–400.

Leggat, S. (2003). Turning evidence into wisdom. *Healthcare Papers, 3*(3), 44–48.

Lindstrom, T., & Rosyik, A. (2003). Ambiguity leads to uncertainty: Ambiguous demands to blood donors. *Scandinavian Journal of Caring Sciences, 17,* 74–77.

Melnyk, B. M. (1999). Building a case for evidence-based practice: inhalers vs. nebulizers. *Pediatric Nursing, 25*(1), 102–103, 101.

Melnyk, B. M., & Fineout-Overholt, E. (2002). Putting research into practice. *Reflections on Nursing Leadership, 28*(2), 22–25, 45.

Novins, P. & Armstrong, R. (1999). Choosing your spots for knowledge management. In *A Blueprint for Change,* Ernst & Young: 45–52.

Oxman, A., Sackett, D, Guyatt, G., & Evidence Based Medicine Working Group. (1993). Users' guides to evidence-based medicine. *JAMA, 270,* 2093–2095.

Rasch, R. & Cogdill, K. (1999). Nurse practitioners' information needs and information seeking: Implications for practice and education. *Holistic Nursing Practice, 13*(4), 90–97.

Sackett, D. L., Straus, S. E., Richardson, W. S., Rosenberg, W., & Haynes, R. B. (2000). *Evidence-based Medicine: How to practice and teach EBM.* Edinburgh: Churchill Livingston.

Shorten, A., & Wallace, M. (1997). Evidence-based practice. When quality counts. *Australian Nursing Journal, 4*(11), 26–27.

Smith, C. A., Ganschow, P. S., Reilly, B. M., Evans, A. T., McNutt, R. A., Osei, A., Saquib, M., Surabhi, S., & Yadav, S. (2000). Teaching residents evidence-based medicine skills: A controlled trial of effectiveness and assessment of durability. *Journal of General Internal Medicine. 15,* 710–715.

Stone, P. (2002). Popping the (PICO) question in research and evidence-based practice. *Applied Nursing Research, 16,* 197–198.

Straus, S., & Sackett, D. (1998). Getting research findings into practice: Using research findings in clinical practice. *British Medical Journal, 317,* 339–342.

chapter 2

37

Finding Relevant Evidence

Ellen Fineout-Overholt, Richard Nollan, Priscilla Stephenson, and Julia Sollenberger

chapter 3

> " He that would have the fruit must climb the tree. "
>
> *Thomas Fuller*

Healthcare knowledge that has been in the journal literature and that has been debated and absorbed into general knowledge is then systematically organized into textbooks. In healthcare, textbooks present established, accepted ideas of diagnostic and therapeutic techniques. However, they are not the best resource for finding current evidence to answer clinical questions because they often take several years to complete. Electronic textbooks may be an improvement in providing a comprehensive resource; however, nearly all electronic versions of textbooks are updated only as often as the print version. Current exceptions are *Harrison's Principles of Internal Medicine* and *UpToDate*.

Tools for Finding the Needle in the Haystack

Given the consistent need for current information in healthcare, frequent review of bibliographic and full-text databases (i.e., any collection of records in an electronic form) that hold the latest studies reported in journals is the best, most current choice for finding relevant evidence to answer compelling clinical questions (Clinical Scenario 3-1).

The use of PICO format (see Chapter 2) to guide and clarify the important elements of the questions is an essential first step toward finding the right information to answer them. Generally, PICO questions are expressed in everyday clinical terminology. Often, in searching for the best evidence to answer a PICO question, databases housing the evidence have their own dialects that can help the searcher navigate the myriad of available studies and articles. Database-specific medical language is often standardized to eliminate or minimize errors that occur because of linguistic usage or spelling. Learning how to navigate different databases is imperative for successfully retrieving relevant evidence. Novices to this type of searching are wise to consult a medical librarian who can assist them in this process.

The next step after formulating a well-built question is to determine the source from which the best evidence is most likely available. Clinicians need peer-reviewed research to answer their questions, and most often the source of that evidence will be a database of published studies. The records in the database are stored, retrieved, and manipulated by the computer.

Databases may contain images, numbers, statistics, or names as in a directory, and they may be as simple or complex as the creators want to make them. They may contain medical history, physical examination, laboratory, or public health data. Databases that contain references to the medical literature often refer to physical objects, such as books or journal publications. Most databases contain specific languages that allow the searcher to negotiate a database more successfully. Choosing the right database and being familiar with its language are essential to a successful, expedient search for answers to a clinical question.

Clinical Scenario 3.1

A 45-year-old mother of three has been newly diagnosed with asthma. She tells you that her friend who has asthma takes a medication that is long-acting. She wonders why the one she has been prescribed is short-acting. She asks you about whether there is support for the medication she has been prescribed (Salbutamol). You searched the literature to help her with the answer. The PICO question for the search is, In adults with asthma (P), how effective is salbutamol (I) compared with salmeterol xinafoate (C) in treating asthma symptoms (O)?

Upon searching the Cochrane Database of Systematic Reviews, you find a systematic review that recommends the longer-acting medication (Walters, Walters, & Gibson, 2003). In an effort to gain more information, you look for an evidence-based guideline in the National Guidelines Clearinghouse database, searching with the key words *short-acting beta agonist*, *long-acting beta agonist*, and *asthma*. The search reveals five guidelines. One is helpful to you as a healthcare provider (Singapore, 2002). On the basis of these two pieces of evidence and your patient's concerns, you discuss the plan of care and the patient's concerns with the healthcare team.

Tool One: Choosing the Right Database

Of the many databases that house healthcare literature, some are available through several vendors at a cost, some are free of charge, and some are available both free of charge and through a vendor for a fee. For example, depending on the search options desired, MEDLINE can be accessed free of charge through the National Library of Medicine's PubMed search system or obtained for a cost in combination with several other databases or via a system such as Ovid. Table 3-1 contains information about access to some of the available databases.

table 3.1   Examples of searchable databases

Database	Description
CINAHL: Cumulative Index of Nursing and Allied Health Literature (1982–present) http://www.cinahl.com/	Studies in nursing, allied health, and biomedicine Individual subscriptions: vary with time you expect to use; student discount http://www.cinahl.com/cdirect/cdirect.htm Institutional subscriptions: contact the CINAHL sales department, e-mail: sales@cinahl.com
MEDLINE: (1966–present) http://www.ncbi.nlm.nih.gov/entrez/query.fcgi? *CMD=Limits&DB=PubMed*	Studies in medicine, nursing, dentistry, psychiatry, veterinary, and allied health Individual subscriptions: free and at a cost, depending on vendor and desired search options Institutional subscriptions: free and at a cost, depending on vendor and desired search options
EMBASE http://www.embase.com/	Biomedical and pharmaceutical studies No individual subscription option found. Institutional subscription: pricing based on number of real users in institution
PsycINFO (1887–present) http://www.apa.org/psycinfo/	Psychology and related healthcare disciplines Must be accessed through a vendor: APA, Ovid Individual pay-as-you-go option http://www.apa.org/psycinfo/products/ individuals.html Institutional subscriptions http://www.apa.org/psycinfo/products/ institutions.html
Cochrane Database of Systematic Reviews *http://www.cochrane.org/*	Full text of regularly updated systematic reviews prepared by the Cochrane Collaboration. Completed reviews and protocols. Available via Internet or CD-ROM. Subscription is to *Cochrane Library*, containing seven databases. Individual subscription: flat fee www.cochrane.org/reviews/clibintro.htm

chapter 3

41

This chapter focuses primarily on six databases:

- Cochrane Database of Systematic Reviews (CDSR)
- National Guidelines Clearinghouse (NGC)
- MEDLINE
- Cumulated Index of Nursing and Allied Health Literature (CINAHL)
- Exerpta Medica online (EMBASE)
- PsycINFO

Most of these databases now provide access to a combination of their own database and MEDLINE citations. These types of databases greatly facilitate access to the biomedical literature; however, using them effectively can present several challenges.

Databases are essential information resources for all healthcare professionals. MEDLINE and CINAHL are among the best known comprehensive databases and can arguably be described as representing the scientific knowledge base of healthcare. However, the amount of information in these databases seems to exceed the mechanisms to contain it. These two broad databases cannot cover all areas of interest to healthcare professionals. In addition to MEDLINE and CINAHL, there are hundreds of databases available today, some of which are highly specialized, and their numbers are growing in response to the desire for more readily available information.

Cochrane Database of Systematic Reviews

The *Cochrane Library* contains several databases, including:

- **Cochrane Database of Systematic Reviews**
- **Cochrane Database of Methodology Reviews**
- **Database of Abstracts of Reviews of Effects**
- Cochrane Central Register of Controlled Trials
- Cochrane Methodology Register
- **NHS Economic Evaluation Database**
- **Health Technology Assessment Database**

The Cochrane Collaboration can be accessed via **http://www.cochrane.org** or **http://www.wileyeurope.com/WileyCDA/Section/id-101093.html**

The CDSR is a valuable source of synthesized evidence (i.e., preappraised) for clinicians. It is a highly esteemed database that includes the full text of the regularly updated **systematic** reviews prepared by The Cochrane Collaboration.

These reviews are syntheses of studies that answer a common clinical question and are conducted using rigorous methods that can be found in the Cochrane Reviewers' Handbook at **http://www.cochrane.dk/cochrane/handbook/hbook.htm**. Abstracts of updated reviews as well as reviews in the current edition of the database are accessible on the Web site. In addition, the Cochrane Library can be searched for abstracts of reviews at **http://www.update-software.com/Cochrane/abstract.htm**.

Full-text systematic reviews currently can be accessed only by subscription.

The Cochrane database houses completed reviews that are prepared and maintained by collaborative review groups, as well as protocols for reviews currently being prepared. All protocols include an expected date of completion. Protocols provide the background, objectives, and methods for reviews in progress. It is important to understand the difference between a protocol and a completed review when searching this database.

The CDSR is a fairly small database, in part because systematic reviews are relatively new in the history of healthcare. Unlike MEDLINE (10 million citations) and CINAHL (3 million citations), the CDSR contains a few thousand citations and is limited to a single publication type—systematic reviews—including meta-analyses. A single word search in the MEDLINE or CINAHL databases will easily result in thousands of *hits* (i.e., articles or studies that contain the searched word). Because it is a small database, the CDSR database has no **controlled vocabulary**; the broadest search is likely to retrieve only a small, manageable number of hits. This makes the database easy to search and to review.

The CDSR is the *first* database that should be searched when seeking to find an answer to a clinical question. If systematic reviews exist that can answer the clinical question, the search for relevant evidence and the critical appraisal process has already been done. The clinician then needs to appraise the systematic review critically. Chapter 5 contains more information on critical appraisal of systematic reviews. If the systematic review is valid and applicable, the clinician is off and running after reading only one study (i.e., the systematic review) versus the potentially numerous ones covered in the review.

National Guidelines Clearinghouse

The next database to search is the NGC that is supported by the Agency for Healthcare Research and Quality (AHRQ).

Guidelines are systematically developed statements about a plan of care for a specific set of clinical circumstances involving a particular population. The best guidelines for clinical practice are based on rigorous scientific evidence (i.e. systematic reviews or randomized controlled trials [RCTs]); however, there are guidelines that can assist in decision making that are based on a consensus of expert opinion.

The NGC houses structured abstracts (summaries) about the guideline and its development; has a condensed version of the guideline for viewing (i.e., summary); has links to full-text guidelines, where available, and/or ordering information for print copies; and has Palm-based personal digital assistant (PDA) downloads of the complete NGC summary for all guidelines represented in the database. In addition, the database provides a guideline comparison so that users can compare across several guidelines. These are just a few of the features of the NGC database. As with all the databases in this chapter, more can be learned from actually using the database to answer a clinical question.

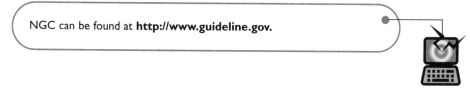

NGC can be found at **http://www.guideline.gov.**

MEDLINE

MEDLINE is produced by the National Library of Medicine and is available free of charge through the PubMed search engine. The MEDLINE database has been widely used. The

PubMed search engine was launched in June 1997, and it received approximately 2 million searches that month. In June 2002, PubMed reported 1.3 million searches per day. Since its inception, there have been numerous improvements to the PubMed pages, including a growing number of subject-oriented journal groups and clinical search filters.

MEDLINE is available 24 hours a day to any computer in the world with Internet access. The National Library of Medicine also leases the MEDLINE file to vendors, such as Ovid. These types of companies load the database into their own user interfaces with an array of additional features beyond those available in PubMed and sell subscriptions to libraries and others. It is important to acknowledge that the original file of indexed citations is the same MEDLINE product in PubMed as in any of these other vendors' versions of the file. It contains citations from more than 4,600 biomedical journals in medicine, nursing, pharmacy, dentistry, and allied health. More than 52% of the articles contain abstracts; 80% are in English; and the database is updated weekly. MEDLINE has worldwide coverage, including many non-English languages, though it tends to focus on North American journal articles. To facilitate complete searches, MEDLINE uses a controlled vocabulary (i.e., a hierarchical arrangement of descriptive terms that serve as mapping agents for searches, often unique to each database) called *medical subject headings*, or MeSH for short. (**Controlled vocabulary** and **controlled thesaurus** are discussed in more detail later.)

The database MEDLINE is available free of charge through the PubMed search engine at **http://www.ncbi.nlm.nih.gov/entrez/query.fcgi.**

Cumulated Index of Nursing and Allied Health Literature

The CINAHL database is produced by Cinahl Information Systems and contains article citations with abstracts, when available, from 13 nursing and allied health disciplines.

Articles are retrieved from journals, books, drug monographs, dissertations, and images that are sometimes difficult to locate in other databases. CINAHL is usually accessed through libraries but can be accessed through a personal CINAHLdirect subscription via the CINAHL Information Systems Web site (http://www.cinahl.com). Several pricing options are available based on an estimate of the online time needed.

A corresponding service, CINAHLexpress, provides document delivery service of articles from the 1,200 items it indexes. In addition, STAT Search is a service that provides a professional searcher to assist you. The CINAHL database includes more than 3 million journal articles from 1982 to present. About 70% of the citations in CINAHL also appear in the MEDLINE database. CINAHL also has a controlled vocabulary. It is an English language database and available through various vendors.

The CINAHL database is available at **http://www.cinahl.com**

Excerpta Medica Online

EMBASE is the major European biomedical and pharmaceutical database indexing in the fields of drug research, pharmacology, pharmaceutics, toxicology, clinical and experimental human medicine, health policy and management, public health, occupational health, environmental health, drug dependence and abuse, psychiatry, forensic medicine, and biomedical engineering/instrumentation. EMBASE currently has more than 9 million records gathered from international journals, including more than 5,000 journal titles from 70 countries. More than 80% of the citations in EMBASE contain full author abstracts.

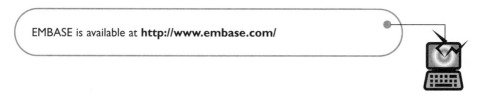

EMBASE is available at **http://www.embase.com/**

PsycINFO

PyscINFO is a bibliographic database that indexes publications as early as the late 1800s.

This database of scholarly literature in behavioral sciences and mental health contains more than 1 million citations, 11% of which are books and 12% dissertations. Professionals in psychology and related fields such as psychiatry, education, neuroscience, nursing, and other healthcare disciplines can find relevant evidence in this database to answer specific clinical questions.

PsycINFO is available at **http://www.apa.org/psycinfo/about/**

Searching the literature can be both rewarding and frustrating, primarily because the volume of literature is huge. The MEDLINE database alone provides reference to 10 million citations, and it cannot cover *all* worldwide health care journals. Searching multiple databases can increase the number of relevant articles in any search. Databases such as MEDLINE, CINAHL, EMBASE, PsycINFO, and others impose organization on the chaos of the journal literature. Each offers coverage that is broad and sometimes overlapping. Knowing which databases to search first and for what information is imperative for a successful, efficient search.

Tool Two: Understanding Database Structure

The kinds of databases most often searched for relevant evidence to answer clinical questions are those that contain either bibliographic data or full-text articles.

Bibliographic Databases

Bibliographic databases contain information about publications, including author, title, journal name, or publisher. Often, they describe the article or study in an abstract, or synopsis. However, these databases do not contain the full-text article. Box 3-1 is an example of a bibliographic database citation that was found in the search for evidence to help answer the question, How do children experience chronic illness? A bibliographic record (i.e., citation) can include many details about the reference, such as author, article title, journal title, and the abstract, if the reference article is published with one. The database can be searched by these details to access the article. The details are sometimes called *access points*.

The usefulness of PsycINFO, MEDLINE, CINAHL, and other bibliographic databases cannot be overestimated. Imposing an organizational matrix on an otherwise amorphous body of disconnected articles, textbooks, and other publications makes retrieval of relevant evidence much simpler. A confusing point can be that some bibliographic databases seem to offer full-text articles. If a full-text article is offered in a citation on a bibliographic database, it is because the vendor or library has chosen to pay for a subscription to the online journal that offers full-text articles. The full-text articles are not housed in the bibliographic database. Rather, mechanisms exist to enable the vendor to link to the full-text article that is displayed along with the database citation.

Full-Text Databases

Full-text databases contain whole articles, including the text, charts, graphs, and other illustrations. They contain article citations as well. The CDSR is a full-text database. Vendors such as Ovid may add hyperlinks to the references of full-text articles, making it easy to identify a key idea and connect to the hyperlink for the cited text. The advantage of this type of hyperlink is that the searcher can follow an idea from one article to the next, identifying a family of articles that focus on a certain idea. Although this can be a very useful tool for finding articles that address similar issues, it also can lead the searcher far afield and interfere with a focused or comprehensive search.

Full-text database records contain the same types of access points as bibliographic databases, with the added capability for searching captions and illustrations. By searching the entire text of the article, the searcher can retrieve an increased number of studies (i.e., the **yield**); however, the likelihood that the studies retrieved may not be relevant to the clinical question also increases. Additionally, full-text databases do not offer controlled vocabulary headings to aid in searching.

The ease of full-text retrieval can tempt clinicians to limit their searches to full-text only in databases such as MEDLINE and CINAHL. A caveat about this technique is that clinicians can miss evidence by limiting their search to only those articles where full text is readily available. Although full-text limiting is a useful tool to get a rapid return on a search, the clinician must keep in mind that there may be relevant studies that are not captured in such a limited search.

Knowing the structure of the database being searched is helpful when trying to find relevant evidence. Full-text articles, when available, are a great resource. Understanding how to navigate the database structure includes identifying problems with jargon and ambiguity. These types of issues can create difficulty in finding relevant evidence. To be successful in finding the desired evidence, it is important to know how to negotiate a database in its language.

Tool Three: Speaking the Database's Language

Databases have their own language that can enable the searcher to find information quickly. When the question is broad and requires a more comprehensive approach, using a database's own language, called a **controlled vocabulary or controlled thesaurus** is an effective approach to searching. For example, a broad brush would be required to gather all relevant evidence to

box 3.1

Example of a PsycINFO Bibliographic Record

Accession Number
Journal Article: 2003-01573-002.

Author
Young, Bridget; Dixon-Woods, Mary; Windridge, Kate C; Heney, David.

Institution
U Hull, Dept of Psychology, Hull, United Kingdom, 1
U Leicester, Dept of Epidemiology & Public Health, Leicester, United Kingdom, 2
U Leicester, Dept of General Practice & Primary Health Care, Leicester, United
   Kingdom, 3
Leicester Royal Infirmary, Children's Hosp, Leicester, United Kingdom, 4.

Correspondence Address
Young, Bridget. Dept of Psychology, U Hull, Hull United Kingdom HU6 7RX,
B.Young@hull.ac.uk.

Title
Managing communication with young people who have a potentially life-threatening chronic illness: Qualitative study of patients and parents.

Source
BMJ (British Medical Journal). Vol 326(7384) Feb 2003, 305–309.
BMJ Publishing Group, United Kingdom

Publisher URL
http://www.bmjpg.com

Journal URL
http://www.bmj.com/

ISSN
0959-8154 (Print)

Language
English

Abstract
Examined young people's and parents' accounts of communication about cancer in childhood. Thirteen families, comprising 19 parents and 13 patients aged 8–17 yrs par-

box 3.1 *(continued)*

ticipated. Most parents described acting in an executive-like capacity, managing what and how their children were told about their illness, particularly at the time of diagnosis. Their accounts were shaped by concerns to manage their identity as strong and optimistic parents and to protect their child's well-being. The patients identified elements of their parents' role that both facilitated and constrained their communication, and while they welcomed their parents' involvement, some expressed unease with the constraining aspects of their parents' role. Some young people described feeling marginalized in consultations and pointed to difficulties they experienced in encounters with some doctors. There are difficulties in managing communication with young people who have a chronic, life-threatening illness. Health professionals need to be aware of how the social positioning of young people and the executive role of parents can contribute to the marginalization of young people and hamper the development of successful relationships between themselves and young patients.

Key Concepts
health professionals; constraining aspects; social positioning; chronic illness; young patients; parents' role

Subject Headings
*Chronic Illness
*Neoplasms
*Parent Child Communication
*Parental Role

Classification Code
Health & Mental Health Treatment & Prevention [3300]; Childrearing & Child Care [2956]

Population Group
Human; Male; Female. Childhood (birth–12 yrs); School Age (6–12 yrs); Adolescence (13–17 yrs); Adulthood (18 yrs & older).

Form/Content Type
Empirical Study

Special Feature
References; Peer Reviewed

Publication Type
Journal Article

Publication Year
2003

box 3.1 (continued) ————————————————————————————

Update Code
20030512

Media Type
Print (Paper)

Number of Cited References
Number of Citations: 23, Number of Citations Displayed: 23

Cited References

1. Cassileth, B. R., Zupkis, R. V., Sutton-Smith, K., & March, V. (1980). Information and participation preferences among cancer patients. *Ann Intern Med*, 92, 832–6.

2. Fallowfield, L., Ford, S., & Lewis, S. (1995). No news is not good news: Information preferences of patients with cancer. *Psycho-oncol*, 4, 197–202.

3. Leydon, G. M., Boulton, M., Moynihan, C., Jones, A., Mossman, J., Boudioni, M., et al. (2000). Cancer patients' information needs and information seeking behaviour: In-depth interview study. *Br Med J*, 320, 909–13.

4. Scott, J. T., Entwhistle, V. A., Sowden, A., & Watt, I. (2002). Communicating with children and adolescents about their cancer. *Cochrane Library* (Issue 4). Oxford: Update Software.

5. British Medical Association. (2001). *Consent, rights and choices in health care for children and young people.* London: BMJ Books.

6. Dixon-Woods, M., Young, B., & Heney, D. (1999). Partnerships with children. *Br Med J*, 319, 778–80.

7. Stewart, T. J., Pantell, R. H., Dias, J. K., Wells, P. A., & Ross, A. W. (1981). Children as patients: A communications process study in family practice. *J Fam Pract*, 13, 827–35.

8. Strong, P. (1979). *The ceremonial order of the clinic.* London: Routledge & Kegan Paul.

9. Davis, A. G. (1982). *Children in clinics.* London: Tavistock.

10. Tates, K., & Meeuwesen, L. (2001). Doctor-parent-child communication. A (re)view of the literature. *Soc Sci Med*, 52, 839–51.[Reference Link].

11. Van Dulman, A. M. (1998). Children's contributions to pediatric outpatient encounters. *Pediatrics*, 102, 563–8.

12. Barnes, J., Kroll, L., Burke, O., Lee, J., Jones, A., & Stein, A. (2000). Qualitative interview study of communication between parents and children about maternal breast cancer. *Br Med J*, 321, 479–82.

13. Claflin, C. J., & Barbarin, O. A. (1991). Does "telling" less protect more? Relationships among age, information disclosure, and what children with cancer see and feel. *J Pediatr Psychol*, 16, 169–91.

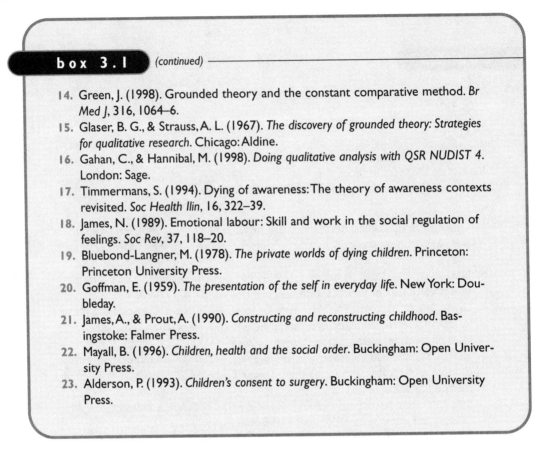

box 3.1 *(continued)*

14. Green, J. (1998). Grounded theory and the constant comparative method. *Br Med J*, 316, 1064–6.
15. Glaser, B. G., & Strauss, A. L. (1967). *The discovery of grounded theory: Strategies for qualitative research.* Chicago: Aldine.
16. Gahan, C., & Hannibal, M. (1998). *Doing qualitative analysis with QSR NUDIST 4.* London: Sage.
17. Timmermans, S. (1994). Dying of awareness: The theory of awareness contexts revisited. *Soc Health Ilin*, 16, 322–39.
18. James, N. (1989). Emotional labour: Skill and work in the social regulation of feelings. *Soc Rev*, 37, 118–20.
19. Bluebond-Langner, M. (1978). *The private worlds of dying children.* Princeton: Princeton University Press.
20. Goffman, E. (1959). *The presentation of the self in everyday life.* New York: Doubleday.
21. James, A., & Prout, A. (1990). *Constructing and reconstructing childhood.* Basingstoke: Falmer Press.
22. Mayall, B. (1996). *Children, health and the social order.* Buckingham: Open University Press.
23. Alderson, P. (1993). *Children's consent to surgery.* Buckingham: Open University Press.

answer the question, What is the best intervention for fall prevention in the elderly? When the clinical question is narrow and requires specific evidence to answer it, the controlled thesaurus can be most helpful, but more care is required in its use. The best way to begin a search is by searching carefully using concepts that are guided by a well-built question. Box 3-2 contains the essential steps of a search strategy.

MeSH Headings

MeSH headings are the National Library of Medicine's thesaurus for MEDLINE's controlled vocabulary. MeSH is a hierarchical arrangement of nearly 22,000 descriptive terms that allows a visual display of related terms. An additional 132,000 terms are in a separate chemical thesaurus. EMBASE has a similar product, EMTREE, with 46,000 drug and medical terms. It incorporates some MeSH terms used by the National Library of Medicine, as well as almost 20,000 Chemical Abstracts Service registry numbers. CINAHL also incorporates a hierarchical structure similar to MeSH, but the thesaurus has some of its own unique terms. Of the 11,500 CINAHL subject headings, about 70% also appear in MeSH. CINAHL adds more than 2,000 terms to reflect the specific needs of nursing and allied health personnel. PsycINFO uses a thesaurus of over 5,000 index terms in its book format, *Thesaurus of Psychological Index Terms* (9th ed., 2001, American Psychological Association).

box 3.2

Essential Steps to a Search Strategy

Step One: Formulate a well-built clinical question without jargon or ambiguity.

Step Two: Determine the type of database that is appropriate for the question.

Step Three: Determine the type of study design that would best answer the question.

Step Four: Enter a subject heading (e.g., MeSH) and/or textword search guided by the PICO components of the question.

Step Five: Begin combining searches to find relevant evidence.

Step Six: Further restrict combined searches for study design, methods, indicators of clinical meaningfulness, or other appropriate, available limits. Consider limiting the search to English and human, depending on the question and searcher.

Step Seven: Apply a priori inclusion and exclusion criteria to studies gathered by the search to find the best available evidence.

MeSH headings are descriptors that range from broad headings such as "vitamins" to specific, such as "ascorbic acid."

MeSH headings can be found at the National Library of Medicine, **http://www.nlm.nih.gov/pubs/factsheets/mesh.html.**

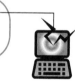

MeSH headings are arranged in alphabetical and hierarchical order. There are always multiple MeSH headings associated with one article. In addition, subheadings are attached to the headings themselves. The searcher can choose to search with individual subheadings, groups of headings, or with all of them, depending on the purpose of the search. Figure 3-1 shows some typical subheadings that are listed under a MeSH heading. For example, if the focus of the search is the adverse effects of a medication, that subheading could be selected and the search narrowed.

It is much harder to search a full-text database than to search one that also includes a controlled vocabulary, such as MeSH headings used in MEDLINE. An advantage of full-text databases is that by using **textwords**, every word in the text and the illustration captions can now be searched. However, it should be noted that the issues with jargon and ambiguity apply here as with any textword search. An idea can be represented with different words by different authors. This ambiguity requires the searcher to choose alternative ways of identifying the idea in the database to obtain all the relevant evidence. For example, *cancer* can be described as a tumor, neoplasm, or mass, or it may be described in compound words beginning with such pre-

Subheadings for: **Amoxicillin**

☐ **Include All Subheadings (2186)**

-- or choose one or more of these subheadings --

ⓘ ☐ /ad - Administration & Dosage (684) ⓘ ☐ /im - Immunology (22)
ⓘ ☐ /ae - Adverse Effects (264) ⓘ ☐ /ip - Isolation & Purification (4)
ⓘ ☐ /aa - Analogs & Derivatives (7) ⓘ ☐ /me - Metabolism (15)
ⓘ ☐ /an - Analysis (38) ⓘ ☐ /pk - Pharmacokinetics (105)
ⓘ ☐ /ai - Antagonists & Inhibitors (1) ⓘ ☐ /pd - Pharmacology (379)
ⓘ ☐ /bl - Blood (45) ⓘ ☐ /re - Radiation Effects (1)
ⓘ ☐ /cs - Chemical Synthesis (8) ⓘ ☐ /st - Standards (1)
ⓘ ☐ /ch - Chemistry (28) ⓘ ☐ /sd - Supply & Distribution (1)
ⓘ ☐ /ct - Contraindications (1) ⓘ ☐ /tu - Therapeutic Use (1222)
ⓘ ☐ /du - Diagnostic Use (6) ⓘ ☐ /to - Toxicity (1)
ⓘ ☐ /ec - Economics (24) ⓘ ☐ /ur - Urine (7)

figure 3.1 Typical MeSH subheadings for a medication. Source: Ovid Technologies

fixes as *onco-* or *carcino-*. With a controlled thesaurus, regardless of how the author stated it in the article, the vocabulary heading will help the searcher find all articles that are related to one another. If used effectively, a controlled thesaurus in a database can save time, reduce frustration, and increase success.

A caveat about PubMed's deceptively plain home page is that this page seems to encourage textword searching, but this approach is most likely not the best option to obtain the desired relevant evidence.

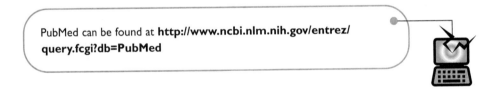

PubMed can be found at **http://www.ncbi.nlm.nih.gov/entrez/ query.fcgi?db=PubMed**

The example in Box 3-3 provides a strategy for using MeSH in PubMed to obtain the desired evidence.

“ *Curiosity is the wick in the candle of learning.* ”

William Arthur Ward

Textwords

Using everyday words and expressions for searches (i.e., key words or textwords) can sometimes lead to good results. This kind of searching is most appropriate when the searcher desires a narrow, focused search yielding a few articles. However, textwords can be ambiguous and jar-

box 3.3

Using MeSH to Narrow a Search in PubMed

In PubMed, locate the MeSH database. If a clinical question is about finding the most effective diagnostic test for breast cancer, the searcher would enter *breast cancer* in the search box and click on the GO button. MeSH will map the term to *breast neoplasms* (MeSH language is neoplasm, rather than cancer). To open the display of available subheadings, the searcher then selects the hyperlink for the subject heading most closely relevant to the concept of the clinical question and chooses the most appropriate subheading(s). At the appropriate area on the screen, the searcher could elect to make the term a major focus of headings, thus narrowing the results.

The next step is to click on the Send To icon. The details box will appear with the search terms in MeSH format. Select the Search PubMed option to obtain the relevant citations. Click on the Limits term to see the displays available to narrow the search and seek the best evidence to answer the question.

gon-laden. Most search engines and databases have addressed the issue of jargon through a built-in mapping system that uses a combination of cross-references and a complicated textword algorithm to map a term to the most likely controlled vocabulary term(s). For example, Tylenol is a common analgesic and is often referred to by its trade name rather than by its generic name. In most search engines, the term *Tylenol* is mapped to the generic term *acetaminophen*, as is the European term *paracetamol*.

Mapping requires extensive cross-referencing of terms. For example, EMBASE's EMTREE mapping provides a controlled vocabulary or thesaurus that has more than 45,000 indexing terms and 190,000 synonyms, including MEDLINE's MeSH headings. Mapping is used in many databases, and although it can be reliable for many common terms, such as Tylenol, there are terms for which mapping is not as straightforward and, therefore, not particularly successful.

Ideally, when the searcher enters a concept from the clinical question into the system, the word or phrase will map to one or more of the controlled thesaurus headings. If none of the offered headings matches the concept entered, the searcher can choose to search that word or phrase in the "text" (title or abstract), rather than searching the controlled vocabulary heading (thus the term *textword*). When a topic is so recent that there is likely to be very little available in the journal literature, using key words or textwords may be the best way to find relevant evidence, because controlled vocabulary for the topic is unlikely.

An example of a textword search for the question, Are people diagnosed with AIDS more likely to acquire pneumonia in the community than the elderly? might start with the word *AIDS*. This search in MEDLINE (1966 to August 2003) resulted in nearly 76,300 hits. Many of the articles were about the disease, but the search also included articles on other types of aids, such as visual aids, aid to dependent children, and hearing aids. In addition, this search retrieved only articles containing the word *AIDS*. Those articles that used "acquired immune deficiency syndrome" or "acquired immunodeficiency syndrome" potentially were missed. When the MeSH heading "acquired immunodeficiency syndrome" was searched, almost 64,000 hits were obtained. The difference is that all of these articles contain information about acquired immunodeficiency syndrome. So although the yield was smaller, the search was more successful in that the number of relevant articles was higher. The techniques of combining and limiting can be used to further reduce the yield to a manageable number and will be discussed later.

This example highlights a very important disadvantage to textword searching: synonymy. Even though AIDS is highly significant and specific to anyone in the healthcare profession, to the computer it is nothing more than an array of letters. When doing a textword search in any database, the computer is comparing the array of letters with what it finds in the database and returning just those records that contain the same array of letters.

A second disadvantage of textword searching is jargon. This involves the natural ability that people have for understanding the meaning of a word because of the linguistic, professional, or social context in which it is used. Computers are relatively helpless to do the same. It will not recognize that "immune deficiency" and "immunodeficiency" mean the same. Across specialties, the same concepts can be expressed with different words.

Searching with textwords can be helpful, especially when no controlled vocabulary term exists to adequately describe the topic searched. For this reason, the importance of carefully formulating the PICO question cannot be overemphasized. Using unambiguous, nonjargon terms to describe the PICO components of the clinical question will assist in obtaining the best search in the shortest time.

Focus and Explode

Two techniques that use a controlled thesaurus to narrow or broaden the search, depending on the need, are the "focus" and "explode" options that are available in some search engines (e.g., Ovid). Focusing is a technique that searches and retrieves only the articles that contain the identified subject heading as a major emphasis of the article. This option may be labeled differently in different databases (e.g., the main point of the article). To answer the question, How effective are supplemental vitamins (I) in improving cognition (O) in the elderly (P) in addition to routine exercise (C), a focused search in CINAHL of the heading "vitamins" retrieved 491 hits, all relevant to vitamins.

Exploding is a technique that searches and retrieves articles with all of the more specific elements of the identified heading, that is, it takes all more specific headings that are under it in the hierarchical thesaurus and makes them available by using one exploded heading. In the vitamin example, exploding provided over 4,579 hits in CINAHL. The exploded vitamin search included a study on the latest innovations in coronary intervention, an article unrelated to the question.

Exploding is advantageous for searches where broad terms are needed; however, it can be disadvantageous because the searcher may find papers that are not necessarily helpful in answering the clinical question. Some search systems (e.g., Ovid) enable the searcher to click on the MeSH heading and see the other headings that are under it in the hierarchical thesaurus.

This option helps the searcher create the most relevant search by making a decision about whether to explode.

Another example of the usefulness of the explode function is a search to find information on the role that NSAIDs (all, not just a single agent) play in hypertension. The MeSH term "nonsteroidal, antiinflammatory agents" is called a *family term*. Using the heading, then exploding it means that the name of each of the NSAID agents is a part of the search without entering each name into the strategy. As can be seen in the examples, these techniques can be powerful searching tools if used effectively. MEDLINE and CINAHL both use these tools, but CDSR does not because it is a relatively small database and does not have a controlled thesaurus.

Not all subjects are represented in the controlled thesauruses of MEDLINE, CINAHL, or any database. Some subjects are so rare, unusual, or new that an index term has not been designated. In cases like this, it makes sense to continue to use textwords to identify articles versus using MeSH headings, which could lead to a less efficient search. For example, although the herb saw palmetto is indexed in CINAHL, it is not indexed in MEDLINE, but "plants, medicinal" is listed as a MeSH heading. A search for articles about saw palmetto (n = 63) would be best using the textword rather than the broader term of "plants, medicinal" (n = 11,918) and would yield better, more efficient results.

Combine and Limit

To start the search, enter each of the key concepts from the PICO components of the question into the search field individually. Remember to make these concepts as unambiguous and jargon-free as possible. Hopefully, these words will map to one or more of the controlled vocabulary headings in the database. If not, the word can be searched as a textword (in titles and abstracts). Review the results of each search. Most likely, the aim of the search will not be satisfied at this point. Once the key concepts have been searched, they can be combined in various groupings. To answer a question most completely, these results may need to be further limited and/or combiined to find the most relevant evidence.

For example, to adequately answer the given question about vitamins, exercise, and elders' cognition, the focused vitamin search (n = 491) would be combined with a focused search of "cognition" (n = 1,566; combined search n = 3), and the focused exercise search (n=3,884) would be combined with the cognition search (combined search n = 15). In Figure 3-2, both of these combined searches were limited to "aged 65–79 years" and "aged 80 and over" to find the most relevant evidence (e.g., Cockle and colleagues' [2000] clinical trial investigating the influence of multivitamins on cognitive function and mood in the elderly and Van Sickle and colleagues' [1996] article on the effects of physical exercise on cognitive functioning in the elderly).

If all three focused searches were combined, there were zero results. However, if each of the headings were exploded, then combined (no age limit), one article on the prevention of Alzheimer's disease was found (Anonymous, 2002)(see Figure 3-3).

If appropriate, there are limitations that can be applied to the final grouping of articles to help reduce the less relevant evidence, such as "human" and "English." Figure 3-4 contains a search strategy in MEDLINE to answer the clinical question, In children (P), is acetaminophen (I) or ibuprofen (C) more effective in reducing fever (O)? As you can see, three of the components of the PICO question were searched. All of these components matched MeSH headings— acetaminophen, ibuprofen, and fever—although this is not always the case. All MeSH headings

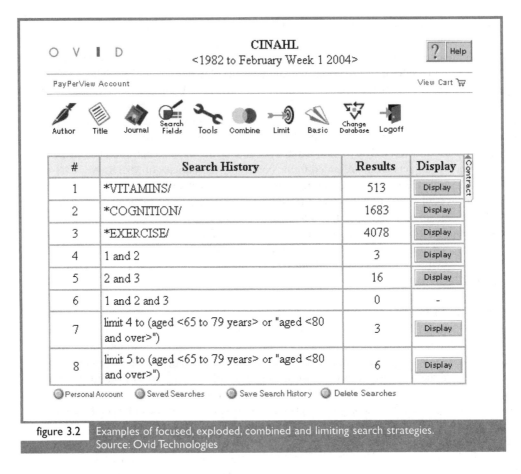

#	Search History	Results	Display
1	*VITAMINS/	513	Display
2	*COGNITION/	1683	Display
3	*EXERCISE/	4078	Display
4	1 and 2	3	Display
5	2 and 3	16	Display
6	1 and 2 and 3	0	-
7	limit 4 to (aged <65 to 79 years> or "aged <80 and over>")	3	Display
8	limit 5 to (aged <65 to 79 years> or "aged <80 and over>")	6	Display

figure 3.2 Examples of focused, exploded, combined and limiting search strategies. Source: Ovid Technologies

were exploded. The subheading "therapeutic use" was chosen for acetaminophen and ibuprofen. All of the subheadings for the MeSH heading "fever" were included to provide the broadest scope. Then the search was limited to children (0–18 years), human, English, and randomized controlled trials (RCTs). The combined and limited search results narrowed a potential 6,854 citations down to an easily reviewable 11 citations.

Ovid offers easily maneuverable limiting and combining options; however, the available limits depend on the database and vendor being searched. Box 3-4 provides one of the MEDLINE citations from the search example. In performing this type of narrow search, if evidence is available, the clinician should have evidence in her/his hands within 3–5 minutes, depending on the quality of computer services available. Keep in mind that having evidence in hand does not guarantee the validity of the evidence. Critical appraisal of evidence is covered in Unit Two of this book.

Inclusion and Exclusion Criteria

Once a search yields a number of potential matches, or "hits," the clinician is wise to have established specific conditions beforehand that will assist in determining which hits are "keepers"

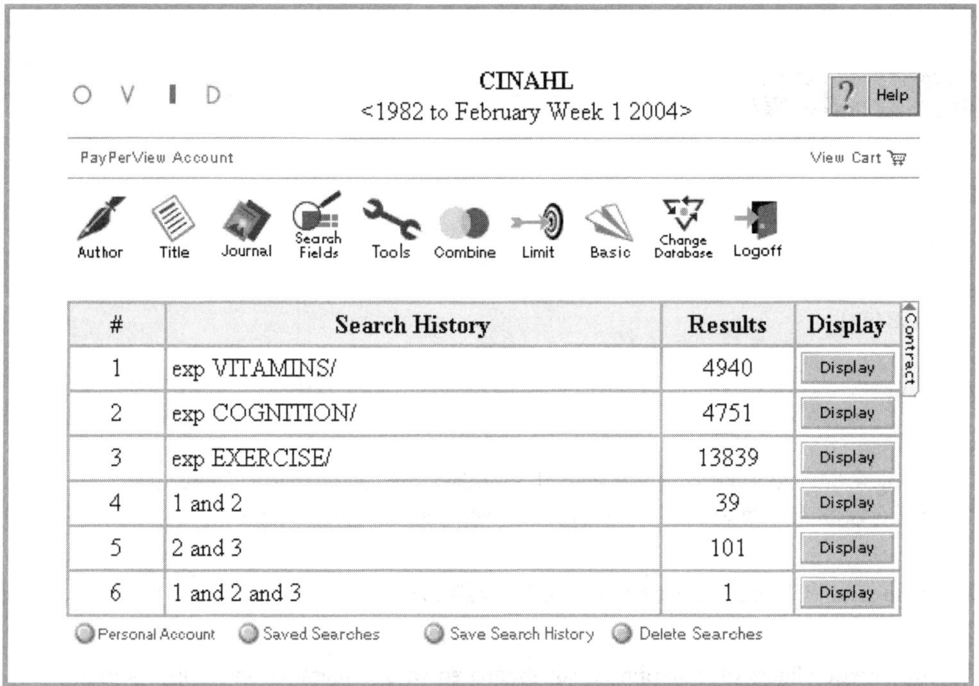

O V I D   **CINAHL**
<1982 to February Week 1 2004>   ? Help

PayPerView Account   View Cart 🛒

Author   Title   Journal   Search Fields   Tools   Combine   Limit   Basic   Change Database   Logoff

#	Search History	Results	Display
1	exp VITAMINS/	4940	Display
2	exp COGNITION/	4751	Display
3	exp EXERCISE/	13839	Display
4	1 and 2	39	Display
5	2 and 3	101	Display
6	1 and 2 and 3	1	Display

◯ Personal Account   ◯ Saved Searches   ◯ Save Search History   ◯ Delete Searches

figure 3.3   Example of exploded and combined search strategies.
Source: Ovid Technologies

O V I D   **Ovid MEDLINE(R)**
<1996 to February Week 1 2004>   ? Help

PayPerView Account   View Cart 🛒

Author   Title   Journal   Search Fields   Tools   Combine   Limit   Basic   Change Database   Logoff

#	Search History	Results	Display
1	exp ACETAMINOPHEN/tu [Therapeutic Use]	604	Display
2	exp IBUPROFEN/tu [Therapeutic Use]	400	Display
3	exp FEVER/	6676	Display
4	1 and 2 and 3	23	Display
5	limit 4 to (human and english language and all child <0 to 18 years> and randomized controlled trial)	11	Display

◯ Personal Account   ◯ Saved Searches   ◯ Save Search History   ◯ Delete Searches

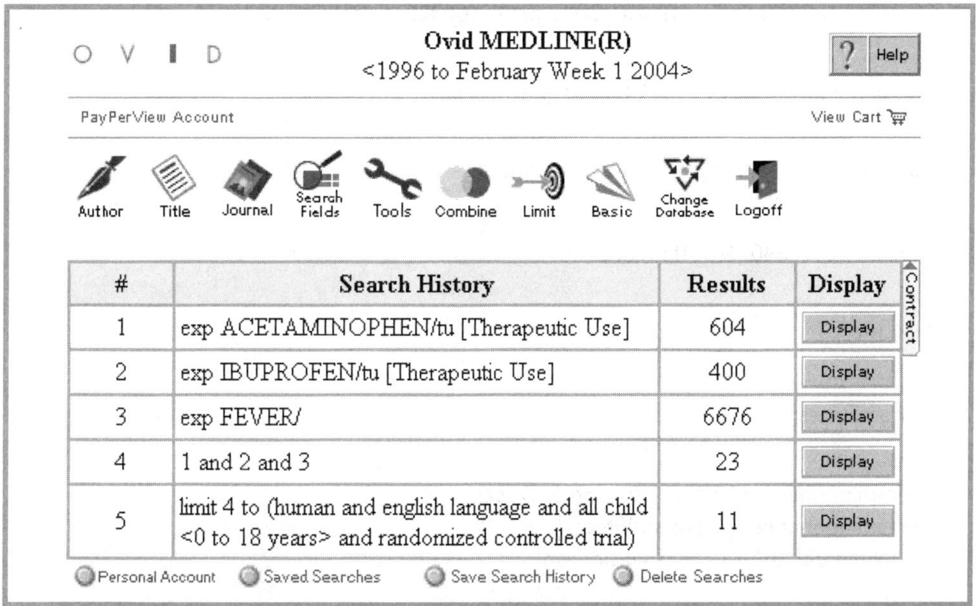

figure 3.4   Example of a typical search strategy.
Source: Ovid Technologies

box 3.4

MEDLINE Record for Search

Unique Identifier
11824173

MEDLINE Identifier
21682821

Record Owner
NLM

Authors
Wong A. Sibbald A. Ferrero F. Plager M. Santolaya ME. Escobar AM. Campos S. S. De Leon Gonzalez M. Kesselring GL. Fever Pediatric Study Group.

Institution
Hospital de Clinicas, University of Sao Paulo, Brazil.

Title
Antipyretic effects of dipyrone versus ibuprofen versus acetaminophen in children: results of a multinational, randomized, modified double-blind study.[comment].

Comments
Comment in: *Clin Pediatr* (Phila). 2001 Jun;40(6):325–6; PMID: 11824174

Source
Clinical Pediatrics. 40(6):313–24, 2001 Jun.

Abbreviated Source
Clin Pediatr (Phila). 40(6):313–24, 2001 Jun.

NLM Journal Code
dhe, 0372606, 8407647, 0372606

Journal Subset
AIM, IM

Country of Publication
United States

MeSH Subject Headings
Acetaminophen/ad [Administration & Dosage]
Acetaminophen/ae [Adverse Effects]
*Acetaminophen/tu [Therapeutic Use]

box 3.4 *(continued)*

Analgesics, Non-Narcotic/ad [Administration & Dosage]
Analgesics, Non-Narcotic/ae [Adverse Effects]
*Analgesics, Non-Narcotic/tu [Therapeutic Use]
Analysis of Variance
Anti-Inflammatory Agents, Non-Steroidal/ad [Administration & Dosage]
Anti-Inflammatory Agents, Non-Steroidal/ae [Adverse Effects]
*Anti-Inflammatory Agents, Non-Steroidal/tu [Therapeutic Use]
*Body Temperature / de [Drug Effects]
Child
Child, Preschool
Comparative Study
Dipyrone/ad [Administration & Dosage]
Dipyrone/ae [Adverse Effects]
*Dipyrone/tu [Therapeutic Use]
Double-Blind Method
Female
*Fever/dt [Drug Therapy]
Human
Ibuprofen/ad [Administration & Dosage]
Ibuprofen/ae [Adverse Effects]
*Ibuprofen/tu [Therapeutic Use]
Infant
Male
Prospective Studies
Sample Size
Time Factors
Treatment Outcome

Abstract

This study compared the antipyretic effectiveness of acetaminophen, ibuprofen, and dipyrone in young children with fever. The results were based on a modified double-blind, randomized, multinational trial that evaluated 628 febrile children, aged 6 months to 6 years. All three drugs lowered temperature in the 555 patients completing the study. Temperature normalization rates in the ibuprofen and dipyrone groups (78% and 82%, respectively) were significantly higher than the acetaminophen group (68%, $P = 0.004$). After 4–6 hours, mean temperature in the dipyrone group was significantly lower than the other groups, demonstrating longer temperature normalization with dipyrone. All three drugs showed comparable tolerability profiles.

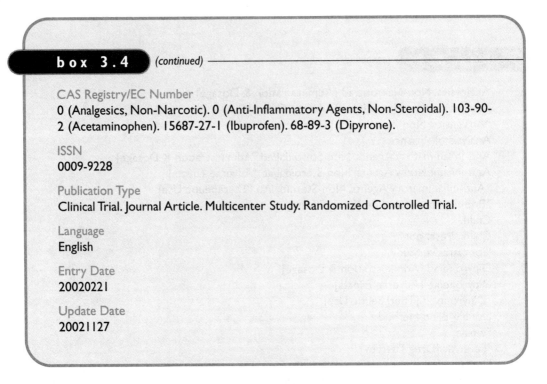

and which will be discarded. These conditions are called **inclusion** and **exclusion criteria**. Often, many of the criteria have been applied in the search strategy as limits. However, there are occasional articles/studies that are not relevant to answering the question and slip through the best search strategy. Stating inclusion and exclusion criteria upon which to judge a study will focus the return of the search to provide the most relevant evidence.

An inclusion criterion for the ibuprofen/acetaminophen example may be that the clinician will accept only studies with samples of children between the ages of 3 and 12 years. An age range this broad may not be available as a single limit. An exclusion criterion may be that the clinician will not accept studies that compare acetaminophen with drugs other than ibuprofen. Often, the bibliographic citation is not adequate to address all of the inclusion and exclusion criteria. The entire study may need to be obtained to determine whether it is a keeper.

The Internet as a Source of Evidence

From a healthcare perspective, the Internet is an amorphous information resource. It is a computer network that can be quite useful if you know where to look for the information you need and if you can discern "good" from "bad" information. Most healthcare consumers do not have such expertise. The healthcare professional must be aware of what relevant healthcare information is posted on the Internet and help the consumer place the information in perspective with the current best scientific evidence available.

Despite the apparent ease of Internet use, several problems accompany using it as a sole resource for finding an answer to a clinical question. However, the ease of accessing information may lead the consumer to believe that the information found on the Internet is valid and reliable. Clinicians must help consumers understand that what they may find about their diagnosis, disease, or healthcare regimen on the Internet may not be of value to them. It may, in fact, mislead them. It is important for practitioners and consumers to consider that there still are many valuable information resources that can be accessed only in paper form and cannot be found via the Internet. In addition, there are as yet no generally accepted *standards* for making healthcare information available on the Internet (Hersh, Gorman, & Sacherek, 1998; Hersh & Hickan, 1998). However, there are texts that assist clinicians to evaluate Web sites (e.g., Fitzpatrick, Romano, & Chasek, 2001) and other Web sites that provide guidelines for evaluating Internet information that can assist both laypersons and clinicians.

For more about evaluating information on the Internet, visit:
http://www.library.jhu.edu/elp/useit/evaluate/
http://www.lib.vt.edu/research/libinst/idle/evaluating.html

Valid science is published primarily in peer-reviewed literature, which is found in databases.

Consumers and healthcare professionals need to keep in mind that anyone can publish a Web page and post whatever he or she likes on the page. Moreover, this can be done more easily and less expensively than publishing on paper. A search of the Internet using a popular search engine such as Google or Yahoo! on any topic may yield several hundred thousand hits, of which only a few will be clinically significant. In addition, a search on any of the popular Internet search engines covers only a small percentage of available Web pages, and the search results rarely, if ever, include hits from high-quality resources, such as MEDLINE or CINAHL. In general, the Internet is not an evidence-based resource.

Finding the right source for evidence to answer clinical questions is only one step in the evidence-based practice (EBP) process. Determining the most appropriate study design to answer the question is of equal importance. These two steps increase the likelihood of an effective search for best evidence.

Tool Four: The Right Knowledge from the Right Source

In any clinical setting, there are numerous information resources to answer a variety of questions about patient care or about clinical procedures and protocols. Patient data, population statistics, medical knowledge, logistic information, and social influences are general clinical information areas (Gorman, 1995). The journal literature is generally where all new ideas first enter the healthcare knowledge base. It contains a number of publication types, including (from most useful to least) systematic reviews, research articles, narrative reviews, discussion articles, news items, editorials, and letters to the editor.

There are many clinical settings where questions may occur, and the answers may be found in a variety of resources. For example, patient data will come from the patient, family, or the patient's chart or medical record. These types of data usually foster questions that can be answered by acquiring a broad background of knowledge about healthcare disorders. For example, a question about how to interpret vital signs requires the practitioner to acquire foundational physiologic knowledge of how the related body systems work and any variations thereof. In addition, practitioners know the basic features of many disorders, such as adult-onset diabetes or primary hypertension. Occasionally, however, professionals need to refresh their knowledge, especially with unusual, seasonal, or rare disorders, such as hemophilia or Rocky Mountain spotted fever. In these cases, a good text will often suffice. There are other occasions when the need is not for general knowledge but for an answer to a specific question. These questions are not generally discussed in textbooks, or if they are, the discussion will be either incomplete or out of date. If there is an answer to be found, it will typically be in the journal literature.

For example, a patient in the Medical Intensive Care Unit is being treated for refractory atrial fibrillation. After exhausting a range of treatment options, a collaborating clinician remembers hearing that clonidine, a well-known antihypertensive medication, has been used successfully elsewhere and wonders whether it would work on this patient. A journal search discloses a recent RCT that reports positive benefits. The practitioner then can evaluate the trial's findings for use with the current patient.

Finding the right information often depends on its source. When answering clinical questions, clinicians must consider what kind of study is best. Many clinicians and researchers have indicated (for various reasons) that RCTs are the best evidence for establishing cause and effect, thereby guiding clinical practice. However, what does a clinician do when a case study is presented in a journal (e.g., skip it and read the RCT instead)? It would be inadvisable to skip a case study that could help answer the clinical question. All evidence should be considered; however, caution must be used when deciding about practice changes that are based solely on evidence that may contain more bias (see Chapter 1, Box 1-2). Clinicians are making this type of inquiry in an effort to obtain the best evidence to answer their clinical questions. See Table 3-2 for a list of different types of studies and examples of corresponding questions.

A caveat about study design is that the clinical question drives the type of answer you seek. If the question is about causality (i.e., the effects of a treatment or intervention on an outcome), an RCT is the best evidence to answer the question. If the question is about how patients experience an illness, a qualitative study will provide the best answer. These two examples seem reasonable; however, the types of studies that are "in-between" are the gray areas and need further clarification.

For example, questions about patients coping with grief can be answered with both qualitative and quantitative research designs ranging from descriptive studies of how patients cope to randomized trials of the effectiveness of coping interventions (see Table 3-2 for more examples). The best source of information is a systematic review in which the relevant studies have been placed or another type of review that will assist in answering the question. Chapter 5 provides information about quantitative studies and the types of questions they may answer, and Chapter 6 provides information about qualitative studies and related questions.

> " *Never give up, for that is just the place and time that the tide will turn.* "
>
> *Harriet Beecher Stowe*

table 3.2 Types of studies to answer clinical questions

Example of a Question	Design
In patients with acute respiratory distress syndrome (ARDS), how effective is prone positioning on weaning parameters compared with supine positioning?	Systematic reviews and meta-analyses Single randomized controlled trials (RCTs)
In pregnant women, what are the effects of prenatal care on a healthy delivery and a healthy baby compared with no prenatal care?	Well-controlled, nonrandomized experimental studies
What is it like to live with a spouse who has Alzheimer's disease?	Qualitative
What are the coping mechanisms of parents who have lost a child to AIDS?	Descriptive studies
What is the national standard (i.e., used across the country) for prevention of wandering in patients with Alzheimer's living in long-term care facilities?	Opinion reports of experts and professional organizations

Preappraised Literature: A Gold Mine in the Haystack

Preappraised literature ranges from meta-analytic systematic reviews to synopses of single studies. These golden nuggets have already been critically appraised for the clinician. This type of synthesis is the heart of EBP (Stevens, 2001). The time from finding the evidence to application can be reduced through this type of resource. The Cochrane Collaboration is a major producer of systematic reviews. AHRQ supports centers that produce systematic reviews. The question is how to locate these nuggets.

Systematic reviews by the Cochrane Collaboration are housed in its own database, the CDSR. Other systematic reviews are housed in general databases, such as MEDLINE. To search for systematic reviews, you can use the textwords *systematic review* and the MeSH heading of *evidence-based medicine*. These searches would be combined with the search generated from your question. The same technique can be used with *meta-analysis* and *guidelines*, which are also MeSH headings.

When searching for guidelines in the NGC database, all searching is done by textword, because this database has no controlled vocabulary. The NGC Web site is easily maneuvered. Type in the key concepts from your question that you want to find in the guideline database. Inquiries about guidelines need not necessarily follow the PICO format because the question is about a treatment regimen or plan of care versus an intervention, prognosis, etiology, and the like. For example, What is the best prescribed plan for treating asthma in adolescents? is a reasonable question that can be answered by a guideline.

A more detailed search may be needed to arrive at the best guideline, and this can be accomplished via **http://www.guidelines.gov/search/detailedsearch.aspx.**

A detailed search using the concepts of *asthma* and *adolescent* reduced the search yield to 4 from a general search yield of 88 potential guidelines, using only the textword *asthma*. One of the four guidelines was relevant, entitled *Asthma from The University of Michigan Health System* (UMHS Asthma Guideline, 2000). More about guidelines can be found in Chapter 9.

Other Evidence: Randomized Controlled Trials (RCTs) to Expert Reports

Questions regarding the effectiveness of certain treatments or interventions on outcomes indicate that RCTs would be the strongest study design that would provide the best answers. For example, two types of questions that require RCTs to answer them are causal inference questions and comparative efficacy questions. The clinical question, In cancer patients (P), is chemotherapy and radiation together (I) more effective than chemotherapy alone (C) in preventing the recurrence of cancer (O)? requires that the researchers report the number of participants in the experimental group and the comparison group of the RCT whose cancer recurred and the number who did not. To find such information for this type of question, the searcher can apply the limit (or controlled vocabulary heading, in some databases) "randomized controlled trial" to the combined search for the appropriate MeSH headings, as seen in Figure 3-5.

Some libraries may house data known as "saved searches." The library at the University of Rochester has predefined filters (referred to as "gold filters") that allow clinicians to filter their searches even further than MeSH headings or textwords and combinations thereof. These saved searches serve to find the most sought-after studies for answering clinical questions (primarily in MEDLINE, but CINAHL has saved searches as well). The sought-after studies are those whose results best reflect valid, scientific evidence.

Using these filters, the clinician develops a subject search, then adds a filter to sift through the list and pull out the "gold," hence the name gold filters. These filter strategies were refined, and updated by the University of Rochester Miner Library Reference librarians from searches developed by Ann McKibbon and Cindy Walker-Dilks of McMaster University. For example, these presearched filters cover treatment, including searches for number needed to treat, risk reduction, outcome, and RCT, among many others. When combined with the MeSH heading and/or textword search, these filters sort through thousands of studies and increase the likelihood that the search will gather all of the relevant evidence.

When experimental studies do not use random assignment or selection, generalizable inferences cannot be made as they can with randomized studies. However, these studies need not be discarded. Searching only for RCTs when a question may be answered by an experimental study without randomization is not wise. Some questions do not ethically allow for a randomized study. An example would be the question, Do patients with acute myocardial infarction (AMI) (P) who are routinely treated with oxygen (I) in the emergency room have less myocardial damage (O) compared with those with AMI who are not treated with oxygen (C)? A study designed to answer this question would have to reflect a comparison that could be randomly assigned; however, to randomly withhold a known therapeutic treatment (e.g., oxygen) would be

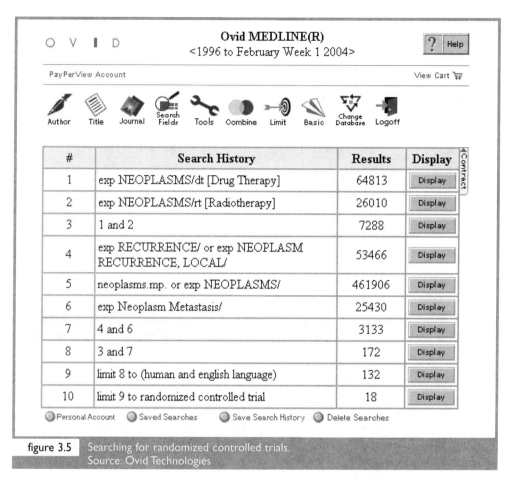

#	Search History	Results	Display
1	exp NEOPLASMS/dt [Drug Therapy]	64813	Display
2	exp NEOPLASMS/rt [Radiotherapy]	26010	Display
3	1 and 2	7288	Display
4	exp RECURRENCE/ or exp NEOPLASM RECURRENCE, LOCAL/	53466	Display
5	neoplasms.mp. or exp NEOPLASMS/	461906	Display
6	exp Neoplasm Metastasis/	25430	Display
7	4 and 6	3133	Display
8	3 and 7	172	Display
9	limit 8 to (human and english language)	132	Display
10	limit 9 to randomized controlled trial	18	Display

figure 3.5 Searching for randomized controlled trials.
Source: Ovid Technologies

unethical. The question also would change to reflect the comparison. For example, Do patients with acute myocardial infarction (AMI) (P) who are routinely treated with oxygen (I) in the emergency room have less myocardial damage (O) compared with those who are routinely treated with oxygen and sublingual nitroglycerin (C)? Limiting searches to a study design is wise if only that type of study can answer the question.

Qualitative and descriptive studies offer perspective and insight into practice and relationships with patients. These types of studies often can answer clinical questions. For example, the question, How does it feel for a child to live with the diagnosis of cancer? cannot be answered with an RCT. To find relevant evidence, the searcher may want to do a search using the MeSH heading or textword *qualitative*, depending on the database (see Figure 3-6). In PsycINFO, qualitative research is not a subject heading; however, it is in MEDLINE, and "qualitative studies" is a heading in CINAHL. In the example from PsycINFO, the most relevant evidence was obtained by combining the results from the textword and thesaurus headings generated from the question. Using this simple technique reduced the search from over 10,500 options to 20 easily reviewed studies.

chapter 3

65

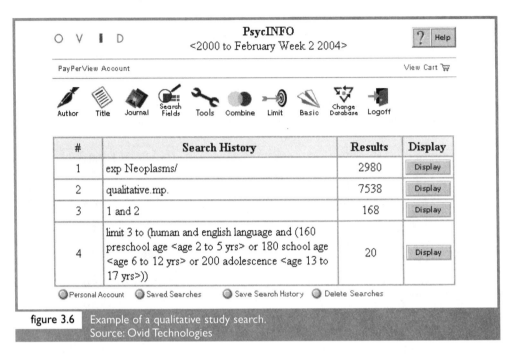

figure 3.6 Example of a qualitative study search.
Source: Ovid Technologies

Expert and professional organization reports can provide valuable information for practice. Sometimes these are evidence-based documents that can be used to generate practice change. In many cases, these are consensus reports that are generated from experts who have a plethora of expertise and some scientific evidence. When using such expert reports or materials generated from a professional organization, exercise caution. Practice changes need to be based on valid scientific evidence, if it exists. However, there are some instances where expert opinion is the best available evidence to answer a clinical question. For example, across the country, what is the national standard for deep vein thrombosis (DVT) prophylaxis in emergency rooms? The answer to the question will not be found in an RCT but may be found in a consensus statement from experts in DVT prophylaxis who gather at a conference to discuss and present relevant evidence on this topic.

When beginning the search for an answer to a clinical question, it is important to discern what type of evidence will offer the best answer. Searching for that kind of evidence using subject headings (e.g., MeSH), textword, or preperformed saved searches enables the clinician to minimize search time and increases the yield of relevant evidence.

A Final Tool: Time and Money

Producing, maintaining, and making databases available is financially costly and time-consuming. Although computer technology has revolutionized the print industry and made it easier to transfer documents and information any time around the world in seconds, the task of producing databases still relies on people to make decisions about what to include and how to index it. Databases produced by government agencies such as MEDLINE are produced with public money and are either very inexpensive or without cost to the searcher. The MEDLINE database is available to anyone in the world who has access to the Internet. The data in MEDLINE are inexpensively available to information vendors and can often be searched on a variety of search engines. Biomedical databases produced by private organizations, such as CINAHL or the CDSR, license their product, usually to libraries but also by subscription to individuals. If there is no in-house library, it is worth the time and effort to locate libraries in the area and find out their access policies.

For clinicians to practice based on evidence, databases are necessary, and costs are associated with them. However, all clinicians with computers can have access to MEDLINE free of charge. In many instances, institutions must make decisions about what databases to house, and these decisions may be based on new databases available and the resources available for purchasing subscription databases. If libraries cannot afford the databases, departments may entertain the idea of independently securing access to databases that they consider to be important. Often, these types of subscriptions to selected databases are costly to acquire and maintain. The cost of a database subscription is not just for the licensing fees but also for the hardware, software, Internet access, and staff to facilitate its use.

Although there is a cost associated with searching databases for relevant evidence, regular searching for answers to clinical questions has been shown to save money. Researchers conducted an outcome-based, prospective study to measure the economic impact of MEDLINE searches on the cost both to the patient and to the participating hospitals (Klein et al., 1994). They found that searches conducted early (i.e., in the first half) in patients' hospital stays resulted in significantly lower cost to the patients and to the hospitals, as well as shorter lengths of stay.

Computerized retrieval of medical information is a fairly complex activity. It begins by considering the kind of information needed, creating an answerable question, planning and executing the search in an appropriate database, and analyzing the retrieved results. Clinicians must remember the costs of both searching and obtaining relevant evidence, as well as the costs of not searching for and applying relevant evidence.

> 66 *Do not go where the path may lead, go instead where there is no path and leave a trail.* 99
>
> *Ralph Waldo Emerson*

How to Know You Have Found the Needle

Successfully searching for relevant evidence is as important as asking a well-built PICO question. Without determining the appropriate database or using controlled database vocabulary, limits, and specified criteria to navigate the database maze; and without considering the cost of not searching for the best evidence, clinicians cannot get the answers enabling them to provide the best care to their patients.

The key to knowing whether the needle has been found is in further evaluation of the selected studies from a successfully executed search. This evaluation method is called *critical appraisal*, the next step in the EBP process. Some journals are dedicated to preappraisal of existing literature. Most of these articles are not syntheses (e.g., systematic reviews) but rather critical appraisals of current single studies. For example, the journal *Evidence-Based Nursing* (*EBN*) reviews 140 general medical, specialist, and nursing journals to identify research that would be clinically meaningful to nurses. Appraisals of 24 studies (both quantitative and qualitative) are published quarterly. The *American College of Physicians (ACP) Journal Club* is another publication dedicated to preappraised literature. More than 100 journals are scanned for evidence relevant to clinicians. Specific criteria are applied to the appraised articles, and the appraisals are published bimonthly in the journal.

These types of journals assist the clinician in reducing the time it takes from asking the question to applying valid evidence in decision making.

> 66*Do what you can, with what you have, where you are.*99
>
> *Theodore Roosevelt*

There needs to be some discussion about when a thorough search to answer a compelling clinical question yields either too little valid evidence to support confident practice change (i.e., inconclusive evidence) or no evidence. In most cases, clinicians are not in positions to do full-scale, multisite clinical trials to determine the answer, and the science may not be at the point to support such an investigation. However, determining what is effective in the clinician's own practice by implementing the best evidence available(i.e., outcomes management) can generate evidence. In addition, generating evidence by conducting smaller scale studies, either individually or with a team of researchers, is an option. Chapters 10–12 address how to generate evidence to answer clinical questions.

references

American Psychological Association (2001). *Thesaurus of Psychological Index Terms*. Washington, DC: American Psychological Association.

Anonymous (2002). Your best bets for preventing Alzheimer's disease. *Harvard Health Letter, 27*(10), 6.

Cockle, S. M., Haller, J., Kimber, S., Dawe, R. A., & Hindmarch, I. (2000). The influence of multivitamins on cognitive function and mood in the elderly. *Aging & Mental Health. 4,* 339–353.

Fitzpatrick, J., Chasek, R., & Romano, C. A. (2001). *Nurses guide to consumer health websites*. New York: Springer.

Gorman, P. (1995). Information needs of physicians. *Journal of the American Society for Information Science, 46*, 729–736.

Harrison, *Principles of internal medicine*. Retrieved March 14, 2004 from Harrisons. accessmedicine.com

Hersh, W. R., Gorman, P. N., & Sacherek, L. S. (1998). Applicability and quality of information for answering clinical questions on the web. *JAMA, 280,* 1307–1308.

Hersh, W. R., & Hickam, D. H. (1998). How well do physicians use electronic information retrieval systems: A framework for investigation and systematic review *JAMA, 280,* 1347–1352.

Klein, M. S., Ross, F. V., Adams, D. L., & Gilbert, C. M. (1994). Effect of online literature searching on lengthy of stay and patient care costs. *Academic Medicine, 69,* 489–495.

National Library of Medicine. Retrieved from http://www.nlm.nih.gov/pubs/factsheets/mesh.html. Accessed on August 18, 2003.

Singapore, (2002). *Management of asthma.* National Medical Research Council (Singapore Ministry of Health)—National Government Agency [Non-U.S.]. 58 pages. NGC:002501, retrieved from www.guidelines.gov on October 13, 2003.

Stevens, K. R. (2001). Systematic reviews: The heart of evidence-based practice. *AACN Clinical Issues: Advanced Practice in Acute and Critical Care, 12*(4), 529–538.

UMHS Asthma Guideline (2000). Ann Arbor (MI): University of Michigan Health System. Retrieved from National Guidelines Clearinghouse at www.guidelines.gov on August, 11, 2003.

UpToDate (2004). Retrieved March 14, 2004 from http://www.uptodate.com

Van Sickle, T. D., Hersen, M., Simco, E. R., Melton, M. A., & Van Hasselt, V. B. (1996). Effects of physical exercise on cognitive functioning in the elderly. *International Journal of Rehabilitation & Health. 2*(2),67–100.

Walters, E. H., Walters, J. A. E., & Gibson, P. W. (2003). Regular treatment with long-acting beta agonists versus daily regular treatment with short-acting beta agonists in adults and children with stable asthma. Cochrane Airways Group, *Cochrane Database of Systematic Reviews*, Section 3.

Step Three: Critically Appraising Evidence

"Knowledge, the object of Knowledge, and the Knower are the three factors which motivate action"

Friedrich von Schiller

Critically Appraising Knowledge for Clinical Decision Making

Kathleen R. Stevens

chapter 4

How does a practitioner know which actions to take in a given clinical care situation? For example, are videotaped orientations effective in decreasing preoperative anxiety or is one-to-one counseling necessary? Each clinical decision made or action taken is based on knowledge. This knowledge derives from a variety of sources, such as research, theories, experience, tradition, trial and error, authority, or logical reasoning.

> 66 *The wisest mind has something yet to learn.* 99
>
> *George Santayana*

Knowledge Sources

The healthcare professions have made major inroads in identifying, understanding, and developing an array of knowledge sources that inform clinical decisions and actions. We now know that systematic inquiry (research) produces the most dependable knowledge upon which to base practice. In addition, practitioners' expertise and patients' choices and concerns must be taken into account in providing effective and efficient healthcare. Research, expertise, and client choices are all necessary evidence but alone are insufficient for best practice.

Initially, most clinical actions were based solely on logic, tradition, or conclusions drawn from keen observation (i.e., expertise). Although effective practices sometimes have evolved from these knowledge sources, the resulting practice has been successful less often than hoped for in producing intended patient outcomes. Additionally, conclusions that are drawn solely from practitioner observations can be biased because such observations usually are not systematic; similarly, non–evidence-based practices (EBP) across caregivers and settings vary widely. The result is that for a given health problem, a wide variety of clinical actions are taken without reliably producing the desired patient outcomes.

It is well recognized that systematic investigation (i.e., research) holds the promise of deepening our understanding of health phenomena, patients' responses to phenomena, and the probable impact of clinical actions on resolving health problems. Following this realization, research evidence has become highly valued as the basis for clinical decisions.

The research utilization (RU) and EBP movements have escalated attention to the knowledge base of clinical care decisions and actions. In the mid-1970s, RU represented a rudimentary approach to using research as the prime knowledge source upon which to base practice. In the early stages of developing research-based practice, RU approaches promoted using results from a single study as the basis for practice.

Several problems arise with this approach, particularly when more than one study on the same topic has been reported. In this case, multiple studies are difficult to summarize and may produce conflicting findings, and large and small studies may hold different conclusions. This understanding of the evidence produced through research has led to more sophisticated and rigorous approaches for moving research knowledge into practice. These approaches are largely embodied in the EBP paradigm.

> 66 *What is important is to keep learning, to enjoy challenge, and to tolerate ambiguity. In the end there are no certain answers.* 99
>
> *Martina Horner*

Weighing the Evidence

The EBP movement catapults the use of knowledge in clinical care to new heights of sophistication, rigor, and manageability. A key difference between the mandate to "apply research results in practice" and today's EBP paradigm is acknowledgement of the relative weight and role of various knowledge sources as the bases for clinical decisions. "Evidence" is now viewed and scrutinized from a clinical epidemiological perspective. This means that the practitioner takes into account the validity and stability of the specific evidence when clinical recommendations are made (Stevens, Abrams, Brazier, Fitzpatrick, & Lilford, 2001). The EBP approach addresses the issues of variation in ways of managing similar health problems and the deficit between scientific evidence and clinical practice. In other words, it makes clear the evidence underlying effective practice (i.e., best practice) and specifies actions to take in the event of insufficient scientific evidence. In addition, EBP methods such as systematic reviews increase our ability to manage the ever-increasing volume of information produced in order to develop best practices.

Best practice is not new to healthcare providers. For example, mandatory continuing education for licensure in many states is regulatory testimony to the value of staying abreast of new developments. However, emphasis on best practice has shifted from keeping current through traditional continuing education to keeping current with the latest and best available evidence that has been critically appraised for quality. Reliance on inexplicit or inferior knowledge sources (e.g., tradition) is rapidly becoming unacceptable practice in today's quality-focused climate of healthcare. Rather, such practices are being replaced with a quality of knowledge said to include certainty.

Certainty and Knowledge Sources

The goal of EBP is to use the highest quality of knowledge in providing care to produce the greatest impact on patients' health status and healthcare. This entails using the following knowledge sources for care:

- Valid research evidence as the primary basis of clinical decisions
- Clinical expertise to best use the research by filling in gaps and tailoring the clinical action to the individual patient's context
- Patient choices and concerns for determining the acceptability of research-based care to the individual patient

In clinical decisions, the key criterion for quality of underlying knowledge is certainty. Certainty is the level of sureness that the clinical action will produce the intended or desired outcome. Because clinical actions are intended to assist patients achieve a health goal, it is important that we can say with high certainty that what we do with patients is likely to move them toward that intended goal. To appraise certainty, the practitioner first must uncover the source of knowledge underlying the contemplated clinical action, then appraise the quality of that knowledge.

66 *The intuitive mind is a sacred gift and the rational mind is a faithful servant.* 99

Albert Einstein

Rating Strength of the Scientific Evidence

EBP experts have developed a number of taxonomies to rate varying levels of "strength of evidence." These assessments of the strength of scientific evidence provide a mechanism to guide practitioners in evaluating research for its applicability to healthcare decision making. Most of these taxonomies are organized around the various research designs. Many refer to the randomized controlled trial (RCT) as a research design of highest order, and most taxonomies include a full range of evidence, from systematic reviews of RCTs to expert opinions.

Grading the strength of a body of evidence should incorporate three domains: quality, quantity, and consistency (Agency for Healthcare Research and Quality [AHRQ], 2002). These are defined as follows:

- Quality: the extent to which a study's design, conduct, and analysis has minimized selection, measurement, and confounding biases (internal validity) (p. 19)
- Quantity: the number of studies that have evaluated the question, overall sample size across all studies, magnitude of the treatment effect, strength from causality assessment, such as relative risk or odds ratio (p. 25)
- Consistency: whether investigations with both similar and different study designs report similar findings (requires numerous studies) (p. 25)

In an AHRQ study (2002), 7 of 19 such rating systems were judged to include all three domains. Four of the seven indicated that systematic reviews of a body of literature represented the strongest level of evidence; five of the seven included "expert opinion" as evidence. Box 1-2 in Chapter 1 presents a sample system for grading strength of evidence.

Appraising Knowledge Sources

"Critical appraisal" of evidence is a hallmark of EBP. Although critical appraisal is not new, it has become a core skill for those who plan to use evidence to support healthcare decisions (Stevens et al., 2001). The evolution of EBP from evidence-based medicine (EBM) has heavily influenced the current emphasis of critical appraisal of evidence. However, EBM leaders did not intend for appraisal of RCTs to be the final point of critical appraisal. Indeed, the most highly developed methodological source for systematic review, the *Cochrane Reviewers' Handbook* (Clarke & Oxman, 2003), states the reason why RCTs are the first focus of current systematic reviews, making explicit that this is an interim situation (Box 4-1).

EBP methodologists are actively developing methods for systematically summarizing evidence generated from a broad range of research approaches, including qualitative research. The group began with RCTs because the 250,000 existing RCTs represent the preponderance of knowledge about effective medical treatment. This does not preclude interest in and valuing of other types of evidence. EBP efforts have quickly expanded to include all health science disciplines and a broad array of healthcare topics, including nursing services, behavioral research, and preventive health (Stevens, 2002).

The meaning of *evidence* is more fully appreciated within the context of best practice, which reflects the following (Stevens, 2002):

- Research evidence
- Clinical knowledge gained via the individual practitioner's experience
- The patient's and practitioner's preferences and situations
- Basic principles from logic and theory

So the first task in EBP is to identify which knowledge is to be considered as evidence for clinical decisions. Knowledge generated from quantitative and qualitative research, clinical judgment, and patient preferences forms the crucial foundation for practice. Depending on the particular source of knowledge, varying appraisal approaches can be used.

The chapters in Unit Two describe appraisal approaches for the main types of evidence and knowledge to guide clinical practice:

- Evidence from quantitative research
- Evidence from qualitative research

box 4.1

RCTs and Systematic Reviews

The Cochrane Collaboration and the *Cochrane Reviewers' Handbook* focus particularly on systematic reviews of RCTs because they are likely to provide more reliable information than other sources of evidence on the differential effects of alternative forms of healthcare (Kunz, Vist, & Oxman, 2003). Systematic reviews of other types of evidence can also help those wanting to make better decisions about healthcare, particularly those forms of care where RCTs have not been done and may not be possible or appropriate. The basic principles of reviewing research are the same, whatever type of evidence is being reviewed. Although we focus mainly on systematic reviews of RCTs, we address issues specific to reviewing other types of evidence when this is relevant. Fuller guidance on such reviews is being developed.

Clarke, M., & Oxman, A. D., (Eds.) (2003). Introduction. Cochrane Reviewers' Handbook 4.2.0 *[updated March 2003]; Section 1. Used with permission.*

- Clinical judgment
- Knowledge about patient concerns, choices, and values

The authors of the following chapters apply generic principles of evidence appraisal to the broad set of knowledge sources used in healthcare. The purpose of critically appraising these sources is to determine the certainty and applicability of knowledge, regardless of source.

> **"** *The beginning of wisdom is found in doubting; by doubting we come to the question, and by seeking we may come upon the truth.* **"**
>
> *Pierre Abelar*

Overviews

About Quantitative Evidence

In Chapter 5, "Critically Appraising Quantitative Evidence," the nature of evidence produced through quantitative research varies according to the particular design utilized. The chapter details the various types of quantitative research designs, including case study, single studies, and RCTs, and concludes with a discussion of reviews. The distinctions among narrative reviews, systematic reviews, and meta-analyses are drawn. Helpful explanations about systematic reviews describe how data are combined across multiple research studies. Throughout, critical appraisal questions and hints are outlined.

About Qualitative Evidence

Given the emphasis on RCTs (experimental research design) in EBP, some have inaccurately concluded that there is no role for qualitative evidence in EBP. Chapter 6, "Critically Appraising Qualitative Evidence," provides a compelling discussion of the ways in which qualitative research results inform practice. The rich understanding of the individual patient that emerges from qualitative research connects this evidence strongly to the elements of patient preferences and values—both important elements in implementation of EBP.

About Clinical Judgment and Patients' Contributions

Chapter 7, "Patient Concerns and Choices, and Clinical Judgment in Evidence-Based Practice" outlines the roles of two important aspects of clinical care decision making: patient choices and concerns, and clinical judgment. The discussion emphasizes patient preferences not only as perceptions of self and what is best but also as what gives meaning to a person's life. The role of clinical judgment emerges as the practitioner weaves together a narrative understanding of the patient's condition, which includes social and emotional aspects and historical facts. Clinical judgment is presented as a historical clinical understanding of an individual patient—as well as of psychosocial and biological sciences—that is to be combined with evidence from scientific inquiry. Three components of clinical judgment are discussed: experiential learning, clinical forethought, and clinical grasp. This discussion represents a significant contribution to EBP; it is one of only a few discussions elucidating the role of clinical expertise and patient values, choices, and concerns in clinical care.

  Critical appraisal of evidence and knowledge used in clinical care is rapidly becoming a requirement in professional practice. These chapters will provide a basis for understanding and applying the principles of evidence appraisal to improve healthcare.

> **"***Knowledge speaks, but wisdom listens.***"**
>
> *Jimi Hendrix*

references

Agency for Healthcare Research and Quality (AHRQ). (2002). Systems to rate the strength of scientific evidence. File Inventory, Evidence Report/Technology Assessment No. 47. AHRQ Publication No. 02-E016. Rockville, MD: AHRQ. Retrieved from http://ahrq.gov/clinic/strevinv.htm.

Clarke, M., & Oxman, A. D. (Eds.) (2003). Introduction. *Cochrane Reviewers' Handbook* 4.2.0 [updated March 2003]; Section 1. Retrieved from http://www.cochrane.dk/cochrane/handbook/hbook.htm. Accessed October 21, 2003.

Kunz, R., Vist, G., & Oxman, A. D. (2003). Randomisation to protect against selection bias in healthcare trials (Cochrane Methodology Review). In *Cochrane Library, 1*. Oxford: Update Software.

Stevens, A., Abrams, K., Brazier, J., Fitzpatrick, R., & Lilford, R. (Eds.) (2001). *The advanced handbook of methods in evidence based healthcare*. London: Sage Publications.

Stevens, K. (2001). The truth, the whole truth...about EBP and RCTs. *Online Journal of Knowledge Synthesis for Nursing*.

Critically Appraising Quantitative Evidence

Linda Johnston

chapter 5

> ❝*Nothing great was ever achieved without enthusiasm.*❞
>
> *Ralph Waldo Emerson*

Clinicians read healthcare literature for various reasons. Some do it solely in an attempt to keep up to date with the rapid changes in delivery of healthcare. Others may have a specific research interest and want to be aware of the current research results in their field.

Increasingly, with the advent of the evidence-based practice (EBP) healthcare movement, clinicians read the literature to help them make informed decisions about managing a particular patient or group of patients in their care (Guyatt et al., 2000).

The big question for the clinician then becomes, How do I critically appraise the strength of evidence produced through **quantitative research** designs? In this chapter, a variety of quantitative designs are explored in relation to the strength of evidence produced. Table 5-1 outlines the study design that generally is most appropriate for the particular clinical question.

table 5.1 The research design to answer the question

Clinical Question	Research Design
Effectiveness of an intervention	Systematic review, RCT, cohort
Diagnostic	Cross-sectional
Prognostic	Cohort
Harm, causation	Case-control, cohort

Hierarchy of Evidence

There are various hierarchies of evidence. However, the majority of them agree with the **hierarchy of evidence** presented in Chapter 1 (See Chapter 1, Box 1-2), which presupposes that a **systematic review** documenting homogeneity in the results (i.e., agreement) of a large number of high-quality **randomized clinical trials** (RCTs; i.e., randomized with concealment, double-blinded, complete follow-up, intention-to-treat analysis) yields the strongest and least biased estimate of the effect of an intervention (Guyatt & Rennie, 2002; Harris et al., 2001; Phillips et al., 2001). Such systematic reviews have been called the "heart of EBP" (Stevens, 2001).

An RCT is the best research design for providing information about cause-and-effect relationships. Thus, the higher a methodology ranks in the hierarchy, the more likely the results of such methods are to represent objective reality and the more certainty the clinician has that the intervention will produce the same health outcomes again. Ranking the evidence helps clinicians temper their clinical decisions with more or less certainty.

Critical Appraisal Principles of Quantitative Studies

There are three questions to consider when appraising any study (O'Rourke & Booth, 2000):

1. Are the results of the study valid? **(validity)**
2. What are the results? **(reliability)**
3. Will the results help locally? **(applicability)**

The critical appraisal process provides clinicians with the means to interpret and determine the applicability of results to their particular patients (Crombie, 1996; O'Rourke & Booth, 2000). When interpreting results presented in quantitative research papers, the reader should always consider that there may be multiple explanations for an effect reported in a study.

When appraising quantitative studies, it is important to recognize which factors of validity and reliability could influence the results and how far from the true result the reported result may be. Nearly every study has some flaws. Therefore, the process of critical appraisal should assist the clinician in deciding whether a study is flawed to the point that it should be discounted as a source of evidence. Interpretation of results requires consideration of the **statistical significance** of the results (including the potential for incorrect analysis), as well as **clinical significance** of the study findings.

Are the Study Results Valid? (Validity)

The **validity of a study** refers to whether the results of the study were obtained via sound scientific methods and needs to be ascertained before the clinician can make any informed assessment of the size and precision of the effect(s) reported. Validity may be compromised by **bias** and/or by **confounding variables.**

Bias

Bias is anything that distorts the study findings (e.g., **nonhomogeneous sample,** researchers' expectations of relationships and outcomes; Polit & Hungler, 1999) and can be introduced at any point in the design of a study. Misleading results—and thus, incorrect conclusions—can result from bias in a study. When critically appraising research, the clinician needs to be aware of possible sources of bias. The selection of participants for a study may be the earliest point at which bias can be introduced. The experimental hierarchy in Figure 5-1 demonstrates multiple points in the process of determining the final study sample where bias may be introduced.

In Figure 5-1, the ideal but often infeasible sample to include in a study is the **reference population,** that is, those people in the past, present, and future to whom the study results can be generalized. Researchers typically utilize a study population that they assume will be representative of the reference population. However, of the study population, there will be those people willing to participate and those who refuse to participate. In studies where potential participants volunteer to be involved, there may be characteristics of that group by virtue of their volunteering that in some way influence the final results. This is particularly so in those studies where people's attitudes or beliefs are being explored because these may be the very characteristics that influence their decision of whether to participate (Crombie, 1996). Evidence users must be aware that despite the best efforts of the investigators to select a sample that is representative

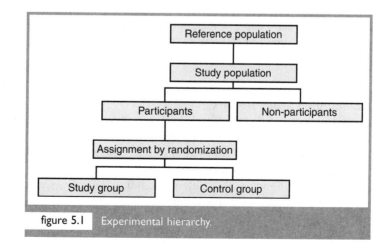

figure 5.1   Experimental hierarchy.

of the reference population, there may be significant differences between their study sample and the general population.

Gatekeeper Effect. Another element known to introduce bias is the well-intentioned person acting as a gatekeeper, particularly in studies involving vulnerable populations. For example, researchers conducting a study with patients receiving palliative care may have difficulty recruiting sufficient numbers of participants because the patients' caregivers may consider it too burdensome to ask patients to participate in research at a difficult time in their lives. *This introduces bias into the study and may ultimately exclude the very people who could benefit from the research.*

Measurement. Measurement bias also may influence study results. *Systematic error* can occur through using an incorrectly calibrated device that gives consistently higher or lower measurements than the actual. Data collectors may deviate from established objective data collection protocols or their individual personality traits may affect the eliciting of information from patients in studies involving interviews or surveys. Studies that rely on patient recall for data also are subject to bias (Crombie, 1996). Recall may be affected by a number of factors. Asking patients with brain tumors about their past use of cellular phones might generate highly accurate or falsely inflated responses because those patients seek an explanation for their disease, compared with patients who do not have tumors and whose recall of phone use may be less accurate in the absence of disease (Muscat et al., 2000).

In longitudinal studies, loss of patients to follow-up also may contribute to measurement bias. Nonreporting of losses to follow-up may mask the real reason for observed differences between the experimental intervention and control groups of patients. Possible reasons for loss of participants (i.e., *study attrition*) could include unforeseen side effects of the intervention or onerous data collection procedures. Such losses lead to noncomparable groups and misleading results.

Contamination is another form of measurement bias. This occurs when participants originally allocated to a particular group or arm of a study are exposed to an alternative group's intervention (i.e., the comparison intervention). For example, in a study of asthmatic school children that compares retention of asthma management information that was given to the children in written form and by video, results may be compromised if those in the video group lend their videos to those in the written information group. In another example, patients in a placebo-controlled trial somehow become aware that they have been assigned to the placebo group and, believing they should be in the intervention arm of the study, find some way to access the intervention.

Confounded Study Results

A study's results may be confounded when a relationship between two variables is actually due to a third, either known or unknown variable (i.e., a confounding variable). The confounding variable relates to both the exposure (i.e., intervention) and the outcome but is not directly a part of the causal pathway between the two.

Lifestyle and health are often interlinked, sometimes making it difficult to determine the confounding influences. For example, a study may report a link between high caffeine intake and insomnia and headaches (Awada & al Jumah, 1999). However, if the study population includes people engaged in shiftwork, it may be the irregular working hours causing the symptoms and not the caffeine itself. Figure 5-2 demonstrates how confounding variables can lead to confusing results. The shiftwork is related to both the exposure (i.e., high caffeine intake) and the outcomes (i.e., headaches and insomnia). However, it is not directly causal (i.e., irregular working hours do not cause headaches or insomnia).

When critically appraising a study, the clinician should judge whether the investigators considered the possibility of confounding variables in the original design as well as in the analysis and interpretation of their results. Minimizing the possible impact of confounding variables on a study's results is best addressed by a design that utilizes a randomization process (i.e., random assignment) to assign participants to a study group (i.e., experimental or control group). In this way, confounding variables, either known or unknown, will equally influence the outcomes of the different groups in the study.

It is possible that confounding variables will influence a study's results despite an investigator's best efforts. Unplanned co-interventions occurring at the same time may have an impact on the observed outcomes. This is often referred to as **history**. As an example, a study is launched for the purpose of determining the effects of an educational program regarding infant nutrition (i.e., the experimental intervention group) in comparison with the usual delivery of information on infant growth and development provided at maternal and child health visits (i.e., the control group). At about the same time as the study commences, the regional health department begins a widespread media campaign to promote child health. Therefore, the confounding historical event of the regional emphasis on education would make it difficult to directly attribute any positive observed outcomes solely to the experimental intervention itself.

What Are the Results? (Reliability)

Having determined the validity of a study's findings, the clinician should then consider the size and precision of the effects reported (i.e., reliability). The **reliability of study findings** refers to whether the effects have sufficient influence on practice, clinically and statistically (i.e., the results can be counted on to make a difference when clinicians apply them to their practices; that

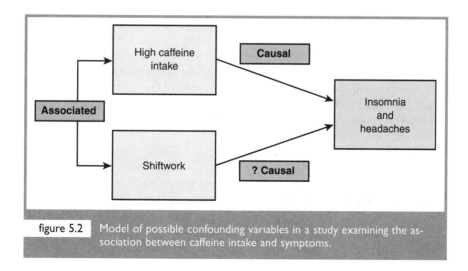

figure 5.2   Model of possible confounding variables in a study examining the association between caffeine intake and symptoms.

is, are the findings reliable?). At this point, an examination of the numerical data reported in the results section of a study is incorporated into the critical appraisal process.

> **❝** *Patience is the companion of wisdom.* **❞**
>
> Saint Augustine

Size and Precision of the Effect: Do the Numbers Add Up?

The number of participants in the study population should be clearly indicated. The total number in each group or arm of a study will usually form the denominator in subsequent critical analyses of results. This is usually referred to and reported as N. The N may be arrived at after prespecified inclusion and exclusion selection criteria for a sample are met. In all studies, the total number of participants approached and the number consenting to participate should be reported. In addition, in the case of RCTs, the final numbers assigned to the intervention and control groups should be reported.

The numerators in the analyses are the participants with the outcome of interest, reported as n. The clinician should check that the numerator total equates with the original N reported. When this is not the case, it is often due to **loss of subjects to follow-up,** (e.g., trial participants dropping out of the study or deaths occurring during the study [**attrition**]). The researchers should account for any difference in final numbers of participants versus the number of subjects who commenced the study. This may provide important qualitative information. For example, a study reporting the effectiveness of depression management that uses frequent individual appointments with a professional may have far fewer numbers of participants at the end of the study than were originally enrolled. The onerous nature of the frequent appointments may mean that although the intervention was effective, its practicability is limited.

Magnitude of the Effect

The **magnitude of effect** refers to the degree of the difference or lack of difference between the various groups (i.e., experimental and control groups) in a study. The effect is essentially the "rate" of occurrence in each of the groups for the outcome of interest. It is helpful when trying to determine the magnitude of effect to use a table, such as Table 5-2. The table can have additional columns and rows for more intervention groups or a larger number of outcome measures. It should be stressed that clinicians do not need nor are they expected to carry statistical formulae around in their heads in order to critically appraise the literature. Some knowledge of commonly used statistical tests and when they should be used is adequate for the appraisal process. However, it is always helpful to keep a health sciences statistics book nearby as a reference when doing a critical appraisal.

The **occurrence rate** can be reported as incidence or prevalence. **Prevalence** refers to the persons in the at-risk population who have the outcome or disorder in a given "snapshot in time." Prevalence is reported as a percentage or proportion (e.g., the proportion of patients who acquire ventilator-associated pneumonia [VAP] to all patients who were at risk for VAP) and is sometimes referred to as the pretest probability of an individual to have an outcome. **Incidence** is the new occurrences of the outcome or disorder within the at-risk population in a specified time frame. Incidence is a true rate.

table 5.2   Measure of effect

Exposure	Outcome Yes (Cases)	No (Controls)	No (Controls)
Yes (Cohort)	a	b	a + b
No (Cohort)	c	d	c + d
Total	a + c	b + d	a + b + c + d

Note. a + b is the denominator, N, i.e., the total number of study participants exposed to the intervention.

a is the numerator, n, i.e., those participants exposed to the intervention who had the outcome of interest.

b is the numerator, n, i.e., those participants exposed to the intervention who did not have the outcome of interest.

c + d is the denominator, N, i.e., the total number of study participants not exposed to the intervention.

c is the numerator, n, i.e., those participants not exposed to the intervention who nevertheless had the outcome of interest.

d is the numerator, n, i.e., those participants not exposed to the intervention and who did not have the outcome of interest.

a + c is the total number of study participants, both exposed and not exposed to the intervention, who had the outcome of interest.

b + d is the total number of study participants in the control and intervention groups who did not have the outcome of interest.

For example, a survey distributed to parents of all school-aged children in a particular region asking whether their children had an audible wheeze in the last week would indicate the prevalence of asthma at the point in time in which the survey was conducted (Akinbami & Schoendorf, 2002). However, if information were being sought on the utility of investing in a large-scale asthma management plan for schools, a study reporting the incidence (45 new cases, or 25% increase) of asthma over a period of time (e.g., the past 5 years) would be more useful (Ronchetti et al., 2001).

Effect measures compare the differences in occurrences of outcomes between groups (Guyatt, Sackett, & Cook, 1994). **Risk** is the probability that a person (currently free from a disease) will develop a disease at some point. Using Table 5-2 as a guide, the risk in the exposed group (Re) of developing the outcome of interest (occurrence rate) is:

$$\text{Risk in exposed (Re)} = a/(a + b)$$

The odds of the outcome of interest occurring in the exposed group are:

$$\text{Odds in exposed} = a/b$$

Similarly, using Table 5-2, the risk in the unexposed group (Ru) of developing the outcome of interest (occurrence rate) is:

$$\text{Risk in }\textit{un}\text{exposed (Ru)} = c/(c + d)$$

The odds of the outcome of interest occurring in the unexposed group are:

$$\text{Odds in }\textit{un}\text{exposed} = c/d$$

The following is an example of the risk of dying from meningitis. In one year, 152 (i.e., a + b) children contracted meningitis. Fifteen (i.e., a) of those children died. The proportion of children who are at risk of dying from meningitis is 15/152 = 9.87%. In other words, there is approximately a 10% chance of dying from contracting meningitis. The odds of dying from meningitis are 15/137 (i.e., a/b) = 1/9.13. In other words, 15 children die for every 137 children with meningitis who survive, that is, the odds of dying are approximately one in nine.

> ❝*One of the greatest discoveries a man makes, one of his great surprises, is to find he can do what he was afraid he couldn't do.*❞
>
> *Henry Ford*

Strength of Association

Risk ratio (*relative risk* [RR]) and *odds ratio* (OR) are reported as measures of association between groups exposed and unexposed to the intervention and the outcome. RR measures the strength of association and is the risk of the outcome in the exposed group (Re) divided by the risk of the outcome in the unexposed group (Ru). RR is used in prospective studies, such as RCTs and cohort studies.

$$Re/Ru = RR = [a / (a + b)] / [c / (c + d)]$$
$$RR = a(c + d) / c(a + b)$$

If the outcome is something we want (e.g., stopping smoking), RR greater than 1 means the treatment is better than control. If the outcome is something we do not want (e.g., death), RR greater than 1 means the treatment is worse than control.

The OR is the odds of a case patient (i.e., someone in the intervention group) being exposed (a/b) divided by the odds of a control patient being exposed (c/d). OR is usually reported in retrospective studies, such as case-control studies where the number of sick and not sick patients is known but not the total number of people. Table 5-2 can again be used here to guide the OR calculation.

$$OR = (a/b) / (c/d)$$
$$OR = ad/bc$$

Whereas RR measures the strength of association, the risk difference (RD) measures the absolute difference between the exposed and unexposed groups' risks (i.e., occurrence in the exposed/intervention group [Re] subtracted from the occurrence in the control group [Ru]). This value also is referred to as the *absolute risk reduction* (ARR).

$$RD = Ru - Re = ARR$$

Interpreting results that are presented as an RR, OR, or RD can be difficult, not only for the clinician but also for the consumer—an essential contributor to the healthcare decision-making process when using best evidence.

Another measure of strength of association, the relative risk reduction (RRR), is the proportion of risk for bad outcomes in the intervention group compared with the unexposed control group.

$$RRR = \{|Re - Ru|/Ru\} \times 100\%$$

A more meaningful way to present the results so that the reader can understand the difference between the treatment or intervention and the control in achieving a specific outcome is through the calculation of the **number needed to treat** (NNT).

$$NNT = 1/\text{Risk difference or ARR}$$
$$NNT = 1/ARR$$

The NNT represents the number of people who would need to receive the experimental therapy to prevent one bad outcome or cause one additional good outcome.

Example. You are a clinician who is working with patients who want to quit smoking. They have friends who have managed to quit by using nicotine chewing gum and wonder whether this also might work for them. You find a trial that measured the effectiveness of nicotine chewing gum versus a placebo (Table 5-3). Of the experimental group, 18.2% quit smoking (Re). However, some participants in the control group also gave up smoking (10.6%) (Ru). The number of extra quitters per 100 people treated therefore was (RD):

$$18.2\% - 10.6\% = 7.6\% \ (7.6\% = 7.6 / 100 = .076)$$

How likely is it that this treatment will help the individual asking you for advice? The NNT is calculated as:

$$1 / .076 = 13.2$$

We need to treat 13 smokers with gum for one additional person to give up smoking. Nicotine gum is a relatively inexpensive and easy-to-use treatment, and given the costs of smoking, treating 13 smokers to help one stop is reasonable.

The size of the NNT, be it very large or very small, will assist in deciding about the use of a treatment. However, other influences on the decision-making process, such as patient preference and resource issues, also need to be taken into account. Sometimes, although a treatment may have a beneficial effect, there also may be negative effects. For example, a medication may be very effective, but side effects also are associated with that medication. Evaluation of the risks (e.g., side effects) and benefits of the medication will help the clinician determine the merit of prescribing it for patients.

chapter 5

87

table 5.3   The effectiveness of nicotine chewing gum

Exposure	Outcome		Total
	Yes (Quit)	No (Not Quit)	
Yes (Nicotine gum)	1149	5179	6328
No (Placebo)	893	7487	8380
Total	2042	12666	

Number needed to harm (NNH) is the number of clients who, if they received an intervention, would result in one additional person being harmed (i.e., having a bad outcome) compared with the patients in the control arm of a study. This important statistic is determined using the increase in risk of a bad outcome in the treatment group (Re) compared with the risk in the unexposed control group (Ru). This is called the *absolute risk increase* (ARI).

Note: Some clinicians use the absolute value of the difference between the occurrence in the exposed/intervention group [Re] and the occurrence in the control group [Ru], using the formula |Re-Ru| for both ARR and ARI

$$NNH = 1 / \text{Risk increase or ARI}$$

$$NNH = 1 / ARI$$

Deciding whether the benefits outweigh the harms is an important, additional component in clinical decision making.

> **"** *Patience and perseverance have a magical effect before which difficulties disappear and obstacles vanish.* **"**
>
> *J o h n   Q u i n c y   A d a m s*

Measures of Clinical Significance

It is very important that the clinician involved in the critical appraisal process consider the results of a study within the context of practice by asking the question, Are the reported results of actual clinical significance? When critiquing a study, the clinician needs to be aware that the way in which the results are reported may be misleading when trying to interpret their significance. Calculation of the ARR retains the concept of the underlying susceptibility of a patient to an outcome and can distinguish between huge and very small treatment effects. In contrast, RRR loses the notion of existing baseline risk and, thus, this analysis of results fails to discriminate between large and small treatment effects.

Re = 0.15	Ru = 0.20
ARR = Ru − Re	0.20 − 0.15 = 0.05
Relative risk = Re/Ru	0.15 / 0.20 = 0.75
RRR = {|Re − Ru|/Ru} × 100	{|.15 − .20| / .20} × 100 = 25%
NNT = 1/ARR	1 / (0.05) = 20

Example One.   In this hypothetical example, the intervention group was women who wore socks and not hose during their shift on the patient unit. The risk of foot odor in the sock-wearing intervention group (Re) was 0.15; sometimes this is called the *experimental event rate* or *occurrence*. The event rate (Ru) of the control group (no socks, just hose) for foot odor was 0.20. The calculated ARR was 5%, a seemingly small effect. That is, wearing socks had a small effect on foot odor. However, the RRR is 25%, which seems like a reasonable effect. In other words, the proportional reduction of those with foot odor in the sock-wearing group was moderate compared with the reduction of foot odor in those who did not wear socks. The ARR is the more clinically meaningful value to assist in decision making. In this example, it would take having 20 people wear socks to prevent one episode of foot odor. It could be argued that 20 people are a reasonable NNT in this situation.

Clinicians must keep in mind that a substantial RRR in an outcome that is very rare means little in terms of impact of an intervention. The example below indicates that the observed risk is clearly very low; in fact, it is 100 times lower than in the data set above.

A study investigated the benefits of wearing shoes in your home. The occurrence of a stubbed toe in the shoe-wearing group (Re) was .0015, a very small effect. The event rate in the no-shoes group was .0020, still a very small effect. The ARR is minuscule at .0005. However, the RRR remains the same as the above example, 25%.

$Re = 0.0015$ $Ru = 0.0020$

$ARR = Ru - Re$ $0.0020 - 0.15 = 0.0005$

$Relative\ risk = Re/Ru$ $0.0015 / 0.0020 = 0.75$

$RRR = \{|Re - Ru|/Ru\} \times 100$ $.0005 / .0020 - 100 = 25\%$

$NNT = 1/ARR$ $1 / (0.0005) = 2{,}000$

These two sets of hypothetical data show that the RR and RRR remain the same despite the 100-fold less risk of the occurrence. However, the NNT is substantially affected. Treating 20 persons versus 2,000 is quite a difference, no matter what the intervention. In the case of rare outcomes, more patients or clients need to be treated to prevent one bad outcome or to cause one additional good outcome.

When critiquing the presentation of RRR data, clinicians must be aware of the lack of perspicacity of the RR and RRR in providing clinically meaningful data.

Example Two.   Suppose that the rate of an occurrence of a disease is 96% in the control group (Ru) and 28% in the intervention group (Re).

$RRR = \{|Re - Ru|/Ru\} \times 100 = \{|28\% - 96\%|/96\%\} \times 100$

$RRR = 71\%$

$ARR = Ru - Re = 96\% - 28\% = 68\%$

On the basis of these reported results, the intervention looks very impressive in terms of its effectiveness in reducing, in this case, the unwanted outcome. But what happens when the rate of occurrence is extremely low to begin with in the population under study? In the following example, the rate of an occurrence in the control group is 0.00096% and in the intervention group 0.00028%.

$RRR = \{|0.00028\% - 0.00096\%|/0.00096\%\} \times 100$

$RRR = 71\%$

$ARR = 0.00096\% - 0.00028\% = 0.00068\%$

The RRR has remained unchanged, but the intervention actually has only a trivial effect when the ARR is reported. The way data are reported may influence the final decision of the patient and clinician with respect to accepting or rejecting a proposed intervention.

Precision of the Measurement of Effect

When critically appraising the results presented in a study, the clinician needs to consider not only the magnitude of the effect but also the precision of the measurement of that magnitude. The degree of precision is related to the degree of **random error** present. When repeated measures of the same outcome are similar in a study, it is presumed that there is low random error. The most frequently reported way of representing the extent to which random error may influence the measure of effect is by **confidence intervals.** The confidence interval (CI) gives us the range in which the real answer lies with a given degree of certainty. It describes an interval around the estimated effect point. In general, research papers will present a 95% CI. A 95% CI for the mean is sometimes loosely described as having a 95% probability of containing the true mean. The formula for calculating the CI is:

$$95\% \text{ CI} = \text{Mean} \pm (1.96 \times \text{standard error})$$

$$\text{Standard error} = \text{standard deviation} / \text{square root of } n$$

It should be reiterated here that a clinician does not need to be able to remember how a CI is calculated. What is important is to understand *what* contributes to the calculation.

Example One. As an example of what a CI means, consider a bag containing a mixture of black and white balls, with 30 total balls. The number of black balls in the bag could be anywhere between 0 and 30. Therefore the $\text{CI}_{[\text{black balls (bb)}]} = 0\text{--}30$. Six balls are removed from the bag, of which 4 are black and 2 are white. We know there must have been at least 4 and no more than 28 black balls originally, so the $\text{CI}_{[\text{bb}]} = 4\text{--}28$. An additional 3 black and 6 white balls are removed, so the $\text{CI}_{[\text{bb}]}$ is now 7--22. Next, 3 black and 5 white balls are removed, so the $\text{CI}_{[\text{bb}]} = 10\text{--}17$. Four black balls are removed with the resulting $\text{CI}_{[\text{bb}]} = 14\text{--}17$. Finally, the last 3 balls are taken out of the bag; 2 black and 1 white. So to begin with, there were 16 black balls in the bag. Notice that as the total sample of balls removed became larger, the CI became smaller. These were absolute CIs because there was a known fixed and finite number of balls that existed in the bag.

However, interventions in healthcare are not predetermined, and the real world of clinical practice is not predictable with any certainty. We can never be absolutely certain whether an intervention will help our patients, but we can try to be reasonably certain. Ninety-five percent CIs provide us with the range in which we can expect the "true" result to lie 95% of the time, meaning that in 1 in 20 studies, on average, the real value will lie outside the CI limits.

The *wider* the CI, the less confident we are about the true result. The width of the CI is greatly dependent on sample size. The larger the sample size in a study, the greater the power is to detect a true result and the more confident we can be about the study findings, resulting in a smaller CI. As the experimental hierarchy showed earlier, the study population is supposed to be representative of the variability inherent in the reference population (see Figure 5-1). A larger sample size is more likely to account for that variability in the measures observed; thus, the more confident we can be about where the true result lies with a subsequently shorter CI surrounding the estimate of true effect.

Remember that OR is a measure of RR (i.e., relative risk), calculated by taking the ratio between two measures of risk. If there is no difference in risk between the two groups, the RR is 1 because the risk in each group is the same, and a number divided by itself is 1. A CI range that includes an RR of 1 suggests that there is a nonstatistically significant difference be-

table 5.4   Outcome of smoking cessation at six months following acupuncture therapy or placebo (sham acupuncture)

| | Outcome | | |
Exposure	Yes (Quit)	No (Not Quit)	Total
Yes (Acupuncture)	5	23	28
No (Sham acupuncture)	4	23	27
Total	9	46	55

Gillams, J., Lewith, G., & Machin, D. (1984). Acupuncture and group therapy in stopping smoking. Practitioner, 228, 341–344.

tween the intervention and the control group. Some examples of CIs and how they relate to sample size and statistical significance follow.

Example Two. Investigators conducted a trial to test the effectiveness of acupuncture for smoking cessation (Gillams, Lewith, & Machin, 1984). The control group participants received sham acupuncture.

The OR can be calculated from the information provided in Table 5-4, and the OR and its associated 95% CI are presented in Figure 5-3. The figure indicates an OR of 1.24 with a CI of 0.30–5.13.

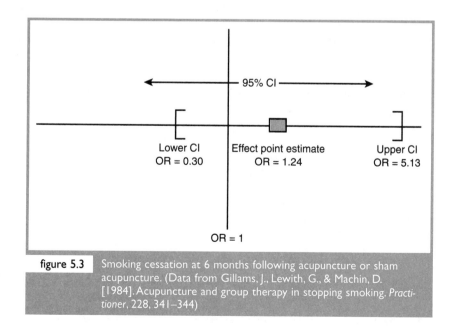

95% CI

| Lower CI | Effect point estimate | Upper CI |
| OR = 0.30 | OR = 1.24 | OR = 5.13 |

OR = 1

figure 5.3   Smoking cessation at 6 months following acupuncture or sham acupuncture. (Data from Gillams, J., Lewith, G., & Machin, D. [1984]. Acupuncture and group therapy in stopping smoking. *Practitioner, 228, 341–344*)

As seen in Figure 5-3, the 95% CI includes the OR of 1.0 (0.30–5.13) so the difference in effectiveness between acupuncture and sham acupuncture in aiding smoking cessation is statistically nonsignificant (i.e., it is just as likely that people would stop smoking if they received acupuncture as it is if they received the placebo therapy).

Example Three.   A number of trials have been conducted to determine the effectiveness of corticosteroid administration in reducing mortality following acute traumatic brain injury. In fact, a systematic review has been done of these trials (Alderson & Roberts, 2002). A small trial conducted in 1987 produced the results shown in Table 5-5 (Chacon, 1987).

Figure 5-4 indicates the calculated OR and 95% CI. The study population numbers provided in Table 5-5 are small; there are only five patients in each arm of the trial. Subsequently, the CI is extremely wide, as indicated in Figure 5-4, from a lower OR of 0.15 to an upper OR estimate of 872.0—off the scale, as indicated by the arrowhead. The small sample size leads to reduced confidence in where the "true" result may lie.

The results of another trial assessing the effectiveness of reducing mortality associated with traumatic brain injury are shown in Table 5-6 (Grumme et al., 1995). Figure 5-5 depicts the calculated OR and 95% CI. From the results presented in Table 5-6, the OR can be calculated. Note the much larger sample size in this study compared with the previous trial. From Figure 5-5, it can be seen that the 95% CI is much tighter. This indicates a greater degree of confidence in where the "true" estimate of effect lies. However, the CI still includes an OR of 1 (CI 0.51–1.34); thus, the difference in outcome between the two groups is not statistically significant.

Many journals that publish healthcare research are requesting that investigators provide CI data rather than the traditional *p* value used to report statistical significance. The aim of statistical analyses is to determine whether an effect observed is true or whether it may have occurred by chance. If an **effect size** (i.e, calculated as the mean of the experimental group minus the mean of the control group divided by the pooled standard deviation) is found to be so large that it is unlikely to have occurred by chance, we say it is statistically significant. By convention, a *p* value of 0.05 or less is considered a statistically significant result. *P* values are the statistical test of the

table 5.5 The effectiveness of corticosteroids for management of acute traumatic brain injury

| | Outcome | | |
Exposure	Yes (Dead)	No (Alive)	Total
Yes (Steroid)	1	4	5
No (Placebo)	0	5	5
Total	1	9	10

Chacon, L. (1987). Edema cerebral en traumatismo craneoencefalico severo en ninos tatados con y sin dexametasona [Brain edema in severe head injury on children treated with and without dexametasone]. Medicina Critica Venezolana, 2, 75–79.

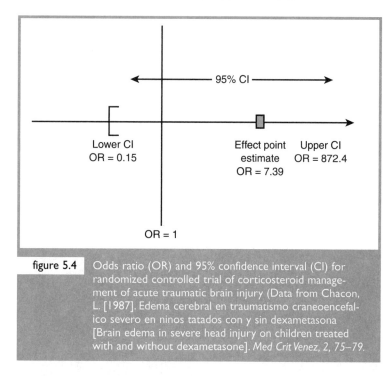

| figure 5.4 | Odds ratio (OR) and 95% confidence interval (CI) for randomized controlled trial of corticosteroid management of acute traumatic brain injury (Data from Chacon, L. [1987]. Edema cerebral en traumatismo craneoencefalico severo en ninos tatados con y sin dexametasona [Brain edema in severe head injury on children treated with and without dexametasone]. *Med Crit Venez, 2,* 75–79. |

assumption that there is no difference between an experimental intervention and a control. *P* values tell us the probability of an event, given the assumption that there is no true difference. *P* values provide a rather arbitrarily set "cut-off" at which we decide that the probability of a result is large or larger than we have observed occurring by chance. But unlike CIs, *p* values do not tell us anything about the precision of the measures or the size of the effect. A small observed effect would suggest that the play of chance could not be excluded as a reason for the result.

table 5.6 Effectiveness of administration of steroid in reducing deaths associated with brain injury

Exposure	Outcome		Total
	Yes (Dead)	No (Alive)	
Yes (Steroid)	38	137	175
No (Placebo)	49	146	195
Total	87	283	370

Grumme, T., Baethmann, A., Kolodziejczyk, D., Krimmer, J., Fischer, M., & Eisenhart Rothe, B. (1995). Treatment of patients with severe head injury by triamcinolone: a prospective, controlled multicenter trial of 396 cases. Research in Experimental Medicine, 195, 217–229.

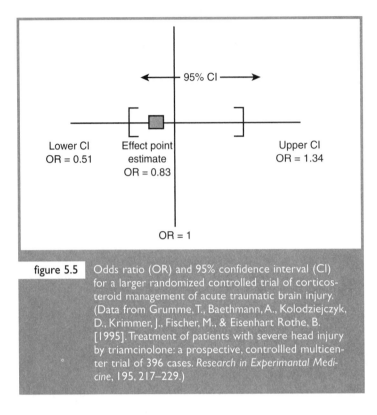

figure 5.5	Odds ratio (OR) and 95% confidence interval (CI) for a larger randomized controlled trial of corticosteroid management of acute traumatic brain injury. (Data from Grumme, T., Baethmann, A., Kolodziejczyk, D., Krimmer, J., Fischer, M., & Eisenhart Rothe, B. [1995]. Treatment of patients with severe head injury by triamcinolone: a prospective, controllled multicenter trial of 396 cases. *Research in Experimantal Medicine*, 195, 217–229.)

But how does a clinician reading a research report know how large or how small an effect size can be and still be true? The size of a result has to be considered in relation to the amount of variation or sampling error expected. This is called the *standard error* (SE). If an effect reported is more than two SE away from zero, the result is considered statistically significant (i.e., it is very unlikely to have occurred by chance). How unlikely? A p value of less than 0.05 means it is very unlikely that the observed result occurred by chance. In fact, there is only a 1 in 20 probability that the result is not the true result and is due to chance.

Power

Confidence about the accuracy and representativeness of the results found in a study is key to successful use of those study findings. Researchers are more confident about their findings when the CI is narrow and does not contain the value of 1. There are many things that influence whether researchers obtain this preferred CI. Investigators in planning, implementing, and analyzing their studies may "get it wrong" for several reasons. Sample size can lead to wrong conclusions and is an obvious factor for both researchers and research consumers to consider. Adequate sample size is best determined by analyzing the power and effect size desired. To fully understand power, there needs to be an understanding of how error can influence the interpretation of a study's findings.

There are two types of error that can occur when drawing conclusions about the effects of an intervention (i.e., **Type 1** and **Type 2 errors**). The **null hypothesis** (H0) means that the experimental and control treatments have the same effect. The assumption is that there is no difference in rates of outcome between the two groups. Investigators test this hypothesis in experimental studies. Table 5-7 describes Type 1 and Type 2 errors, the two possible errors that can occur in making conclusions. Type 1 error occurs when researchers conclude from an experiment that a difference does exist between treatments, when in truth it does not. Type 2 error occurs when the investigators conclude from their results that no difference exists between the groups, when in fact there is a difference.

Sample size is a component of **power**. Appropriate sample size is determined by addressing power (1-β; probability of making Type 1 error), effect size (expected strength of the relationship), and significance level (α; probability of making Type 2 error). Larger sample size means greater power to detect a true effect. When critiquing a study, one needs to determine whether an a priori (i.e., determined beforehand) power calculation was done by the researchers; that is, before they commenced their study, did they calculate the sample size required to detect important differences if they occurred?

Type 1 error can be inflated by repeated analyses of the data, making multiple treatment comparisons, or measuring multiple outcomes. This is sometimes referred to as "data dredging." The power of a study (1-β) is the ability of the study to detect a clinically important difference. Ideally, studies should be designed to have 80–90% power. Eighty percent power means the investigators will find a result, if there is one, 80% of the time. Studies are often underpowered, mainly because of inadequate sample size.

A research consumer appraising a study should consider whether a negative finding was reported. A failure to find a significant difference does not mean that one does not exist. The failure to find significance may result from the researchers not addressing power issues. In other words, the study may not have had sufficient power to detect important differences.

Sensitivity and Specificity

Although it is true that clinicians are interested in the effectiveness of interventions, other types of questions arise in clinical practice on a daily basis. One such question is about diagnostic tests. For example, does routine blood glucose testing in asymptomatic adults result in early identification of type 2 diabetes mellitus and a reduction in associated morbidity? Or as another example, does the presence of what and/or how many symptoms suggest acute sinusitis requiring antibiotic therapy? Assessing the accuracy of a diagnostic test is usually achieved through a **cross-sectional study** design that compares a test classification of a disorder with a **gold standard** or reference test.

table 5.7　The two possible errors in hypothesis testing

	H1 is True	H0 is True
	A real difference exists	There is no difference
Yes	Correct decision	Type 1 error
No	Type 2 error	Correct decision

Sensitivity refers to the proportion of people who have positive test results and who really have the disease. **Specificity** refers to the people who do not have the disease and whose test results are negative. If a diagnostic test has a specificity of 1.0 and a sensitivity of 1.0, it is said to be a perfectly accurate and valid test. There are four possible groups of people when conducting diagnostic testing (Table 5-8):

- Group a: disease positive and test result positive
- Group b: test result positive but do not actually have the disease (**false positive**)
- Group c: disease positive but test negative (**false negative**)
- Group d: disease negative and test result is negative

$$\text{Sensitivity} = a / (a + c)$$

$$\text{Specificity} = d / (b + d)$$

Likelihood ratios (LRs) are used to assess how good a diagnostic test is and to help the clinician decide what tests to undertake (Jaeschke, Guyatt, & Sackett, 1994). LR, which is equivalent to RR in other studies, is less likely to change with the prevalence of a disorder and can also be used to combine the results of a number of diagnostic tests. The LR is the likelihood that a given test result would be expected in a person with the disease of interest compared with the likelihood that the same result would be seen in someone without the disease. There are LRs for a positive test result and LRs for a negative test result.

$$\text{LR} + = \text{sensitivity} / (1\text{-specificity})$$

$$\text{LR} - = (1\text{-sensitivity}) / \text{specificity}$$

Example. In a study of 201 patients by Lindboek and colleagues (1996), patients presented with acute sinusitis, as evidenced by a variety of symptoms. In the study, four symptoms were significantly associated with the presence of infection as diagnosed by CT scan. These were:

1. purulent secretions in cavum nasi
2. purulent rhinorrhea
3. two phases in the illness history
4. an erythrocyte sedimentation rate (ESR) greater than 10 mm/hr

Table 5-9 gives the results of the CT scans done in patients presenting with all four symptoms versus no symptoms. The sensitivity of the four symptoms together is approximately 95% (43

table 5.8 Calculating specificity and sensitivity

Target Disorder			
Diagnostic test result	Present	Absent	Total
Positive	a	b	a + b
Negative	c	d	c + d
	a + c	B + d	a + b + c + d

table 5.9 The diagnostic value of symptom presentation for acute sinusitis

	Target Disorder	
Number of signs and symptoms present	Sinusitis present on CT scan	Sinusitis absent on CT scan
Four	43	1
Nil	2	14
Total	45	15

Lindboek, M., Hjortdahl, P., & Johnsen, U. (1996). Use of symptoms, signs, and blood tests to diagnose acute sinus infections in primary care: Comparison with computed tomography. Family Practice, 28, 183–188.

/ 45), and the specificity is approximately 93% (14 / 15). The LR+ is 13.5, and the LR− is 0.05. Thus, in this example, the presence of all four symptoms is highly predictive of acute sinusitis.

The Centre for Evidence Based Medicine in the United Kingdom has developed two mnemonics for remembering the difference between sensitivity and specificity:

- **SnNout:** When a test has a high *Sen*sitivity, a *N*egative result rules *out* the diagnosis
- **SpPin:** When a test has a high *Sp*ecificity a *P*ositive result rules *in* the diagnosis.

A very high LR (above 10) rules in the disease, whereas a very low LR (below 0.1) virtually rules out the chance that the patient has the disease.

Many clinicians find appraising diagnostic studies a difficult and confusing task. Keeping a health statistics text handy and using questions found in Box 5-1 may be helpful in deciding the value of a study.

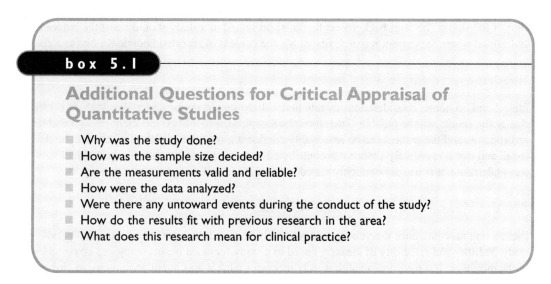

box 5.1

Additional Questions for Critical Appraisal of Quantitative Studies

- Why was the study done?
- How was the sample size decided?
- Are the measurements valid and reliable?
- How were the data analyzed?
- Were there any untoward events during the conduct of the study?
- How do the results fit with previous research in the area?
- What does this research mean for clinical practice?

> 66*Patience, persistence and perspiration make an unbeatable combination for success.*99
>
> *Napolean Hill*

Additional Questions to Ask in a Critical Appraisal

A general convention is followed when laying out a quantitative research paper and presenting results. Similarly, there is an accepted layout for the critical appraisal process. It includes standard critical appraisal questions to ask (Box 5-1), with minor differences suggested by the various experts in the critical appraisal of research and evidence-based healthcare (Oxman, Sackett, & Guyatt, 1993).

Developed for particular research study designs or for specific members of the healthcare professions, many critical appraisal checklists are available (Evidence-Based Health Care, 2002; Greenhalgh, 1997). Some are available at various Web sites, for example:
http://www.med.ualberta.ca/ebm/ebm.htm and
http://www.cebm.net/downloads.asp.

Why Was the Study Done?

A clear explanation of why the study was carried out is crucial. Usually, this is summarized in the aims of the study. The brief background literature presented in a study should assist the reader to understand where the current research fits within the context of reported knowledge on the topic.

How Was the Sample Size Decided?

Ethical and economic considerations dictate that a study should not be undertaken if there is little chance the results will be reliable. Therefore, the sample size should be sufficient enough that the investigators and the readers can be reasonably confident a true effect, if there is any, can be detected and that it is unlikely chance has contributed to the result. If an a priori power calculation was undertaken, it is usually explicitly stated in the methods section of the research report.

Are the Measurements Valid and Reliable?

Factors that may influence the validity and reliability of a study's results were discussed previously. **Validity** and reliability of measures used in a study focus on the accuracy and consistency of the measures. If a measure is valid, it truly measures what it was intended to measure. For example, if an instrument is valid and is said to measure anxiety, it should not measure depression. A reliable instrument is one that is stable over time and is comprised of individual items/questions that all consistently measure the same construct. There are several statistical techniques that can be applied to instrument results to determine reliability (e.g. **Cronbach's alpha**).

Systematic or **random error** can be introduced at any point during a study's design. The validity and reliability of measures used in a study will be discussed in the methods section of the published report. Any acknowledgment on the part of investigators that validity and/or reliability may be an issue influencing their results will usually be presented in the discussion section of the research report.

How Were the Data Analyzed?

A subsection of the methods section of a quantitative research study should describe the statistical methods used to analyze the data. The clinician need not be familiar with a large number of complex approaches to analysis; an understanding of which tests are generally used with which types of data is sufficient. However, there are a few tips that those new to critical appraisal and statistical analyses may find helpful.

- Try to discern whether the test chosen for analyzing the data was chosen because it gave a significant *p* value. A statistical test should be chosen on the basis of its appropriateness for the type of data collected, not because it gives the answer for which the investigators had hoped.
- A second concern should be whether a large number of analyses were undertaken on the same data. This is often referred to as "data dredging" because the greater the number of analyses, the more likely that a significant although specious result will be found.

Were There Any Untoward Events During the Conduct of the Study?

A number of problems may arise during a study and may influence the final results. These may be unpredictable and occur by chance or they may be secondary to a flaw or flaws in the original study design. One such problem is loss to follow-up (i.e., study attrition), which results in missing data and introduction of bias.

How Do the Results Fit with Previous Research in the Area?

The literature review at the beginning of a research report sets the scene for the current research and should be framed in such a way that the clinician will understand the purpose of the research. The discussion section of the report should discuss the research findings in light of what is already known and how those findings complement or contradict previous work.

What Does this Research Mean for Clinical Practice?

The point of critical appraisal and evidence-based decision making in healthcare is to utilize research findings to improve clinical practice. Thus, asking what the research means for clinical practice is one of the most important questions to ask during critical appraisal. Clinicians should look at the study population and ask whether the results can be extrapolated to *their* patients. Additionally, the size of the effect reported has to be assessed for its clinical importance. There are additional specifically relevant appraisal questions that should be addressed, depending on the study design.

Critical Appraisal of Case Studies

Case reports are historically ranked lower in the hierarchy of evidence (Chapter 1, Box 1-2) because of their lack of objectivity. Thus, they are possibly least useful in making patient management decisions about a large group of patients. Case reports describe the history of a single patient (or a small group of patients), usually in the form of a story. These publications are often of great interest to clinicians because they are usually written in a way that appeals to those who are not experts in research and have a strong clinical focus.

These types of studies have recently gained greater respectability because they often provide information that would not necessarily be reported in the results of a clinical trial or survey. In addition, they may alert health professionals to rare and/or adverse events. Publications reporting a clinician's experience and a discussion of early indicators and possible preventive measures can be an extremely useful addition to the clinician's knowledge base. A case series would present a number of patients with similar complications and their outcomes. Statistical analyses would rarely, if ever, be conducted within the context of a case report or case series because the participant numbers are small or singular, and the purpose of such studies is not to make inferences about the general population.

What the Literature Says: Answering a Clinical Question

You find the following recent case study that describes a similar complication to one you have just experienced (Clinical Scenario 5-1): Johnston, L. & McKinley, D. (2000). Cardiac tamponade after removal of atrial intracardiac monitoring catheters in a pediatric patient: Case report. *Heart & Lung, 29,* 256–261.

Clinical Scenario 5.1

You are caring for an infant four days after cardiac surgery in the pediatric intensive care unit. Platelets and albumin were administered the night before because of the infant's abnormal clotting profile. In consultation with the healthcare team, you remove the pulmonary artery catheter. You notice continuous ooze from the site and a marked deterioration in the patient's condition. Cardiac tamponade is diagnosed, and the patient requires a reopening of the sternotomy and removal of 200 mL of blood from the pericardial sac. At the end of your shift, you wonder how rare such a complication is in this patient population and decide to look at the literature.

It is not a research study, but it does have a useful description of the pathophysiology of tamponade. There also is a reference to the frequency with which this complication occurs (a rate of 0.22%). The authors also report their experience with a single patient and provide some recommendations for limiting the potential for bleeding complications in this patient population. You take a copy of the paper to your unit for discussion and go on to develop an addition to your unit protocol manual with regard to awareness of possible complications arising from removal of monitoring catheters.

N-of-1 Studies

A variation on the case study is the *N*-of-1 study where *N* equals the number of patients or clients in the study. Large-scale RCTs may not always be the appropriate research method for a particular disorder. In this case, an *N*-of-1 approach, also known as a "single case experiment," may be more feasible (Chow, Penberthy, & Goodchild, 1998). An *N*-of-1 trial design is usually associated with the delivery in random order of a treatment to an individual patient for a period of time, followed by a treatment period with an alternative therapy or a placebo. Both the clinician and patient should be blinded to the treatment. Symptom management is a frequent outcome assessed in such a trial. An *N*-of-1 trial is done to find the best treatment for an individual patient, not the average patient. We neither know nor are concerned with what the implications of the results of such a trial are with respect to generalizability to other patients with similar problems. Therefore, these types of studies are similarly categorized toward the lowest level of evidence, along with case reports, and do not usually contain statistical analyses.

Critical Appraisal of Case-Control Studies

Case-control studies are an appropriate research approach when asking questions about harm or causation or rare events (e.g., brain tumors). These types of studies investigate why some people develop certain types of diseases or why clients behave the way they do. Examples of such questions might be, Is there a relationship between use of cellular phones and development of a particular type of brain tumor? or Why do adolescents with cystic fibrosis fail to comply with their medication regimen?

The investigators try to identify factors that explain, at least in part, or act as markers or variables for identifying the cause of disease or reason for the behavior. The case-control method relies on a comparison of characteristics of individuals with the disease or observed behavior with characteristics of a group of control individuals. The assumption underpinning this methodological approach is that any difference found will be a likely indicator of why the "cases" become "cases."

One cannot determine the incidence or prevalence of a particular disease or behavior using a case-control methodology because the number of cases and controls is determined by the sample size chosen by the investigator(s), rather than the proportion in the population. However, a **case-control study** design can provide an estimate of the strength of an association between a variable and an outcome.

Rapid Appraisal Questions for Case Control Studies

There are three rapid appraisal questions for case-control studies that can assist the clinician in quickly determining if a study is worthy of consideration (see Box 5–2.)

How Were the Cases Obtained?

When appraising a case-control study, the clinician first asks the question, How were the cases identified? The investigator(s) should provide an adequate description or definition of a case that often includes the diagnostic criteria, any exclusion criteria, and an explanation of how the cases were obtained (e.g., from a specialist center, such as an oncology unit, or from the general population).

The source of the cases has important implications for the appraisal of the study. Recruitment of patients from an outpatient chemotherapy unit could include patients with well-established and managed disease and not those who are newly diagnosed. Bias could be introduced where cases are recruited from a general population because the potential participants could be at various stages in their disease or have a degree of the behavior of interest. Similarly, bias may arise if some of those cases sought are not included in the study for whatever reason. It is well recognized that there are certain characteristics in patients who choose to be involved in research studies versus those who avoid inclusion.

Were Appropriate Controls Selected?

Selection of controls should be based on the premise that the controls will be similar to the cases in all respects except that they do not have the disease or observed behavior of the cases. They, too, may be selected from a specialist source or from the general population. The controls in case-control studies may be concurrent (i.e., they are recruited into the study contemporaneously with the cases). Alternatively, they may be what are referred to as *historical controls* (i.e., the person's past history is examined). Case-control studies with historical controls are generally viewed as lower on the hierarchy of evidence than those studies with concurrent controls because there is more likelihood of bias.

Were Data Collection Methods the Same for the Cases and Controls?

Data collection is another potential generator of bias in a case-control study because of the retrospective approach to determining the possible predictive factors for developing the disease or behavior. Recall bias needs to be considered. For example, the people (cases) who have developed brain tumors may have spent a considerable amount of time thinking about why they developed the disease and recall in great detail their past cellular phone use.

In contrast, the controls who have probably not considered the possibility of brain tumor development may have difficulty in accurately recalling phone use. The data should ideally be collected in the same way for both the case and control groups. Blinding of the data collector to either the case or the control status or to the risk factors of interest assists in reducing the inherent bias in a case-control approach and thus provides more accurate information.

Additional Considerations

The possibility of confounding variables needs to be considered when interpreting a case study. As discussed earlier, confounding variables are extrinsic factors that are associated with the predictor variable and the real cause of the outcome variable.

Case-control studies also commonly report risk data. Often, when thinking about discrete measures of disease outcomes, we consider the notion of **risk**. Risk refers to the probability that a person (free from the disease) will develop it at some point during a time period. Measures of disease may be discrete or continuous. Discrete measures of disease are "yes/no" measures reported in a study, such as alive or dead, diagnosis of a disease, or experience of an event, such as an acute myocardial infarction. Examples of continuous measures of outcomes reported in studies are blood pressure, quality of life, or pain scores.

What the Literature Says: Answering a Clinical Question

The following study may help to answer questions generated from the family member in your practice (Clinical Scenario 5-2): Inskip, P., Tarone, R., Hatch, E., Wilcosky, T., Shapiro, W., and Selker, R. et al. (2001) Cellular telephone use and brain tumors. *New England Journal of Medicine, 344*, 79–86.

Enrolled in the study were 782 case participants with histologically confirmed glioma, meningioma, or acoustic neuroma. Participants came from a number of hospitals. The control participants were 799 patients admitted to the same hospitals as the case participants but with nonmalignant conditions. The predictor measured was cellular phone use, which was quantified using a personal interview to elicit information regarding duration and frequency of use. Once the details of the study are established, the general critical appraisal questions are answered. In addition, the questions in Box 5–2 can assist in critically appraising this study to determine its value to this particular patient and family.

Are the Results of the Study Valid? (Validity)

Inskip and colleagues describe in detail how cases were ascertained from patients with first diagnosis of tumor and the number of eligible patients who agreed to participate. Control patients were concurrently recruited from the same healthcare centers and were frequency matched for age, sex, and ethnic group. A research nurse administered a computer-assisted personal interview with the patient or his/her proxy if the patient was too ill, functionally impaired, or had died. Participants were asked about frequency of cellular phone use. Patients were matched on certain demographic variables, which adds to the validity of the study findings. However, there

Clinical Scenario 5.2

A concerned relative follows you into the hall from the room of a family member who has just been diagnosed with a rare brain tumor. He tells you he recently saw a program on television that described research linking cellular phone use to the development of some forms of cancer. His relative has used a cellular phone for many years, and he wonders whether that may have caused his relative's tumor. It is a valid question, and you would like to know what the research literature has to say about this issue.

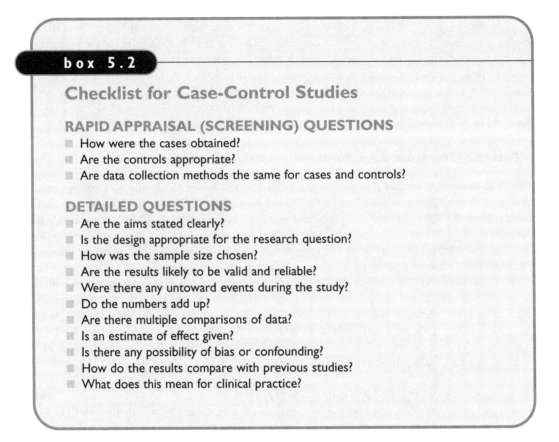

may be other variables unaccounted for that influence the outcome. In addition, recall bias may threaten the validity of the study. The clinician can have some confidence in the validity of this study's findings; however, complete confidence is not possible.

What Are the Results? (Reliability)

As compared with never or very rarely using a cellular phone, the relative risks associated with cumulative phone use for more than 100 hours were 0.9 for glioma (95% CI 0.5–1.6), 0.7 for meningioma (95% CI 0.3–1.7), 1.4 for acoustic neuroma (95% CI 0.6–3.5), and 1.0 (95% CI 0.6–1.5) for all types of tumors combined. The CI reported gives us an estimate of the precision of the measurement of effect in this study. All CIs contain 1, so all of these results are not statistically significant. For example, from this study's findings, for 100 hours of cell phone use, a person is just as likely (0.9) to have a glioma as someone who has not used a cell phone. The sample size is moderate to large, so we would expect the narrower CIs found in this study. The tighter CI in association with a nonsignificant result reflects that there really was no difference between the groups.

Will the Results Help Locally? (Applicability)

The data analysis does not support the hypothesis that recent cellular phone use causes brain tumors. However, possible inaccuracies in patient recall or in misclassification of levels of exposure with different types of cellular phones may indicate that the results are not conclusive. In addition, the widespread use of cellular phones is a relatively recent phenomenon, so the findings provide only an estimate of risk at an early stage in the use of this technology. As a result of these caveats, the study is a good starting place for further research on this issue, but the findings have been potentially influenced by too much bias to make any practice changes based on the results.

Critical Appraisal of Cohort Studies

The **cohort study** design is especially suitable for asking questions about prognosis (Box 5-3) (Laupacis et al., 1994). A *cohort* refers to a study population sharing a characteristic or group of characteristics. For example, a cohort could be adolescents experiencing their first episode of psychosis or all school-aged children in a region who have had audible wheezing in the last six weeks. The study population in this example shares the characteristics of being adolescent or school-aged and experiencing psychoses or having a wheeze. Cohort studies generally follow people over a period of time to determine outcomes, perhaps in response to particular interventions or therapies or as a natural progression of a disease. Assignment of participants to exposure or comparison control groups is based on the measurement of these factors; participants are not randomly allocated. Thus, cohort studies are a "nonexperimental" research design. As previously mentioned, cohort studies are longitudinal in that participants are studied over a period of time. Cross-sectional studies are similar to cohort studies except that the outcomes are measured in a snapshot of time.

chapter 5

105

box 5.3

Checklist for Cohort Studies

RAPID APPRAISAL (SCREENING) QUESTIONS
- What are the characteristics of the patient population under study?
- Is there a control group and if not, is its absence appropriate?
- Is the approach to and duration of follow-up appropriate for the research question being asked?

DETAILED QUESTIONS
- Is the design appropriate for the research question?
- Are objective outcome criteria used?
- How precise are the estimates of likelihood?
- Are the study participants similar to your own patients?
- Can the results of the study assist you in choosing an intervention in your practice setting?

Rapid Appraisal Questions for a Cohort Study

There are three rapid appraisal questions for cohort studies that can assist the clinician in quickly determining if a study is worthy of consideration (see Box 5–3.)

What Were the Characteristics of the Patient Population Under Study?

When appraising a cohort study, establishing the characteristics of the patients or clients under study is important. The characteristics of the patients included in a cohort study, such as the degree of severity of symptoms or point in the illness trajectory, will determine at least to some extent the impact an intervention may have on the patient's condition or the outcomes resulting from a condition. A suitably detailed description of the population is necessary for the clinician to draw any conclusions about the validity of the results and whether they are generalizable to other populations.

Was There a Control Group, and, If Not, Was the Absence of Such Appropriate?

A clinician will have difficulty drawing conclusions from prospective cohort studies reporting outcomes if a control group has not been included for comparison. For example, assessing the impact of congenital heart disease (CHD) on an infant's cognitive and motor development could be best undertaken in a study that matched a cohort of infants with CHD with a similar control cohort without disease or with an unrelated condition (e.g., gastroenteritis). In contrast, a cohort study that seeks to describe the clinical and/or social course of a disease such as schizophrenia and the severity of symptoms experienced with increasing age would not require a control group.

Was the Approach to and Duration of Follow-Up Appropriate for the Research Question Being Asked?

In appraising a cohort study, the clinician should consider the approach to follow-up. Patients enrolled in a cohort study, particularly over a long time, may be lost to follow-up. Additionally, the condition of interest in a cohort study may "predispose" patients to incomplete or noncompliant participation in a study. For example, this is commonly found in studies of patients with a terminal or end-stage illness in which death during the study and before follow-up data are completely collected is quite likely. The extent of loss to follow-up may bias the study results.

The clinician also should integrate clinical expertise with appraisal skills when thinking about the measurement of the outcome(s) of interest. Objective measures will be based on a gold standard, such as a biochemical test or clinical interview conducted by a psychologist. Self-reporting by a patient or arrival at a diagnosis by a clinician may be outcome measures that are subject to an element of bias. The length of follow-up will depend on the outcome(s) of interest. Wound breakdown as a consequence of an early discharge program after surgery would require a shorter follow-up period than a study examining hospital admissions for management of acute asthma subsequent to an in-school education strategy.

What the Literature Says to Answer A Clinical Question

The following study may help to answer the question about adolescents and schizophrenia (Clinical Scenario 5-3): Hafner, H, Hambrecht, M, Loffler, W, Munk-Jorgensen, P., & Riecher-

Clinical Scenario 5.3

You have been working in a community mental health program for a number of years. A large proportion of your client base is young people who have experienced their first episode of schizophrenia. Your colleagues have suggested there may be differences in the disease and social course of schizophrenia depending on age at onset. You volunteer to find a paper for the next journal club that investigates the influence of age on the symptom-related course of the disease.

Rossler, A. (1998). Is schizophrenia a disorder of all ages? A comparison of first episodes and early course across the life-cycle. *Psychological Medicine, 28,* 351–365. Using the general critical appraisal questions, this study will be critically appraised to determine whether it provides valid, relevant evidence.

The participants in the study were 1,109 patients first admitted to a mental health institution with a broad diagnosis of schizophrenia at either age 12–20 years, 21–35 years, or 36–59 years. The timing of follow-up for the course of symptoms was at six months and at one, two, three, and five years after first admission. The outcomes measured were symptom severity as measured by scores on the symptom-based Present State Examination, using a computer program to arrive at diagnostic classifications (PSE-CATEGO). The higher the score on the PSE-CATEGO, the more severe the illness.

Are the Results of the Study Valid? (Validity)

Symptomatology, functional impairment, and social disability were assessed by clinically experienced, trained psychiatrists and psychologists using previously validated instruments. Onset and course before first admission were assessed retrospectively with a standardized instrument. Ensuing symptoms and social consequences were prospectively followed over five years. Given these methods, the study findings are valid and can help in determining practice.

What Are the Results? (Reliability)

Patients with early-onset schizophrenia, especially men, presented with higher PSE-CATEGO scores than did patients with late-onset disease. In men, symptom severity decreased with increasing age of onset. In women, symptom severity remained stable, although there was an increase in negative symptoms with late onset. Disorganization decreased with age, but delusions increased markedly across the whole age of onset range.

The main determinant of social course was level of social development at onset. There is no explanation of why a five-year follow-up period was chosen, nor is there any information on any losses to follow-up. Inferential statistics were used to determine any differences between groups, and *p* values were reported.

Will the Results Help Locally? (Applicability)

Some of the study participants are similar in age and social development to those in your clinic population. Although much of the data show trends rather than statistically significant differences, the authors of the study developed some suggestions about why any differences exist. You and your colleagues could use this information to plan early intervention programs with the goal of limiting the negative consequences of schizophrenia in young people. This study is applicable to your practice and should be used to assist you in making decisions. Always keep in mind, however, that any time you use evidence to make clinical decisions, evaluation of the difference the evidence makes in your own practice is essential.

Critical Appraisal of Randomized Controlled Trials

By virtue of their methodology and strength in establishing cause and effect, RCTs are generally considered the most appropriate research design to answer questions of effectiveness of interventions. They rank as Level II evidence in the hierarchy of evidence as a result of the minimal amount of bias introduced in a well-conducted study (See Chapter 1, Box 1-2). An RCT compares the effectiveness of different treatments to determine which is better. RCTs are experimental designs whereby participants are *randomly* allocated or assigned to a particular treatment, often referred to as the "arms" of a study. An RCT may have two arms: a treatment/intervention arm and a control arm. The control may be a placebo or usual care. RCTs may have more than two arms when more than two different interventions are being compared. RCTs also are longitudinal in that participants are studied over a period of time to assess the effects of an intervention or treatment on outcomes over time.

In crossover trials, participants are randomly assigned to study arms that consist of a sequence of two or more random treatments given consecutively. These trials allow the participants' response to treatment A to be compared with their response to treatment B. In this type of design, there will usually be a "washout" period between the treatments to allow the effects of the first treatment to subside (Sibbald & Roberts, 1998).

RCTs are sometimes considered to be an "artificial" representation of real clinical practice because of the control the investigators have over most aspects of the study. Predetermined inclusion and exclusion criteria provide a **homogeneous study population.** The investigator(s) carefully structures the intervention and the control before conducting the study. The outcomes of interest also are predetermined. One could suggest that the results of a trial are really only generalizable to the particular population studied in that trial because of this "artificiality." Notwithstanding this criticism, RCTs remain the most valid study design for assessing benefits or harms of an intervention.

Although all the issues and standard appraisal questions discussed earlier in this chapter apply to RCTs, additional questions are specific to trial methodology.

> "*Patience and perseverance have a magical effect before which difficulties disappear and obstacles vanish.*"
>
> *John Quincy Adams*

Rapid Appraisal Questions for RCTs

There are rapid appraisal questions for RCTs that can assist the clinician in quickly determining if a study is worthy of consideration (see Box 5–4.)

Randomization

Because the purpose of an RCT is to determine the effectiveness of an intervention in producing an outcome, the groups allocated to either the experimental treatment or the control need to be equivalent. This is best achieved through random allocation or assignment to a treatment or condition (Altman & Bland, 1999; Roberts & Sibbald, 1998; Roberts & Torgerson, 1998). If the clinician chooses which patients should receive which treatments or if the patients self-select the treatment they will receive, there are likely to be important demographic and clinical differences between the groups (Roberts & Torgerson, 1999).

The process of random assignment will be reported in the methods section of the published research report and could be determined by a random number-generating table or a simple toss of a coin. The clinician needs to be wary of a "randomization" process that reports allocation of the intervention on the basis of such criteria as the day of the week, the participants' dates of birth, or a particular clinic. This is referred to as *pseudo-* or *quasi-randomization* because something may be systematically different about the study participants presenting on a particular day of the week or at a particular clinic. This convenience approach could result in groups that are not comparable at baseline.

The above refers to simple randomization, but there also are variations and extensions to the randomization process. One method employs *cluster randomization*, whereby a group of participants is randomized to the same treatment together. The unit of measurement in such a study is the experimental unit, such as the clinic as a whole rather than the individual participant (Kerry & Bland, 1998; Torgerson, 2001). Block randomization is when participants from groups with characteristics that cannot be manipulated (e.g., age, gender), the blocking variable, are randomly assigned to the intervention and control groups in equal numbers (i.e., 40 men out of a group of 100 men and 40 women out of a group of 100 women). Stratified randomization ensures an equal distribution of certain patient characteristics (e.g., gestational age or severity of illness) across the groups.

Concealment of Allocation

The point at which the treatment is allocated is another opportunity for bias to enter the study (Torgerson & Roberts, 1999). Randomization should be concealed, ideally by using a service independent of the study investigators, such as a central research facility where clinicians can phone or fax the enrollment of a new participant—a process called *distance randomization*. The central facility can determine the treatment allocation and inform the healthcare provider. A commonly used method of concealment that is described in the methods section of a research paper is the use of sealed, opaque envelopes containing pieces of paper with the randomly generated treatment allocation. However, this process is susceptible to bias because clinicians, seeking the treatment they believe would most benefit their patients, may open envelopes in advance or even hold them up to a light to read when enrolling participants in a study.

Blinding

Blinding is undertaken to eliminate the bias that could arise from a subjective assessment of outcomes (Day & Altman, 2000). Most clinicians are familiar with the term *double blind*, which refers to keeping the study participants, the clinicians caring for the participants, and the investigators or those collecting and analyzing the data unaware of which treatment was assigned to which patient. Without that knowledge, there is less likelihood that the expectations of those involved in the study will influence the results observed. The degree of blinding utilized in a study partly depends on the intervention being studied and the outcome of interest.

For example, death as an outcome is objective and unlikely to be influenced by knowledge of the intervention. However, quality of life or pain scores are relatively subjective measures and may be influenced by knowledge of the treatment on the part of the participant, if self-reporting, or the health professionals involved in the study, if they are collecting the data.

The placebo or control intervention is another method used for blinding. Investigators go to lengths to be sure that the placebo, if a drug, looks, smells, and tastes like the experimental drug and is given via the same mode of delivery. In the past, trials investigating outcomes related to a particular type of surgery have been controlled by "sham surgery," a practice now considered unethical.

Blinded assessment of an outcome can be performed even if the intervention is not blinded. For example, patients with burns could be allocated a dressing type used in current practice or an experimental bioengineered dressing. The patients and their caregivers would be aware of who received which treatment. However, healing as an outcome could be measured objectively in a blinded fashion by taking photos of the wounds at various time points and asking burn experts not associated with the study to score degree of healing from the photos. When an intervention is a different style of patient management, such as home versus hospital care, blinding is impossible.

Loss to Follow-Up

Researchers conducting RCTs prospectively follow people over a period of time, sometimes for years. When critiquing such studies, the research consumer needs to consider the original number of participants enrolled in the study and compare that number with the final numbers comprising the data set at measurement of outcomes. There is a concern if the number of participants who drop out of a study is very high. Depending on the study question, by convention, a dropout rate of 20% or less is considered acceptable. The longer the period of study, the higher the dropout rate is likely to be. If studies report a dropout rate of more than 20%, it is important that the investigators state whether the subjects who dropped from their study were similar in demographic variables than the subjects who remained in the study. If not, one must carefully question the study's findings.

Additional Questions to Ask When Appraising an RCT

The above rapid appraisal questions serve as a suitable screening mechanism for the busy clinician to use when deciding whether the results of an RCT should form the basis for a change in or support for clinical practice. However, there are additional trial-specific appraisal questions that the clinician needs to consider (see Box 5-4).

What Were the Inclusion and Exclusion Selection Criteria for the Study Participants?

The study population needs to be relevant to the problem the study is trying to address. Sufficient information about how the participants were selected should be provided in the research paper, usually in the methods section, so the reader can decide whether the results reported will

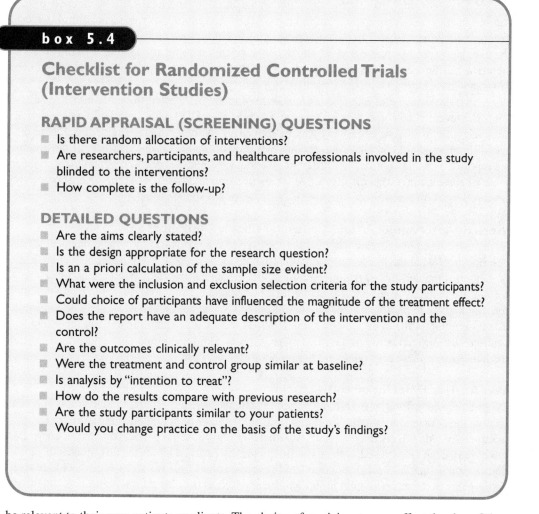

box 5.4

Checklist for Randomized Controlled Trials (Intervention Studies)

RAPID APPRAISAL (SCREENING) QUESTIONS
- Is there random allocation of interventions?
- Are researchers, participants, and healthcare professionals involved in the study blinded to the interventions?
- How complete is the follow-up?

DETAILED QUESTIONS
- Are the aims clearly stated?
- Is the design appropriate for the research question?
- Is an a priori calculation of the sample size evident?
- What were the inclusion and exclusion selection criteria for the study participants?
- Could choice of participants have influenced the magnitude of the treatment effect?
- Does the report have an adequate description of the intervention and the control?
- Are the outcomes clinically relevant?
- Were the treatment and control group similar at baseline?
- Is analysis by "intention to treat"?
- How do the results compare with previous research?
- Are the study participants similar to your patients?
- Would you change practice on the basis of the study's findings?

111

be relevant to their own patients or clients. The choice of participants may affect the size of the observed treatment effect. For example, an intervention delivered to people with advanced disease and cared for in a specialist center may not be as effective for or relevant to those with early-stage disease managed in the community.

Was Randomization Successful?
In addition to noting whether allocation to the intervention or control arm of the study was randomized, the reader should be able to find information that demonstrates the randomization was successful with characteristics of both groups similar at baseline. This is often the first data reported in the results section of a research paper and can include demographic variables of the groups, such as age and gender, stage of disease, or illness severity scores.

Investigators generally indicate where there were statistically significant differences in variables between the groups. The clinician needs to decide whether these differences were clinically meaningful, albeit statistically significant.

As an example, researchers may undertake a trial to determine the effectiveness of oral sucrose in alleviating procedural pain in infants. The intervention (sucrose) and control (water) groups are randomized and are not significantly different for gestational age, birth weight, and the like. However, by chance and despite the appropriate randomization, there is a statistically significant difference in the severity of illness scores between the two groups and in the number of infants in each group who use a pacifier as a comfort measure.

If the outcome of interest was incidence of infection, these differences may be irrelevant. However, an outcome such as lower pain scores associated with a procedure as a result of administration of sucrose could very well be influenced by these variables and, thus, the baseline differences should be taken into account when reporting the observed effects. If the groups are reported as being significantly different on certain baseline variables, it is important to determine whether the investigators controlled for those baseline differences in their statistical analyses through use of certain procedures (e.g., analysis of covariance tests).

Were the Intervention(s) and Control(s) Clearly Described?

If treatments used in a research study are to be used in the real world of clinical practice, a clear description of what the intervention and control entailed is needed. If the detail is unclear, it is possible that the delivery of the interventions differed among the study population, thereby resulting in an altered observed treatment effect. For example, drug dosages, detail of written information given to participants, or number of clinic visits should all be adequately described. The description of the interventions in the methods section also should report any other interventions that differed between the two groups, such as additional clinic visits, telephone calls, or the like because these may confound the reported results.

Was Analysis by Intention to Treat?

Despite the best efforts of investigators, some patients assigned to a particular group may not receive the allocated treatment throughout the entire study period. Noncompliance with the treatment or side effects may arise or, for whatever reason, some participants in the control group may even be exposed to the experimental intervention. One of the advantages of randomization is that, as a result of comparable groups at baseline, it becomes just as likely that participants in the experimental group will be exposed to the control intervention as it is that those in the control group will be exposed to the intervention under study. Patients who change treatment or drop out of a study may be systematically different from those who do not. Exclusion of these patients from analysis would mean that comparison of treatments was inequitable. If the comparability of groups is to be maintained through the study, the data should be analyzed according to the group to which the patient was originally allocated. This is known as "intention-to-treat" analysis. This conservative approach may minimize Type 1 error, in which investigators conclude that a difference does exist between treatments when it really does not. In contrast, this form of analysis has been criticized as too conservative and more susceptible to Type 2 error, which results in the conclusion that no difference exists when in fact there is one.

Sometimes it is acceptable to exclude patients from final data analysis. This includes patients who were actually ineligible to be enrolled in the trial and who were mistakenly randomized, as well as patients who were prematurely enrolled in a trial but who never received the intervention.

Excluding large numbers of patients from analysis may not introduce bias but because it will reduce the sample size, it may reduce the power of the study to detect important differences (Fergusson et al., 2002).

Are the Outcomes Measured Clinically Relevant?

EBP requires integration of clinical expertise with the best available research evidence and patient values, concerns, and choices. Clinicians need to utilize their own expertise at this point in the critical appraisal process to decide whether the outcomes measured in a study were clinically appropriate. They also need to assess whether the timing of outcome measurement in relation to the delivery of the intervention was appropriate (Roland & Torgerson, 1998). For example, it may be important to measure the effectiveness of an intervention, such as corticosteroid administration in the management of traumatic brain injury, by measuring survival to discharge from the intensive care unit. However, if wanting to determine the effectiveness of a cancer therapy, survival to five years for study participants may be a more relevant time frame. Outcome measures such as mortality would appear appropriate in these examples but would not likely be relevant in trials with patients having dementia or chronic back pain. Quality of life scores or days lost from work might be more useful measures in studies with these types of participants.

Investigators may be interested in more than one outcome when designing a study, such as lowered pain scores and an improved quality of life score. Researchers should designate the primary outcome of interest in their research report, and they should clarify what outcome formed the basis for the a priori power calculation, if one was carried out. This ensures the minimizing of repeated measures or data dredging until a significant result is found.

How Were the Size and Precision of Effect Reported?

As discussed earlier in this chapter, trials should report the total number of study participants assigned to the groups, the numbers available for measurement of outcomes, and the occurrence or event rates in the groups. If these data are not reported, the measures of effect, such as RR and OR, cannot be calculated. CI and/or p values (or the information required to calculate these) should also be included in the results presented in order to identify the precision of the estimates of effect.

The reader has to decide on the usefulness or clinical significance of any differences observed. For example, an antihypertensive medication may reduce mean blood pressure in the experimental group by 2 mm Hg, and it is reported as statistically significant. However, such a decrease would not be meaningful in clinical practice. If the CI is wide and includes the point estimate of no effect, such as an RR of 1 or a reported p value of greater than 0.05, the precision of the measurement is likely to be inadequate. A question the clinician must then ask is, Did the study have sufficient power to detect a true difference? If the results are nonsignificant and the CI is wide, it is possible that the sample size was not large enough. A tighter CI in association with a nonsignificant result would more likely reflect that there really was no difference between the treatments.

Increasingly, trials are conducted across a large number of healthcare sites. In such studies, it is important for the clinician to consider whether results obtained were similar among the different settings. Homogeneity of the effects of the treatment in different settings would suggest a result that the clinician could be confident was the true result.

Clinical Scenario 5.4

At a recent meeting of the surgical division managers of your hospital, the budget was discussed. An idea was proposed that a cost-cutting measure may be found in the earlier discharge of women after surgery for breast cancer. Debate about the advantages and disadvantages of such a change to health service provision continued until it was decided to investigate the available evidence.

What the Literature Says: Answering A Clinical Question

The following study may help to answer the question about early discharge after surgery for breast cancer (Clinical Scenario 5-4): Bundred, N., Maguire, P., Reynolds, J., Grimshaw, J., Morris, J., and Thomson, L. et al. (1998) Randomised controlled trial of effects of early discharge after surgery for breast cancer. *British Medical Journal, 317,* 1275–1279. Using the general critical appraisal questions, the clinician can critically appraise this study to determine whether it provides valid, relevant evidence.

The participants in the study were 100 women who had early breast cancer and who were undergoing mastectomy and axillary node clearance (20) or breast conservation surgery (80). The intervention and comparison were early discharge program versus routine length of stay. The outcomes measured were physical illness (i.e., infection, seroma formation, shoulder movement) and psychological illness (i.e., depression and anxiety scores). The timing of follow-up was first preoperatively, then one and three months postoperatively.

Are the Results of the Study Valid? (Validity)

Patients were randomized in clusters for each week of admissions when a research nurse opened a sealed envelope containing the randomization code. A flow diagram was provided in the report to identify the recruitment, participation, and follow-up patient numbers. A power calculation was undertaken a priori, and intention-to-treat analysis was used. The patients were not blinded to the intervention but there is no mention of whether the investigators assessing outcomes were blinded. A detailed description of the intervention and the control management is given. The groups were similar at baseline. Based on these methods, the study results should be considered valid.

What Are the Results? (Reliability)

Results are expressed as OR with 95% CI, and *p* values are provided where there was statistical significance. Women discharged early had greater shoulder movement (OR 0.28, 95% CI 0.08–0.95) and less wound pain (OR 0.28, 95% CI 0.10–0.79) at three months, compared with the standard length of stay group. Symptom questionnaire scores were significantly lower in the early discharge group at one month. It is difficult to determine whether there were clinically meaningful differences in the psychological measures because a total of six tools were used to measure psychological illness. Multiple measurements in themselves are more likely to lead to significant results.

Will the Results Help Locally? (Applicability)

The results presented in this research paper are those of a planned interim analysis. The total number of patients required for the study is 200 but interim analysis was done to confirm no adverse consequences of early discharge. This is a reasonable approach to take but it would be useful to read the results of the full study when completed. It would appear that early discharge might be appropriate if women are given sufficient support and resources. However, there was no costing analysis undertaken, so research that addressed this point may need to be appraised before making any final decisions about changing an entire health service model. Based on these issues, this evidence will assist clinicians to consider early discharge but will not answer the clinical question of whether it is the best option for most women who have had surgery for breast cancer.

Critical Appraisal of Systematic Reviews

A systematic review (also often referred to as an *evidence synthesis*, *overview*, *integrative review*, or *meta-analysis*; see Table 5-10) is a compilation of like studies to address a specific clinical question. To conduct a review, a detailed search strategy is employed to find the relevant evidence to answer a clinical question. The researcher(s) determine beforehand what inclusion and exclusion criteria are going to be used to filter the found studies. Systematic reviews of RCTs, considered Level I evidence, are found at the top of the hierarchy of evidence (Melnyk, 2003) (see Chapter 1, Box 1-2). The systematic review methodology is the most rigorous approach to minimization of bias.

table 5.10 Definitions of different types of reviews

Review	Definition
Systematic review (often called an *overview* or *evidence synthesis*)	A compilation of like studies to address a specific clinical question using a detailed, comprehensive search strategy and rigorous appraisal methods for the purpose of summarizing, appraising, and communicating the results and implications of contradictory results or otherwise unmanageable quantities of research. Systematic review is the most rigorous approach to minimization of bias.
Meta-analysis	A statistical approach to synthesizing the results of a number of studies that produces a larger sample size and thus greater power to determine the true magnitude of an effect. Used to obtain a single-effect measure (i.e., a summary statistic) of the summarized results of all studies included in a review.
Integrative review	A systematic review that does not have a summary statistic because sample sizes cannot be summarized in an integrative review (usually due to heterogeneous studies/samples).
Narrative review	A review that includes published papers that support an author's particular point of view; serves as a general background discussion of a particular issue. How papers are found is not systematic.

A systematic review is not the same as a literature review or "narrative review." The methods used in a systematic review are specific and rigorous, whereas a narrative review usually includes some published papers that support an author's particular point of view or serve as a general background discussion of a particular issue. A systematic review is a scientific method used to summarize, appraise, and communicate the results and implications of contradictory results or otherwise unmanageable quantities of research.

Few research trials have a large enough sample size to provide a conclusive answer to questions about clinical effectiveness. Archie Cochrane, an epidemiologist after whom the Cochrane Collaboration is named, recognized that the increasingly large number of RCTs of variable quality and differing results hampered the implementation of improved practice: "It is surely a great criticism of our profession that we have not organised a critical summary, by specialty or subspecialty, adapted periodically, of all relevant randomized controlled trials" (Cochrane, 1979, p. 9). Thus, the systematic review methodological approach was adopted to assist healthcare professionals in making sense of the overwhelming amount of information available. To appraise studies' relevance to clinical decision making, the method of undertaking a systematic review needs to be understood.

> ❝*If your determination is fixed, I do not counsel you to despair. Few things are impossible to diligence and skill. Great works are performed not by strength, but perseverance.*❞
>
> *Dr. Samuel Johnson*

The Process of a Systematic Review

The process of undertaking a systematic review comprises several phases and is detailed, time-consuming, and often costly (Dissemination, 1996). In Phase 1 of the process, the individuals undertaking the review have to decide on the clinical practice question they want to answer, then assess the volume and type of literature available to answer that question. Particular outcomes of interest need to be identified and their relevance to the question confirmed.

Phase 2 of a review involves developing criteria for inclusion of particular study types and determining how the validity of those studies will be assessed. A protocol is developed to predetermine the way in which the review will be conducted. As such, it is the first means of limiting bias.

Phase 3 is the search for and retrieval of both published and unpublished literature related to the research question. Rigorous standards for searching the literature result in locating research findings across disciplines and languages. Multiple automated databases (e.g., MEDLINE, CINAHL, EMBASE) are searched. Specific criteria are indicated to determine which studies will be retained and which will be discarded.

The assessment of the quality of the studies retrieved is undertaken in Phase 4. In Phase 5, the validity of those studies is assessed. Data are extracted from the individual studies in Phase 6. Phase 7 includes both a narrative overview of the included studies in terms of the participants and settings, and a quantitative synthesis of the results of the studies where possible. This statistical approach to synthesizing the results of a number of studies is referred to as **meta-analysis**.

Overviews or integrative reviews do not apply statistical analyses to the results across studies. Phases 8–10 include peer review of the results of a review and dissemination to clinicians.

A major advantage of a systematic review is the combining of multiple study results. In meta-analyses, combining the results of a number of studies produces a larger sample size and thus greater power to determine the true magnitude of an effect. Because of the strength of this type of evidence, this relatively new methodology has become a hallmark of EBP (Stevens, 2001).

Example

You are thinking of establishing an early discharge program for first-time mothers but are concerned that such a program may be associated with unplanned readmissions for breast-feeding related problems. You find three RCTS with different sample sizes. The smallest study ($n = 50$) reports there is no difference in readmissions between the early discharge and routine length of stay groups. A study with a larger sample size ($n = 100$) reported an increase in readmissions in the experimental group. The study with the largest sample size ($n = 1,000$) reports an increase in readmissions in the control group. All three studies are rigorously conducted trials with very similar patient demographics. Which study results do you believe and use to make a decision regarding instituting such a program?

Intuitively, and hopefully after reading this chapter, you would place greater faith in the study with the largest sample size. The larger sample size is more likely to capture the variation in the reference population and thus represent the real effect of such a program. But ideally, you would like to find a meta-analysis that combines the results of all three studies. This would provide a sample size of 1,150 and be even more likely, as a result of greater power, to detect an important difference.

A systematic review is a form of *secondary research* because it uses previously conducted studies. The study types discussed previously in this chapter would be *primary research* studies. Because it is such an obviously different research approach, it requires unique critical appraisal questions to address the quality of a review (Oxman, Cook, & Guyatt, 1994).

Rapid Appraisal Questions for Systematic Reviews

There are three rapid appraisal questions for systematic reviews that can assist the clinician in quickly determining if a systematic review is worthy of consideration (see Box 5–5).

Identification of the Literature

One reason the systematic review is considered to be the least biased research methodology is the way in which the literature pertaining to the research question is identified and obtained. The research literature comprises the raw data for a review. When appraising a systematic review, the clinician looks for a detailed description of the databases accessed, the search strategies used, and the search terms. The databases should be specified, as should the years searched. The authors should indicate whether retrieved information was limited to English language studies only. MEDLINE and CINAHL are probably the best known healthcare publication databases for such studies. Although these databases index thousands of journals, not all journals are indexed by any certain database (Zielinski, 1995). If reviewers limit their search to English language sources, they are presenting a biased view of the research pertaining to that particular research question. EMBASE is a European language database of healthcare research, but the cost of access to this database and translation of non-English language papers may be prohibitive.

Search terms used should be clearly described so the reader can make an informed decision about whether all relevant publications were found. For example, a review of antibiotic therapy for otitis media may identify the search terms *otitis media* and *glue ear*. However, *red ear* also is a commonly used term for this disorder, and omission of the term from the search strategy may lead to a failure to identify all the literature.

Both published and unpublished research should be identified and retrieved where possible because of the issue of "publication bias," which occurs when publication of a study's results is based on the direction ("positive" or "negative") or significance of the findings (Dickersin, 1990). It should be stressed that studies reporting significant or positive results are not more likely to be published because journal editors think they will sell more copies but because investigators whose study results are nonsignificant are less likely to submit their studies for publication. To the extent that publication bias exists, results of systematic reviews or meta-analyses that include only published results would be misleading.

"Grey literature" refers to publications such as brochures and conference proceedings. Attempts also should be made to retrieve these sources of information. Reviewers will commonly report hand-searching relevant journals and examining the reference lists of previously retrieved papers for possible studies. In addition, a review will usually specify whether researchers in the field of interest were contacted to identify other studies. Additionally, authors of retrieved studies may be contacted if there is insufficient information provided in the publication to make a decision regarding inclusion. This process of literature retrieval is obviously costly, and the reader needs to consider whether the absence of such an exhaustive search affects the conclusions drawn in the review.

Assessment of Quality for Inclusion

The critical appraisal process itself suggests that the research may be of varying quality. A rigorous, high-quality review will be based on the sole inclusion of high-quality studies. A clear description of the basis for quality assessment should be included in the review. This is usually done using a checklist. Although a review with a rigorous methodology that includes only RCTs is considered the highest level of evidence, there are clinical questions (e.g., questions of prognosis) that are not appropriate for an RCT design. In such cases, other study types, such as cohort studies, may be reviewed.

The quality of studies to be included is decided independently by at least two members of the review team. The independent assessment further reduces the possibility of bias influencing the final studies included. This process is usually described in the review, and the process for resolution of disagreement should also be reported.

Synthesis of Results

When appraising a systematic review, the clinician also examines the studies that were included and excluded. They are usually presented in a table format and provide the reader with information about the study populations, setting, and outcomes measured. Ideally, included studies should be relatively homogenous with respect to these aspects. Reasons for exclusion, such as study design or quality issues, also are included in a table. The information presented in these tables assists the reader to decide whether it was appropriate to combine the results of the studies.

Meta-analysis

Meta-analysis is the statistical method used to obtain a single-effect measure of the summarized results of all studies included in a review. It should be stated here that it is not necessary for the clinician to have a sound or even moderate understanding of the mathematics involved in such methods. The meta-analysis of a number of trials gives due weight to the sample size of the studies included and provides a precise estimate of treatment effect. The "forest plot" (colloquially called a "blobbogram," see Figure 5-6) is a diagrammatic representation of the results of trials, along with their CIs. Earlier in this chapter, there was a discussion of measures of effect and precision of estimates with an explanation of OR and CI. You may want to revisit that section now and when appraising a review. The "blob," or square, is the measure of effect of the particular study, and the horizontal line through it is the CI. The size of the square reflects the size of the study effect. Each blob gives the result of a trial and shows how effective the treatment was compared with the control. The white diamond is the cumulative treatment effect of all studies.

If the outcome is the same for the treatment and control group, the resulting OR is 1.0 (i.e., the treatment makes no difference). If the CI crosses the line of no treatment effect (OR = 1.0), the study is not statistically significant.

If the outcome is something you do not want (e.g., death, pain, or infection), a square to the right of the line means that the treatment was worse than the control in the trial (i.e., there were more deaths in the treated group). A square to the left of the line means that the treatment was better. The opposite is true for outcomes you want (e.g., stopping smoking or continuation of breast-feeding).

Return now to Figure 5-3, which displayed the results of a study of acupuncture for smoking cessation. The square (OR = 1.24) is to the right of the line, meaning that the treatment (acupuncture) was better than the control (sham acupuncture) for smoking cessation, a desired outcome. Now go back to Figure 5-5, which displayed the results of a trial of corticosteroid therapy for reducing mortality associated with traumatic brain injury. The square lies to the left of the

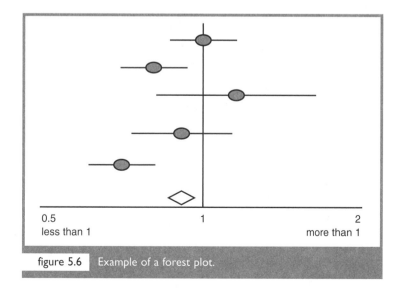

0.5	1	2
less than 1		more than 1

figure 5.6   Example of a forest plot.

line (OR = 0.83). The outcome of interest (i.e., death) is not desired. Therefore, in this case, the treatment (i.e., steroids) is better than the control (i.e., placebo).

Although bringing together all of the studies around a particular clinical question provides important information, in some cases, the studies are too dissimilar for it to make any sense to combine the results in any statistical way. In such a review, there is no attempt made on the part of the reviewers to provide a quantification of the effectiveness of the intervention under study. Alternatively, the studies may not be of sufficient quality to combine. The bias inherent in very small studies is inflated by combining their results.

Additional Questions to Ask When Appraising a Systematic Review

Box 5-5 presents additional questions for appraising a systematic review. Careful consideration of these and the following questions will provide the practitioner with valid, reliable evidence to answer compelling clinical questions.

Was the Heterogeneity of the Included Studies Investigated?
Obviously, by chance, there will be some variation in the results of individual studies that examine the same question. However, the differences or heterogeneity in effect reported can be due to study design. Formal statistical methods can be used to test whether there is significant hetero-

---

box 5.5

Checklist for Appraising a Systematic Review

RAPID APPRAISAL (SCREENING) QUESTIONS
- Are all relevant papers identified?
- How is the quality of the papers assessed?
- How are results summarized?

DETAILED QUESTIONS
- Does the review address a clearly focused research question?
- What are the inclusion and exclusion criteria for studies?
- Are the interventions similar between studies?
- Are outcome measures similar between studies?
- Is it reasonable to combine the studies?
- What measures of occurrence or exposure are reported in each study?
- Are magnitude and precision of the effects reported?
- Are participants in the review studies similar to your patients?
- Are all important outcomes considered?
- Would you consider a change in practice based on the results?

geneity among the studies that precludes their being combined. Generally, reviewers report using such a test. However, as with all statistical tests, statistical significance is not the same as clinical significance. The reader needs to assess each report included in an analysis and make a qualitative decision about whether they are similar enough to be combined. For example, the question under review may be the effectiveness of colloid versus crystalloid in volume replacement therapy. A study examining the differences in outcome in a population of sick neonates is obviously different in a number of ways from a study of the effectiveness of these therapies in a sample of adults with extensive burns. Both populations require volume replacement but the differences in age as well as the physiologic need for such therapy makes it meaningless to combine the studies to estimate a true effect.

The reader can make an informed guess as to whether the studies are not sufficiently homogeneous in terms of the size of effect by looking at the forest plot. A forest plot with estimates of effect scattered all over, with their associated CI, suggests wide variation in the measure and precision of effect.

Was the Possibility of Publication Bias Explored?

Studies reporting a positive result have a higher chance of being published. Thus, inclusion of only published studies may result in a biased reporting of the effect of an intervention. The reader needs to be reassured that all reasonable attempts were made to retrieve both published and unpublished studies. When unpublished studies are not included, the size of any effect is likely to be overestimated. One way to detect whether selection bias is present is through the use of another statistical test, the **"funnel plot."** The sample size is plotted against the effect size in such a plot. Smaller studies have more chance variability than bigger studies, so a symmetrical inverted funnel is expected. An asymmetrical plot may indicate selection bias through the absence of some studies.

Was the Subgroup Analysis Performed Appropriately?

Reviewers may be tempted to analyze by subgroups if no overall effect is found. Study subsets may be analyzed on the basis of particular patient demographics or methodologic quality of the included studies. However, in such analysis, the purpose of the initial randomization to treatment and control groups in the underlying studies is essentially lost because this balance does not extend to groupings after the fact.

Was a Sensitivity Analysis Done?

A sensitivity analysis helps determine how the main findings may change as a result of pooling the data. It involves first combining the results of all the included studies. The studies considered of lowest quality or unpublished studies are then excluded, and the data is reanalyzed. This process is repeated sequentially, excluding studies until only the studies of highest quality are included in the analysis. An alteration in the overall results suggests how sensitive the conclusions are to the quality of the studies included.

Have the Reviewers Justified Their Conclusions?

EBP requires integrating the best evidence with clinical expertise and patient values, choices, and concerns. Clinicians are cautioned that there are poor-quality systematic reviews, just as there are poor-quality primary studies. The clinician needs to ask whether the interpretations of the reviewers on the strength of the evidence are justified and valid.

Clinical Scenario 5.5

Nursing staff on your unit in a residential elder care facility have just completed an audit of falls in the previous 12 months. A total of 45 falls were documented during that period, and it is possible the actual number was even higher. Interested and concerned clinicians meet to discuss the results and consider options for reducing this incidence. A few people bring copies of trials with them that discuss the efficacy of various interventions. All the trials look like high-quality studies but they all show different results. Which one to believe? It would be nice to have one study that summarizes all the available evidence for you and presents the implications for clinical practice.

What the Literature Says: Answering a Clinical Question

The following study may help determine interventions are needed to decrease the incidence of falls (Clinical Scenario 5-5): Gillespie, L., Gillespie, W. J., Robertson, M., Lamb, S., Cumming, R., & Rowe, B. (2002). Interventions for preventing falls in elderly people. (*Cochrane Review*) The *Cochrane Library, 4*, Oxford: Update Software.

In this systematic review, the objective was to assess the effects of interventions designed to reduce the incidence of falls in elderly people (i.e., living in the community, in institutional care, or in hospital care). The search strategy was designed and conducted by the Cochrane Musculoskeletal Group specialized register. Databases of MEDLINE (1966–2001), EMBASE (1988–2001), CINAHL (1982–2001), National Research Register, and Current Controlled Trials were searched. A hand search of reference lists of articles was conducted, and field researchers were contacted. The selection criterion was that studies were randomized trials of interventions designed to minimize the effect of or exposure to risk factors for falling in elderly people. Main outcomes of interest were the number of fallers or falls. Trials reporting only intermediate outcomes were excluded. The data collection and analysis methods involved two reviewers independently assessing trial quality and extracting data. Data were pooled using the fixed effect model where appropriate. The **fixed effect model** is based on the "traditional assumption is that the event rates are fixed in each of the control . . . and treatment groups. Any variation in the observed event rates is then attributed to random chance. If the trials being combined are truly clinically homogeneous and have been designed properly (for example, with balanced arms), which is the situation that will commonly pertain, then in this (and only in this) case it is appropriate to pool raw data" (Moore, Gavaghan, Edwards, Wiffen, & McQuay, 2002).

The main results were that interventions of benefit include muscle strengthening, group exercise, home hazard assessment and modification, withdrawal of psychotropic medication, and multidisciplinary, multifactorial risk factor screening. Interventions of unknown effectiveness include nutritional supplementation, pharmacologic therapies, hormone replacement therapy, fall prevention programs in institutional settings, and interventions using a cognitive/behavioral approach alone.

The reviewers' conclusions were that interventions to prevent falls that are likely to be effective are now available. Costs per fall prevented have been established for four of the interventions. Some potential interventions are of unknown effectiveness, and further research is indicated.

Are the Results of the Study Valid? (Validity)

Only RCTs that met quality inclusion criteria were included in the review. A large number of databases were searched, and both English and non-English language sources were searched. Two reviewers independently assessed the quality of trials and extracted the data. Tables of included and excluded studies were provided. These methods produced valid results.

What Are the Results? (Reliability)

RR and 95% CI were given for interventions likely to be of benefit, such as a program of muscle strengthening (RR 0.80, 95% CI 0.66–0.98) and home hazard assessment and modification (RR 0.64, 95% CI 0.49–0.84). Pooled study results were tested for heterogeneity, and the authors acknowledged that cluster randomized study results could not be pooled with individually randomized study results, because a falsely narrow CI would be calculated.

Will the Results Help Locally? (Applicability)

Although there was variation in the study settings, types of patients, and interventions included in this review, the authors provided a description of the circumstances in which a particular intervention may be beneficial. Economic outcomes were not reported, and there were no trials of reducing the serious consequences of falls. Given the clinical question of reducing falls in an elder care facility, the evidence is applicable.

Conclusion

Evidence-based healthcare decision making requires the integration of clinical expertise with the best available research evidence and the patients' values, concerns, and choices. To do this, the clinician must develop skills in appraising available research findings. An understanding of study design principles and how different designs are used to investigate different clinical questions is the precursor to utilizing research for practice. Accessing and using one of the many critical appraisal skills guides available on a regular basis will help the clinician learn more about the scientific basis for health management and lead to more informed decision making and better patient outcomes.

> *In the confrontation between the stream and the rock, the stream always wins—*
> *not through strength but by perseverance.*
>
> H. Jackson Brown

references

Akinbami, L. J., & Schoendorf, K. C. (2002). Trends in childhood asthma: Prevalence, health care utilization, and mortality. *Pediatrics, 110,* 315–322.

Alderson, P., & Roberts, I. (2002). Corticosteroids for acute traumatic brain injury (Cochrane Review). *Cochrane Library, 4* (Oxford: Update Software).

Altman, D., & Bland, J. (1999). Treatment allocation in controlled trials: Why randomize? *British Medical Journal, 318,* 1209.

Awada, A., & al Jumah, M. (1999). The first-of-Ramadan headache. *Headache, 39*(7), 490–493.

Bundred, N., Maguire, P., Reynolds, J., Grimshaw, J., Morris, J., Thomson, L., Barr, L., & Baildam, A. (1998). Randomised controlled trial of effects of early discharge after surgery for breast cancer. *British Medical Journal, 317,* 1275–1279.

Chacon, L. (1987). Edema cerebral en traumatismo craneoencefalico severo en ninos tatados con y sin dexametasona [Brain edema in severe head injury on children treated with and without dexametasone]. *Medicina Critica Venezolana, 2,* 75–79.

Chow, T., Penberthy, A., & Goodchild, C. (1998). Ketamine as an adjunct to morphine in postthoracotomy analgesia: An unintended N-of-1 study. *Anesthesia and Analgesia, 87*(6), 1372–1374.

Cochrane, A. (Ed.). (1979). *A critical review, with particular reference to the medical profession.* London: Office of Health Economics.

Crombie, I. (1996). *The pocket guide to critical appraisal.* London: BMJ Publishing Group.

Day, S., & Altman, D. (2000). Blinding in clinical trials and other studies. *British Medical Journal, 321,* 504.

Dickersin, K. (1990). The existence of publication bias and risk factor for its occurrence. *Journal of the American Medical Association, 263,* 1385–1389.

Dissemination, N. C. f. R. a. (1996). *Undertaking systematic reviews of research on effectiveness.* York: University of York.

Evidence-Based Health Care. (2002) *An open learning resource for health care practitioners.* (2nd ed.). London: Critical Appraisal Skills Programme (CASP).

Fergusson, D., Aaron, S., Guyatt, G., & Hebert, P. (2002). Post-randomisation exclusions: the intention to treat principle and excluding patients from is. *British Medical Journal, 325,* 652–654.

Gillams, J., Lewith, G., & Machin, D. (1984). Acupuncture and group therapy in stopping smoking. *Practitioner, 228,* 341–344.

Gillespie, L., Gillespie, W., Robertson, M., Lamb, S., Cumming, R., & Rowe, B. (2002). Interventions for preventing falls in elderly people (Cochrane Review). *Cochrane Library, 4* (Oxford: Update Software).

Greenhalgh, T. (1997). *How to read a paper: The basics of evidence based medicine.* London: BMJ Publishing.

Grumme, T., Baethmann, A., Kolodziejczyk, D., Krimmer, J., Fischer, M., & Eisenhart Rothe, B. (1995). Treatment of patients with severe head injury by triamcinolone: A prospective, controlled multicenter trial of 396 cases. *Research in Experimental Medicine, 195,* 217-229.

Guyatt, G. H., Haynes, R. B., Jaeschke, R. Z., Cook, D. J., Green, L., Naylor, C. D., Wilson, M. C., & Richardson, W. S. (2000). Users' guides to the medical literature: XXV. Evidence-based medicine: Principles for applying the users' guides to patient care. Evidence-Based Medicine Working Group. *Journal of the American Medical Association, 284*(10), 1290–1296.

Guyatt, G. H., Sackett, D. L., & Cook, D. J. (1994). Users' guides to the medical literature. II. How to use an article about therapy or prevention. B. What were the results and will they help me in caring for my patients? Evidence-Based Medicine Working Group. *Journal of the American Medical Association, 271*(1), 59–63.

Guyatt, G., & Rennie, D. (2002). *Users' guides to the medical literature.* American Medical Association: AMA Press.

Hafner, H., Hambrecht, M., Loffler, W., Munk-Jorgensen, P., & Riecher-Rossler, A. (1998). Is schizophrenia a disorder of all ages? A comparison of first episodes and early course across the life-cycle. *Psychological Medicine, 28*(2), 351–365.

Harris, R. P. , Hefland, M., and Woolf, S. H., et al. (2001). Current methods of the U.S. Preventive Services Task Force: A review of the process. *American Journal of Preventive Medicine, 20,* 21–35.

Inskip, P., Tarone, R., Hatch, E., Wilcosky, T., Shapiro, W., Selker, R., Fine, H., Black, P., Loeffler, J., & Linet, M. (2001). Cellular-telephone use and brain tumours. *New England Journal of Medicine, 344*(2), 79–86.

Jaeschke, R., Guyatt, G. H., & Sackett, D. L. (1994). Users' guides to the medical literature. III. How to use an article about a diagnostic test. B. What are the results and will they help me in caring for my patients? The Evidence-Based Medicine Working Group. *Journal of the American Medical Association, 271*(9), 703–707.

Johnston, L., & McKinley, D. (2000). Cardiac tamponade after removal of atrial intracardiac monitoring catheters in a pediatric patient: Case report. *Heart and Lung, 29*, 256–261.

Kerry, S., & Bland, J. (1998). Analysis of a trial randomised in clusters. *British Medical Journal, 316*, 54.

Laupacis, A., Wells, G., Richardson, W. S., & Tugwell, P. (1994). Users' guides to the medical literature. V. How to use an article about prognosis. Evidence-Based Medicine Working Group. *Journal of the American Medical Association, 272*(3), 234–237.

Lindboek, M., Hjortdahl, P., & Johnsen, U. (1996). Use of symptoms, signs, and blood tests to diagnose acute sinus infections in primary care: Comparison with computed tomography. *Family Practice, 28*, 183–188.

Melnyk, B.M. (2003). Critical appraisal of systematic reviews: A key strategy for evidence-based practice. *Pediatric Nursing,29* (2), 125, 147–149.

Muscat, J., Malkin, M., Thompson, S., Shore, R., Stellman, S., McRee, D., Neugut, A., & Wynder, E. (2000). Handheld cellular telephone use and risk of brain cancer. *The Journal of the American Medical Association, 284*(23), 3001–3007.

Moore, R., Gavaghan, D., Edwards. J., Wiffen, P., & McQuay, H. (2002). Pooling data for number needed to treat: No problems for apples. *BMC Medical Research Methodology, 2*. Retrieved on October 15, 2003 from http://www.biomedcentral.com/1471-2288/2/2.

O'Rourke, A., & Booth, A. (2000). *Unit 4: Critical appraisal and using the literature.* Research Training Programme Literature Review and Critical Appraisal Module. School of Health and Related Research, University of Sheffield. Retrieved October 8, 2001, from http://www.shef.ac.uk/~scharr/ir/units/.

Oxman, A. D., Cook, D. J., & Guyatt, G. H. (1994). Users' guides to the medical literature. VI. How to use an overview. Evidence-Based Medicine Working Group. *Journal of the American Medical Association, 272*(17), 1367–1371.

Oxman, A. D., Sackett, D. L., & Guyatt, G. H. (1993). Users' guides to the medical literature. I. How to get started. The Evidence-Based Medicine Working Group. *The Journal of the American Medical Association, 270*(17), 2093–2095.

Phillips, B., Ball, C., Sackett, D., Badenoch, D., Straus, S., Haynes, B., & Dawes, M. (2001). *Levels of evidence.* Oxford Centre for Evidence-Based Medicine. Retrieved July 27, 2001, from http://minerva.minervation.com/cebm/docs/levels.html.

Roberts, C., & Sibbald, B. (1998). Randomising groups of patients. *British Medical Journal, 316*, 1898–1900.

Roberts, C., & Torgerson, D. (1998). Randomisation methods in controlled trials. *British Medical Journal, 317*, 1301–1310.

Roberts, C., & Torgerson, D. (1999). Baseline imbalance in randomised controlled trials. *British Medical Journal*, 185, 319.

Roland, M., & Torgerson, D. (1998). What outcomes should be measured? *British Medical Journal, 317*, 1075–1080.

Ronchetti, R., Villa, M. P., Barreto, M., Rota, R., Pagani, J., Martella, S., Falasca, C., Paggi, B., Guglielmi, F., & Ciofetta, G. (2001). Is the increase in childhood asthma coming to an end? Findings from three surveys of schoolchildren in Rome, Italy. *European Respiratory Journal, 17*(5), 881—886.

Sibbald, B., & Roberts, C. (1998). Crossover trials. *British Medical Journal, 316*, 1719–1720.

Stevens, K. R. (2001). Systematic reviews: The heart of evidence-based practice. *AACN Clinical Issues: Advanced Practice in Acute and Critical Care, 12*, 4, 529–538.

Torgerson, D. (2001). Contamination in trials: is cluster randomisation the answer? *British Medical Journal, 322*, 355–357.

Torgerson, d., & Roberts, C. (1999). Randomisation methods: Concealment. *British Medical Journal*, 319, 375–376.

Zielinski, C. (1995). New equities of information in an electronic age. *British Medical Journal, 310*, 1480–1481.

Critically Appraising Qualitative Evidence

Bethel Ann Powers

chapter 6

All scientific evidence is important to clinical decision making, and all evidence must be critically appraised to determine its contribution to that decision making. Part of critical appraisal is applying the clinician's understanding of a field of science to the content of the report. Qualitative research may not be as familiar to practitioners as quantitative research, especially in terms of how it can be useful in guiding practice. Therefore, this chapter provides information to help clinicians with:

● **Language and concepts that will be encountered in the qualitative literature**

● **Aspects of qualitative research that are known to have raised concerns for readers less familiar with different qualitative methods**

● **Issues surrounding the use of evaluative criteria that, if not understood, could lead to their misuse in the appraisal of studies and subsequent erroneous conclusions**

With adequate knowledge, practitioners can extract what is good and useful to clinical decision making by applying appropriate method-specific and general evaluative criteria to qualitative research reports. Glossary boxes are provided throughout the chapter to assist the reader in understanding common terms and concepts that support and structure the chapter discussion.

It is important for clinicians to gain knowledge and an ability to appreciate qualitative research as sources of evidence for clinical decision making. As with all knowledge, application is the best way to gain proficiency. To further hone skills in the appraisal of qualitative research, an appendix demonstrates how to use the appraisal guide at the end of the chapter with a variety of sample articles. Reading these articles is the best way to fully appreciate how to apply the guide. First-hand appraisal of qualitative studies requires active engagement with the evidence. The purpose of this chapter is to prepare clinicians to engage with and move beyond the material presented to applying it when appraising the literature in their particular fields of practice.

> ❝*Anything that we have to learn we learn by the actual doing of it.*❞
>
> *Aristotle*

Carrying Coals to Newcastle: The Contribution of Qualitative Research to Decision Making

Qualitative approaches are becoming more sophisticated and increasingly visible in cross-disciplinary literature. Therefore, discussing the validity of using qualitative research evidence for decision making in healthcare practice would seem a bit like "carrying coals to Newcastle" (i.e., bringing coal to coal-mining country) except for the need to address its role in evidence-based practice (EBP) frameworks not designed to accommodate it. And herein lie both the challenge and the opportunity to expand the concept of what counts as evidence and thereby call attention to the relevance of qualitative research for EBP.

Expanding the Concept of Evidence

Clinical trials and other types of intervention research have been the primary focus of EBP from its inception as a clinical learning strategy used at McMaster Medical School in the 1980s to its global recognition via the systematic reviews provided by the Cochrane Collaboration. Typically, selection of studies to be evaluated in EBP reviews is guided by evidence hierarchies that sustain and extend this focus on treatments and their reported effects by differentiating among research designs according to the strength of their predictive abilities. Compared with quasi-experimental and nonexperimental (i.e., comparative, correlational, descriptive) designs, randomized clinical trials (RCTs) easily emerge as the designated gold standard for determining that the effectiveness of a treatment is not overestimated (Jennings & Loan, 2001). Because of the extent to which "rules of evidence" (i.e., determination of weakest to strongest evidence with a focus on support of the effectiveness of interventions) tend to dominate discussions within the EBP movement, the position of qualitative studies has remained unclear. Qualitative studies most often are ranked lower in a hierarchy of evidence, along with descriptive, evaluative, and case studies as weaker forms of evidence compared with other research designs (i.e., RCTs) that examine interventions. However, applying the same linear framework used to evaluate intervention studies hardly fits the divergent purposes and nonlinear nature of qualitative research traditions and designs.

Expanding the concept of evidence beyond narrow, dogmatic interpretations is a priority for EBP (Pearson, 2002). Work groups have formed to determine how qualitative research may be evaluated and included more in systematic reviews (Giacomini & Cook, 2000a, 2000b; Jennings & Loan, 2001; Pearson, 2002).

Additionally, qualitative outcome analysis (QOA) has been suggested as a method to advance some projects beyond identification of potentially helpful approaches in clinical situations to implementing and evaluating such proposed interventions in practice (Morse, Penrod, & Hupcey, 2000). At the same time, a need to balance scientific knowledge gained through empirical research with non–research-based evidence in clinical decision making has been noted to be part of the work of expanding the concept of evidence. That is, for "a more comprehensive description of evidence-based . . . practice[,] . . . evidence must extend beyond the current emphasis on empirical research and randomized clinical trials, to the kinds of evidence also generated from ethical theories [e.g., based on standards, codes, and philosophies], personal theories [e.g., derived from autobiographical experience and insights], and aesthetic theories [e.g., represented by examples of aesthetic criticism and the creative arts]" (Fawcett et al., 2001, p. 118).

Efforts to expand the concept of evidence are not inconsistent with some articulations of fundamental tenets of the EBP movement. A clear example is in the introduction to Sackett and colleagues' (2000) text on *Evidence-Based Medicine*, where the goal of EBP is represented as the successful integration of three elements of clinical care:

- Best research (i.e., clinically relevant) evidence
- Clinical expertise
- Patient preferences

Research evidence is the portion of the EBP paradigm that has received the most attention, possibly because it represents "a profound paradigm shift for both medical education and medical practice [that served to] lower the value of authority opinion and raise the value of data-based studies and research critiques" (Jennings & Loan, 2001, p. 122). Consequently, much of the current literature focuses on helping practitioners develop their skills in retrieving, critically appraising, and synthesizing databased studies and research critiques.

However, stressing the importance of interventions based on best research evidence (i.e., scientific ways of knowing) does not diminish the need for integrating the remaining elements into clinical decision making. The best blend of science and art is when we also "use our clinical skills and past experience" (i.e., ethical, personal, and aesthetic ways of knowing) and consider "the unique preferences, concerns, and expectations each patient brings to a clinical encounter" (i.e., a human science perspective) to better serve our patients and their families. "When [all] three elements are integrated, clinicians and patients form a diagnostic and therapeutic alliance which optimizes clinical outcomes and quality of life" (Sackett et al., 2000, p. 1).

Recognizing Research Relevant to Practice

Before clinicians can critically appraise qualitative research, they must have an appreciation for and basic knowledge of its methodologies and practices. Science and art come together in the design and execution of qualitative studies. Qualitative research comprises many methodologies and research practices rooted in the social and human sciences. Questions asked by qualitative researchers are influenced by these traditions' focus on in-depth understanding of human experiences and the contexts in which the experiences occur.

In the health sciences, knowledge generated by qualitative studies may contain the theoretical bases for explicit interventions. However, studies that promote better understanding of what health and illness situations are like for people, how they manage, what they wish for and expect, and how they are affected by what goes on around them also may influence practice in other ways. For example, heightened sensitivity or awareness of life from others' vantage points may lead to changes in how persons feel about and behave toward one another, as well as prompt reflection on and discussions about what practical actions might be taken on an individual basis or a larger scale.

The significant growth in qualitative health science literature from 1980 to 1990 occurred at least in part because these approaches were capable of addressing many kinds of questions that could not be answered by quantitative (including quantitative descriptive) research methods. Because of the expansion and evolution of qualitative methods, clinicians across disciplines will encounter a more varied mix of articles on different clinical topics. Therefore, to keep up to date on the latest developments in their fields, practitioners need to be able to recognize and judge the validity of relevant qualitative as well as quantitative research studies.

> *The heights by great men reached and kept were not obtained by sudden flight. But they, while their companions slept, were toiling upward in the night.*
>
> *Thomas S. Monson*

Separating Wheat from Chaff

When we critically appraise a study, we act as the wind that blows away the chaff (i.e., imperfections) so that what is good and useful remains. There are no perfect studies. So the task becomes one of sifting through and deciding whether good and useful elements outweigh a study's shortcomings.

To critically appraise qualitative research reports, the reader needs a sense of the diversity that exists within this field (i.e., a flavor of the language and mindset of qualitative research) to appreciate what is involved in using any set of criteria to evaluate whether a study is valid and useful. This decreases the possibility of misconstruing such criteria because of preconceived notions about what they signify and how they should be used. Brief overviews of how qualitative approaches differ and a synthesis of basic principles for evaluating qualitative studies follow.

Managing Diversity

Qualitative research designs and reporting styles are very diverse. In addition, there are many ways to classify qualitative approaches. Therefore, it is necessary to be able to manage this diversity through an awareness of different scientific traditions and associated research methods and techniques used in qualitative studies.

External Diversity Across Qualitative Research Traditions

Qualitative research traditions have origins within scientific disciplines (e.g., anthropology, sociology, psychology, philosophy) that influence the theoretical assumptions, methods, and styles of reporting used to obtain and convey understanding about human experiences. Therefore, despite similarities in techniques for data gathering and management, experiences are viewed through different lenses, studied for different purposes, and reported in language and writing styles consistent with the research tradition's origins. Among qualitative traditions commonly used in health sciences research are ethnography, grounded theory, phenomenology, and hermeneutics.

Ethnography. Ethnography involves the study of a social group's **culture** through time spent combining **participant-observation** (see Box 6-1) and in-depth interviews in the informants' natural setting. This appreciation of culture—drawing on anthropologic theory and practice—provides the context for a better understanding of answers to specific research questions. For example, cultural understanding may help answer questions about:

- People's health/illness beliefs and practices
- Work-world issues of concern to members of caregiver subcultures (e.g., home healthcare aides, family members, parish nurses)
- Individuals' experiences in certain types of settings (e.g., community center, emergency room, nursing home)

Fieldwork is the term that describes all research activities taking place in or in connection with work in the study setting (i.e., field). These activities include the many social and personal skills required when gaining entry to the field, maintaining field relationships, collecting and analyzing data, resolving political and ethical issues, and leaving the field. Researchers may have **key informants** (in addition to other informants) who assist them in establishing rapport and learning about cultural norms. Research reports are descriptions and interpretations that attempt to capture study informants' **"emic"** points of view balanced against the researcher's **"etic"** analytic perspectives. These efforts to make sense of the data also may provide a basis for generating theory (Coffey & Atkinson, 1996).

---

box 6.1

Ethnography Research Terms

Culture: Shared knowledge and behavior of people who interact within distinct social settings and subsystems.

Participant-observation: Observation and participation in everyday activities in study informants' natural settings.

Fieldwork: All research activities carried out in and in relation to the field (informants' natural settings).

Key informant: A select informant/assistant with extensive or specialized knowledge of his/her own culture.

Emic and etic: Contrasting "insider" views of informants (emic) and the researcher's "outsider" (etic) views.

Grounded Theory. The purpose of grounded theory, developed by sociologists Glaser and Strauss (1967), is to generate theory about how people deal with life situations that is "grounded" in empirical data and describes the processes by which they move through experiences over time. Movement often is expressed in terms of stages or phases (e.g., stages/phases of living with a chronic illness, adjusting to a new situation, or coping with loss). This tradition involves the study of social processes from the perspective of **symbolic interaction** (see Box 6-2). Data collection and analysis procedures are similar to those of ethnographic research, but the focus is on symbolic meanings conveyed by people's actions in certain circumstances, resultant patterns of interaction, and their consequences.

The goal is to discover a core variable through procedures of **constant comparison** (i.e., coding, categorizing, and analyzing incoming data while continually seeking linkages by constantly comparing informational categories with one another and with new data) and **theoretical sampling** that directs data gathering toward **saturation** of categories (i.e., completeness). The *core variable*, or **basic social process** (BSP), is the basis for theory generation. It recurs frequently, links all the data together, and describes the pattern followed, regardless of the various conditions under which the experience occurs and different ways in which persons go through it. In the literature, the reader may encounter terms that are used to further describe types of BSP (e.g., a basic social psychological process (BSPP); a basic social structural process (BSSP). Researchers typically will describe what these terms mean within the context of the study.

Phenomenology. Phenomenology is the study of **essences** (i.e., meaning structures; see Box 6-3) intuited or grasped through descriptions of **lived experience**. Husserl's philosophy described lived experience (i.e., the lifeworld) as understandings about life's meanings that lie outside of a person's conscious awareness. Thus, in studying the meaning, or essence, of an experi-

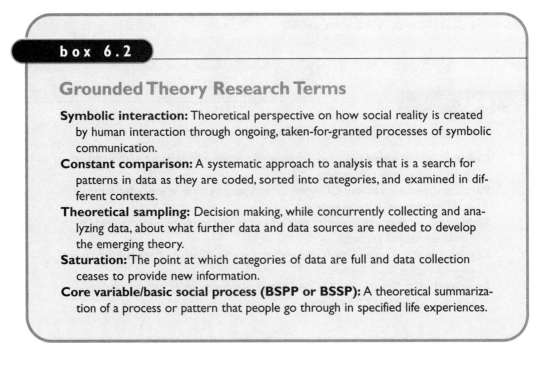

box 6.2

Grounded Theory Research Terms

Symbolic interaction: Theoretical perspective on how social reality is created by human interaction through ongoing, taken-for-granted processes of symbolic communication.

Constant comparison: A systematic approach to analysis that is a search for patterns in data as they are coded, sorted into categories, and examined in different contexts.

Theoretical sampling: Decision making, while concurrently collecting and analyzing data, about what further data and data sources are needed to develop the emerging theory.

Saturation: The point at which categories of data are full and data collection ceases to provide new information.

Core variable/basic social process (BSPP or BSSP): A theoretical summarization of a process or pattern that people go through in specified life experiences.

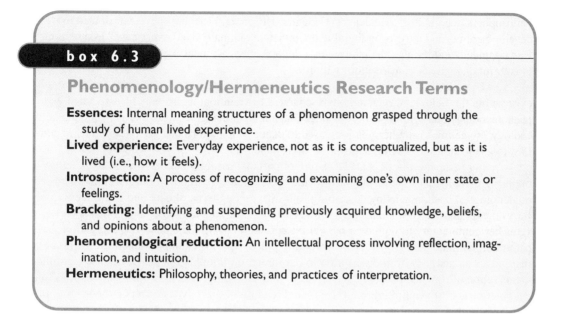

box 6.3

Phenomenology/Hermeneutics Research Terms

Essences: Internal meaning structures of a phenomenon grasped through the study of human lived experience.

Lived experience: Everyday experience, not as it is conceptualized, but as it is lived (i.e., how it feels).

Introspection: A process of recognizing and examining one's own inner state or feelings.

Bracketing: Identifying and suspending previously acquired knowledge, beliefs, and opinions about a phenomenon.

Phenomenological reduction: An intellectual process involving reflection, imagination, and intuition.

Hermeneutics: Philosophy, theories, and practices of interpretation.

ence (phenomenon), researchers need to recognize their own personal feelings (**introspection**) and suspend their beliefs about what the experience is like (**bracketing**). Interpretive insights are derived by collecting experiential descriptions from interviews and other sources and engaging in intellectual analytic processes of reflection, imagination, and intuition (**phenomenological reduction**). A certain philosopher's perspective may be used to direct this analysis (e.g., Husserl, Heidegger, Merleau-Ponty).

Phenomenology, represented as schools of thought within philosophy, offers perspectives shaped through ongoing intellectual dialogues rather than explicit procedures. Descriptions of research processes have come from outside of the parent discipline of philosophy. Processes often cited are:

- The philosophically, language-oriented, descriptive-interpretive phenomenology of educator Max van Manen (the German Dilthey-Nohl and the Dutch Utrecht schools of phenomenological pedagogy)
- The empirical descriptive approaches of the Duquesne school of phenomenological psychology (i.e., Giorgi, Colaizzi, Fischer, and van Kaam).

Examples of phenomena of interest to clinical researchers include what various illness experiences are like for persons or how a sense of hope, trust, or being understood is realized in their lives. Insights offered through research reports range in style from lists of themes and straightforward descriptions (i.e., empiric descriptions) to philosophical theorizing and poetizing (i.e., interpretations).

Hermeneutics. Hermeneutics has a distinct philosophical history as a theory and method of interpretation (originally associated with the interpretation of Biblical texts). However, various philosophers (e.g., Dilthey, Heidegger, Gadamer, Hirsch, and Ricoeur) have contributed to its development beyond a focus on literal texts to viewing human "lived experience" as a text that is to be understood through the interpreter's dialogical engagement (i.e., thinking that is like a thoughtful dialogue or conversation) with life.

There is not a single way to practice hermeneutics. A variety of theories and debates exist within the field. However, although separated by tradition, it also may be associated with phenomenology and certain schools of phenomenological thought. Thus, "hermeneutic phenomenology" sometimes is the terminology used to denote orientations that are interpretive, in contrast to, or in addition to being descriptive (van Manen, 1990).

For instance, Chesla's (1994) study of parents' caring practices with schizophrenic offspring demonstrates the results of drawing on hermeneutic tradition in interpretive phenomenology. Chesla begins by describing four different patterns of care and using them to reflect on existing theories about how families care for schizophrenic members; then she elevates her commentary to include a radical interpretation of how the observed caregiving patterns illuminate dominant societal parenting practices. This example illustrates the process that moves an analysis from description to interpretation in the hermeneutic tradition. A fuller appreciation of how the process contributes to understandings that have implications for clinical practice is best acquired through first-hand reading of these types of reports, engaging reflectively with the actual words of the written text, and experiencing the total effect of the narrative.

Internal Diversity Within Qualitative Research Traditions

Qualitative research traditions vary internally as well as externally. For example, there are several reasons why ethnographic, grounded theory, or phenomenologic accounts may assume a variety of forms, including:

- When a tradition acts as a vehicle for different representational styles and theoretical or ideological conceptualizations
- When historical evolution of a tradition results in differing procedural approaches
- When studies differ individually in terms of their focus on description, interpretation, or theory generation

Representation and Conceptualization.   **Representation** of research findings (i.e., writing style, including authorial voice and use of literary forms and rhetorical devices) should not be a matter of dictate or personal whim. Rather, it is part of the analytic process. Ethnography and phenomenology, in particular, are traditions that exhibit a great variety of representational styles. There are many issues and debates about representation in qualitative research, with articles and entire texts devoted to the topic (Atkinson, 1992; Richardson, 1990; van Manen, 1990; Sandelowski, 1998b; Van Maanen, 1988; Wolcott, 1990). Suffice it to say that the issue for the researcher is to be true to the data and to the reader of the research. Thus, qualitative research reports may be conversational dialogues. They may contain researchers' personal reflections and accounts of their experiences; poetry, artistic, and literary references; hypothetical cases; or fictional narratives and stories that are based on actual data, using study informants' own words in efforts to increase sensitivity and enhance understanding of a phenomenon.

box 6.4

General Qualitative Research Terms

Representation: Part of the analytic process that raises the issue of providing a truthful portrayal of what the data represent (e.g., essence of an experience; cultural portrait) that will be meaningful to its intended audience.

Case study: An intensive investigation of a case involving a person or small group of persons, an issue, or an event.

Biography: An approach that produces an in-depth report of a person's life. Life histories and oral histories also involve gathering of biographical information and recording of personal recollections of one or more individuals.

Critical inquiry: Theoretical perspectives that are ideologically oriented toward critique of and emancipation from oppressive social arrangements or false ideas.

Feminist epistemologies: A variety of views and practices inviting critical dialogue about women's experiences in historical, cultural, and socioeconomic perspective.

On the one hand, researchers should not abuse artistic license by "producing emotional or aesthetic effects simply for the sake of producing them" (Coffey & Atkinson, 1996, p. 129). On the other hand, readers should not see a research report as unconventional if that report is enriched by using an alternative literary form as a faithful representation that best serves a legitimate analytic purpose. In addition, if the representation is meaningful to the reader, it meets a criterion of analytic significance in keeping with these traditions' scholarly norms. For example, in "A Portrait: Magdalena's Dream," Averill (2002) presents a brief creative composite vignette, a story told from the vantage point of a hypothetical individual that draws on analysis from an elsewhere-reported ethnographic study. Together with other types of reports of Averill's research, this representation offers insights on what life can be like for rural older Hispanic persons.

Some standard forms of representation also are used with ethnographic, phenomenological, and grounded theory designs to bring out important dimensions of the data. For example, actual **case studies** and biographical accounts can be used effectively to exemplify life in a particular culture or to illustrate social realities and human experiences in more detailed and personal ways. Creswell (1998) discussed how case studies and biographies, although they may serve as helpful adjuncts to other studies, also are traditions in their own right.

Major qualitative traditions also may be vehicles for distinctive theoretical or ideological concepts. For example, a critical ethnography combines ethnographic methods with methods of **critical inquiry** or cultural critique. The result has been described as "conventional ethnography with a political purpose" (Thomas, 1993, p. 4). The reader should expect to find an integration of empirical analysis and theory related to a goal of emancipation from oppressive circumstances or false ideas. For example, Resnick's (1996) critical ethnography of motivation in geriatric rehabilitation discusses how study-based insights about negative beliefs and patients' feelings of domination were used to facilitate dialogue and encourage improvements in the research fieldwork setting, benefiting both patients and staff.

Similarly, a feminist grounded theory involves empirical analysis guided by a feminist perspective. Again, the reader should expect to be informed about the nature of the critique, because there are many different **feminist epistemologies** (i.e., ways of knowing and reasoning). Epistemologic issues invite critical dialogue about women's experiences and the historical, social, cultural, and economic determinants of those experiences. For instance, Wuest's (1998) study of women's caring strategies reveals how women who care experience personal growth and demonstrate "reciprocity, commitment, love, and obligation" through prioritizing and establishing boundaries in response to "competing and changing demands of caring within [the context of their] current health and social structures"(pp. 39–40).

Historical Evolution. Use over time may refine, extend, or alter and produce variations in the practice of a research tradition. One example of this within anthropology is the developing interest in **interpretive ethnography** (see Box 6-5). This occurred as researchers crossed disciplinary boundaries to combine theoretical perspectives from practices outside of the discipline (e.g., phenomenology, hermeneutics, **semiotics**, **sociolinguistics**, and **critical theory**) to inform their work. Examples include:

- Good's (1994) critique of medical knowledge and practice
- Csordas's (1994) cultural phenomenologic examination of embodiment as a metaphor that may be applied to topics as diverse as pain, ritual healing, dietary customs, and political violence
- Peacock's narrative "life-story" approach to understanding historical, psychocultural, and psychosocial events (Peacock & Holland, 1993)

Another example of historical evolution within a tradition is the controversy between Glaser and Strauss, the originators of grounded theory. Many of the differences center on Glaser's (1992) objections to Strauss and Corbin's (1990) addition of *axial coding* as a procedure not featured in earlier books about the method (Glaser & Strauss, 1967; Chenitz & Swanson, 1986; Glaser, 1978). Axial coding involves the use of a prescribed coding paradigm with predetermined subcategories (e.g., causal conditions, strategies, context, intervening conditions, and consequences) intended to help researchers pose questions about how categories of their data relate to one another. Glaser (1992) objected to forcing data into a fixed model. He argued that his examples of 18 different coding families that may be used to systematically link categories of data (Glaser, 1978) illustrate but do not limit possibilities for analysis where coding should be driven by conceptualizations about data. These and other concerns (e.g., inattention to earlier developed ideas about BSPs and saturation of categories) led Glaser to assert that Strauss and Corbin's model is a new method called "full conceptual description," indicating that he felt it was no longer oriented to the discovery, or **emergence**, of theory (i.e., grounded theory method as originally conceived by himself and Strauss) (Melia, 1996).

These developments in grounded theory offer clear choices between Straussian or Glaserian methods of analysis (Stern, 1994). However, as Kendall (1999) indicates, some re-

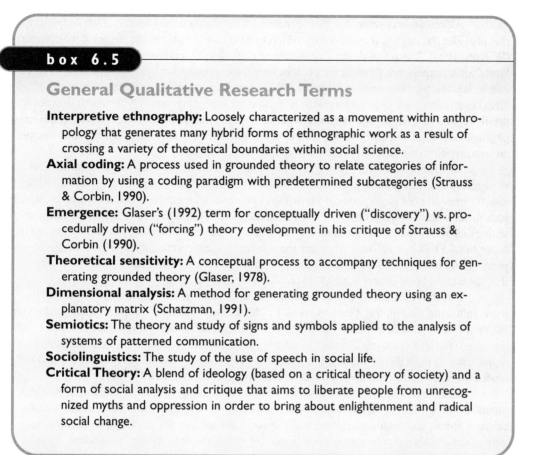

box 6.5

General Qualitative Research Terms

Interpretive ethnography: Loosely characterized as a movement within anthropology that generates many hybrid forms of ethnographic work as a result of crossing a variety of theoretical boundaries within social science.

Axial coding: A process used in grounded theory to relate categories of information by using a coding paradigm with predetermined subcategories (Strauss & Corbin, 1990).

Emergence: Glaser's (1992) term for conceptually driven ("discovery") vs. procedurally driven ("forcing") theory development in his critique of Strauss & Corbin (1990).

Theoretical sensitivity: A conceptual process to accompany techniques for generating grounded theory (Glaser, 1978).

Dimensional analysis: A method for generating grounded theory using an explanatory matrix (Schatzman, 1991).

Semiotics: The theory and study of signs and symbols applied to the analysis of systems of patterned communication.

Sociolinguistics: The study of the use of speech in social life.

Critical Theory: A blend of ideology (based on a critical theory of society) and a form of social analysis and critique that aims to liberate people from unrecognized myths and oppression in order to bring about enlightenment and radical social change.

searchers appear not to be aware that they need to choose and identify the approach they believe is more applicable or useful in their work. The development over time of complex sets of procedures intended to lead researchers through the theory-generating process (Glaser, 1978; Strauss, 1987; Strauss & Corbin, 1990) instead gradually have served to raise more questions and concerns (Robrecht, 1995). Difficulties encountered by researchers have encouraged some to search for alternative methods, such as Schatzman's (1991) **dimensional analysis** model, that retain the ideas intrinsic to grounded theory but provide new frameworks for analytic processes (Robrecht, 1995).

Description, Interpretation, and Theory Generation. Qualitative researchers amass many forms of data: recorded observations (fieldnotes), interview tapes and transcripts, documents, photographs, and collected or received artifacts from the field. There are numerous ways to approach these materials.

All researchers write descriptively about what data analysis reveals. Detailed description provides the empirical evidence on which to base interpretations and theory development (Wolcott, 1994). The act of describing necessarily involves researchers' interpretations of the "facts" of an experience through the choices they make about what to report and how to represent it. Researchers also refer to Geertz's (1973) notion of "**thick description**" (as opposed to "thin description"; see Box 6-6) as what is needed for interpretations. Thick description not only details reports of what people say and do but also incorporates the textures and feelings of the physical and social worlds in which people move and—always with reference to that context—an interpretation of what their words and actions mean.

Describing meaning in context is important because it is a way to try to understand what informants already know about their world. Informants do not talk about that which they take for granted (i.e., tacit, personal knowledge) because their attention is not focused on it. And sometimes what they do is different from what they say because everyday actions in familiar settings also draw on tacit understandings of what is usual and expected. Thick descriptions attempt to take this into account. They are the researchers' interpretations of what it means to experience life from certain vantage points through written expression that is "artful and evocative" as well as "factual and truthful" (Van Maanen, 1988, p. 34).

It is the researcher's choice to report research findings in more factual, descriptive terms (allowing the empirical data to speak for themselves) or more interpretive terms (drawing out the evidence that illuminates circumstances, meanings, emotions, intentions, strategies, motivations). But this mostly is a matter of degree for researchers whose work in a designated tradition tends to push them toward more in-depth interpretation. Additionally, the venue and intended audiences influence decisions about how to represent research findings.

Theory generation also is a proper goal in ethnography and an essential outcome in grounded theory. In these traditions, theories are empirical evidence-based explanations of how cultural, social, and personal circumstances account for individuals' actions and interactions with others. Analyzed data supply the evidence in which the theories are "grounded." Results from individual studies are *substantive theories* that account for situation-specific areas of inquiry, such as processes used by families caring for elders (Phillips & Rempusheski, 1986) or

unit 2

138

---

box 6.6

General Qualitative Research Terms

Thick description: Description that does more than describe human experiences by beginning to interpret what they mean.

(Grounded) Substantive theory: A systematic explanation of a situation-specific human experience/social phenomenon.

(Grounded) Formal theory: A systematic explanation of an area of human/social experience derived through meta-analysis of substantive theory.

for persons with AIDS (Brown & Powell-Cope, 1991), or by individuals dealing with postpartum depression (Beck, 1993), drug addiction (Kearney, Murphy & Rosenbaum, 1994), or domestic violence (Newman, 1993). As theory-generating studies accumulate, there is rising awareness of the need for synthesizing multiple researchers' substantive theories about diverse but related phenomena (metasynthesis) to produce *formal theories* (a higher level of conceptualization) (Benoliel, 1996; Kearney, 1998; Morse, 2000b; Morse & Johnson, 1991; Sandelowski, Docherty, & Emden, 1997). For example, subjecting a number of related theories such as those above to metasynthesis could produce more encompassing and hence more useful formal theories that could apply in a variety of situations, such as family processes of adaptation or passages and processes of vulnerable people (Benoliel, 1996). Theory generation is not expected in phenomenologic or hermeneutic approaches. The purpose of these studies is to understand and interpret human experience, not to explain it.

Qualitative Descriptive Studies. "Descriptive research is a type of quantitative research that is usually preliminary to more controlled experimental or correlational research" (Powers & Knapp, 1995, p. 42). "[It] typically entails surveys or other pre-structured means to obtain a common dataset on pre-selected variables, and descriptive statistics to summarize them" (Sandelowski, 2000b, p. 336). However, there is another kind of descriptive research that is more qualitative in nature. It uses qualitative researchers' favored research techniques and may have "overtones . . . the look, sound, or feel of [ethnographic, grounded theory, or phenomenological] approaches" (Sandelowski, 2000b, p. 337).

Qualitative descriptive studies (see Box 6-7) serve to summarize factual information about human experiences with more attention to the feel of the data's subjective content than tends to be found in quantitative description but with less of the reading into, between, and over data required of the more interpretive traditions (Poirier & Ayres, 1997). Some reports confuse their association with qualitative traditions by mislabeling of the work, inappropriate referencing, and misapplication of terms to describe research methods as though they were examples of those traditions. But there is no need for such affectation. Sound, qualitative descriptive studies

---

box 6.7

General Qualitative Research Terms

Qualitative description: Description that "entails a kind of interpretation that is low-inference [close to the "facts"] or likely to result in easier consensus [about the "facts"] among researchers" (Sandelowski, 2000b, p. 335).

Naturalistic research: Commitment to the study of phenomena in their naturally occurring settings (contexts).

Field studies: Studies involving direct, first-hand observation and interviews in informants' natural settings.

can have practical significance in themselves and may also be an important source of ideas and hypotheses for future research.

Sandelowski (2000b) suggests that researchers "name their method as qualitative description [and] if . . . designed with overtones from other methods, they can describe what these overtones were, instead of inappropriately naming or implementing these other methods" (p. 339). Another approach to labeling would be to highlight the research technique, such as an *observation study* or *interview study*. Some use **naturalistic research** (Lincoln & Guba, 1985) as a label, although what this largely signifies is the intellectual commitment to studying phenomena in the natural settings or contexts in which they occur. **Field study** is another generic term for research that involves direct, first-hand observations and interviews in the informants' natural settings. Lofland and Lofland (1995) and other references provide guides to data collection and analysis activities needed for such studies. Labels such as "exploratory" or "cross-sectional" may be used, although these are concepts that have quantitative design connotations.

Qualitative Evaluation and Action Research Studies. Some studies that use qualitative research techniques need to retain their unique identities. For example, evaluation of educational and organizational programs, projects, and policies may use qualitative research techniques of interviewing, observation, and document review to generate and analyze data (Patton, 1990).

Also, various forms of **action research,** including **participatory action research** (PAR; see Box 6-8), may use field techniques of observation and interviewing as approaches to data collection and analysis. These research projects relate to distinct sets of methods and ideological perspectives that involve politics and the power and use of knowledge. For example, in education and organization research, the goal of PAR is to improve existing conditions for socially oppressed groups or communities through participation of all those involved. Another example might be physician-anthropologist Farmer's (1999) professional autobiographic field account of battling modern plagues (e.g., AIDS, TB) among the poor of rural Haiti and urban Peru. In this work, he challenges accepted beliefs and practices of epidemiology and international health, arguing that "excuses" based on "cost-effectiveness" and explanations citing patient "noncompliance" inevitably lead to blaming the victims and are symptomatic of deeper social ills.

Favored Research Techniques

Favored techniques used in qualitative research reflect the needs of particular study designs. Although they cannot be wholly disentangled from the theories and the scientific traditions that give rise to them, it is appropriate for them to appear last in a discussion of methods because techniques do not drive research questions and designs. They are the servants, not the masters. By themselves, they are not what makes a study qualitative. Nevertheless, a secure knowledge of techniques and their uses has important consequences for successful execution and evaluation of studies.

Observation and Fieldnotes. In fieldwork, observation, combined with other activities, moves back and forth along a *continuum* according to the needs of the research across time. Spradley (1980) described different points on the continuum as complete observer, observer as participant, participant as observer, and complete participant. **Participant-observation** (i.e., active engagement of the researcher in settings and activities of people being studied; Box 6-9) encompasses all of these social roles with less time spent at the extremes. Most time is spent in

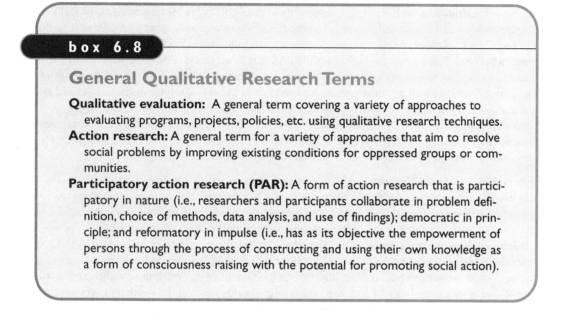

the middle where distinctions between observer as participant and participant as observer are blurred. This is similar to everyday life in which the emphasis shifts back and forth as people take more or less active roles in interactions (e.g., speaking and listening, acting and watching, taking the initiative and standing by), depending on the situation.

box 6.9

General Qualitative Research Terms

Participant-observation: The active engagement of the researcher in settings and activities of people being studied.

Observation continuum: A range of social roles encompassed by participant-observation and ranging from complete observer to complete participant at the extremes.

Field notes: Self-designed observational protocols for recording notes about field observations.

Analytic notes: Notes that researchers write to themselves to record their thoughts, questions, and ideas as a process of simultaneous data collection and data analysis unfolds.

Fieldnotes are self-designed observational protocols for recording notes about field observation. Most are not actually recorded in the field, where researchers may only be able to do "jottings" (e.g., phrases and key words as memory aids) until it is possible to compose an expanded account. Field notes are highly detailed records of all that can be remembered of observations, as well as researcher actions and interactions. They may include maps and drawings of the environment, as well as conversations and records of events. **Analytic notes** (also called *reflective notes* or *memos*) are notes researchers write to themselves about ideas for analysis, issues to pursue, persons to contact, questions, personal emotions, understandings, and confusions brought into focus by writing and thinking about the field experience. This process illustrates how data collection and analysis occur simultaneously throughout the study.

Interviews and Focus Groups. Although a variety of interview forms and question formats are used in qualitative research, their common purpose is to provide ways for informants to express and expand on their own thoughts and remembrances, reflections, and ideas. Informal conversational interviews that occur in the natural course of participant-observation are of the **unstructured, open-ended** type (Box 6-10). Formal interviews, however, often involve use of interview guides that list or outline in advance the topics and questions to be covered. Interviews remain conversational, and the interviewer has flexibility in deciding sequence and wording of questions on the basis of how the conversation is flowing, but the **semistructured interview** approach makes data collection more comprehensive and systematic from informant to informant.

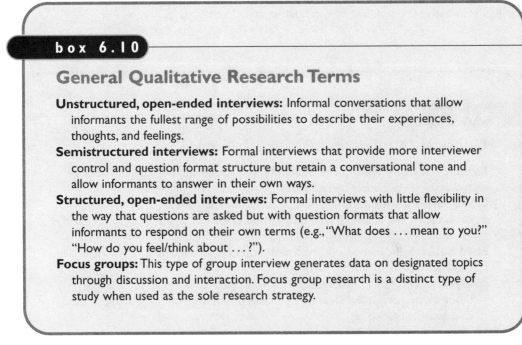

box 6.10

General Qualitative Research Terms

Unstructured, open-ended interviews: Informal conversations that allow informants the fullest range of possibilities to describe their experiences, thoughts, and feelings.

Semistructured interviews: Formal interviews that provide more interviewer control and question format structure but retain a conversational tone and allow informants to answer in their own ways.

Structured, open-ended interviews: Formal interviews with little flexibility in the way that questions are asked but with question formats that allow informants to respond on their own terms (e.g., "What does . . . mean to you?" "How do you feel/think about . . . ?").

Focus groups: This type of group interview generates data on designated topics through discussion and interaction. Focus group research is a distinct type of study when used as the sole research strategy.

Some studies also use **structured, open-ended** question formats where informants answer the same exactly worded question(s) but are free to describe their experiences in their own words and on their own terms. Although this discussion covers several interview methods, it does not exhaust possible interview approaches.

Group interviews may be used in addition to individual interviews in field research. In recent years, **focus groups** have been used in combination with other forms of data collection in both qualitative and quantitative research studies to generate data on designated topics through discussion and interaction. Group moderators direct interaction in structured or semistructured ways, depending on the purpose of the interview.

When used as the sole research strategy, the focus group interview represents a distinct type of study with a history in marketing research. Thus, researchers should limit their naming of the method to "focus group" and refer to primary sources for information on specific focus group strategies when planning to use this as the central data collection technique (e.g., Krueger, 1994; Morgan, 1993).

Narrative, Discourse, and Content Analysis.

Analysis in qualitative research involves extracting themes, patterns, processes, essences, and meanings from "textual data"(i.e., written materials such as field notes, interview transcripts, and various kinds of documents). But there is no single way to go about this. For instance, narrative, discourse, and content analysis are examples of broad areas (paradigms) within which researchers work; each comprises many different approaches.

Narrative analysis is concerned with generating and interpreting stories about life experiences. It is a specific way to understand interview data, representing it in the form of "truthful fictions" (Sandelowski, 1991, p. 165). Kleinman's (1988) *The Illness Narratives* is a well-known example in the medical literature, cited by *JAMA* (on the book's back cover) as "a major contribution to the care techniques for the chronically ill" and by the *New England Journal of Medicine* as "thought-provoking . . . touching . . . much needed by practicing physicians."

This Harvard psychiatrist and anthropologist drew extensively on quotations from interviews with patients and his own clinical notes to construct stories of pain, suffering, and healing to represent what readers need to understand about the illness experience in close-up, emotional human terms. Gubrium's (1993) *Speaking of Life: Horizons of Meaning for Nursing Home Residents* is another example of using personal narratives to answer questions about quality of life issues for persons in institutional settings. Although qualitative researchers commonly deal with stories of persons' experiences, narrative analysis is a particular way of dealing with stories. Therefore, the term should not be used casually to refer to any form of analysis that involves narrative data.

Discourse analysis is a general term covering various approaches to the analysis of recorded talk. Conversation analysis is one such approach that focuses on the details of ordinary, everyday talk to reveal unspoken norms and ways that speakers collaborate to create meaning. Some examples are Labov and Fanshel's (1977) *Therapeutic Discourse: Psychotherapy as Conversation* and Mishler's (1986) *Research Interviewing: Context and Narrative*. Forms of conversation and discourse analysis are related to traditions within sociology (ethnomethodology, the study of how knowledge is socially constructed or the study of how people "do" everyday things), anthropology (ethnoscience—semantic ethnography), and semiotics (theory and study of signs and symbols applied to the analysis of systems of patterned communication). These various microanalytic techniques emphasize linguistic principles and semantics. Current examples from clinical literature are sparse.

Qualitative **content analysis** is most commonly mentioned in research reports in connection with procedures that involve breaking down data (e.g., coding, comparing, contrasting, and categorizing bits of information), then reconstituting them in some new form, such as description, interpretation, or theory. Ethnographers refer to this as *working data* to tease out themes and patterns. Grounded theorists describe *procedural sequences* involving different levels of coding and conceptualization of data. Phenomenologists also may use **thematic analysis** as one of many analytic strategies. To avoid confusion, it should be noted that there are forms of **quantitative** content analysis that use very different principles to deal with narrative data in predetermined, structured ways.

Sampling Strategies. *Sampling* decisions involve choices about study sites or settings and persons who will be able to provide information and insights about the study topic. A single setting may be chosen for in-depth study, or multiple sites may be selected to enlarge and diversify samples or for purposes of comparison. Some studies of human experiences are not specific to a particular setting. Within and across sites, researchers must choose activities and events that, through observation and interview, will yield the best information. For example, if in a study of elderly persons' adjustment to congregate living, data gathering is limited to interviews in individuals' private quarters, there will be a loss of other persons' perspectives (e.g., family members, service providers) and the ability to observe how participants interact with others in different facets of community life.

Choice of participants (i.e., informants or study subjects in qualitative studies) is based on a combination of criteria, including the nature and quality of information they may contribute (i.e., **theoretic interest**), their willingness to participate, their accessibility, and their availability. A prominent qualitative sampling strategy is purposeful.

Purposeful sampling (Box 6-11) enables researchers to select informants who will be able to provide particular perspectives that relate to the research question(s). In grounded theory, this is called **theoretical sampling** (i.e., sampling is used in specific ways to build theory). **Nominated**, or **snowball sampling** also may be used, in which informants assist in recruiting other people they know to participate. This can be helpful when informants are in a position to recommend persons who are well informed on a topic and can provide a good interview. **Volunteer samples** also are used when researchers do not know potential informants and solicit for participants with the desired experience who meet study inclusion criteria. With all types of sampling, researcher judgment and control are essential to be sure that study needs are met.

Researchers' judgments, based on ongoing evaluation of quality and quantity of different types of information in the research database, determine the number and variety of informants needed. Minimum numbers of informants needed for a particular kind of study may be estimated, based on historical experience. For example, 30–50 interviews typically meet the needs of ethnographic and grounded theory studies, whereas six may be an average sample size for a phenomenologic study (Morse, 1994). However, if a study involves multiple interviews of the same persons, fewer informants may be needed. And if the quality of information that informants supply is not good or sufficient to answer questions or saturate data categories, more informants will be needed. Decisions to stop collecting data depend on the nature and scope of the study design; the amount, richness, and quality of useable data; the speed with which types of data move analysis along; and the completeness or saturation (Morse, 2000a).

---

box 6.11

General Qualitative Research Terms

Purposeful/theoretical sample: A sample intentionally selected in accordance with the needs of the study.

Nominated/snowball sample: A sample obtained with the help of informants already enrolled in the study.

Volunteer sample: A sample obtained by solicitation or advertising for participants who meet study criteria.

Theoretic interest: A desire to know or understand it better.

An adequate sample size . . . is one that permits—by virtue of not being too large—the deep, case-oriented analysis that is a hallmark of all qualitative inquiry, and that results in—by virtue of not being too small—a new and richly textured understanding of experience (Sandelowski, 1995, p. 183).

Random sampling, used in quantitative studies to achieve statistically representative samples, does not logically fit with purposes of qualitative designs (i.e., to seek out persons who will be the best sources of information about an experience or phenomenon). In addition, relying on random sampling would delay saturation in qualitative studies (i.e., possibly producing too much of some and not enough of other needed data) and result in oversaturation (i.e., unmanageable volume) that also would not serve (Morse, 1998b).

Data Management and Analysis. Qualitative studies generate large amounts of narrative data that need to be managed and manipulated. Personal computers and word processing software facilitate data management (Box 6-12), including:

- Data entry (e.g., typing fieldnotes and analytic memos, transcribing recorded interviews)
- "Cleaning," or editing
- Storage and retrieval (e.g., organizing data into meaningful, easily located units or files)

Data manipulation involves coding, sorting, and arranging words, phrases, or data segments in ways that advance ongoing analysis. Various types of specialized software have been developed to support management and manipulation of textual data. There is no inherent virtue in using or not using qualitative data analysis software (QDAS). It is wise to consider the advantages and disadvantages (Richards, 1998; St. John & Johnson, 2000). Most important to remember is that QDAS packages, unlike statistical software, may support but do not perform data analyses. And users need to be certain that the analyses they must perform do not suffer as a result of inappropriate fit with the limits and demands of a particular program or the learning curve that may be involved.

---

box 6.12

General Qualitative Research Terms

Qualitative data management: The act of designing systems to organize, catalogue, code, store, and retrieve data. (System design influences, in turn, how the researcher approaches the task of analysis.)

Computer-assisted qualitative data analysis: An area of technological innovation that in qualitative research has resulted in uses of word processing and software packages to support data management.

Qualitative data analysis: A variety of techniques that are used to move back and forth between data and ideas throughout the course of the research.

Data analysis occurs throughout data collection to ensure that sampling decisions produce an appropriate, accurate, and sufficiently complete and richly detailed data set to meet the needs of the study. Also, to manage the volume of data involved, ongoing analysis is needed to sort and arrange data while developing ideas about how to reassemble and represent them as descriptions, theories, or interpretations.

Sorting may involve making frequency counts, coding, developing categories, formulating working hypotheses, accounting for negative cases (instances that contradict other data or do not fit hypotheses), or identifying concepts that explain patterns and relationships among data. Research design and specific aims determine which of many analytic techniques will be used (e.g., phenomenological reduction, constant comparison, narrative analysis, content analysis).

Similarly, the results of data analysis may take many forms. A common example is thematic analysis that systematically describes recurring ideas or topics (i.e., themes) that represent different yet related aspects of a phenomenon. Data may be organized into tables, charts, or graphs or presented as narratives using actual quotes from informants or reconstructed life stories (i.e., data-based hypothetical examples). Data also may be presented as typologies or taxonomies (i.e, classification schemes) that serve explanatory or heuristic (i.e., illustrative and educational) purposes (Powers, 1988, 2001). Researchers also may use drama (Bluebond-Langner, 1978; Ellis & Bochner, 1992), self-stories (Paget, 1993; Olson, 1993), and poetry (Richardson, 1992) to immerse the reader in the informants' world, decrease the distance between author and reader, and more vividly portray the emotional content of an experience (Denzin, 1997).

Blurred Genres and Mixing Methods. It is unhelpful to view qualitative research as a singular entity that can be divorced from the assumptions of the traditions associated with different methods or reduced to an assemblage of data collection and analysis techniques. Misunderstandings about it have paralleled its rising popularity—a direct outcome of increased recognition of its usefulness in answering questions that other research approaches cannot answer. Such rapid proliferation and dispersion of qualitative perspectives and methods has taken place across disciplines that Geertz (1983) described the resulting intellectual climate of the 1970s to mid-1980s as one of "blurred genres." And Denzin and Lincoln (1994) described the current "historical moment" as one distinguished by an unprecedented number of choices: "There have never been so many paradigms, strategies of inquiry, or methods of analysis to draw upon and utilize" (p. 11).

Because there are so many choices that necessarily involve multilevel (e.g., paradigm, method, and technique; Box 6-13) commitments (Sandelowski, 2000a), seasoned researchers have cautioned against nonreflective, uncritical mixing of qualitative perspectives, language, and analytic strategies to produce a "haphazard" or "sloppy mish mash" that does not meet rigorous scholarly standards (Coffey & Atkinson, 1996, p. 193; Morse, 1991, p. 15). This is coupled with a concern about researchers who rely on textbooks or survey courses for direction in lieu of expert mentorship. The concern is that their ability to recognize within- and across-method subtleties and nuances, identify decision points, and anticipate consequences involved in the research choices they make may be compromised as a result of the insufficient depth of understanding afforded by these limited knowledge bases (Morse, 1991, 1997a; Stern, 1994). Novice readers of qualitative research (and beginning researchers) are advised first to learn about pure methods so that they will be able to proceed with greater knowledge and confidence, should they later encounter a hybrid (combined qualitative) or mixed-method (combined qualitative and quantitative) approach.

---

box 6.13

General Qualitative Research Terms

Paradigm: A world view or set of beliefs, assumptions, and values that guide all types of research by identifying where the researcher stands on issues related to the nature of reality (ontology), relationship of the researcher to the researched (epistemology), role of values (axiology), use of language (rhetoric), and process (methodology) (Creswell, 1998).

Method: The theory of how a certain type of research should be carried out (i.e., strategy, approach, process/overall design, and logic of design). Researchers often subsume description of techniques under a discussion of method.

Techniques: Tools or procedures used to generate or analyze data (e.g., interviewing, observation, standardized tests and measures, constant comparison, document analysis, content analysis, statistical analysis). Techniques are method-neutral and may be used, as appropriate, in any research design—either qualitative or quantitative.

Appraising Individual Qualitative Studies

A variety of method-specific and general criteria have been proposed for evaluating qualitative studies. In fact, there is a large variety of rules related to quality standards, but there is no agreed-upon terminology or preset format that bridges the diversity of methods enough to be able to dictate how researchers communicate about the rules they followed. And only part of the judgment involves what researchers say they did. The other part is how well they represent research results, the effect of the presentation on readers, and reader judgments about whether study findings seem credible and useful.

Method-Specific Evaluative Criteria

The concept of "scientific rigor" in qualitative research encompasses "multiple criteria of evaluation [that] now compete for attention in this field" (Denzin & Lincoln, 1994, p. 11). Some specifically relate to central purposes and characteristics of traditional methods. For example, ethnography's emphasis on understanding human experience in cultural context is reflected by six variables proposed by Homans (1955) to evaluate the adequacy of field studies: *time, place, social circumstance, language, intimacy,* and *consensus.*

Elaboration on these variables relates to values placed on prolonged close engagement of the researcher with study participants, active participation in daily social events, communication, and confirmation of individual informant reports by consulting multiple informants. Appraisals of an ethnographic/field study's accuracy (credibility) may be linked to how well values such as these appear to have been upheld.

Similarly, the ultimate goal of grounded theory-influenced evaluative criteria was summarized by Glaser and Strauss (1967) as: *fit, grab, work,* and *modifiability* (see Box 6-14).

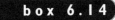

box 6.14

Glaser and Strauss' Grounded Theory-Influenced Evaluative Criteria

- **Fit:** Categories must be indicated by the data.

- **Grab:** The theory must be relevant to the social/practice world.

- **Work:** The theory must be useful in explaining, interpreting, or predicting the study phenomenon.

- **Modifiability:** the theory must be adaptable over time to changing social conditons van Manen's (1990) pedagogic, semiotic/language-oriented approach to phenomenology is reflected in his four conditions or evaluative criteria of any human science text. The text must be *oriented*, *strong*, *rich*, and *deep* (see Box 6-15).

When reading a phenomenological report that meets these criteria, the reader can be confident that the text fulfills its purpose as "a critical philosophy of action" that leads to "tactful thoughtfulness: situational perceptiveness, discernment, and depthful understanding" (van Manen, pp. 155–156).

The above are just a few examples of how active researchers working within specific traditions have conceptualized their craft. Because there is such diversity in qualitative inquiry, no single set of criteria can serve all qualitative approaches equally well. But there have been efforts to articulate criteria that may more generally apply to diverse qualitative research approaches. The method-specific criteria to some extent drive these general criteria. However, the primary driver for the variety of attempts to develop general criteria has been perceived communication gaps between qualitative and quantitative researchers whose use of language and world views often differ. Despite these attempts, there is not agreement among qualitative researchers about how or whether it is appropriate to use the general appraisal criteria.

General Criteria for Evaluating Qualitative Studies

Examples of general evaluative criteria are those proposed by Lincoln and Guba (1985) that offer qualitative equivalents to quantitative concepts of validity and reliability. These help to explain the scientific rigor of qualitative methods to quantitatively oriented persons. But it has been argued that by framing discussion on the basis of the belief structures of quantitative researchers and drawing attention away from other criteria of equal importance, the criteria fail to address paradigmatic differences. The differences reflected by qualitative researchers' world view are in the ways they perceive reality as subjective and multiple (i.e., the ontological issue); the way they view the relationship between the researcher and the researched as close and col-

---

box 6.15

van Manen's Phenomenologic Evaluative Criteria

- **Oriented:** Answers a question of how one stands in relation to life/how one needs to think, observe, listen, and relate

- **Strong:** Clear and powerful

- **Rich:** Thick description/valid, convincing interpretations of concrete experiences

- **Deep:** Reflective/instructive and meaningful

laborative (i.e., the epistemologic issue); the belief that all research is value laden, and biases that are naturally present need to be dealt with openly (i.e., the axiologic issue); the conviction that effective use of personal and literary writing styles are key to meaningful representation of research results (i.e., the rhetorical issue); and the ways in which inductive logic is used to draw out and encourage development of emerging understanding of what the data mean (i.e., the methodologic issue) (Creswell, 1998).

Thus, Guba and Lincoln (1994) acknowledge that although their criteria "have been well received, their parallelism to positivist criteria makes them suspect . . . [and, therefore,] the issue of quality criteria . . . is not well resolved" (p. 114).

Trustworthiness Criteria

When appraising qualitative research, applying Lincoln and Guba's (1985) trustworthiness criteria can be helpful. These criteria include *credibility, transferability, dependability*, and *confirmability* (see Box 6-16).

Credibility. Credibility (paralleling internal validity) is demonstrated by accuracy and validity that is assured through documentation of researcher actions, opinions, and biases; negative case analysis (e.g., accounting for outliers/exceptions); appropriateness of data (e.g., purposeful sampling); adequacy of the database (e.g., saturation); and verification/corroboration by use of multiple data sources (e.g., triangulation), validation of data and findings by informants (e.g., member checks), and consultation with colleagues (e.g., peer debriefing).

Some caveats about the above indicators of credibility merit mentioning. Member checks can be problematic when researchers' findings uncover implicit patterns or meanings of which informants are unaware. Thus, they may not be able to corroborate findings and may need to reexamine the situation and "check-out results for themselves" (Morse, 1994, p. 230).

Also, member checks are seldom useful for corroborating reports that are a synthesis of multiple perspectives because individuals are not positioned well to account for perspectives beyond their own. Therefore, member checks should be seen as an ongoing process for assuring that informants' recorded accounts accurately and fairly reflect their perceptions and experiences. But as an ultimate check on the final interpretation of data, they are not required; it is up to the researcher to decide when and how they may be useful (Morse, 1998a; Sandelowski,

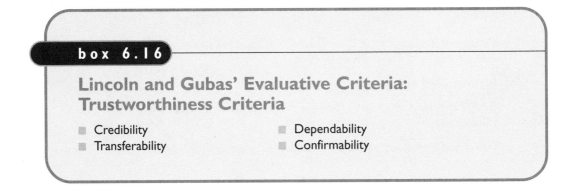

box 6.16

Lincoln and Gubas' Evaluative Criteria: Trustworthiness Criteria

- Credibility
- Transferability
- Dependability
- Confirmability

1993, 1998a). As a result, when reading a qualitative report, member checks may or may not be present.

Peer debriefing involves seeking input (substantive or methodological) from knowledgeable colleagues as consultants, soliciting their reactions as listeners, and using them as sounding boards for the researcher's ideas. It is up to the researcher to decide when and whether peer debriefing will be useful. It is important to distinguish peer debriefing from quantitative researchers' use of multiple raters and expert panels. In qualitative research, it is not appropriate to use individuals outside of the research to "validate" the researcher's analyses and interpretations because these are arrived at inductively through closer contact and understanding of the data than an outside expert could possibly have (Morse, 1994, 1997b, 1998a; Sandelowski, 1998a). Because peer debriefing may not always be useful, the reader should not expect to encounter this credibility criterion in every qualitative report.

Transferability.   Transferability (paralleling external validity) is demonstrated by information that is sufficient for a research consumer to determine whether findings are meaningful to other people in similar situations (analytic or theoretical vs. statistical generalizability). The practical usefulness of a qualitative study is judged by its:

- Ability to represent how informants feel about and make sense of their experiences
- Effectiveness in communicating what that information means and the lessons that it teaches

Is has been thought that because qualitative studies did not meet generalizability standards for quantitative studies, the results were not generalizable. However, the extent to which research-based understandings can be applied to experiences of individuals in similar situations (i.e., transferability) defines a study's generalizability. Therefore, it is misleading to say that results of qualitative studies are not generalizable (Sandelowski, 1996). When the reader holds this idea or encounters it in the literature, it usually means that there is a lack of understanding about the differences between statistical generalization and analytic or theoretic generalization. The former pertains to mathematically based probabilities with which implications of study findings can be extended to a larger population, consistent with the purposes of quantitative research designs. The latter pertains to logically and pragmatically based possibilities with which implications of study findings can be extended to a larger population, consistent with the purposes of qualitative research designs.

Dependability.   Dependability (paralleling reliability) is demonstrated by a research process that is carefully documented to provide evidence of how conclusions were reached and whether, under similar conditions, a researcher might expect to obtain similar findings (i.e., the concept of the audit trail).

Confirmability.   Confirmability (paralleling objectivity) is demonstrated by providing substantiation that findings and interpretations are grounded in the data (i.e., links between researcher assertions and the data are clear and credible).

Other general criteria are linked to concepts of credibility and transferability but relate more to the effects that various portrayals of the research may have. For example, a second set of criteria developed by Guba and Lincoln (1989) have overtones of a critical theory view that when the goal of research is to provide deeper understanding and more informed insights into human experiences, it also may prove to be empowering (Guba & Lincoln, 1994, p. 114).

Authenticity Criteria

Box 6-17 lists Guba and Lincoln's (1989) evaluative *authenticity criteria. Fairness* is the degree to which informants' different ways of making sense of experiences (i.e., their "constructions") are evenly represented by the researcher. *Ontological authenticity* is the scope to which personal insights are enhanced or enlarged. *Educative authenticity* is the extent to which there is increased understanding of and appreciation for others' constructions. *Catalytic authenticity* is how effectively the research stimulates action. *Tactical authenticity* is the degree to which persons are empowered to act.

Ontological and educative authenticity, in particular, are at the heart of concerns about how to represent research results. That is, to transfer a deeper understanding of a phenomenon to the reader, researchers may strive for literary styles of writing that make a situation seem more "real" or "alive." This also is called making use of *verisimilitude*, an important criterion of traditional validity (Creswell, 1998; Denzin, 1997). It refers to any style of writing that *vicariously draws readers into the multiple realities of the world that the research reveals*, seen from both informant and researcher perspectives.

Integrity and Synthesis

Within the EBP movement, conversations among researchers and practitioners (largely those most oriented to quantitative research) about the relative merits of different forms of inquiry have focused on "gold standards" of excellence in the design of individual studies and the ultimate gold standard in terms of a hierarchy of evidence. Two interrelated dilemmas that this situation poses for qualitative researchers and practitioners may be explained in terms of *competing goods*. Competing goods are values that are balanced in such a way that satisfying one poses some difficulty in satisfying the other. For example:

> It is good to adhere to method-specific standards of excellence versus it is good to be able to communicate about those standards in ways that are understandable to persons less familiar with the methods.

The reason that many quantitative researchers and practitioners appreciate Lincoln and Guba's (1985) trustworthiness criteria is that they are understandable and seek to impose a sense of order and uniformity on a field that is diverse and difficult to understand. Thus, some readers

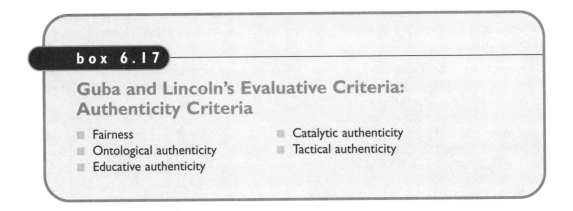

box 6.17

Guba and Lincoln's Evaluative Criteria: Authenticity Criteria

- Fairness
- Ontological authenticity
- Educative authenticity

- Catalytic authenticity
- Tactical authenticity

unit 2

152

readers have greater confidence in qualitative reports that cite these criteria. But that does not mean that reports that do not cite them are necessarily deficient. Many qualitative researchers and practitioners resist parallelism (i.e., using words that mirror the concepts and values of quantitative research) because they think that it may detract from better method-specific explanations of their research (a matter of training and individual preference). Some also think it could undermine the integrity of qualitative methods themselves (a matter of principle). Furthermore, they know that examples of procedures to ensure quality and rigor are more or less appropriate for different kinds of qualitative studies and, therefore, attempts to talk about the general properties of qualitative designs and findings pose many constraints. As a result, there is a threat to integrity if general criteria come to be viewed as rigid rules that must apply in every instance. Therefore, it is incumbent upon nonqualitative researchers and practitioners to assimilate more details about the differences, similarities, and nuances of this large field of research than they might at first prefer in order to conduct a fair and accurate appraisal of qualitative reports.

A second competing good is:

> It is good to pursue answers to relevant research questions with studies best designed to answer them versus it is good to agree on the sources of strongest evidence for making practice-based decisions.

This dilemma reflects a debate within a debate. At its most superficial levels, the debate is about what research methods provide the strongest sources of evidence for answering critical practice-related questions. At its deeper levels, the debate is about what counts as a critical practice-related question. Typically, the research questions that qualitative researchers ask cannot be answered by and are not necessarily preliminary to current EBP conceptions of strongest evidence (quasi-experimental studies and clinical trials). They may dovetail with related questions best answered by broad-based quantitative approaches, but answers to qualitative questions come from a different vantage point. Other forms of research cannot match their purposes or replicate the in-depth specificity of their focus on individual cases and circumstances. That is their particular strength. Thus, pragmatically, identifying sources of strongest evidence depends on the clinical question, not on where research approaches stand in a hierarchy.

The key to agreement on the sources of strongest evidence for making practice-based decisions is identifying what the practitioner needs to know to improve approaches to caregiving and understanding the interplay between the researcher's answers (whether statistically or analytically/theoretically generalizable) and the practitioner's view of best evidence based on need. Because no single research study or set of approaches can capture the whole picture in any clinical area that would be of concern to caring practitioners, some narrow hierarchical thinking about sources of best evidence may need to give way to broader notions of synthesis across available research approaches (qualitative, quantitative, and mixed method).

Walking the Walk and Talking the Talk: Critical Appraisal of Qualitative Research

This chapter began by comparing critical appraisal of individual research reports with separating wheat from chaff. Separating out the chaff involves applying the reader's understanding of the diversity within the field of qualitative research to the content of the report. Then extracting what is good and useful involves applying the appropriate method-specific and general evaluative criteria to the research report. Using the guide in Box 6-18 to appraise qualitative research studies depends on a degree of familiarity with the preceding introduction to the diversity of characteristics, language, concepts, and issues associated with this field.

The guide adopts the EBP format of basic quick appraisal questions followed by questions of a more specific nature. However, there are caveats. One is that no individual study will contain the most complete information possible about everything in the appraisal guide. Sometimes, as in quantitative reports, the information really is there, built into the design itself but dependent on reader knowledge of the method. At other times, because the volume of data and findings may require a series of reports that focus on different aspects of the research, authors sometimes direct readers to introductory articles that are more focused on methods and broad overviews of the study. Also, space limitations and a journal's priorities determine the amount of detail that an author may provide in any given section of the report.

> 66 *Nothing in the world can take the place of persistence. . . . Persistence and determination alone are omnipotent.* 99
>
> *Calvin Coolidge*

Putting Feet to Knowledge: Walking the Walk

It is time to put feet to the knowledge the reader has gained through this chapter. The reader is encouraged to use Appendix B that demonstrates one approach to the application of the appraisal guide for qualitative evidence. The appendix contains 25 exemplars of qualitative research reports from the clinical literature. The selection process first involved a period of time spent in the stacks of a medical center library, discovering what clinicians in different fields of practice are reading and researching. Exploration validated the appropriateness of the preceding section. That is, it confirmed that clinical researchers across professions and specialty areas are "walking the walk and talking the talk" with regard to using a variety of qualitative approaches with attendant methodologies, terms, and concepts as discussed and defined above.

Choices resulting in the sampling presented here were guided by the following criteria:

- A mix of recent articles (2001–2002) representing a variety of concerns across different clinical areas
- A range of qualitative research designs that illustrate the achievement of valid results
- A range of research purposes that illustrate a variety of ways in which results may help readers care for their patients
- A variety of publication sources—clinical specialty as well as research journals, and interdisciplinary as well as nursing journals

Exemplars are arbitrarily grouped into three clusters of studies related to:

1. Care in different practice settings
2. Family issues and personal relationships

box 6.18

Guide to Critical Appraisal of Qualitative Research

QUICK QUESTIONS

What were the results of the study?

1. Is the phenomenon (human experience) clearly identified?
2. Does the research approach fit the purpose of the study?
3. Are conclusions consistent with reported study findings?

Are the results valid?

1. How were study participants chosen?
2. How were accuracy and completeness of data assured?
3. Do findings fit the data from which they were generated?

Will the results help me in caring for my patients?

1. Are findings relevant to people in similar situations?
2. Are the reader's insights enhanced or enlarged?
3. How may the research stimulate action?

DETAILED QUESTIONS

How does the researcher identify the study approach?

1. Are language and concepts consistent with the approach?
2. Are data collection and analysis techniques appropriate?

Is the significance/importance of the study explicit?

1. Does review of the literature support a need for the study?
2. What is the study's potential contribution?

Is the sampling strategy clear and guided by study needs?

1. Does the researcher control selection of the sample?
2. Do sample composition and size reflect study needs?

Are data collection procedures clear?

1. Are sources and means of verifying data explicit?
2. Are researcher roles and activities explained?

(continued)

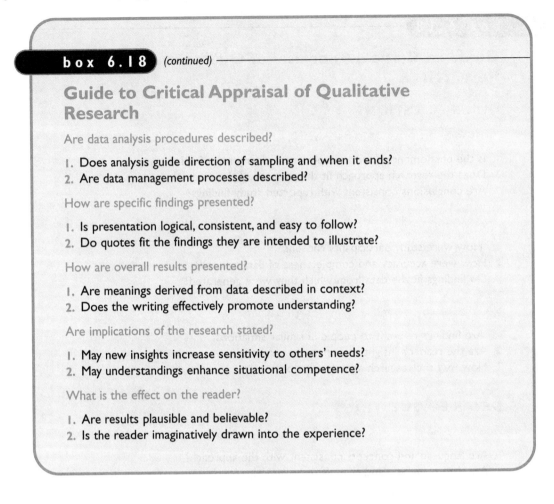

box 6.18 (continued)

Guide to Critical Appraisal of Qualitative Research

Are data analysis procedures described?

1. Does analysis guide direction of sampling and when it ends?
2. Are data management processes described?

How are specific findings presented?

1. Is presentation logical, consistent, and easy to follow?
2. Do quotes fit the findings they are intended to illustrate?

How are overall results presented?

1. Are meanings derived from data described in context?
2. Does the writing effectively promote understanding?

Are implications of the research stated?

1. May new insights increase sensitivity to others' needs?
2. May understandings enhance situational competence?

What is the effect on the reader?

1. Are results plausible and believable?
2. Is the reader imaginatively drawn into the experience?

3. Individual human experiences

Each is organized with a summarization of research questions, designs, and methods, using the quick appraisal format:

- What were the results of the study?
- Are the results valid?
- Will the results help me in caring for my patients?

These studies are all relatively good and typical examples of different types of qualitative work that span a variety of specialties. Factors that may affect reader response to the summaries are:

1. Individual preference: In the real world, persons choose the topics that interest them.
2. The ease with which the report submits to summarization: Appreciation and understanding of qualitative reports depend on individual reading of and engagement with the report in its en-

tirety. Therefore, the articles lose some of their communicative and evocative qualities when parsed apart and retold.

The results of the summarization process combined with individual preference may affect the studies' initial appeal. Because in every case evaluations of an article's plausibility and generalizability (transferability) require the use of independent reader judgments, first-hand reading is recommended.

It should be pointed out, as well, that under the criterion *assessing validity*, the author has tried to identify elements in the article that speak to Lincoln and Guba's (1985) trustworthiness criteria (credibility, dependability, confirmability, and transferability). This is done to show how portions of a report may convey the appropriate information without resorting to the use of this terminology. This is important because many scientifically sound reports do not refer to these criteria. Most of the ones selected for the appendix did not. Therefore, the reader needs to become comfortable with the method-specific criteria that authors elect to present. In the meantime, the approach taken here may help them to identify the many ways in which these more general references to trustworthiness and validity may be inherent in reports that by their nature will not use that specific language or be uniform in format and narrative style.

> 66 *Changes may not happen right away, but with effort even the difficult may become easy.* 99
>
> *Bill Blackman*

Keeping it Together: Synthesizing Qualitative Evidence

In EBP, there is support for the notion that "best practice should reflect the whole range of [research] evidence available—both quantitative and qualitative" (Pearson, 2002, p. 21). However, strategies for systematically and procedurally keeping the two together are at an early evolutionary stage.

There are, of course, examples of mixed-method studies that combine qualitative and quantitative approaches in different ways. For example, Creswell (2003) discusses mixed-method models that involve variations of several procedural strategies:

- Sequential—in "which the researcher seeks to elaborate on or expand the findings of one method with another method," beginning with either a qualitative or a quantitative approach
- Concurrent—in "which the researcher converges quantitative and qualitative data in order to provide a comprehensive analysis of the research problem"
- Transformative—in "which the researcher uses a theoretical lens as an overarching perspective within a design that contains both qualitative and quantitative data"(p. 16)

Although certain kinds of questions may effectively be pursued by combining qualitative and quantitative approaches in a single study, this does not make findings more valid, credible, or robust. And if care is not taken, a study could be weaker and less credible as a result of an uncritical, inappropriate use of mixed methods. When evaluating a research approach, readers need to be sure that the research questions are what lead the researchers to the most appropriate methods. It also should be understood that the advantages of combining methods in a single study are specific to that study. It would be too simplistic to think of mixed methods as a metaphor or as a symbol of how, in general, qualitative and quantitative research should come together in the minds of researchers or research consumers.

Keeping qualitative and quantitative research contributions together as alternative ways to understand the complexities of phenomena within clinical practice fields involves appreciation for how the strengths of each of these sets of approaches answer different questions and illuminate different aspects of clinical issues and concerns. More visibly drawing qualitative research into an EBP environment together with quantitative research is likely to be advanced by efforts at synthesizing bodies of qualitative evidence and incorporating qualitative evidence in systematic reviews.

Apart from and prior to the emergence of EBP, qualitative researchers have expressed the need to identify and synthesize critical masses of qualitative findings. These efforts focused on evaluation of the relative contributions of individual studies and elevation of the level of analysis of qualitative study findings. The result of qualitative secondary analysis or metasynthesis would be a formal theory or a new refined interpretive explanation of the phenomenon (Kearney, 1998; Sandelowski, Docherty, & Emden, 1997). Although there are examples of qualitative metasynthesis in the literature (Barroso & Powell-Cope, 2000; Beck, 2002; Jensen & Allen, 1994; Kearney, 2001; Morse & Johnson, 1991), there is a lack of clear direction or agreed-upon techniques for conducting such a study. This needs to be addressed, because there are numerous procedural issues to be overcome, including:

- How to characterize the phenomenon of interest when comparing conceptualizations and interpretations across studies
- How to establish inclusion criteria and sample from among a population of studies
- How to compare studies that have used the same or different qualitative strategies
- How to reach new understandings about a phenomenon by seeking consensus in a body of data where it is acknowledged that there is no single "correct" interpretation (Jenson & Allen, 1996)

Qualitative metasynthesis is a type of systematic review that "is firmly based in the interpretive paradigm, unlike quantitative meta-analysis techniques of statistically aggregating or averaging data" (Jensen & Allen, 1996, p. 554). Thus, metasynthesis is a holistic translation, based on comparative analysis of individual qualitative interpretations, which seeks to retain the essence of their unique contributions. Although individual studies can provide useful information and insights, they cannot give the most comprehensive answers to clinical questions. A benefit of the metasynthesis method is that it provides a way for researchers to build up bodies of qualitative research evidence that are relevant to clinical practice.

Incorporating Qualitative Evidence in Systematic Reviews

Because the focus of much of the EBP movement has been on determining the effectiveness of various interventions based on quantitative research findings, it is not clear how research findings from different methodological and epistemological research traditions can be synthesized and incorporated (Estabrooks, 1998; Pearson, 2002). In the quantitative domain, there are instruments to measure research quality and procedures for extracting numbers, such as means or standard deviations, to be subjected to statistical testing. But qualitative studies cannot be reduced to statistics. And because of the nature of qualitative data and the way they are produced, concerns about how to evaluate quality and do justice to multiple interpretations of a phenomenon introduce an element of complexity to the task. Fortunately, researchers are hard at work developing instruments and processes for appraising a set of qualitative studies.

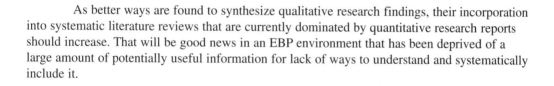

Examples include the work of The Joanna Briggs Institute for Evidence-Based Nursing and Midwifery in Australia (Pearson, 2002) at **http://www.joannabriggs.edu.au/services/sumariinfo.php** and The Qualitative Metasynthesis Project (Sandelowski & Barroso, 2002, 2003) at **http://nursing.unc.edu/research/current/qualitative_metasynthesis.html.**

As better ways are found to synthesize qualitative research findings, their incorporation into systematic literature reviews that are currently dominated by quantitative research reports should increase. That will be good news in an EBP environment that has been deprived of a large amount of potentially useful information for lack of ways to understand and systematically include it.

chapter 6

159

> **"***You will come to know that what appears today to be a sacrifice will prove instead to be the greatest investment that you will ever make.***"**
>
> *Gorden B. Hinkley*

references

Atkinson, P. (1992). *Understanding ethnographic texts*. Newbury Park, CA: Sage.

Averill, J. B. (2002). A portrait: Magdalena's Dream. *Public Health Nursing, 19*, 156–160.

Barroso, J., & Powell-Cope, G. M. (2000). Metasynthesis of qualitative research on living with HIV infection. *Qualitative Health Research, 10*, 340–353.

Beck, C. T. (1993). Teetering on the edge: A substantive theory of postpartum depression. *Nursing Research, 42*, 42–48.

Beck, C. T. (2002). Postpartum depression: A metasynthesis. *Qualitative Health Research, 12*, 453–472.

Benoliel, J. Q. (1996). Grounded theory and nursing knowledge. *Qualitative Health Research, 6*, 406–428.

Bluebond-Langner, M. (1978). *The private worlds of dying children*. Princeton, NJ: Princeton University Press.

Brown, M. A. & Powell-Cope, G. M. (1991). AIDS family caregiving: Transition through uncertainty. *Nursing Research, 40*, 338–345.

Chenitz, W. C., & Swanson, J. M. (1986). *From practice to grounded theory*. Menlo Park, CA: Addison-Wesley.

Chesla, C. A. (1994). *Parents' caring practices with schizophrenic offspring*. In P. Benner (Ed.), Interpretive phenomenology: Embodiment, caring, and ethics in health and illness (pp. 167–184). Thousand Oaks, CA: Sage.

Coffey, A., & Atkinson, P. (1996). *Making sense of qualitative data.* Thousand Oaks, CA: Sage.

Creswell, J. W. (1998). *Qualitative inquiry and research design: Choosing among five traditions.* Thousand Oaks, CA: Sage.

Creswell, J. W. (2003). *Research design: Qualitative, quantitative, and mixed methods approaches* (2nd ed.), Thousand Oaks, CA: Sage.

Csordas, T. J. (1994). *Embodiment and experience: The existential ground of culture and self.* Cambridge, England: Cambridge University Press.

Denzin, N. K. (1997). *Interpretive ethnography: Ethnographic practices for the 21st century.* Thousand Oaks, CA: Sage.

Denzin, N. K. & Lincoln, Y. S. (1994). Introduction. In N. K. Denzin & Y. S. Lincoln (Eds.) *Handbook of qualitative research* (pp. 1–17). Thousand Oaks, CA: Sage.

Ellis, C., & Bochner, A. P. (1992). Telling and performing personal stories: The constraints of choice in abortion. In C. Ellis & M. G. Flaherty (Eds.), *Investigating subjectivity: Research on lived experience* (pp. 79–101). Newbury Park, CA: Sage.

Estabrooks, C. A. (1998). Will evidence-based nursing practice make practice perfect? *Canadian Journal of Nursing Research, 30,* 15–36.

Farmer, T. J. (2002). The experience of major depression: Adolescents' perspectives. *Issues in Mental Health Nursing, 23,* 567–585.

Fawcett, J., Watson, J., Neuman, Walker, & Fitzpatrick, J. J. (2001). On theories and evidence. *Journal of Nursing Scholarship, 33,* 115–119.

Geertz, C. (1973). *The interpretation of cultures.* New York: Basic Books.

Geertz, C. (1983). *Local knowledge.* New York: Basic Books.

Giacomini, M. K. & Cook, D. J. (2000a). Users' guides to the medical literature. XXIII. Qualitative research in health care. A. Are the results of the study valid? *JAMA, 284,* 357–362.

Giacomini, M. K. & Cook, D. J. (2000b). Users' guides to the medical literature. XXIII. Qualitative research in health care. B. What are the results and how do they help me care for my patients? *JAMA, 284,* 478–482.

Glaser, B. G. (1978). *Theoretical sensitivity.* Mill Valley, CA: Sociology Press.

Glaser, B. G. (1992). *Emergence vs. forcing: Basics of grounded theory analysis.* Mill Valley, CA: Sociology Press.

Glaser, B. G., & Strauss, A. L. (1967). *The discovery of grounded theory: Strategies for qualitative research.* New York: Aldine.

Good, B. J. (1994). *Medicine, rationality, and experience: An anthropological perspective.* Cambridge, England: Cambridge University Press

Guba, E. G., & Lincoln, Y. S. (1989). *Fourth generation evaluation.* Newbury Park, CA: Sage.

Guba, E. G., & Lincoln, Y. S. (1994). Competing paradigms in qualitative research. In N. K. Denzin & Y. S. Lincoln, *Handbook of qualitative research,* (pp. 105–117), Thousand Oaks, CA: Sage.

Gubrium, J. F. (1993). *Speaking of life: Horizons of meaning for nursing home residents.* New York: Aldine De Gruyter.

Homans, G. C. (1955). *The human group.* New York: Harcourt Brace.

Jennings, B. M., & Loan, L. A. (2001). Misconceptions among nurses about evidence-based practice. *Journal of Nursing Scholarship, 33,* 121–127.

Jensen, L. A., & Allen, M. N. (1994). A synthesis of qualitative research on wellness-illness. *Qualitative Health Research, 4,* 349–369.

Jensen, L. A., & Allen, M. N. (1996). Meta-synthesis of qualitative findings. *Qualitative Health Research, 6,* 553–560.

Kearney, M. H. (1998). Ready-to-wear: Discovering grounded formal theory. *Research in Nursing & Health, 21,* 179–186.

Kearney, M. H. (2001). Enduring love: A grounded formal theory of women's experience of domestic violence. *Research in Nursing & Health, 24,* 270–282.

Kearney, M. H., Murphy, S., & Rosenbaum, M. (1994). Learning by losing: Sex and fertility on crack cocaine. *Qualitative Health Research, 4,* 142–162.

Kendall, J. (1999). Axial coding and the grounded theory controversy. *Western Journal of Nursing Research, 21,* 743–757.

Kleinman, A. (1988). *The illness narratives: Suffering, healing & the human condition.* New York: Basic Books.

Krueger, R. A. (1994). *Focus groups: A practical guide for applied research.* Thousand Oaks, CA: Sage.

Labov, W., & Fanshel, D. (1977). *Therapeutic discourse: Psychotherapy as conversation.* Orlando, FL: Academic Press

Lincoln, Y. S., & Guba, E. G. (1985). *Naturalistic inquiry.* Beverly Hills, CA: Sage.

Lofland, J., & Lofland, L. H. (1995). *Analyzing social settings* (3rd ed.), Belmont, CA: Wadsworth.

Melia, K. M. (1996). Rediscovering Glaser. *Qualitative Health Research, 6,* 368–378.

Mishler, E. G. (1986). *Research interviewing: Context and narrative.* Cambridge, MA: Harvard University Press.

Morgan, D. L. (1993). *Successful focus groups.* Newbury Park, CA: Sage.

Morse, J. M. (1991). Qualitative nursing research: A free-for-all? In J. M. Morse (Ed.) *Qualitative nursing research: A contemporary dialogue* (pp. 14–22). Newbury Park, CA: Sage.

Morse, J. M. (1994). Designing funded qualitative research. In N. K. Denzin & Y. S. Lincoln (Eds.), *Handbook of qualitative research* (pp. 220–235), Thousand Oaks, CA: Sage.

Morse, J. M. (1997a). Learning to drive from a manual? *Qualitative Health Research, 7,* 181–183.

Morse, J. M. (1997b). "Perfectly healthy, but dead": The myth of inter-rater reliability. *Qualitative Health Research, 7,* 445–447.

Morse, J. M. (1998a). Validity by committee. *Qualitative Health Research, 8,* 443–445.

Morse, J. M. (1998b). What's wrong with random selection? *Qualitative Health Research, 8,* 733–735.

Morse, J. M. (2000a). Determining sample size. *Qualitative Health Research, 10,* 3–5.

Morse, J. M. (2000b). Theoretical congestion. *Qualitative Health Research, 10,* 715–716.

Morse, J. M., & Johnson, J. L. (1991). *The illness experience: Dimensions of suffering.* Newbury Park, CA: Sage.

Morse, J. M., Penrod, J., & Hupcey, J. E. (2000). Qualitative outcome analysis: Evaluating nursing interventions for complex clinical phenomena. *Journal of Nursing Scholarship, 32,* 125–130

Newman, K. D. (1993). Giving up: Shelter experiences of battered women. *Public Health Nursing, 10,* 108–113.

Olson, C. T. (1993). *The life of illness: One woman's journey.* Albany, NY: State University of New York Press.

Paget, M. A. (1993). *A complex sorrow* (M. L. DeVault, Ed.). Philadelphia: Temple University Press.

Patton, M. Q. (1990). *Qualitative evaluation and research methods,* 2nd ed., Newbury Park, CA: Sage.

Peacock, J. L., & Holland, D. C. (1993). The narrated self: Life stories in process. *Ethos, 21,* 367–383.

Pearson, A. (2002). Nursing takes the lead: Redefining what counts as evidence in Australian health care. *Reflections on Nursing Leadership, 28*(4), 18–21.

Phillips, L. R., & Rempusheski, V. F. (1986). Caring for the frail elderly at home: Toward a theoretical explanation of the dynamics of poor quality family caregiving. *Advances in Nursing Science, 8*(4), 62–84.

Poirier, S. & Ayres, L. (1997). Endings, secrets, and silences: Over reading in narrative inquiry. *Research in Nursing & Health, 20,* 551–557.

Powers, B. A. (1988). Social networks, social support, and elderly institutionalized people. *Advances in Nursing Science, 10*(2), 40–58.

Powers, B. A. (2001). Ethnographic analysis of everyday ethics in the care of nursing home residents with dementia: A taxonomy. *Nursing Research, 50,* 332–339.

Powers, B. A., & Knapp, T. R. (1995). *A dictionary of nursing theory and research.* Thousand Oaks, CA: Sage.

Resnick, B. (1996). Motivation in geriatric rehabilitation. Image: *Journal of Nursing Scholarship, 28,* 41–45.

Richards, L. (1998). Closeness to data: The changing goals of qualitative data handling. *Qualitative Health Research, 8,* 319–328.

Richardson, L. (1990). *Writing strategies: Reaching diverse audiences.* Newbury Park, CA: Sage.

Richardson, L. (1992). The consequences of poetic representation: Writing the other, rewriting the self. In C. Ellis & M. G. Flaherty (Eds.), *Investigating subjectivity: Research on lived experience* (pp. 125–137). Newbury Park, CA: Sage.

Robrecht, L. C. (1995). Grounded theory: Evolving methods. *Qualitative Health Research, 5,* 169–177.

Sackett, D. L., Straus, S. E., Richardson, W. S., Rosenberg, W., & Haynes, R. B. (2000). *Evidence-based medicine: How to practice and teach EBM* (2nd ed.), Edinburgh: Churchill Livingstone.

Sandelowski, M. (1991). Telling stories: Narrative approaches in qualitative research. *Image: Journal of Nursing Scholarship, 23,* 161–166.

Sandelowski, M. (1993). Rigor or rigor mortis: The problem of rigor in qualitative research revisited. *Research in Nursing & Health, 16,* 1–8.

Sandelowski, M. (1995). Sample size in qualitative research. *Research in Nursing & Health, 18,* 179–183.

Sandelowski, M. (1996). One is the liveliest number: The case orientation of qualitative research. *Research in Nursing & Health, 19,* 525–529.

Sandelowski, M. (1998a). The call to experts in qualitative research. *Research in Nursing & Health, 21,* 467–471.

Sandelowski, M. (1998b). Writing a good read: Strategies for re-presenting qualitative data. *Research in Nursing & Health, 21,* 375–382.

Sandelowski, M. (2000a). Combining qualitative and quantitative sampling, data collection, and analysis techniques in mixed-method studies. *Research in Nursing & Health, 23,* 246–255.

Sandelowski, M. (2000b). Whatever happened to qualitative description? *Research in Nursing & Health, 23,* 334–340.

Sandelowski, M., & Barroso, J. (2002). Reading qualitative studies. *International Journal of Qualitative Methods, 1*(1), Article 5. Retrieved January 11, 2003 from http://www.ualberta.ca/~ijqm.

Sandelowski, M., & Barroso, J. (2003). Toward a metasynthesis of qualitative findings on motherhood in HIV-positive women. *Research in Nursing & Health, 26,* 153–170.

Sandelowski, M., Docherty, S., & Emden, C. (1997). Qualitative metasynthesis: Issues and techniques. *Research in Nursing & Health, 20,* 365–371.

Schatzman, L. (1991). Dimensional analysis: Notes on an alternative approach to the rounding of theory in qualitative research. In D. R. Maines (Ed.), *Social organization and social process: Essays in honor of Anselm Strauss* (pp. 303–314). New York: Aldine De Gruyter.

Spradley, J. P. (1980). Participant observation. New York: Holt, Rinehart and Winston.

St. John, W. & Johnson, P. (2000). The pros and cons of data analysis software for qualitative research. *Journal of Nursing Scholarship, 32,* 393–397.

Stern, P. N. (1994). Eroding grounded theory. In J. Morse (Ed.), *Critical issues in qualitative research methods* (pp. 212–223). Thousand Oaks, CA: Sage.

Strauss, A. L. (1987). *Qualitative analysis for social scientists.* New York: Cambridge University Press.

Strauss, A. L., & Corbin, J. (1990). *Basics of qualitative research: Grounded theory procedures and techniques.* Newbury Park, CA: Sage.

Thomas, J. (1993). *Doing critical ethnography.* Newbury Park, CA: Sage.

van Manen, M. (1990). *Researching lived experience.* London, Ontario: University of Western Ontario & State University of New York Press.

Van Maanen, J. (1988). *Tales of the field.* Chicago: University of Chicago Press.

Wallace, D. C., Tuck, I., Boland, C. S., & Witucki, J. M. (2002). Client perceptions of parish nursing. *Public Health Nursing, 19,* 128–135.

Wolcott, H. F. (1990). *Writing up qualitative research.* Newbury Park, CA: Sage.

Wolcott, H. (1994). *Transforming qualitative data.* Thousand Oaks, CA: Sage.

Wuest, J. (1998). Setting boundaries: A strategy for precarious ordering of women's caring demands. *Research in Nursing & Health, 21,* 39–49.

The author wishes to thank Mary T. Dombeck, PhD, DMin, RN, and anonymous reviewers for reading and commenting on earlier drafts of this chapter.

unit 2

162

Patient Concerns, Choices, and Clinical Judgment in Evidence-Based Practice

Patricia Benner and Victoria Wynn Leonard

chapter 7

> " *The right to search for truth implies also a duty: One must not conceal any part of what one has recognized to be true.* "
>
> *Albert Einstein*

Nursing like medicine, involves a rich, socially embedded clinical know-how that encompasses perceptual skills, transitional understandings across time, and understanding of the particular in relation to the general. Clinical knowledge is a form of engaged reasoning that follows modus operandi thinking, in relation to patients' and clinical populations' particular manifestations of disease, dysfunction, response to treatment and recovery trajectories. Clinical knowledge is necessarily configurational, historical . . . [(i.e.,] the immediate and long-term histories of particular patients and clinical populations), contextual, perceptual, and based upon knowledge gained in transitions. . . . [Through articulation], clinical understanding becomes increasingly articulate and translatable at least by clinical examples, narratives and puzzles encountered in practice" (Benner, 1994c, p. 139).

The use of research-based evidence in clinical practice is nearly as old as clinical practice itself. To qualify as a self-improving practice rather than a closed practice, it has always been incumbent on the practitioner to bring the latest and most accurate scientific information into any decision made on a patient's clinical problem. To improve or change tradition, nursing must demonstrate ongoing knowledge development and critical evaluation of science and practice.

In simpler times, there was little controversy about the "best" practice because scientific research was yet to proliferate into the multibillion-dollar enterprise that it has now become. "Evidence" was hard to come by and usually anecdotal. The most effective clinicians were keen observers who knew their patients and communities well, often caring for them over long periods of time.

What is new about the current evidence-based practice (EBP) movement in this time of expanding scientific research and information is the attempt to aggregate data in ever larger meta-analytic studies for application by responsible but hurried practitioners who often are working in impersonal practice settings and caring for large numbers of patients they seldom know well.

This enterprise of aggregating data relieves practitioners of some of the time-consuming reading, evaluating, and weighing of all of the published research relevant to their clinical practices. The body of health literature is expanding exponentially and is expected to double in 19 years. Clinicians' feelings of being overwhelmed by research "evidence" will certainly grow along with the literature, as will the need for a way to "digest" it. But the myth that enough "scientific evidence" exists to completely drive practice creates its own set of problems. That is why a critical evaluation of the strengths and weaknesses of the available evidence for any particular patient situation is so crucial to effective EBP.

Best Evidence: Research and Patient Concerns

Although the concept of applying "best evidence" in a clinical decision seems straightforward, it is actually very complex. Skillful critical thinking is needed to evaluate the evidence for its robustness and scientific rigor. Moreover, it needs to be considered in light of the patient's concerns and preferences. The patient's concerns and preferences are crucial because most clinical situations are underdetermined (i.e., knowledge and information are incomplete), and the particular patient and circumstance are changing across time. The patient's diagnosis may be imprecise and the degree of pathophysiology uncertain, and the patient's responses to particular interventions will vary.

Good clinical judgment requires the most critical and up-to-date appraisal of existing science and application of this evidence where it is most relevant to a particular patient's concerns and disease trajectory.

In thinking critically about EBP, a two-pronged approach is useful. First the validity of the evidence itself needs to be examined carefully. This involves assessing the way the research was conceived and funded as well as how the findings were disseminated (or not). Second, how the evidence is applied to clinical decision making must be examined because expert clinical decision making is a much more nuanced and multidimensional process than the straightforward application of evidence. Clinical decision making and application of evidence requires good clinical judgment that includes the patient's concerns, preferences, and choices.

If clinical judgment could be reduced to a 1:1 application of evidence to particular cases, practice could be completely standardized and applied in a strictly technical manner, accomplishing exact replication and reproduction of findings from the general to the particular case (to be discussed as "techne" later in this chapter).

Clinical trials constitute a high level of "best evidence" in EBP. Other levels of relevance include basic empirical bench and epidemiological science, narrative inquiry on illness experience and disease trajectories, case studies, and other qualitative research (discussed in other chapters). Even if clinical trials alone provided best evidence for a particular patient, the reliability of the trial must be critically evaluated, just as is required in all science (see Box 7-1 for an in-depth discussion of potential flaws in research evidence). To enhance good clinical judgment and to have confidence in clinical practice guidelines generated by "best evidence," we need "better evidence" as urgently as we require the "best" of what evidence is available to us. System reforms need to be directed upstream—where research and evidence generation begins—rather than midstream, where EBP tries to make the best of a situation at a point where critical biases are already anchored. Reconceiving research to eliminate upstream biases and to enhance clinical judgment will require restructuring the way we execute clinical research.

Even if the universe of clinical trials were perfect and meta-analysis could generate a perfect summary of what is known about treatment of a particular problem, practitioners would still have to proceed with caution. The logic of EBP provides a static snapshot of a conclusion based on aggregate evidence about one general condition to produce a yes or no decision. The clinician still must make a clinical judgment about a particular patient, usually with a complex particularized medical history and patterns of responses.

The practitioner must judiciously consider relevant patient particularities and concerns in making clinical decisions, such as gender, age, socioeconomic class, and illness experiences. In the patient's narrative, the particular clinical history, the social concerns, and the lifeworld concerns are revealed in ways that get covered over with just straight clinical information gathering.

Scannell (2002) argues that EBP "strives to be a little too much of everything . . . by proposing a system of medical knowledge that tries to eliminate subjective bias on one hand (in data collection and analysis) while invoking it on the other (through clinical applications that incorporate the subjective values of patients and the clinical judgments of physicians)" (p. 7). This is wonderfully illustrated in a *New York Times* article entitled "When Doctors Say Don't and the Patient Says Do" (Siegel, October 29, 2002).

Marc Siegel describes a determined 93-year-old woman who is a tap dancer and a former teacher of dance at Julliard. For the past 50 years, she was an avid tap dancer at amateur shows and recitals, until it was discovered that she had a "bulging disc in her neck and tissue so inflamed that it encroached on the space intended for the spinal cord, the crucial super-highway of the nervous system" (p. 7, Section F, Col. 1). All scientific evidence on prognosis for someone of her age undergoing spinal surgery unanimously showed that the risks outweighed the benefits, even though this particular patient's heart was in excellent health and she was also in excellent physical condition. When the risks of surgery were enumerated and weighed against the almost certain continued pain and incapacitation without the surgery, the woman asked, "Can the surgery make me dance again?" The physician replied, "It's possible." "Then," the woman responded, "I'll take my chances." A neurosurgeon who was willing to do the surgery was obtained. When the patient returned to the physician's office after surgery, she appeared to be a vigorous woman whose vitality was returning. Her walking had already progressed beyond her presurgical capacities.

Several weeks later, the physician received an invitation to her first postsurgical tap dancing recital. The woman explained, "You see, we patients are not just statistics. We don't always behave the way studies predict we will."

box 7.1

Thinking Critically About Clinical Trials

When evaluating evidence generated by randomized controlled trials (RCTs), practitioners need to consider increasing threats to valid results caused, for example,
by dropout rates and by several other factors:

- Exclusivity—the exclusion of women, children, minorities, elderly people, and individuals with mixed diagnoses and/or comorbid conditions from most clinical
  trials
- Conflicts of interest—on the part of the investigators
- Inappropriate involvement of research sponsors—in the design and management of RCTs
- Publication bias in disseminating trial results

Exclusivity

The exclusion of women, children, minorities, and those with complex chronic
medical problems from most clinical trials raises very basic issues of justice and
fairness, in addition to issues of validity of generalization of findings. These excluded populations constitute most of the population being treated with clinical
practice guidelines generated by "best evidence." Until clinical trials can become
more inclusive, the argument that patients are being treated based on the best evidence *for them* is usually not technically true.

Conflicts of Interest

Currently, between $300 and $600 million is needed to develop a single new drug.
This cost is rising as pharmaceutical companies look for new drugs for chronic
conditions. Trials to establish efficacy *of drugs* for chronic conditions require large
subject pools and lengthy study periods. They must be conducted at multiple centers to ensure statistical validity. Approximately 70% of the money for clinical drug
trials in the United States comes from industry rather than from the National Institutes of Health (NIH; Bodenheimer, 2000). In fact, the majority of NIH funding is
directed toward basic science research (DeAngelis, 2000). Thus, pharmaceutical
companies are conducting the lion's share of clinical research in the United States.
The threat of conflict of interest to the development of unbiased clinical practice
guidelines is a significant problem that must be addressed squarely by clinicians
who use good clinical judgment in evaluating evidence for clinical decisions for
particular patients.

Inappropriate Involvement of Research Sponsors

The vested interests of corporate sponsors of research are in the favorable review
of their products leading approval by the U.S. Food and Drug Administration (FDA)
and the ability to profitably market their products to both clinicians and consumers.
This vested interest shapes which products are chosen for development

(continued)

box 7.1 *(continued)*

Thinking Critically About Clinical Trials

(this is the reason for the moniker *orphan* for drugs with limited profitability) and how the evidence for their use is generated.

A significant outcome of sponsor involvement may be exemplified in clinical practice guidelines. These guidelines provide specific clinical recommendations for particular diagnostic entities. In a study designed to quantify the extent and nature of interactions between authors of clinical practice guidelines and the pharmaceutical industry, Choudhry et al. (2002) found that 87% of authors had some form of interaction with the pharmaceutical industry, and 59% had relationships with companies whose drugs were considered in the guidelines they authored. Some 55% indicated that the guideline creation process with which they were involved had no formal process for declaring these relationships. This is why critical appraisal of the relevant evidence is a central part of the practitioner's clinical judgment.

Publication Bias in Disseminating Trial Results

Marcia Angell (2000) in a *New England Journal of Medicine* editorial entitled "Is Academic Medicine for Sale?" reports that the *Journal* requires that guest editorial writers have no important financial ties to companies that make products related to the issues they discuss. Because of this relatively stringent attempt to prevent bias in the *Journal*, Angell reports, they routinely encounter difficulty in finding experts to write editorial reviews who do not have financial relationships with corporations producing products related to the reviews. This is especially true, she reports, in disciplines that involve the heavy use of expensive drugs and devices. Brennan (1994), also in a *New England Journal of Medicine* editorial ("Buying Editorials"), recounts being approached by a public relations firm asking whether she would be interested in writing an editorial for a medical journal. More accurately, the firm proposed that its editorial staff write the editorial for her review before submission under her name. The caller told Brennan that the entire project would be funded by a pharmaceutical manufacturer; her firm was merely the intermediary. She would be paid $2,500 for her time.

Traditionally, pharmaceutical companies contracted with academic research scientists to conduct clinical trials. Increasingly, though, corporate funding is now being channeled into contract research organizations (CROs). CROs are for-profit, independent contractors whose sole purpose is to coordinate and expedite clinical trials. During the 1990s, pharmaceutical companies increased the use of CROs from 40% to 80% (Rettig, 2000). At the same time, clinical study grant funding grew by more than 20% annually (CenterWatch, 2002). The result is a major shift in the way clinical research is being funded and conducted.

Academic centers continue to lose research dollars. They currently participate in about 50% of trials, down from 80% five years ago (Association of Clinical Research Professionals, 2002). With the movement of clinical research away

(continued)

box 7.1 (continued)

Thinking Critically About Clinical Trials

from academic centers, there is also a shift in the oversight of research. The more public and regulated space of academic research centers, where objectivity has always been the goal of research, is being replaced by the private, profit-driven, largely unexamined culture of CROs. This shift becomes more troublesome when one considers the expansion of CROs into activities such as medical writing for journals, including the ghost writing of "guest editorials" for peer-reviewed journals.

The validity of inferences made from any study sample depends on knowing that the sample is representative of the relevant population. Making valid inferences from meta-analytic synthesis requires that the sample of studies reviewed be representative of all studies that have been carried out.

Evidence-based practice (EBP) requires the practitioner to search for all available evidence, published and unpublished. That is why EBP is made easier by meta-analyses or integrative reviews that have done that work for the practitioner One criteria to discern an overview article's "worth" is if the authors speak to whether or not they have covered ALL the relevant studies, published and unpublished.

Many welcome the expansion of links between the private and public sectors. Some see it as the inevitable result of the growth of technology and the need for its dissemination and the reality of funding streams for clinical research. Others are understandably cautious. These relationships have the potential to both extend and despoil the growing body of clinical knowledge.

Clinical Judgment in Evidence-Based Practice

This story reveals the inextricable links between ethical and clinical decision making and the problematic implications of applying population-based research findings to individual patients. Good clinical judgment requires that the clinician discern what is good in a particular situation. The patient never offers an average statistical life to a possible medical intervention. Each patient has only one particular life and is concerned with his or her particular chances.

Every clinical judgment has ethical aspects about the goods and potential harms in a particular situation. The clinician must engage in a fiduciary relationship with the patient—acting in the patient's best interests and doing as little harm and as much good as possible. Scientific medicine separates the social from the medical in ways that nursing and doctoring particular patients never can. This patient presented clinical evidence that she experienced an exceptional health and fitness level, far different from projections based on the "average" 93-year-old person. One can imagine many different age-based scenarios with 30- or 60-year-olds who may be in extremely fragile health and who would require adjusted decisions based on their lower fitness and health levels. Social aspects, however, weighed in heavily in this decision, as in most other clinical decisions. The patient explained that tap dancing was her life. She literally could not imagine a life without tap dancing. She also had a robust confidence in her physical and emotional ability to withstand the surgery successfully. It is her life and her choice, and in the end, her outcomes proved that she was right.

This illustrates EBP at its best, where the science is there and indicates one path for treatment, but the patient's concerns and a realistic estimate of what is possible (for this exceptionally fit and active older woman) guides choices and decision making. Good clinical judgment always includes notions of good practice and a fiduciary relationship with the patient. The clinician used good clinical judgment in evaluating the medical feasibility of the woman's preferred decision and helped her find a surgeon who also found the risks acceptable. In the end, all clinicians learned from this exceptional patient. Including patients' central concerns, their history and information, preferences, and values in clinical decision making is a key to proficient EBP.

Nurses and doctors point out that they weave together a narrative understanding of their patients' condition that includes social and emotional aspects as well as many relevant current and historical clinical facts of the case (Benner, 2001; Benner et al., 1996; Tanenbaum, 1994; Cassel, 1991; Hunter, 1991; Wulff et al., 1990).

Elements of Good Clinical Judgment

Clinical judgment requires knowing the patient (Tanner et al., 1993) and entails reasoning across time about the particular through changes in the patient's condition and/or changes in the clinician's understanding of the patient's situation (Benner, Hooper, Kyriakidis & Stannard, 1999, p. 10–11). Clinicians use evidence based on psychosocial sciences and basic sciences (e.g., physiology, anatomy, biochemistry, pharmacology, genetics), reasoning across time about the patient's transitions and history, an understanding of the patient's particular concerns, and evidence that draws on a comparative analysis of research, not only on the results of randomized clinical trials (RCTs). It is a dangerous simplification to imagine that evidence from clinical trials could apply directly to a particular patient care decision without evaluating the validity of the clinical trial and its relevance for that particular patient. The evidence must always be interpreted by the clinician in terms of what she or he knows about the way the evidence was obtained and in light of the clinician's interpretations of the patient's concerns, history, family and cultural context, and disease trajectory.

Summary results of comparative evidence from clinical trials must also be critically evaluated. As noted earlier, crucial questions about possible flaws in the research must be considered. Were there biased commercial influences in the design, presentation, or dissemination of the research? What is the credibility of the research and how well can it be directly applied to particular patients? Sometimes the research is robust and convincing; at other times, it is weaker and more conflicted. Still at other times, the relevant clinical trial research for a particular patient has not yet been done. Practice patterns, skills, and clinical insights are never infallible; they need constant clarification (i.e., thoughtful questioning and reflection about particular patient outcomes and a careful review of the basic science and its effectiveness).

Clinical Judgment and Self-Improving Practices

To continuously improve a practice, different clinical interventions and consequent outcomes must be compared. The goal is for a practice to be a self-improving practice through science and experiential clinical learning and correction, rather than a closed or deteriorating tradition that repeats errors. A self-improving practice can be compared with a closed traditional practice that depends only on past patterns rather than correction from experiential learning and science. A self-improving clinical practice depends on experiential learning and clinical inquiry of every practitioner in the everyday course of their practices.

Experiential Learning

Experience, as noted by Gadamer (1976), is never a mere passage of time or exposure to an event. To qualify as experience, it requires a turning around of preconceptions, expectations, sets, and routines or adding some new insights to a particular practical situation. Experiential learning is at the heart of improving clinical judgment.

Experiential Learning: Techne and Phronesis

Joseph Dunne (1997) revisits the distinction that Aristotle made between *techne* and *phronesis*. In EBP, techne (i.e., the art or skill involved in deliberately producing "something") involves producing outcomes by a means-ends strategy, whereby the *maker or producer* governs the outcome by mastering the means of its production. When nurses talk about establishing prespecified outcomes, they are talking about outcomes that can be the only predictable outcomes of techne; for example, known blood pressure parameters in the responses of a particular patient to specific drug dosages within a narrow time frame. When influence, persuasion, patient concerns, preferences, fear, or other emotions are involved, outcomes cannot be prespecified because the outcomes depend on mutual agreements and situated possibilities for the patient and clinician, and on too many complex variables.

By contrast, phronesis, which is good judgment applied to human conduct (or to clinical practice), cannot rely strictly on a means-ends rationality determined by preset norms, standards, or separation of means and ends. Phronesis involves reasoning across time about changes in the particular patient's condition and changes in the clinician's understanding. For instance, a clinical guideline that specifies outcomes without identifying means for achieving the outcome for a particular patient is a good example of separating means and ends. Therefore, phronesis involves ethical comportment, clinical judgment, and a respectful fiduciary relationship with the patient and family. Phronesis depends on a patient-clinician relationship that allows discernment of the human concerns at stake and encourages a patient to disclose the concerns with confidence and trust in the safety of the relationship. Good patient-clinician relationships can guide actions and treatments that are in tune with the needs, concerns, and autonomy of the patient.

When means and ends are radically separated, both can be distorted and understanding lost about which good ends are worthy and how to create them. For example, one cannot separate the means of respectful and trustworthy communication with a patient from the ends of respect for the patient's autonomy and concerns. Nursing and medicine are compelled by safety and efficiency to use techne in situations where outcomes are predictable and reliable. However, it is false logic to assume that a clinical problem is amenable to simple standardized technical applications (techne) when reasoning about the *particular* (i.e., the patient's condition and/or changes in the clinician's understanding and/or patient/family notions of good) may alter technical and statistical prescriptions, as they did in the case of the tap dancer who did not fit the statistical profiles.

It is wise to establish solid scientific direction that can alleviate the uncertainty and risk of human judgments when possible. However, it is unwise to mistake a situation that requires clinical judgment about a particular patient and inappropriately apply a standard guideline that does not fit the situation because of clinical, ethical, social, or psychological reasons. Again, the woman who wanted to continue her rewarding life as a tap dancer had good reason to risk surgery, and it would have been less than good ethical and clinical judgment to deny her request.

Risks and Cautions

A risk of practice that depends on outcomes research based on the evaluation of clinical trials is that the practice works best in remedial situations in which current practices achieve below average outcomes for the patient populations. Practice that achieves lower than average success rates in light of evidence from multicenter clinical trials can guide practice improvement. However, in some situations, outcome success exceeds standardized expected success rates because of innovations and advanced practice skills in the local situation. In such cases, practice based on evidence from the multicenter trials must be critically evaluated to avoid degrading above-standard practice to the average success rates.

If an excellent center of practice is developing new lines of therapy and the level of skillfulness achieves what other centers do not, it is counter-productive to bring the outcomes down to the "standard" of practice when they are above the standard. Variation below the standard must be brought up to the standard. This is the remedial work of benchmarking. But practice that achieves above-standard outcomes should not be lowered to the standard; otherwise, the practice would cease to be innovative and self-improving.

Kierkegaard called this a dangerous form of leveling that results when public averages are used to adjust practice to fit public norms, regardless of the level of a particular practice. A self-improving practice needs to meet minimal standards, be engaged in ongoing improvements and experiential learning, raise standards in everyday practice, and evaluate intermittent external updates from scientific studies and practice guidelines.

Technical cure and restorative care cannot be mutually exclusive for the clinician. Basic natural sciences, evidence from clinical trials and other research, psychosocial sciences, and clinical judgment are partnered with the patient's concerns and changing condition, and all are implicated in discerning the best course of action in particular clinical situations. When nursing, medicine, and other healthcare practices are understood as *practices* that encompass more than the science and technologies they use to effect cures, all types of relevant knowledge can be brought to bear on the relational, particular, and ethical dimensions of the patient/family and healthcare. Notions of good are intrinsic to nursing as a socially organized practice. For example, accuracy, not error; attentiveness, not neglect; recognition practices, not depersonalization are notions of good that are internal to being a good nurse.

In most cases, good and poor nursing care can be recognized by nurses, even though it would be impossible to list formally all the precise behaviors and comportments of excellent nursing care. Kassirer (1992) noted that in medicine, "Controlled studies guide us in the right direction, but only occasionally do patients match the study population precisely. The art of medicine involves interpolating between data points" (p. 60).

Tanenbaum (1994), drawing on Kassirer, notes, "The experienced physician reworks patient, intervention, and outcome variables to set his expectations for the case at hand" (p. 37). It is not possible to list or formalize explicitly all aspects or features of an underdetermined social practice such as nursing, law, or social work. Philosophers call this problem the "limits of formalization" (Dreyfus, 1992). Likewise, the practical knowledge embedded in the traditions of science cannot be made completely formal and explicit (Lave & Wenger, 1991; Polanyi, 1958). Every complex social practice has a combination of formal theoretical knowledge and skilled practical know-how. Practical skilled know-how includes tacit and explicit knowledge.

Clinical Expertise

Everyday practical comportment of nurses includes a foreground of focused attention and a background that guides their perception and action. Science and technology formalize the reasoning and knowledge associated with scientific experiments to the extent possible. But even scientists have social influences that shape their practices and practical skilled know-how that escapes notice and formalization. It sometimes mistakenly appears that thinking within a particular scientific discipline is restricted to what can be made "formalizable," that is, turned into formal models, lists of formal criteria, or operational definitions. However, as Thomas Kuhn (1970) demonstrated through historical examples, every scientific community (such as clinical practitioners) has tacit, social, and nonrationalizable aspects to its scientific work. These aspects, for example, may include the use of metaphors, insights about what constitutes an interesting scientific problem, skillful know-how in conducting experiments, and other particularized practices, to name a few.

The practice of a particular discipline such as nursing or a science such as biochemistry contains the ethos or notions of what counts as good nursing or good scientific practice. In practice disciplines such as nursing and medicine, the ethos (i.e., ethics or notions of good) of practice influences what is considered relevant science, just as advances in scientific knowledge influence practice.

Experiential learning in clinical practice is a way of knowing, and it contributes to knowledge production. It also should influence the development of science. Viewing practitioners who actively learn from their practices as contributors to knowledge production further illustrates a nontechnological understanding of what constitutes a practice. That is, even though the practitioners use technology, they do not imagine that simple mechanical or production processes are all that is involved. Practitioners must use skillful attunement, discernment, interaction, and judgment in a facilitating relationship with the patient (Dunne, 1993).

Physicians also describe their clinical work as coming to know a patient (Tanner et al., 1993) and gaining a good clinical grasp, as described by Tanenbaum (1994) in an ethnographic study of everyday doctoring:

> The doctors I studied also did interpretive work. Virtually every senior physician spoke of the volume and complexity of medical information. "The number of complicating factors—parameters per patient—is unbelievable." And I observed attending physicians work and rework what they knew in order to make sense of an individual case. Doctors would find it "bothersome," or would be "confused" when they could not get a patient's pieces to "fit": "I don't put him together very well." They frequently used a visual metaphor in which their work was to discern "an emerging picture." One attending physician likened knowing a patient to viewing a canvas, arguing that computer manipulation of patient data "is like describing a painting," not incorrect exactly, but incomplete. According to this informant, the physician, like the viewer, comprehends a whole that is greater than the sum of its parts, and this grasp of a meaningful medical whole has been documented elsewhere—as perceiving a gestalt, getting a joke (Wartofsky, 1986), or calling up a prototype (Groen & Patel, 1985, p. 32).

Ethical and clinical perceptual acuity and good clinical judgment are central to safely practicing evidence-based nursing. Good clinical judgment depends on knowing the patient, understanding his or her concerns, preferences, history, and understanding of the illness, as well as the best relevant scientific knowledge (Benner & Wrubel, 1982; Blum, 1994; Vetleson, 1994). Theoretical and scientific knowledge alone are not sufficient to ensure that nurses will form helpful relationships with patients or that nurses will notice and correctly identify early signs and symptoms or therapy, anxiety, or suffering. This is true even though the nurse may know theoretically what the formal characteristics of these patient conditions are. The most formal measurements cannot replace the perceptual skills of the nurse in recognizing when a measurement is relevant and what the measurement means, which are at the center of good clinical judgment.

In addition, following the *course* of the patient's development of signs and symptoms (i.e., the trajectory or evolution of signs and symptoms) informs the clinician's understanding of the relevance of the signs and symptoms. The context and temporal unfolding of signs and symptoms are important. This creates the need for reasoning about the patient's transitions, not just considering a static list of signs and symptoms. The practitioner who applies algorithms or makes particular clinical judgments based on aggregate outcomes data alone ignores, at great peril, the clinical know-how, relational skills, and the need for reasoning across time that are essential for effective patient care (Halpern, 2001).

The value of EBP depends on the ongoing development of good clinical discernment and judgment combined with valid scientific evidence in actual practice. The Dreyfus Model of Skill Acquisition (Benner, 2001; Dreyfus, 1979) is based on determining the level of expertise in practice that is evident in particular situations. It elucidates strengths in the practice situation, as well as omissions or problems. Situated practice capacities (i.e., expertise as enacted in a particular situation) are described rather than traits or talents of the practitioners (i.e., these traits and talents exist separate from a particular situation).

At each stage of experiential learning (novice, advanced beginner, competent, proficient, expert), clinicians can perform at their best. For example, one can be the best advanced beginner possible, typically during the first year of practice. However, no practitioner can become more skilled without experience, despite the necessary attempts to make practice as clear and explicit as possible through care guidelines and clear instructions. If the nurse has never encountered a particular clinical situation, support from other clinicians, additional information, and experiential learning are required to accurately assess and manage the clinical situation. For example, referring to critical pathways is not the same as recognizing when and how these pathways are relevant or must be adapted to particular patients. Experiential learning that leads to individualization and clinical discernment is required to render critical pathways sensible and safe. Such individualization requires clinical discernment based on experience with past whole concrete clinical situations. This ability to make clinical comparisons between whole concrete clinical cases without decomposing the whole situation into its analytical components is a hallmark of expert clinical nursing practice. Each patient/clinician encounter requires understanding the particular patient's illness experience. Such an understanding of the particular patient is required for all health care practitioners. Such humanistic values are, as Eric J. Cassel (condensed and cited by Frankford, 1994) argues, essential also to good doctoring:

Proponents of medical humanism have stressed that good doctoring involves more than attending to disease. Illness is simply greater than a biomedically conceived problem. For example, when pneumonia develops in an elderly, grieving, socially isolated widower, in part because his inflamed arthritic knee has reduced his level of activity and led to malnourishment, it does little good simply to diagnose and treat that pneumonia and then send him back to the life-context from which he came. Diagnosis and treatment of the pneumonia is essential, of course, but alone it is insufficient because the cause of the illness is not only the pneumococcus that invaded his lungs. Rather cause derives from a unique and personal and social context: From the standpoint of the process that is an illness, it is artificial to stop at the boundaries of the body. The story of the old man includes the social facts of his solitude, the personal matter of his bereavement, his living conditions, his bad knee, his failure to maintain proper nutrition, the invasion of the pneumococcus, its progress in his lungs, his worsening infection, collapse, being discovered, being brought to the hospital, antibiotics, respirator support, and so on (Cassell, 1991, p. 13).

Accordingly, as Cassell has shown, good doctoring must consist of attending to this entire story of illness, and it must be a process of inserting values and treating the whole person. Instead of reducing patients to a few variables, whether stipulated by biomedical or social scientific positivism, doctors must be encouraged to contextualize their patients' problems because "clinicians treat particular patients in particular circumstances at a particular moment in time, and thus they require information that particularizes the individual and the moment" (Cassell, 1991, as cited by Frankford, 1994, p. 769).

A renewing, coherent, recognizable professional identity requires that practitioners develop notions of good that are constantly being worked out and extended through experiential learning in local and larger practice communities. These notions of good guide the judicious use of a range of sciences, ethics, and humanities used in their practices. Practice is a way of knowing, as well as a way of comporting oneself in practice (Ruddick, 1989; Taylor, 1993; Taylor, 1994). A self-improving practice directs the development, implementation, and evaluation of science and technology. Clinical judgment requires moral agency (i.e., the ability to affect and influence situations), relationship, perceptual acuity, skilled know-how, and narrative reasoning across time about particular patient transitions. As Joseph Dunne notes (1997):

> A practice is not just a surface on which one can display instant virtuosity. It grounds one in a tradition that has been formed through an elaborate development and that exists at any juncture only in the dispositions (slowly and perhaps painfully acquired) of its recognized practitioners (p. 378).

How Narratives Inform Clinical Understanding

A narrative mode of description best captures clinical judgment and experiential learning because a narrative can capture chronology, the concerns of the actor, and even the ambiguities and puzzles as the story unfolds (Benner, 1984; Benner, Tanner, & Chesla, 1996; Hunter, 1991).

Jane Rubin (1996) points out that the agent/actor's concerns organize how the story is told, what is included or left out, and even where the story begins and ends. Nurses' clinical narratives can reveal their taken-for-granted clinical understandings. Articulating those understandings verbally and in writing can assist in making innovations and experiential learning in practice accessible to others, thereby opening the possibility of making clinical knowledge cumulative and collective, as well as generating new questions and topics for research. Innovations and new clinical understandings occur in practice, but they will remain hidden if they are not articulated and made visible so that they can be evaluated and improved. Practicing nurses develop clinical knowledge and their own moral agency as they learn from their patients and families.

Experiential learning in most work environments—particularly in high-risk settings—requires courage and supportive learning environments. Nurses' stories can reveal the particular, nuanced, and ethically driven care that nurses elaborate in the course of taking care of particular patients. Embedded in these stories is clinical wisdom that other nurses can identify with and appropriate for their own clinical practices. Local practice communities develop distinct clinical knowledge and skills.

Collecting, reflecting on, and interpreting narratives both in practice and in academic settings can uncover new knowledge and skills and identify areas of excellence as well as impediments to good practice. One way to accomplish this is through telling and writing narratives in the first person about clinical situations in which the clinician learned something new. Teaching nurses and other clinicians to think reflectively about these narratives will help clinicians not only to identify the concerns that organize the story but also to see the notions of good embedded in the story. Reflective thinking also will enhance relational, communicative, and collaborative skills and articulation of newly developing clinical knowledge.

The goal of capturing experiential learning is to articulate new clinical knowledge, which involves the forming of the story, the concerns that shape the story, and how the story ends, as revealed in the dialogue and perceptions of the storyteller. Narratives reveal contexts, processes, and content of practical moral reasoning. Thus, stories create moral imagination (i.e., the ability to perceive when ethical issues are involved and to imagine how to respond to perceived ethical demands, even as they expose knowledge gaps and paradoxes).

Narratives about experiential learning reveal moral agency and changes in the storyteller's perceptions. Moreover, they reveal shifts in styles of practice. Because all research must be evaluated and implemented by the practitioner, ways are needed to capture this process of understanding and experiential learning inherent in translating research findings into practice. Often, storytelling about experiential learning occurs in shift reports or other oral reports between clinicians. For example, "the patient transitioned into a full-blown pulmonary edema with specific changes in hemodynamic parameters." Or, first-person, experience near narratives may be systematically gathered from clinicians who participate in interpreting the narratives. Experience near, first-person narratives provide the storyteller's direct first person account of an actual clinical situation. The following interview excerpt is taken from a naturalistic study of actual clinical situations in intensive care units (ICUs). In this interview, an advanced practice nurse (APN) illustrates clinical grasp and clinical forethought, as well as experiential learning:

> **APN**: A man was admitted to the ICU on a mechanical ventilator with a status post cardiac arrest. He had been intubated, on full ventilatory support for less than a day. . . . He did not appear to have any problems initially, at least in terms of ventilation and oxygenation, with ruling in for an MI. He was basically in a stabilization period of support. He was not instrumented with a PA catheter. He was awake, cognitively aware, at least as best as we could tell. . . . I remember getting a call late in the afternoon and the staff nurse thought that the patient seemed to be working a little bit harder on the ventilator, and she had approached the intern and the resident. I work in a teaching facility, and they looked at the patient, didn't really notice, particularly, that the patient was struggling with his breathing, or that there was a slight increase in the respiratory rate that seemed to be sustained. The nurse also had reported to me that the heart rate had been elevated, but the patient didn't appear to be hemodynamically compromised, so she wasn't too worried about it, but she was wondering if the ventilator settings were appropriate. . . . One of the first things that I noticed when I went in the room was that the patient wasn't breathing very rapidly, but he was using a lot more respiratory effort on each breath. . . . He was using more accessory muscles, and he was actively exhaling. The breathing appeared paradoxical, meaning he wasn't using the diaphragm; he was using accessory muscles. But there really wasn't a marked tachypnea pattern. And again, I

looked at the ventilator sheets to see again how long the patient had been on the ventilator. I was wondering if it was just . . . maybe . . . an agitation situation... maybe he needed some sedation, or [to figure out] what was going on. The nurse also remarked that in the last 20 minutes, the patient's mentation had deteriorated. Where he had been a little more responsive, he was now less responsive, and so she was even more nervous. So the three us—I believe it was either the senior resident or the junior assistant resident, myself, and the staff nurse—talking in the patient's room, or looking at the ventilatory parameters, and clearly the patient's mentation had deteriorated, breathing appeared to be more labored. So, I asked them if they had taken a recent chest x-ray, or if there was anything new going on with the patient that was important, and they said, "No, the patient had a chest x-ray in the morning as a part of a routine check, but there hadn't been any follow-up." I asked the nurse if there had been any change in breath sounds, and she said, "No." And the JR [junior resident], who was in the room, said he noticed no differences as well. So I took a listen, and the chest was really noisy, but I . . . I thought that the breath sounds were a little more diminished on the right side as opposed to the left side. So I asked if there was any indication to repeat the chest x-ray, or if that was their finding as well. Now with breath sounds, often there isn't symmetry necessarily and . . . but there wasn't anything outward in terms of chest excursion . . . and by visual inspection it looked like it would be symmetric. But nevertheless, I went ahead and looked at the ventilator parameters. The ventilatory support settings appeared to be appropriate. Possibly the backup rate could have been a little higher, but the patient wasn't really assisting much over the control rate. The patient had a pulse oximeter. Those settings were fairly stable, in the low 90s, as I recall, and the patient was not hypotensive
. . . was a little more tachycardic though than what the nurse had led me to believe over the phone, during our telephone conversation . . . somewhere around 120s, 130s . . . something like that. But the patient wasn't exhibiting signs of, you know, EKG changes or hypotension associated with that. He was on no vasoactive drugs at the time. There was a slight increase in the airway pressures, but it wasn't high enough that would really warn me that I felt that there was a marked change in compliance at that time. The patient appeared to be returning most of the tidal volume that was being delivered by the ventilator.

So I stayed in with the nurse, and we were talking and going over what the plan was and things we might be looking for in the evening, because it was late afternoon, and I was going to be getting ready to go home. So, right before I left—the nurse had temporarily left the room—I noticed, and at first I wasn't sure if it was just the room lighting, or, if there was a true color change. Subsequently there was a color change in the patient. But I noticed that the patient's upper torso looked a little duskier to me, especially the head and neck area. And I pulled his gown down. And I noticed there was a clear demarcation and color, and this was sort of in the midchest area, up to the neck and to the head. I listened to the breath sounds again and noticed that they appeared even more diminished on the right side, as opposed to the left side. So I was thinking that this was . . . maybe a pneumothorax. Again, the patient's mentation had not improved. When I brought this up to the JR, and actually the cardiology fellow was up there as well, in the latter part of the afternoon, they didn't think it was a pneumothorax because the patient was returning most of the exhaled volume. And they thought that under positive pressure, this would be a tension pneumothorax, and we should see a decrease in exhaled volumes or marked increase in airway pressures. And I know from the literature—and at least my own experience—it isn't always so clear-cut like that. So the chest x-ray was ordered, and not . . . probably 10 or 15 minutes from the time that I get this curb side-consult with the fellow and even before Radiology came up, this patient dropped his blood pressure, his heart rate went up, and when we listened to his breath sounds, it was clear the patient's breath sounds had decreased even more.

And there happened to be an attending over on the MICU in the coronary care unit attending a postarrest who came over, and emergently inserted a chest tube and clearly it was a big pneumothorax. And I guess what sort of stood out in my mind was that people were really looking at a lot of the classic parameters that they're taught that you should see. And I don't know if it was necessarily because of what I've read, or I think a lot of it has to do with what I've seen clinically, and I try to incorporate at least what I know from knowledge and what I've seen in practice, is that it isn't always so clear-cut. I mean, it just isn't. And sometimes you really have to kind of go on physical exam findings and not necessarily— it's important to pay attention to the things you anticipate, but sometimes the things that aren't so obvious can be very clinically significant.

This narrative account of experiential learning about clinical manifestations of a tension pneumothorax contains much practical knowledge about interpreting ambiguous clinical signs and symptoms, advocating for a needed diagnostic test (i.e., chest x-ray), negotiating different interpretations by getting different opinions, and finally responding quickly to a dramatic change in the patient's rapidly changing condition. It is a good example of the kind of modus operandi (MO) thinking involved in clinical judgment. MO thinking is the kind of thinking a detective uses in solving a case. Transitions, trajectories, and evidence are studied as they are uncovered—often narratively. The patient's trajectory matters in interpreting clinical signs and symptoms, but the story also illustrates two pervasive habits of thought and action in clinical practice: **clinical grasp** and **clinical forethought**.

Clinical Grasp

Clinical grasp describes clinical inquiry in action. Clinical grasp includes problem identification and clinical judgment across time about the particular transitions of particular patient/family clinical situations. Four aspects of clinical grasp include:

- Making qualitative distinctions
- Engaging in detective work
- Recognizing changing clinical relevance
- Developing clinical knowledge about specific patient populations

Making Qualitative Distinctions

Qualitative distinctions refer to those distinctions that can be made only in a particular, contextual, or historical situation. In the clinical example above, the nurse was listening for qualitative changes in the breath sounds, changes in the patient's color, and changes in the patient's mental alertness. Clinical appreciation of the context and sequence of events—the way a clinical situation changes over time—is essential for making qualitative distinctions. Therefore, it requires paying attention to transitions in the patient. Many qualitative distinctions can be made only by observing differences in the patient or patient's situation through touch, sound, or sight, as in skin turgor, color, and capillary refill (Hooper, 1995).

Engaging in Detective Work and More

Clinical situations are open-ended and underdetermined. MO thinking keeps track of the particular patient, the way the illness unfolds, and the meanings of the patient's responses as they have occurred in the particular time sequence. It requires keeping track of what has been tried and what has or has not worked with the patient. In this kind of reasoning-in-transition, gains and losses in understanding are understood by the clinician in a narrative form that culminates in the best possible clinical decisions for the patient (Benner et al., 1999; Elwyn & Gwyn, 1999). However, in the example, the clinician also thinks of the possibility of a pneumothorax. A second comparative chest x-ray is needed. Later in the interview, he states:

> **APN**: I guess it could have been a pulmonary embolus. But I was really sort of focused in the differences and the fact that it was fairly similar appearance, which can happen with pulmonary emboli. The heart rhythm pattern had not changed, although it was elevated. There was some tachycardia. But it sort of was leading me to believe that this was more sort of a pulmonary problem, as opposed to a pulmonary circulation problem, you know?

The clinician is guessing that this is a problem of physically moving air in and out rather than an obstruction in pulmonary circulation. The clinical evidence from the patient's signs and symptoms is subtle, so the clinician stays open to disconfirmation but proceeds with trying to get the chest x-ray and is prepared to recognize the sudden change in the patient's respiratory status when that occurs.

Another qualitative distinction was the judgment of whether the patient's change in mental status and agitation was due primarily to anxiety or to hypoxia. With MO thinking, sequencing and context are essential to making judgments. MO thinking uses the global understanding of the situation and operates within that situated understanding. The clinician was always focusing on some respiratory problem. The overall grasp of the clinical situation determines the approach used in MO thinking.

Recognizing Changing Clinical Relevance

Recognizing changes in clinical relevance of signs and symptoms and the patient's concerns is an experientially learned skill that enables clinicians to change their interpretations of patient data and concerns based on changes in the patient's condition. The meanings of signs and symptoms are changed by sequencing and history. For example, the patient's mental status and color continued to deteriorate, and his breath sounds diminished. Once the chest tubes were in place, there was a dramatic change in the patient's color. Clinical evaluation of each of these changes in the patient's signs and symptoms were made by examining the transitions in time and sequence as they occurred.

Developing Clinical Knowledge About Specific Patient Populations

Because this clinician has had the opportunity to observe both pulmonary circulation problems and mechanical breathing problems, he can recognize a kind of "family resemblance" with other mechanical breathing problems (as opposed to pulmonary circulation problems) that he has noticed with other patients.

Refinement of clinical judgment is possible when nurses have the opportunity to work with specific patient populations. Understanding the characteristic patterns of a particular patient population well can assist with recognizing shifts in a patient's disease trajectory that do not mesh with usual patterns and that, therefore, may signal a problem.

Clinical Forethought

Clinical forethought is another pervasive habit of thought and action in nursing practice evident in the narrative example. Clinical forethought plays a role in clinical grasp because it structures the practical logic of clinicians. Clinical forethought refers to at least four habits of thought and action:

- Future think
- Clinical forethought about specific patient populations
- Anticipation of risks for particular patients
- Seeing the unexpected

Future Think

Future think is the practical logic of the practitioner situated in practice (Bourdieu, 1990). In the example, the APN states, "So I stayed in with the nurse, and we were talking and going over what the plan was and things we might be looking for in the evening." Anticipating likely immediate future events assists with making good clinical judgments and with preparing the environment so that the nurse can respond to the patient's immediate needs in a timely fashion. Without this lead time or the developing sense of salience for anticipated signs and symptoms and the subsequent preparation of the environment, essential clinical judgments and timely interventions would be impossible in rapidly changing clinical situations.

Future think influences the nurse's response to the patient. Whether in a fast-paced ICU or a slower-paced rehabilitation setting, thinking and acting with patients' anticipated futures in mind guides clinical thinking and judgment. Future think captures the way judgment is suspended in a predictive net of thoughtful planning ahead and preparing the environment for likely eventualities.

Clinical Forethought About Specific Patient Populations

This habit of thought and action is so second nature to the experienced nurse that he or she may neglect to tell the newcomer the "obvious." Clinical forethought includes all the anticipated actions and plans relevant to a particular patient's possible trends and trajectories that a clinician prepares for in caring for the patient (Benner et al., 1999). Clinical forethought involves much local specific knowledge, such as who is a good resource and how to marshal support services and equipment for particular patients. The staff nurse used good judgment in calling the APN to assist in solving the puzzle when she was unable to convince the less clinically experienced JR. The APN made use of all available physicians in the area. Part of what made a timely response possible was the actual planning involved in closely monitoring the patient and mashaling other clinician resources in this situation that changed rapidly.

Examples of preparing for specific patient populations abound in all settings. For instance, anticipating the need for a pacemaker during surgery and having the equipment assembled and ready for use saves essential time. Another example might be forecasting an accident victim's potential injuries when intubation or immediate surgery might be needed for the accident victim.

Anticipation of Risks for Particular Patients

The narrative example is shaped by the foreboding sense of an impending crisis for this particular patient. The staff nurse uses her sense of foreboding about the changes in the patient's breathing to initiate her problem search. This aspect of clinical forethought is central to knowing the particular patient, family, or community. Nurses situate the patient's problems almost like a map or picture of possibilities. This vital clinical knowledge that is experientially learned from particular patients needs to be communicated to other caregivers and across care borders. Clinical teaching can be improved by enriching curricula with narratives from actual practice and by helping students recognize commonly occurring clinical situations.

For example, if a patient is hemodynamically unstable, managing life-sustaining physiologic functions will be a main orienting goal. If the patient is agitated and uncomfortable, attending to comfort needs in relation to hemodynamics will be a priority. Providing comfort measures turns out to be a central background practice for making clinical judgments and contains within it much judgment and experiential learning (Benner et al., 1996).

When clinical learning is too removed from typical contingencies and strong clinical situations in practice, nurses will lack practice in active thinking-in-action in ambiguous clinical situations. With the rapid advance of knowledge and technology, nurses need to be good clinical learners and clinical knowledge developers. One way to enhance clinical inquiry is by increasing experiential learning, which requires open learning climates where transitions can be discussed and examined—including false starts or misconceptions in actual clinical situations. Focusing only on performance and on "being correct" and not on learning from breakdown or error dampens the curiosity and courage to learn experientially.

Learning from experiential learning is central to developing one's moral agency as a clinician. One's *sense* of moral agency as well as *actual* moral agency in particular situations changes with the level of skills acquired (Benner et al., 1996). Experiential learning is facilitated or hampered by learning how to relate to patients/families and engage the clinical problems at hand. Those nurses who do not go on to become expert clinicians have some learning difficulty associated with skills of involvement (i.e., communication and relationship) and consequently, difficulty making clinical judgments, particularly qualitative distinctions (Benner et al., 1996). Experienced, nonexpert nurses saw clinical problem solving as a simple weighing of facts, or rational calculation. They did not experience their own agency (i.e., their ability to influence situations). They failed to see qualitative distinctions linked to the patient's well-being.

Seeing the Unexpected

One of the keys to becoming an expert practitioner lies in how the person holds past experiential learning and background habitual skills and practices. If nothing is routinized as a habitual response pattern, practitioners cannot attend to the unexpected, particularly in emergencies. However, if expectations are held rigidly, subtle changes from the usual will be missed, and habitual, rote responses will rule.

The clinician must be flexible in shifting between what is in the background and the foreground of his or her attention. This is accomplished by staying curious and open. The clinical "certainty" associated with perceptual grasp is distinct from the kind of "certainty" achievable in scientific experiments and through measurements. It is similar to recognizing faces or family resemblances. It is subject to faulty memory and mistaken identities; therefore, such perceptual grasp is the *beginning* of curiosity and inquiry—not the end.

In rapidly moving clinical situations, perceptual grasp is the starting point for clarification, confirmation, and action. The relationship between foreground and background of attention needs to be fluid so that missed expectations allow the nurse to see the unexpected. For example, when the rhythm of a cardiac monitor changes, the nurse notices the change in the rhythm's sound, and what had been background or tacit awareness becomes the foreground of attention (i.e., focal awareness). A hallmark of expertise is the ability to notice the unexpected (Benner et al., 1996). Background expectations of usual patient trajectories form with experience. These background experiences form tacit expectations that enable the nurse to notice subtle failed expectations and to pay attention to early signs of unexpected changes in the patient's condition.

Polanyi (1958), a physician and philosopher, wrote about the distinction between focal and tacit awareness. Tacit awareness operates at a perceptual level, usually as a result of a skilled embodied takeover of experiential learning. A tacit awareness allows one to notice changes without explicitly directing attention to the potential change until it happens. Clinical expectations gained by caring for similar patient populations form a tacit clinical forethought that enables the experienced clinician to notice missed expectations. Alterations from implicit or explicit expectations from a range of scientific studies, ethical concerns, and clinical experience set the stage for experiential learning, depending on the openness of the learner.

Conclusion

EBP must be contextualized by the nurse in particular clinical settings and particular patient-nurse relationships, concerns, and goals. EBP can provide guidelines and intelligent dialogue with the best practice options in particular situations. It cannot be assumed that the flow of knowledge is only from science to practice; it results also from direct experiential learning in practice. Patient/family and healthcare values and concerns, as well as practice-based knowledge, must also be central to the dialogue between patient and clinician that incorporates the patients' values, concerns, and choices. In patient situations, EBP also incorporates developing expertise and using clinical judgment in conjunction with valid science to provide the best possible care.

References

Angell, M. (2000). Is academic medicine for sale? *New England Journal of Medicine, 342,* 1516–1518.

Association of Clinical Research Professionals (2002). *White paper on future trends.* Retrieved from http://www.acrpnet.org/index_fl.html. Accessed November 24, 2002.

Benner, P. (1984; 2001). *From novice to expert: Excellence and power in clinical nursing practice.* Menlo Park, CA: Addison-Wesley.

Benner, P. (1994). The role of articulation in understanding practice and experience as sources of knowledge in clinical nursing. In Tully, J. & Wenstock, D. M. (Eds.). *Philosophy in an age of pluralism. The Philosophy of Charles Taylor, 9,* 136–155.

Benner, P., Hooper-Kyriakidis, P., & Stannard, D. (1999). *Clinical wisdom and interventions in critical care: A thinking-in-action approach.* Philadelphia: W.B. Saunders.

Benner, P., Tanner, C. A., & Chesla, C. A. (1996). *Expertise in nursing practice: Caring, clinical judgment, and ethics.* New York: Springer.

Benner, P., & Wrubel, J. (1982). Clinical knowledge development: The value of perceptual awareness. *Nurse Educator, 7,* 11–17.

Blum, L. (1994). *Moral perception and particularity.* Cambridge, England: Cambridge University Press.

Bodenheimer, T. (2000). Uneasy alliance: Clinical investigators and the pharmaceutical industry. *New England Journal of Medicine, 342,* 1539–1544.

Bourdieu, P. (1990). *The logic of practice.* (R. Nice, Trans.) Stanford, CA: Stanford University Press.

Brennan, T. A. (1994). Buying editorials. *New England Journal of Medicine, 331,* 673–675.

Cassel, E. J. (1991). *The nature of suffering and the goals of medicine.* New York: Oxford University Press.

Choudhry, N. K., Stelfox, H. T., & Detsky, A. S. (2002). Relationships between authors of clinical practice guidelines and the pharmaceutical industry. *JAMA, 287,* 612–617.

CenterWatch Newsletter, 9(9), September 2002.

DeAngelis, C. D. (2000). Conflict of interest and the public trust. *JAMA, 284,* 2237–2238.

Dreyfus, H. L. (1992). *What computers still can't do: A critique of artificial reason.* Cambridge, MA: MIT.

Dreyfus, H. L. (1979). *What computers can't do: The limits of artificial intelligence* (Rev. ed.). New York: Harper & Row.

Dunne, J. (1997). *Back to the rough ground, practical judgment and the lure of technique.* Notre Dame, IN: University of Notre Dame Press.

Dunne, J. (1993). *Back to the rough ground, practical judgment and the lure of technique.* Notre Dame, IN: University of Notre Dame Press.

Frankford, D. M. (1994). Scientism and economism in the regulation of health care. *Journal of Health Politics, Policy and Law, 19,* 773–799.

Gadamer, H. G. (1976). *Truth and method.* Barden G., Cumming J. (Eds. and Trans.). New York: Seabury.

Groen, G. J., & Patel, V. L. (1985). Medical problem-solving: Some questionable assumptions. *Medical Education, 19,* 95–100.

Halpern, J. (2001). *From detached concern to empathy. Humanizing medical care.* London: Oxford University Press.

Hooper, P. L. (1995). Expert titration of multiple vasoactive drugs in post-cardiac surgical patients: An interpretive study of clinical judgment and perceptual acuity. Unpublished doctoral dissertation, University of California at San Francisco, San Francisco.

Hunter, K. M. (1991). *Doctors' stories: The narrative structure of medical knowledge.* Princeton, NJ: Princeton University Press.

Kassirer, J. P. (1992). Clinical problem-solving–A new feature in the journal. *New England Journal of Medicine, 326,* 60–61.

Kierkegaard, S. (1962 Trans.). *The present age.* New York: Harper & Row.

Kuhn, T. S. (1970). *The structure of scientific revolutions.* (2nd ed.). Chicago: University of Chicago.

Lave, J. & Wenger, E. (1991) *Situated learning: Legitimate peripheral perspectives (Learning in doing: Social, cognitive and computational perspectives.)* Cambridge, England: Cambridge University Press.

Polanyi, M. (1958). *Personal knowledge: Towards a post-critical philosophy.* New York: Harper & Row.

Rettig, R. A. (2000). The industrialization of clinical research. *Health Affairs, 19,* 129–146.

Rubin, J. (1996). Impediments to the development of

clinical knowledge and ethical judgment in critical care nursing. In P. Benner, C. A. Tanner, & C. A. Chesla (Eds.). *Expertise in nursing practice: Caring, clinical judgment, and ethics* (pp. 170–192). New York: Springer.

Ruddick, S. (1989). *Maternal thinking: Toward a politic of peace.* New York: Ballantine.

Scannell, K. (2002). Interrogating the bodies of evidence: Patients and the foundations of evidence-based medicine. Kaiser Permanente: *Ethics Rounds, 11*(1), 8.

Siegel, M. (2002). When doctors say don't and the patient says do. *New York Times* (Science). Oct. 29, p. D7.

Tanenbaum, S. J. (1994). Knowing and acting in medical practice: The epistemological politics of outcomes research. *Journal of Health Politics, Policy and Law, 19*(1), 31–44.

Tanner, C. A., Benner, P., Chesla, C. A., Gordon, D. R. (1993). The phenomenology of knowing the patient. *Image, 25,* 273–280.

Taylor, C. (1993). Explanation and practical reason. In M. Nussbaum & A. Sen (Eds.). *The quality of life.* Oxford, England: Clarendon.

Taylor, C. (1994). Philosophical reflections on caring practices. In S. S. Phillips & P. Benner (Eds.). *The crisis of care: Affirming and restoring caring practices in the helping professions* (pp. 174–187.). Washington, DC: Georgetown University Press.

Vetleson, A. J. (1994). *Perception, empathy, and judgment: An inquiry into the preconditions of moral performance.* University Park, PA: Pennsylvania State University Press.

Wartofsky, M. W. (1986). Clinical judgment, expert programs, and cognitive style: A counter-essay in the logic of diagnosis. *Journal of Medicine and Philosophy, 11,* 81–92.

Wulff, H. R., Pederson, S. A., & Rosenberg, R. (1990). *Philosophy of medicine: An introduction.* Oxford, England: Blackwell Scientific.

Acknowledgment

This chapter draws heavily on two chapters in *Clinical wisdom and Interventions in Critical Care: A Thinking-in-Action Approach.* Philadelphia: W. B. Saunders, 1999. Chapter Two, "Clinical Grasp and Clinical Inquiry: Problem Identification and Clinical Problem Solving," pp. 23–61, was developed primarily by Patricia Hooper-Kyriakidis, RN, PhD. Chapter Three, "Clinical Forethought: Anticipating and Preventing Potential Problems," pp. 63–87, was developed primarily by Patricia Benner, RN, PhD.

unit three

Steps Four and Five: Applying the Evidence

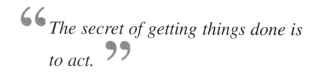

" *The secret of getting things done is to act.* "

Dante Alighieri

Using Models and Strategies for Evidence-Based Practice

Donna Ciliska, Alba DiCenso, Bernadette Mazurek Melnyk, and Cheryl Stetler

chapter 8

- Continuous caregiver support during labor reduced the frequency of episiotomy and cesarean delivery, the need for intrapartum analgesia, and the proportion of infants with an Apgar score lower than 7 at 5 minutes (Hodnett, 2002).

- Placing mechanically ventilated adults in a semirecumbent position rather than in a supine position reduced the rate of nosocomial pneumonia (Drakulovic et al., 1999).

- An educational-behavioral intervention provided to mothers shortly following their premature infants' admissions to the neonatal intensive care unit improved infant cognitive development at 6 months corrected age (Melnyk et al., 2001).

Each intervention cited above is within the scope of clinical practice for healthcare providers. Evidence from these studies indicates their positive impact on patient outcomes and their likely economic benefits for the healthcare system. However, are nurses and other healthcare professionals aware of these studies? How do they learn about them? How can healthcare providers keep up to date with new knowledge that relates to their practices? Once they acquire new knowledge, how do healthcare providers change their own practices and influence others to change practice behaviors within their organizations? Are evaluations conducted to determine whether evidence-based changes in clinical practice result in beneficial outcomes? All of these questions are important in determining the best method for implementing **evidence-based practice** (EBP) (Box 8-1).

The Positive Impact of Interventions on Patient Outcomes

Studies indicate that many nurses as well as other healthcare providers do not actively incorporate research findings into practice. Bostrum and Suter (1993) found that only 21% of 1,200 practicing nurses had implemented a new research finding in the previous 6 months. Furthermore, a qualitative study that explored community nurse decision making in the United Kingdom determined that nurses had an awareness of research but did not perceive it as informing practice (Luker & Kenrick, 1992). Despite these findings, many nurses and other healthcare providers are strongly motivated to become evidence-based practitioners. As a result, there is a paradigm shift from traditional and intuition-driven practice to EBP (Hallas & Melnyk, 2003; Rosswurm & Larrabee, 1999). An important question now is how this shift can be further facilitated.

In the past, nurses and other healthcare providers translated research findings into practice via the **research utilization** movement, which led to the implementation of some research-based findings into practice.

---

box 8.1

Definition of Evidence-Based Practice

EBP is the conscientious use of current best evidence in making decisions about patient care (Sackett, Straus, Richardson, Rosenberg, & Hayes, 2000). It is a problem-solving approach to practice that incorporates:

- A systematic search for and critical appraisal of the most relevant evidence to answer a burning clinical question
- One's own clinical expertise
- Patient preferences and values

Note: *An overview of the steps in EBP is highlighted in Chapter 1.*

Although the terms *research utilization* and *EBP* are often used interchangeably, they are distinguished from each other in this book. Research utilization is the use of research knowledge, often based on a single study, in clinical practice, whereas EBP involves a larger skill set that takes into consideration all of the following factors:

- Best evidence from a thorough search and critical appraisal of all relevant studies
- Context (Kitson, Harvey, & McCormack, 1989)
- Healthcare resources
- Practitioner skills
- Patient status and circumstances
- Patient preferences and values (DiCenso, Cullum, Ciliska, & Guyatt, in press)

This chapter will highlight selected models developed to advance research utilization and EBP, both from individual and organizational perspectives, and will discuss a more general and inclusive model of research dissemination and utilization for healthcare policy and practice. Barriers to EBP and strategies implemented by individuals and organizations to overcome these barriers are discussed. Finally, innovative but not formally evaluated strategies for implementing evidence-based practices will be presented to stimulate ideas for further research.

Models of Evidence-Based Practice and Research Utilization

There has been and continues to be clouding of the boundaries between research utilization and EBP. The models developed by Funk and colleagues (1989) and Stetler (1994) were important historically for promoting practice that deemphasized ritual and isolated, unsystematic clinical experiences based on ungrounded opinion and tradition as well as for raising awareness about the importance of applying research findings in nursing practice.

Funk's Model of Research Dissemination

Funk and colleagues (1989) developed a model for the dissemination of research. The three major components of the model include:

1. Qualities of the research—encompasses the topic, relevance, applicability, and availability of research; the level of control practitioners have over the practice; and the gap between research and practice
2. Characteristics of the communication—use of nontechnical language, emphasis on implications, clarification of limits on **generalizability** (i.e., the ability to say that a study's findings will be applicable to patients in other practice settings), strategies for implementation, demonstration of new techniques, broad dissemination, and discussion between researchers and clinicians
3. Facilitation of utilization—reinforcement of new knowledge, ongoing dialogue between researchers and clinicians, updates on research in the area, sharing of experiences, and giving of support during implementation experiences

Thus, this model considers a number of barriers and facilitators to the utilization of research and gives suggestions for strategies to optimize the uptake of evidence for individuals as well as for organizations.

Stetler Model of Research Utilization and Evidence-Based Practice

The Stetler/Marram model for research utilization, published in 1976, was created to fill a void in existent research textbooks. Specifically, although those textbooks described components of the research process and its importance for the nursing profession, they provided little guidance for progressing from the critique of published findings to application in practice. Since 1976, the Stetler/Marram research utilization model has been revised twice, although its core focus on critical thinking has not changed (Stetler, 1994a, 2001a). When its utilization-related actions are implemented and sustained in the practice setting, the result is EBP (Stetler, 2001a, 2001b).

Overview of the Stetler Model

The Stetler model (Figure 8-1) outlines a prescriptive series of steps to assess and use research findings, thereby facilitating safe and effective EBP. Over the years of its evolution, the phases within the model have shifted from three to six to five. The model grew in complexity in 1994. Since then, it has provided greater guidance for using critical utilization concepts and the details and options involved in applying research to practice in the real world.

The Stetler model has long been known as a "practitioner-oriented" model because of its focus on critical thinking and use of findings by the individual, knowledgeable practitioner (Stetler & Marram, 1976; Kim, 1999). The 2001 version clarified that this guided problem-solving process also applies to groups of practitioners engaged in research utilization projects. Yet it maintains the bottom line that even prepackaged, research-based recommendations are applied to patients, staff members, or other targets of use at the skilled-practitioner level. Without targeted critical thinking at that level, application of research may become a task-oriented, mechanistic routine that can lead to inappropriate, ineffective, and non-EBP.

Definitions of Terms in the Stetler Model

The term *evidence* first appeared in the model in 1976 and, at that stage, referred only to research findings. It was used in the context of *substantiating evidence,* one of four criteria used to determine the applicability of acceptable findings. However, in 1994, the concept of substantiating evidence was broadened to include additional sources of information because "experiential and theoretical information are more likely to be combined with research information than they are to be ignored" (Stetler, 1994a, p. 17).

By 2001 (Stetler, 2001a, 2001b), the concept of evidence had become a key element of the model, appearing 19 times within the two-page "visual" model (see Figure 8-1A and B). Key to understanding the multifaceted meaning of evidence within the current version of the model are the following (Stetler, 2001a, 2001b; Stetler et al., 1998):

- Evidence, within the context of healthcare, is defined as information or facts that are systematically obtained (i.e., obtained in a manner that is replicable, observable, credible, verifiable, or basically supportable) (Stetler, 2002).

Evidence, within the context of healthcare, can come from different sources and can vary in the degree to which it is systematically obtained and, thus, the degree to which it is perceived as basically supportable for safe and effective use.

Different sources of evidence can be categorized as external and internal. *External evidence* comes primarily from research. Without research findings, there would be no EBP movement. However, where research findings are lacking, the consensus opinion/experience of widely recognized experts is considered to be supportable evidence and will often be used to supplement "research-based recommendations" for practice.

Internal evidence comes primarily from systematically but locally obtained facts or information. This includes data from local performance, planning, quality, outcome, and evaluation activity. This also includes the evaluative data collected by research utilization models. In addition, it includes the *consensus* opinion and experience of local groups, as well as *experiential information* from individual healthcare professionals. Another type of internal evidence would be affirmed experience. Although an individual professional's isolated, unsystematic experience and related opinion is not considered to be credible evidence (Stetler, 2001a; Stetler, 1998a; also see Rycroft-Malone, Kitson, Harvey, McCormack, Seers, et al., 2002), those experiential observations or information that have been reflected on, externalized, or exposed to explorations of truth and verification from various sources of data affirm clinicians' experiences and are considered valid evidence in the model.

Haynes (2002) notes the importance of "evidence of patients' circumstances and wishes" (p. 3). Patient wishes are commonly included in EBP definitions, usually labeled as "patient preferences," and should be considered internal evidence (Goode & Piedalue, 1999; Haynes, Sackett, Gray, Cook, & Guyatt, 1996).

Using the Stetler Model

The basic "how to" of research utilization is divided into the following five progressive categories or phases of activity. Figure 8-1 and related publications provide specific guidance and rationale for each of these steps (Stetler, 1994a, 2001a).

1. Preparation: Getting started in research utilization by defining and affirming a priority need, reviewing the context in which research utilization would occur, organizing the work if more than an individual practitioner is involved, and systematically initiating a search for relevant research evidence
2. Validation: Assessing a body of evidence by systematically critiquing each study with a utilization focus in mind, then choosing and summarizing the collected research that relates to the identified need
3. Comparative evaluation/decision making: Making decisions about use after synthesizing the body of summarized evidence by applying a set of utilization criteria, then deciding whether and, if so, what to use in light of the identified need
4. Translation/application: Converting findings, planning their application, and putting the plan to use by defining operational details of how to use the acceptable findings, then implementing use with an evidence-based change plan (Stetler, 2001a)
5. Evaluation: Evaluating the plan in terms of the degree to which it was implemented and whether the goals for using the evidence were met

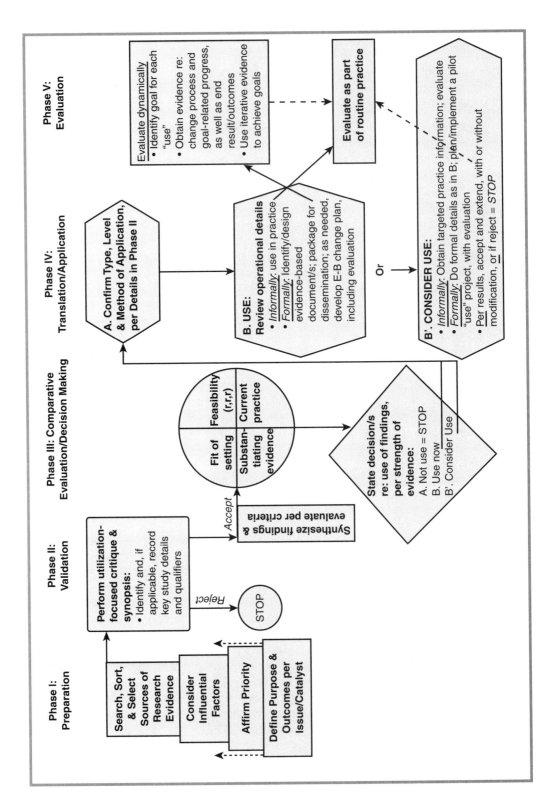

Phase I: Preparation	Phase II: Validation	Phase III: Comparative Evaluation/Decision Making	Phase IV: Translation/Application	Phase V: Evaluation

Phase I: Preparation

Purpose, Context, & Sources of Research Evidence:

- **Potential Issues/Catalysts**
  = a problem, including unexplained variations or less-than-best practice; or routine update of knowledge; or validation/routine revision of procedure, policy, etc; or innovative program goal
- **Affirm perceived problems, with internal evidence**
- **Focus on high priority issues**
- **Decide if need to form a team or involve formal "structures"/key stakeholders**
- **Consider other influential internal and external factors, such as beliefs, resources, or timelines**
- **Define desired, measurable outcome/s**
- **Seek out systematic reviews**
- **Determine need for an explicit type of relevant evidence, if relevant**
- **Select research sources with conceptual fit**

Phase II: Validation

Credibility of Findings & Potential for/Detailed Qualifiers of Application:

- **Critique & synopsize essential components, operational details, and other qualifying factors, per source**
  ◦ See instructions for use of utilization-focused review tables to facilitate this task; fill in the tables for group decision making or potential future synthesis
- **Critique systematic reviews**
- **Re-assess fit of individual sources**
- **Rate the level & quality of each evidence source per a "table of evidence"**
- **Differentiate statistical and clinical significance**
- **Eliminate non-credible sources**
- **End the process if there is no evidence or there is clearly insufficient credible research evidence that meets your needs**

See Stetler, Morsi, Rucki, et al. Appl Nurs res 1998; 11(4):195–206 for noted tables, reviews, & synthesis process.

Phase III: Comparative Evaluation/Decision Making

Synthesis & Decisions/Recommendations per Criteria of Applicability:

- **Synthesize the cumulative findings:**
  ◦ Logically organize & display the similarities and differences across multiple findings, per common aspects or sub-elements of the topic under review
  ◦ Evaluate degree of substantiation of each aspect/sub-element; reference any qualifying conditions
- **Evaluate degree & nature of other criteria:** feasibility (r,r,r = risk, resources, readiness); pragmatic fit; & current practice
- **Make a decision whether/what to use:**
  ◦ Can be a personal practitioner-level decision or a recommendation to others
  ◦ Judge the strength of this decision; and indicate if primarily "research-based" or, per use of supplemental information, "evidence-based"; qualify the related level of strength of decision/recommendations per related table
  ◦ For formal recommendations, determine degree of stakeholder consensus
- **If decision = "Not use" research findings:**
  ◦ May conduct own research or delay use till additional research done by others
  ◦ If still decide to act now, e.g., on evidence of consensus or another basis for practice, STOP use of model but consider need for planned change and evaluation.
- **If decision = "Use/Consider Use," can mean a recommendation for or against a specific practice**

Phase IV: Translation/Application

Operational Definition of Use/Actions for Change:

- **Types** = cognitive, symbolic &/or instrumental
- **Methods** = informal or formal; direct or indirect
- **Levels** = individual, group or department/organization
- **Direct instrumental use:** change individual behavior (vis-à-vis assessment; plan/intervention options; implementation details; &/or evaluation); **or** change policy, procedure, protocol, algorithm, program components, etc.
- **Cognitive use:** validate current practice; change personal way of thinking; increase awareness; better understand or appreciate condition/s or experience/s
- **Symbolic use:** develop position paper or proposal for change; or persuade others regarding a way of thinking
- **CAUTION: Assess whether translation/product or use goes beyond actual findings/evidence:**
  ◦ Research evidence may or may not provide various details for a complete policy, procedure, etc.; indicate this fact to users, and note differential levels of evidence therein
- **Formal dissemination & change strategies should be planned per relevant research** (Include Dx analysis):
  ◦ Simple, passive education is rarely effective as an isolated strategy. Consider multiple strategies, e.g., interactive education, opinion leaders, educational outreach, audit, etc.
- **Consider need for appropriate, reasoned variation**
- **WITH B, where have made a decision to use in the setting:**
  ◦ With formal use, may need a dynamic evaluation to effectively implement & continuously improve/refine use of best available evidence
- **WITH B', where have made a decision to consider use & thus obtain additional, pragmatic information before a final decision**
  ◦ With formal consideration, need a pilot project
  ◦ With a pilot project, must assess if need IRB review, per relevant institutional criteria

Phase V: Evaluation

Alternative Types of Evaluation:

- **Evaluation can be formal or informal, individual or institutional**
- **Consider cost-benefit of various evaluation efforts**
- **Use RU-as-a-process to enhance credibility of evaluation data**
- **For both dynamic & pilot evaluations, include two types of evaluative information:**
  ◦ formative, regarding actual implementation & goal progress
  ◦ summative, regarding Phase I outcomes and goal results

NOTE: Model applies to all forms of practice, i.e., educational, clinical, managerial, or other

figure 8.1   The Stetler Model has five phases (A, pictured and B, described): preparation, validation, comparative evaluation/decision making, translation/application, and evaluation. (From Stetler, C. B. [1994a]. Refinement of the Stetler/Marram model for application of research findings to practice. Nursing Outlook, 42, 15–25; and Stetler, C. B. [2001a]. Updating the Stetler model of research utilization to facilitate evidence-based practice. Nursing Outlook, 49, 272–278. With permission from Elsevier Science.)

Despite the appearance that research utilization is a linear, clear-cut process, it is more fluid in practice. Figure 8-1B has serrated lines between the phases, or columns, to indicate this fluidity and the need to occasionally revisit decisions (e.g., the relevance of specific studies, the fit of various findings, and the nature of current practice). Despite the model's complex appearance, its steps and concepts can be integrated into a professional's way of thinking about research utilization and EBP. This in turn influences how one routinely reads research and applies related findings (Stetler, 1994b).

Critical Assumptions and Model Concepts

To optimize use of this research utilization model, key underlying assumptions must be understood (Stetler, 1994a, 2001a). These assumptions generate the critical thinking and "practitioner" orientation of the model.

The model assumes that both formal and informal use of research findings can occur in the practice setting. Formal, organization-initiated and sanctioned research utilization activity is most frequently discussed in the nursing research utilization literature. Often, this activity results in new policies, procedures, protocols, programs, guidelines, and standards. After the formal documents are disseminated, individuals are expected to use these translated and packaged findings. Individual, research utilization-competent practitioners (i.e., those who are skilled in the process of research utilization, such as in their ability to critique and appropriately use research findings to improve their practices) also can use the model's process in their routine practice and interactions with others (Cronenwett, 1994; Stetler, 1994a, 1994b). These practitioners may use research findings to substantiate or improve a current practice, change their way of thinking about an issue or routine, expand their repertoire of assessment or intervention strategies, or change a colleague's way of thinking about a treatment plan or issue. In this case, the assumption that the user possesses a certain level of knowledge and skills specifically related to research utilization is critical (Stetler, 2001a, 2001b). The knowledge and skills for the safe, appropriate, and effective use of findings include (Stetler, 2001a, pp. 273–274):

- Knowledge of basic concepts of research
- Research utilization and EBP knowledge and skills, including use of tables of evidence and a set of applicability criteria to determine the desirability and feasibility of using a credible study (e.g., the potential risks involved)
- Knowledge and interpretive skills regarding inferential statistics and the applicability of findings at the individual level, including appropriate versus inappropriate variation
- Knowledge of the substantive area under consideration

Advanced-level healthcare practitioners (e.g., master's and doctorally prepared clinicians) are most likely to fulfill these expectations and are also more likely to routinely integrate research findings into their practices. However, with sufficient educational and skills preparation, baccalaureate-prepared healthcare providers also can implement research-based care. Research utilization-competent practitioners also may use an isolated study to meet a particular need (Cronenwett, 1994; Stetler, 1994a, 1994b). Advanced-level clinicians are able to do so because of their critical thinking skills and advanced knowledge of their specialty areas—knowledge that provides them with a *body of evidence* with which to comparatively evaluate the study under consideration for application in their practices.

Another of the model's underlying assumptions is that research findings may be used in multiple ways. Practitioners use findings directly in observable ways to change how they behave or provide care through assessments, clinical procedures, and behavioral interventions. They also use findings indirectly or conceptually, which is not so easy to observe but is very important to EBP. This can involve using findings to change how one thinks about a patient or an issue. It also can involve adding research evidence to one's body of knowledge, merging it with other information, and using it in the future. This can "result in a gradually emerged behavior, as Weiss (1980) suggests, at some unknown point in time due to what she calls 'knowledge creep and decision accretion" (Stetler, 1994a, p.). Finally, research findings can be used symbolically (i.e., strategically) to influence the thinking and behavior of others.

Other key assumptions for the model include the following:

- Contextual and personal factors can influence an individual's or group's use of research evidence and should be recognized up front by the user.
- Research and evaluative data provide probabilistic information, not absolutes, about each individual for whom the evidence is believed to generally "fit." As Geyman suggests, EBP "requires the integration, patient by patient, of . . . clinical expertise and judgment with the best available relevant external evidence" (1998, pp. 46–47). This may require "reasoned individualization" (Stetler, 2001a, p. 275) in the context of a patient's characteristics, clinical circumstances, and preferences.

As EBP has evolved, the scope of EBP models has broadened beyond research utilization to incorporate more complex skills and contributors to the outcome of the model—best practice.

A Model of Evidence-Based Practice for Individual Practitioners

A model adapted from Haynes and colleagues (2002) sets the use of research findings in the context of an evidence-based decision-making framework (DiCenso, Cullum, Ciliska & Guyatt, 2004). Evidence-based decision making is the integration of best research evidence with the patient's clinical status and circumstances, the patient's preferences and action, healthcare resources, and clinical expertise when deciding on treatments/interventions or the type of care to deliver (see Figure 8-2). Evidence-based practice includes the following processes:

- Formulating a clinical question;
- Systematically searching for relevant research evidence;
- Critically appraising the relevance, quality, and applicability of the evidence;
- Making an evidence-based decision regarding implementation by considering the research evidence along with the practitioner's clinical expertise, healthcare resources, and the patient's clinical status, circumstances, preferences, and actions; and depending on the decision,
- Implementing of the practice change and
- Evaluating the change in practice

Making and Implementing Evidence-Based Decisions

To illustrate how the Dicenso and colleagues' model can be implemented, consider the following examples. For many years, public health nurses have been visiting at-risk postpartum moth-

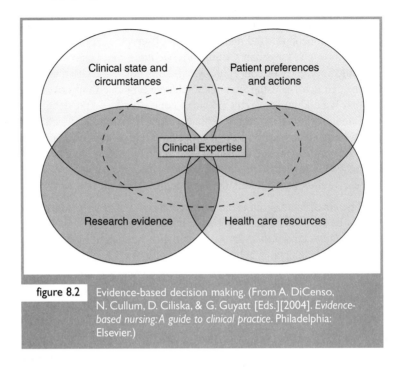

figure 8.2   Evidence-based decision making. (From A. DiCenso, N. Cullum, D. Ciliska, & G. Guyatt [Eds.][2004]. *Evidence-based nursing: A guide to clinical practice*. Philadelphia: Elsevier.)

ers in their homes to provide education and support. The nurses have the clinical expertise; the funding is available to the health department to support this nursing intervention; and the evidence shows that it has produced positive outcomes, both for the mothers and for their children (Ciliska, Mastrilli, Ploeg, Hayward, Brunton, & Underwood, 2001). However, when the community health nurse calls some clients to arrange a home visit, the clients are reluctant to agree and sometimes refuse to be visited. Patient preferences and actions will be the dominant element in this decision regarding a home visit. Optimally, patient values and preferences are based on careful consideration of information that provides an accurate assessment of the patient's condition and possible treatments, as well as the likely benefits, costs, and risks. In this way, clients can make informed decisions based on the best current knowledge.

In addition to patient preferences, clinical decision making requires clinicians to consider the patient's clinical state and circumstances. For example, patients who live in remote areas may not have access to the same diagnostic tests or interventions as those who live near a tertiary care medical center. Also, the effectiveness of some interventions may vary, depending on the patient's stage of illness or symptoms.

Another component of healthcare decisions is resources. Sometimes, even the best evidence cannot be utilized because the intervention is too costly. Now return to the example, where the local health department would like to replace some of the community health nurses with paraprofessionals (lay home visitors) in hopes of delivering similar education and support and achieving comparable outcomes at a lower cost. The nurse manager conducts a literature search and finds an article by Olds and colleagues (2002), which concludes that although nurses achieved significant and important effects on numerous maternal and infant outcomes, paraprofessionals achieved small effects that were rarely statistically significant. Though armed with this research evidence, the health department no longer has the resources to continue the home visiting program using only community health nurses, and it begins to hire and train paraprofessionals. Resources become the dominant element in this decision.

Compiling Evidence.   The ideal situation is for research evidence to be the primary element in the decision. When this is the case, we look for relevant and high-quality studies that address the clinical question.

Consider an in-hospital example in which nurses are concerned about the high rate of intravenous catheter dislodgment. They currently use gauze dressings on the catheter sites, and one nurse, who recently moved to this setting from another institution, notes that there seemed to be far fewer dislodgments where she previously worked when transparent dressings were used. This nurse offers to search the literature for research studies that compare the two types of dressings. She finds a study by Trepepi-Bova and colleagues (1997) and reviews it with the clinical instructor on the unit. Together, they conclude that it is a high-quality study in terms of its methods (**internal validity**) and that the population and setting of the study are sufficiently similar to theirs so that they can apply the results in their unit (**external validity**). From the study's findings, the clinicians conclude that transparent polyurethane dressings on peripheral IV sites may result in fewer catheter dislodgments than gauze dressings with no increase in rates of phlebitis or site infiltration.

Planning a Change.   The nurses talk to their administrator about changing from using gauze dressings to using transparent polyurethane dressings. Their administrator agrees but encourages them to evaluate whether the new type of dressing actually results in a reduction in catheter dislodgments by recording the number of dislodgments for 2 months before and after switching to transparent polyurethane dressings.

Integrating Skills and Experience.   Evidence-based decision making (i.e., using evidence to make decisions about clinical practice) is influenced by the practitioner's experience and general basic skills of clinical practice. Clinician skills include the expertise that develops from multiple observations of patients and how they react to certain interventions. Clinical expertise is essential for avoiding the mechanical application of care maps, decision rules, and guidelines.

Consider an example in which healthcare professionals who work in a psychiatric outpatient facility are wondering whether they are providing the best possible care to their patients with schizophrenia. One of these providers offers to search the literature and finds a recent systematic review reporting that social skills training supported employment programs and that cognitive behavior therapy improved some outcomes in patients with schizophrenia (Bustillo et al., 2001).

In considering these interventions, the healthcare providers believed that they had the expertise to conduct social skills training, as well as access to employment programs to which they could refer their clients. However, they believed that they did not currently have the skills to provide cognitive behavior therapy. As a result, the healthcare providers decided to investigate avenues for learning this skill. Then they presented a proposal to the clinic director that summarized the research evidence and outlined a plan for their continuing education and program development.

In the EBP model, clinical expertise is the mechanism that provides for integration of the other model components. For example, the practitioner's clinical expertise will influence the:

- Quality of the initial assessment of the client's clinical state and circumstances
- Problem formulation
- Decision about whether the best evidence and availability of healthcare resources substantiate a new approach
- Exploration of patient preferences
- Delivery of the clinical intervention
- Evaluation of the outcome for that particular patient

The following scenario exemplifies integrating the best available scientific evidence with clinical expertise. The local school board is concerned about the string of suicides in the high schools in the last year. It asks the school nurses and counselors to implement a suicide prevention program for the students in the next school year. The schools are very supportive of the program, the school nurses and counselors have the skills to implement this program, and resources are sufficient to mount the program. However, the nurses and counselors search the literature and find a high-quality systematic review that shows some evidence that male students who participated in such interventions were more likely to engage in negative coping strategies and possibly suicide than were the males who did not participate in such programs (Ploeg et al., 1996). The school nurses and counselors recommend that the suicide prevention program not be offered but that instead, the school board participate in the evaluation of a "healthy school" approach, which includes an ongoing curriculum in self-esteem enhancement, conflict resolution, and positive relationship building.

The factors in the EBP model will vary in their extent of influence in clinical decision making, depending on the decision to be made. In the past, EBP has been criticized for its "cookbook approach" to patient care. Some believe that it focuses solely on research evidence and in so doing, ignores patient preferences and wishes in decision making. Figure 8-2 shows that research evidence is only one factor in the evidence-based decision-making process and is always considered within the context of the other factors. Depending on the decision, the primary determining factor will vary. One of the advantages of this model is that nurses and other healthcare providers have not traditionally considered research evidence in their decision-making process (Estabrooks, 1998), and this model serves as a reminder to them that such evidence should be one of the factors they consider in their decision making.

Models for Organizations

Four organizational models will now be described:

1. The Iowa model (Titler, 2002)
2. Rosswurm and Larrabee's model (1999)
3. The Advancing Research and Clinical practice through close collaboration (ARCC) model (Melnyk & Fineout-Overholt, 2002a)
4. Kitson's model (1999)

These models differ from the previously described individual practitioner-focused models in that they acknowledge the considerable impact that the organization has on EBP.

The Iowa Model

The Iowa Model of EBP is an organizational model that incorporates the conduct and use of research and other forms of evidence (Figure 8–3) (Titler, 2002).

This model is a revision of the Iowa Model of Research-Based Practice to Promote Quality Care (Titler et al., 1994). Knowledge and problem-focused "triggers" lead clinicians to question practice and search the literature for related research to answer their questions. If high-quality studies are not found, a study is conducted and findings are combined with other knowledge to inform practice. If it is not feasible to conduct a study, other types of evidence (e.g., case reports, expert opinions, theories) are used. EBP guidelines are developed using available evidence. Recommended practice is compared with current practice, and a decision is made about whether the current practice should be changed. If warranted, the changes are implemented using a process of planned changed:

- The practice is pilot tested with a small group of clinicians and clients.
- The guideline is revised based on this pilot, then implemented on a larger scale.
- Outcome data are then collected from staff, clients, and administration.
- Decision points are clearly identified in the process and occur when deciding whether the identified problem is a priority for the organization, whether there is a sufficient research base for the change, and whether the proposed change is appropriate for adoption in practice.

The Iowa model describes how the infrastructure to support research use must involve every level of the organization, from high-level management to front-line clinicians. Roles related to research utilization are included in job descriptions, EBP is linked to quality assurance, and appropriate education is provided. Reward and recognition programs are implemented to recognize staff who use research to solve clinical problems. Clinicians are given time and resources to be involved in research utilization, including problem identification, assessment of evidence, change planning, implementation, and evaluation of change. The organization from the top down places a high priority on research utilization. The utilization of the Iowa model gives a strong message to the organization about its role in the support of EBP.

Rosswurm and Larrabee Model

Rosswurm and Larrabee (1999) developed their model based on theoretical and research literature related to EBP, research utilization, standardized language, and change theory. This model guides practitioners through the entire process of EBP, beginning with the assessment of the need for change and ending with integration of an evidence-based protocol. The model has been used in primary care settings (Rosswurm & Larrabee, 1999) and was adopted as a standard of care delivery in acute care settings (A. Mohide, personal communication, 2002). Organizations that have adopted this model have done so because nurses in the clinical setting find it easy to understand, possibly because they see the stages of the model as similar to the nursing process (A. Mohide & B. King, personal communication, 2002). The steps of the Rosswurm and Larrabee model are shown in Figure 8-4.

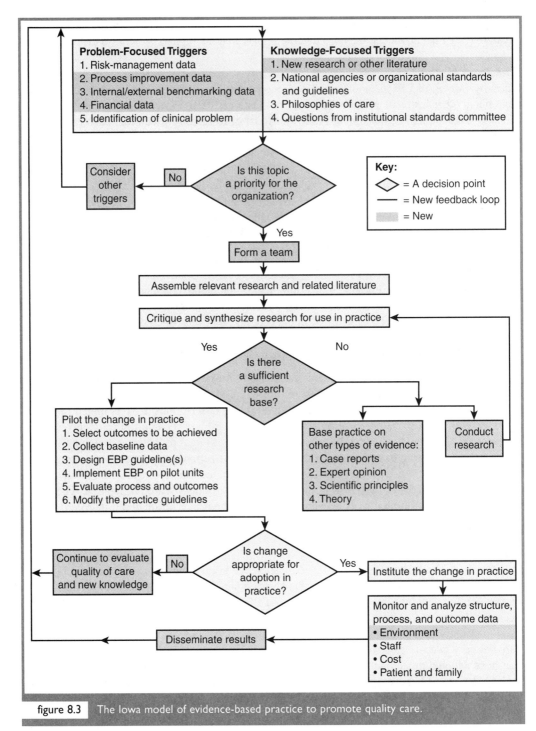

figure 8.3   The Iowa model of evidence-based practice to promote quality care.

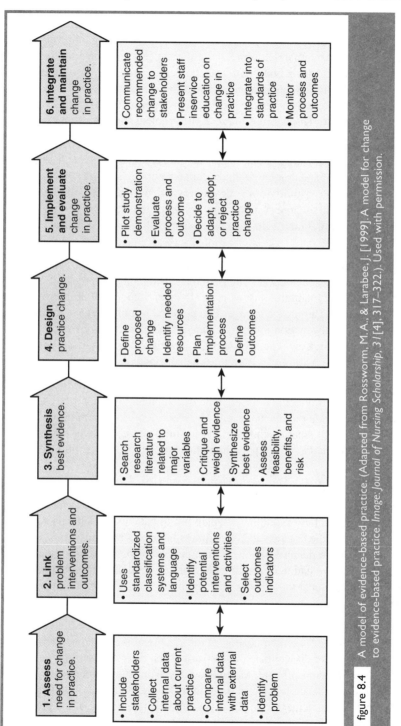

figure 8.4 A model of evidence-based practice. (Adapted from Rossworm, M.A., & Larabee, J. [1999]. A model for change to evidence-based practice. *Image: Journal of Nursing Scholarship, 3 [4]*, 317–322.). Used with permission.

Step 1: Assess Needs of Stakeholders. Step 1 of the Rosswurm and Larrabee model, which is "Assess need for change in practice," suggests identifying and including relevant stakeholders. Any relevant internal data about current practice should be collected, collated, and integrated into a form that is familiar to stakeholders . These data also should be compared with any relevant benchmark or comparative information from similar-sized institutions or units. The comparison of internal and external data may support current practice or indicate a need for change in practice. Through this process, the problem statement can be identified.

Step 2: Build Bridges, Make Connections. Step 2 is "Link problem interventions and outcomes." The authors suggest that one of the links to be made is with a nursing classification or diagnostic system and argue that this will make nursing activities visible, in comparison with the usually greater visibility of medical interventions. Another link to be made is that of identifying potential nursing interventions and activities that can then serve as process indicators for quality monitoring. Finally, the interventions need to be linked with selected patient outcome indicators.

Step 3: Synthesize the Evidence and Determine Relevancy. Step 3 requires that the group "synthesize the best evidence." The search needs to consider potential interventions and outcomes. Retrieved literature must be critically appraised to determine whether the strength of the evidence warrants a practice change. Preappraised resources can be utilized when available from sources such as abstraction journals, *Clinical Evidence*, the *Cochrane Library*, or the Agency for Healthcare Research and Quality (AHRQ). The benefits, risks, costs, and feasibility of the practice change in the particular setting must be considered.

Step 4: Plan the Practice Change. Step 4 is "Design the practice change." The proposed change must be fully defined through the development of a standard care plan, map, policy, or procedure. The required resources must be identified. Also, implications of the change in practice for nurses and other disciplines in terms of the complexity of the desired practice change should be identified to develop the implementation plan. In addition, desired outcomes should be defined.

Step 5: Implement and Evaluate the Practice Change. Step 5 is to "Implement and evaluate the change in practice." The authors suggest a pilot study to demonstrate the feasibility of the change in practice, including acceptability to patients and clinicians. The pilot study should address whether the practice change requires increased resources (e.g., new equipment, personnel), alterations in documentation, or administrative approvals and should provide process and outcome data. Evaluation of the change in process and outcomes facilitates the decision about whether to implement the practice change on a larger and more permanent basis in the unit or agency.

Step 6: Integrate and Maintain the Practice Change. Step 6 is "Integrate and maintain the change in practice." Communication of the change to stakeholders needs to occur, and the information needs to be disseminated to the staff. Then the practice change must be integrated into protocols or standards of care. Multiple strategies must be implemented that involve the frontline staff in the change process in order to overcome barriers within the climate of the organization. When the implementation phase is complete, monitoring of the process and outcomes must be ongoing.

Although the Rosswurm and Larrabee (1999) model appears to cease with Step 6, the last phase of monitoring the process and outcomes may lead to the identification of new problems that would require cycling through the process again. This stepwise, cyclical process was identified by Grol (1997) in his five-step process for changing clinical practice:

- Develop a change proposal.
- Identify obstacles.
- Link change in interventions to obstacles.
- Develop a plan.
- Carry out and evaluate the plan.

The evaluation then identifies a further need for the practice change. The change proposal is further developed, identifying additional obstacles that have arisen, planning for and implementing the plan to overcome the obstacles, and evaluating once more.

The ARCC Model

The ARCC model was founded through a major strategic-planning initiative at the University of Rochester School of Nursing in the spring of 1999, which involved faculty, School of Medicine and Dentistry faculty, individuals representing nursing practice at the academic health center, and community leaders (Melnyk & Fineout-Overholt, 2002a). Through the strategic planning process, the need to strengthen the unification of practice and research in the form of evidence-based care was identified as a high priority. Benchmarking with other leaders at schools of nursing and academic health centers throughout the country also revealed a tremendous national need for the advancement of EBP.

Strategic Planning for ARCC.   The dean and associate dean of research at the School of Nursing met with the director of nursing practice at the University of Rochester Medical Center to determine the amount of financial and staff support that both entities would be willing to contribute to support this new initiative. It was decided that the School of Nursing and Nursing Practice would provide equal contributions to support an associate director position in the newly named Center for Research and Evidence-Based Practice (CREP). This associate director would assist the associate dean for research and director of the CREP in EBP initiatives throughout the medical center. The School of Nursing committed additional resources to support a second associate director to the Center whose responsibility would be to assist the associate dean for research in advancing EBP throughout the greater Rochester healthcare community. The initial primary purposes of the ARCC model were to better integrate research and clinical practice throughout Rochester's academic health center and community and to advance EBP locally as well as nationally.

Survey Results Guide Further Development.   In developing the ARCC model, a survey was first conducted by targeting APNs within the medical center to determine their knowledge and skills regarding EBP, barriers to its implementation, as well as their EBP and scholarly development needs. Findings from this survey disclosed that the APNs identified the following as the major factors that would influence their undertaking an EBP approach to clinical care:

- Use of the CREP
- Mentorship in EBP
- Assistance with outcomes management
- Assistance with scholarly work (Melnyk & Fineout-Overholt, 2002).

Resources, the development of efficient computer search strategies, and time to conduct EBP activities also were identified as important factors that would influence their implementation of evidence-based care. Although the survey's respondents revealed that implementing EBP was important to them, perceived major barriers to successful implementation included heavy patient care demands and administrative responsibilities.

Goals of the ARCC Model.   Specific goals for the ARCC model were established and included the following:

- Promote the use of EBP among APNs and nurses locally and nationally.
- Establish a network of clinicians to support EBP.
- Obtain funding for ARCC.
- Disseminate the best evidence from well-designed studies that could be used in an evidence-based approach to clinical care.
- Conduct an annual conference on EBP.
- Conduct studies to evaluate the effectiveness of the ARCC model on the process and outcomes of clinical care.

Many of these goals have been achieved. In the first 2 years of the model, the ARCC team assisted 35 APNs with EBP initiatives. They also assisted three community agencies with outcomes management projects. In areas where evidence was inadequate to guide practice, ten research grant requests to answer burning clinical questions were developed and submitted, of which four requests were funded. Fifteen nurses also were assisted in preparing their EBP work for regional and national professional meetings. In addition, a local listserve for APNs was established to disseminate information to facilitate EBP. Furthermore, evidence-based rounds were regularly implemented in clinical sites so that the best and latest evidence was available to assist APNs and nurses in answering their burning clinical questions.

Along with the local dissemination of evidence and working knowledge of EBP, the ARCC team has been very active in disseminating evidence from well-designed studies in national publications, including a state-of-the-science article (Melnyk et al., 2000) and ongoing publications focused on the key steps for implementing EBP (Melnyk, 2002, Melnyk & Fineout-Overholt, 2002b). The director of CREP also initiated and regularly edits a journal column in *Pediatric Nursing* entitled "Evidence-Based Practice." The column presents the latest and best evidence to pediatric practitioners to guide best practices with children, youth, and their families. Examples of recent EBP articles include the most effective interventions to guide clinical practice with low-birth-weight premature infants and parents (Melnyk, Feinstein, & Fairbanks, 2002), early predictors of long-term outcomes in hospitalized children (Small, 2002), and effective interventions to prevent comorbidities in overweight/obese children and adolescents (Jerum & Melnyk, 2001). In addition, the ARCC team has conducted multiple workshops and training sessions on EBP, as well as presenting conference keynotes and plenary sessions at local, regional, and national conferences.

Funding to further support and develop the ARCC team's initiatives also has been obtained. AHRQ funded the third and fourth EBP conferences, which were national in scope. The purpose of the annual EBP conference is to develop practitioners' skills in EBP, as well as to bring the best and latest evidence to them in the areas of high-risk children and youth, acute and critical care, aging, and mental health. Funding from AHRQ facilitated the videotaping of conference sessions to disseminate key EBP information nationally on videotapes and CD-ROMs.

The Helene Fuld Health Trust also funded the ARCC model, specifically to assist bedside nurses with evidence-based care and to better integrate EBP into the existing curricula across all educational programs at the University of Rochester School of Nursing, including new accelerated baccalaureate and master's programs for non-nurses and an accelerated master's/doctoral program. The grant from the Helene Fuld Health Trust also is supporting two pilot projects currently in progress. The purpose of these pilot studies is to test the effects of two versions of the ARCC model (i.e., ARCC standard and ARCC enhanced) on patient and staff outcomes in acute care and home settings. The ARCC standard intervention is providing nurses with educational information on EBP and access to an EBP mentor through e-mail communication. In addition to providing educational information on EBP, the ARCC enhanced intervention is providing an EBP mentor on site to teach and guide nurses in these settings in evidence-based care.

The ARCC model is an excellent example of how focused efforts between a school of nursing and nursing practice within an academic health center can accelerate the speed at which research evidence is translated into best practices. Although it has existed for only a few years, the ARCC model has made tremendous strides in facilitating EBP locally and nationally, which is expected to result in quality improvements in the process and outcomes of clinical care.

Kitson's Framework

A fourth model that places more emphasis on the organization is one developed by Kitson and colleagues (Kitson, Harvey, & McCormack, 1989; Kitson, 1999). Kitson's model acknowledges that context is of central importance in effective EBP. This conceptual framework describes the implementation of EBP as a function of the relationship between the nature of the evidence, the appropriateness of the context in which the change is to be implemented, and the characteristics of the facilitation mechanism used to introduce the change. The framework arose from the equation SI = f (E,C,F), where *SI* = successful implementation, *E* = evidence, *C* = context, and *F* = facilitation. Each component is depicted on a three-dimensional matrix having the evidence, context, and facilitation of change on each axis of the cube, with all of these contributing to the success of implementing research findings (Figure 8-5). Although the model does not ignore the importance of individual attributes, it emphasizes that the organization often plays a greater role in research utilization decisions than do these individual attributes.

In Kitson's model, *context* refers to elements of the organization, such as the systems in place for problem solving and monitoring, social networks and the amount of contact with outside organizations, hospital culture, and leadership. Context also includes the individual characteristics of clinicians, such as role, status, power base, education, and attitudes toward using research findings. Novelty and degree of discrepancy from current practice are examples of characteristics of *evidence* that determine implementation. *Facilitation* includes the manner in which the research findings are communicated to individuals. *Successful implementation* occurs when the evidence is strong, the context is receptive to change, and the change process is appropriately facilitated (Kitson et al., 1989). When one or two of the three components are weak, the remaining component(s) must be particularly strong. For example, when the context of the organization cannot change to assist in implementing EBP, translating research findings into practice can be eased by communicating the findings to clinicians in a way that is easily understood and readily applicable (i.e., providing higher levels of support through the facilitation element) (Kitson et al., 1989).

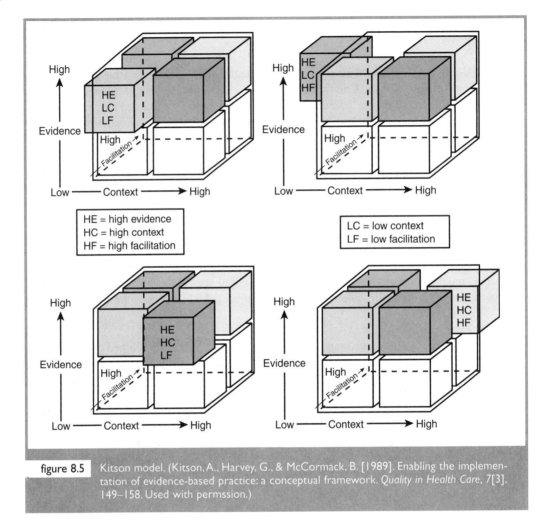

figure 8.5   Kitson model. (Kitson, A., Harvey, G., & McCormack, B. [1989]. Enabling the implementation of evidence-based practice: a conceptual framework. *Quality in Health Care*, 7[3], 149–158. Used with permssion.)

    Careful planning of the practice change with supportive strategies, such as using opinion leaders, role models, interactive inservice education, guidelines, and incentives are all strategies to increase facilitation. Kitson's model can be used much like the "situational analysis" (Cochrane Review Group on Effective Practice and Organization of Care, 1999) to assess potential barriers and facilitators within the elements of the evidence, context, and facilitation.

A Broader Dissemination Framework

A comprehensive framework of research dissemination and utilization for health policy and practice (Dobbins et al., 2002) was developed by integrating Rogers Diffusion of Innovations theory (Rogers, 1995) with organizational behavior, culture, and decision making from the management field with research dissemination, utilization, and EBP from the health field. The framework illustrates that the process of **adoption of research evidence** into decision making is a complex one that occurs across the five stages of innovation (i.e., knowledge, persuasion, decision, implementation, and confirmation). The framework shows that this five-stage process is influenced by characteristics of the individual, the organization, and the environment (Figure 8-6). An advantage of this model is the integration of the diffusion of innovations theory with other relevant organizational and research utilization models.

Strategies to Promote Evidence-Based Practice

Survey results (Champion & Leach, 1989; Kajermo, Nordstrom, Krusebrant, & Bjorvell, 1998; Melnyk & Fineout-Overholt, 2002a; Parahoo, 2000; Retsas & Nolan, 1999) have repeatedly disclosed that major barriers to functioning as evidence-based practitioners include:

- Lack of time
- Difficulty accessing research studies
- Difficulty understanding the language or implications of research
- Lack of skills in critical appraisal
- Lack of autonomy, authority, or control over one's own practice

Because various healthcare professionals seldom function alone, their decision to change a clinical practice cannot be made in isolation of healthcare administrators and other practitioners (e.g., physicians). For example, we now know that placing mechanically ventilated adults in a semirecumbent position rather than in a supine position reduces the rate of nosocomial pneumonia (Drakulovic et al., 1999). However, a decision to position patients in this way in an intensive care unit may often require the cooperation of the entire healthcare team.

Several strategies have been developed to overcome the barriers identified above and to facilitate EBP. They include learning to access systematic reviews, abstraction journals, and clinical practice guidelines. Facilitators also include strategies for institutions to support individuals in EBP, such as providing access to library resources and practice guidelines, ensuring administrative support, and creating a culture of research conduct and utilization.

Strategies for Overcoming Barriers to Evidence-Based Practice

> 66 *Most of our obstacles would melt away if, instead of cowering before them, we should make up our minds to walk boldly through them.* 99
> —*Orison Swett Marden*

Initiate Systematic Reviews

Much of healthcare research has reached a point where more than one study addresses similar important questions. Consider the large number of studies regarding hormone replacement ther-

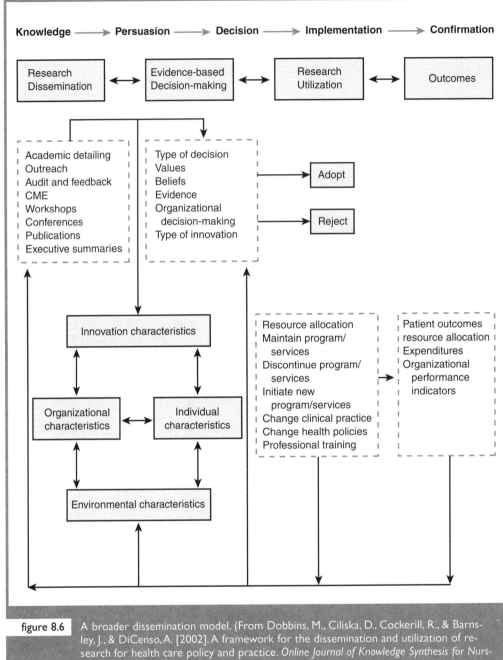

figure 8.6   A broader dissemination model. (From Dobbins, M., Ciliska, D., Cockerill, R., & Barnsley, J., & DiCenso, A. [2002]. A framework for the dissemination and utilization of research for health care policy and practice. *Online Journal of Knowledge Synthesis for Nursing, 9,* 7. Used with permisson from Sigma Theta Tau, International.)

apy (HRT). A quick search of PubMed combining key words *estrogen* and *progestin* and limiting the search to *randomized trials* published in English in 2002 yielded 27 hits. Reading only one or two of these studies may give an unbalanced view of HRT risks and benefits, especially if the high-quality studies are not chosen for review. A synthesis of all research evidence on HRT would provide a balanced view of its benefits and risk for a broader sample population. These types of syntheses are called *systematic reviews*.

Systematic reviews are summaries of evidence, typically conducted by an expert or expert panel on a particular topic, that use a rigorous process for identifying, appraising, and synthesizing studies to answer a specific clinical question and draw conclusions about the data gathered. As such, they are able to overcome the potential biases of a traditional literature review (See Chapter 5 for a more complete description). These reviews offer more complete answers to clinical questions, which should result in better clinical decisions. The process of conducting a systematic review includes:

- Identification of a clear clinical question
- Comprehensive identification of studies
- Review of study relevance
- Evaluation of the methodological quality of individual studies included in the review
- Extraction of data from each study
- Analysis of data, which may include a meta-analysis (i.e., a process of using quantitative methods to summarize the results from the multiple studies, which typically yields an overall summary statistic that represents the effect of the intervention across multiple studies)
- Drawing of conclusions
- Writing and dissemination of the report

At each stage, there is an attempt to overcome possible bias. Usually two or more people who are interested in conducting a systematic review on a clinical topic are involved in identifying a question. Having identified the specific question they desire to address, they conduct a search to verify that a high-quality, up-to-date systematic review does not already exist on the same question.

It is helpful for at least one librarian to be involved in developing the search strategy. Multiple electronic databases are searched by using appropriate key words that are combined in a way to maximize the opportunity of finding all relevant articles. Frequently, relevant journals may be hand-searched to overcome the possibility of missing some studies in bibliographic databases. Experts are contacted to identify any published and unpublished studies that address the clinical question. Ignoring unpublished research risks publication bias, especially if studies that have failed to find statistically significant differences in outcomes have been conducted but not published.

The searchers then review all output from the search and retrieve any articles that the title and abstract screening suggest are appropriate. If there is any doubt about the relevance of an article, it is retrieved. Next, using preset criteria, the searchers independently review each retrieved article for relevance. Again, using preset criteria, the searchers review the relevant articles for their methodological quality (validity). Then, using a pretested tool, at least two individuals conducting the review independently extract relevant data from each study. At the end of each step, the two individuals compare their ratings or data and resolve discrepancies by consensus or by taking the disagreements to a third party for a final decision.

Depending on the type of data reported in the studies, some systematic reviews can include a meta-analysis in which outcome data from each study are statistically combined into a summary estimate of effect, with confidence intervals that indicate the precision of the estimate. Precise results are increased through the combination of data from all studies, and confidence in the results can be greater than with any one study that was included in the meta-analysis.

The final step of a systematic review involves interpreting the results, deriving conclusions, and preparing the written report. The process is rigorous, and understanding the rigor allows one to be more confident in the use of a systematic review. Finding a high-quality, recent systematic review overcomes many of the barriers to using research in clinical decision making, such as lack of access to the journals, lack of money to pay for retrieving articles, lack of time to retrieve and critically appraise studies, and weak critical appraisal skills. Meta-analyses can be quickly identified as a methodologic limit within PubMed; however, the PubMed limit term *review* does not consider whether the article is a meta-analysis.

The *Cochrane Library*

The Cochrane Library (2002) has a database of more than 1,500 systematic reviews, some of which include meta-analyses, where appropriate, and protocols for more than 1,100 other reviews that are in process. The Cochrane Collaboration, an international voluntary group of healthcare researchers dedicated to producing and disseminating systematic reviews, produces this database. In addition, the Cochrane Library contains more than 2,900 reviews summarized and appraised by the Center for Review and Dissemination at the University of York (England) and citations for more than 345,378 controlled trials. All of these databases can be searched within the Cochrane Library in one step. The Cochrane Library includes not only medical and pharmacological data but also information on broader healthcare issues relevant to many disciplines. It is available for searching abstracts of reviews online at no charge. Full-text reviews are accessible through some institutional licensing arrangements or through individual subscriptions, either online or on CD-ROM. Some examples of reviews include one that has examined the effectiveness of nursing interventions for smoking cessation (Rice & Stead, 2002), another that has compared high-frequency jet ventilation versus conventional ventilation for respiratory distress syndrome in preterm infants (Bhuta & Henderson-Smart, 2002), and yet another that has examined the effects of caregiver support for women in labor (Hodnett, 2002).

Agency for Healthcare Research and Quality (AHRQ)

Another source of systematic reviews is the AHRQ. To date, there are 63 evidence reports that are extensive systematic reviews, in addition to several technical methods papers (AHRQ, 2002) produced by the associated Evidence-Based Practice Centers funded through AHRQ. Examples of reviews from AHRQ include management of cancer symptoms, mind-body interactions for gastrointestinal conditions, and modifying dietary behavior related to cancer risk (AHRQ, 2002). These reviews are available in full text online at no cost. Other sources of reviews include the Evidence-Based Practice Centers and other nursing research centers that are involved in the conduct, dissemination, and utilization of systematic reviews.

Search for Evidence-Based Clinical Practice Guidelines and Abstraction Journals

Chapter 9 describes the use of evidence-based **clinical practice guidelines**. They are briefly included here as part of an overview of strategies to overcome the barriers to EBP. Clinical practice guidelines are statements that have been systematically developed to assist practitioners and patients in making decisions about care. At their best, they allow for the integration of research with the clinical context, specific patient circumstances, and patient values. Ideally, guideline development consists of a systematic review of the literature and consensus of a group of decision makers (administrators, policy makers, clinicians, and consumers) who consider the evidence and make recommendations.

A repository of practice guidelines is searchable online through the National Guideline Clearinghouse at **http://www.guideline.gov/** and is sponsored by the AHRQ.

In addition, several specialist groups in nursing have developed clinical practice guidelines. The National Association of Neonatal Nurses (2002), for example, provides online access to its guidelines on peripherally inserted central catheters, pain assessment and management in neonates, and neonatal skin care. Another example is the Registered Nurses Association of Ontario (RNAO, 2002) that has guidelines on assessing and managing pain, assessing and managing Stage 1–IV pressure ulcers, and enhancing healthy adolescent development.

Clinical practice guidelines can overcome the barriers to research utilization by reducing the need to access and critically appraise the literature and make general conclusions and recommendations. They do not eliminate clinical judgment that is required regarding how well particular clients fit with the target population for the practice guideline.

Thomas and colleagues (2000) conducted a systematic review of the use of practice guidelines by allied health professionals. They found 18 studies, 17 of which focused on the use of practice guidelines by nurses. Of the five studies that considered the process of care, three reported an improvement when practice guidelines were used, and in the eight studies that evaluated the outcomes of care, six recorded improvement with the utilization of practice guidelines.

Electronic Guidelines

The RNAO has developed a toolkit to facilitate the implementation of clinical practice guidelines in healthcare settings (DiCenso et al., 2002). The toolkit is based on a conceptual model that depicts six essential components of practice guideline implementation:

1. Selecting the guideline
2. Identifying, analyzing, and engaging stakeholders
3. Assessing environmental readiness
4. Deciding on implementation strategies
5. Evaluating success
6. Considering resources

The toolkit is available on the RNAO Web site at **www.rnao.org.**

Abstraction Journals and Services

Other resources that provide ready access to methodologically filtered studies are the *abstraction journals,* such as *Evidence-Based Medicine, Evidence-Based Mental Health, Evidence-Based Health Policy and Management*, and *Evidence-Based Nursing*. The purpose of these journals is to summarize high-quality, clinically useful studies and present them along with a commentary from an expert clinician summarizing the strengths, limitations, and clinical implications of the study. To identify relevant studies for abstraction in *Evidence-Based Nursing*, every issue of more than 150 healthcare journals is reviewed. Studies that pass quality criteria standards are then rated for relevance to nursing practice. A structured abstract is written and the commentary added. These abstraction journals allow clinicians to keep up with advances in practice.

Abstraction journals are available in print and online through individual or institutional subscriptions. An advantage of electronic access to *Evidence-Based Nursing*, for example, is that although over 1,000 studies per year pass the quality criteria, only 96 of these are abstracted and published. The others are kept in an online searchable database at **www.evidence-basednursing.com.**

This again allows access to preappraised, high-quality literature. Subscribers will soon be able to register their areas of clinical interest and receive electronic notification of new papers in those areas. This database is updated weekly so that within a month of the publication of a new, high-quality, relevant study, subscribers would have notification.

Another abstraction tool, *Clinical Evidence* (2002), is organized around common primary care or hospital-based problems. It presents the current state of knowledge about prevention and treatment of a wide variety of clinical conditions based on thorough literature searches and critical appraisal. *Clinical Evidence* uses information from the abstraction journals and the *Cochrane* Library to highlight existing evidence for questions such as, What is the most effective intervention for the prevention and treatment of pressure sores?

Another tool for finding quality articles is PubMed (**www.ncbi.nlm.nih. gov./PubMed/),** a free, Web-based, public MEDLINE search interface. It includes linkages to full-text journals of participating publishers and will also search "related articles" that are easily accessed. One benefit of PubMed is that users do not need to be familiar with the medical subject heading (MeSH) terms that are the basis of MEDLINE searching.

PubMed's Clinical Queries function acts as a filter to identify only the methodologically sound studies that meet evidence-based standards for four types of research: treatment (e.g., evaluations of clinical interventions), diagnosis (or assessment), etiology (or causation), and prognosis. Searches also can be limited to systematic reviews. In addition, searches can be more sensitive (a broader search with larger number of relevant citations by including those that are less relevant) or more specific (a narrower search with fewer retrieved citations but more likely to be relevant) (Zaroukian, 2001).

Innovative Strategies to Promote Evidence-Based Nursing

This section will describe some strategies that focus on ways to develop EBP skills. For the most part, these strategies are untested and are ripe for evaluation. Once again, the strategies focus on individuals and organizations.

Strategies for Individual Nurses

If your organization or your local educational institution does not yet provide skill development in EBP, there are several ways to cultivate abilities on your own or with a colleague. These include the development of a reflective, inquiring approach to practice, the willingness to use studies conducted in other centers, and self-education in EBP.

Adopt a Reflective, Inquiring Approach

One of the basic building blocks in the development of EBP skills is an inquiring, reflective approach to practice. As Rosswurm and Larrabee (1999) state, stimulation to think about a change in practice can come from patient preferences and dissatisfactions, quality improvement or evaluation data, practitioner dissatisfaction, and queries or new research data. Titler (2002) calls these "triggers." Practitioners need to take the time to think about their patients' reactions to their interventions, as well as to formulate questions about current practices and potential alternatives to management of patient care. Communicating these questions to a librarian or to colleagues with research expertise may be the first step to finding the literature or, if none exists, to recommending a study on your clinical question. Also, communicating the question accompanied by the appropriate literature may lead to quality improvement initiatives and patient care plans/maps, guidelines, or protocols. The first step, however, is an inquisitive, inquiring approach to one's own practice.

> 66 *Asking the right questions takes as much skill as giving the right answers.* 99
>
> *— Robert Half*

Consider Research from Other Centers

Some practitioners are reluctant to use studies conducted in other centers as evidence that might be applied to their own *clinical practice settings*. However, research studies are expensive and time-consuming to conduct. One approach is to consider the reasons why a study might not be applicable, such as a different staffing mix, different patient types, or different resources. There-fore, an important strategy is to assess the inclusion/exclusion criteria of a study and consider how closely your patients match the patients in the study. A better approach may be to ask your-self why the results should not be applied to your patient(s) (Guyatt, Cook, Devereaux, Meade, & Strauss, 2002). If a compelling reason cannot be found, the study results can be applied to your patient population, and you can use a variety of measures to evaluate the effect of the change at your particular practice site.

Librarians or colleagues experienced in searching are crucial to finding evidence that is relevant to your practice. Including librarians in EBP initiatives assists in overcoming initial barriers of unfamiliarity with electronic searching and accessing relevant studies. Searching the preappraised literature described above, such as that in the *Cochrane Library* or *Evidence-Based Nursing*, will overcome the need for highly developed critical appraisal skills.

Educate Yourself

Several good online resources are available for learning the steps of EBP. The *Evidence-Based Nursing* journal hosts an editorial series on critical appraisal of research articles.

Innovative Organizational Strategies

Develop Centers for Evidence-Based Practice

Several research and EBP centers have developed around the world, including Germany, Canada, the United Kingdom, Australia, New Zealand, and the United States. The primary pur-pose of these centers is to advance EBP. Although specific goals of the centers differ, their activ-ities often include the conduct and dissemination of evidence-based resources, such as system-atic reviews and clinical practice guidelines; and the education of healthcare professionals in EBP through formal credit courses, including one-day or intensive one-week workshops. The educational programs seek to develop EBP skills, such as conducting systematic reviews, devel-oping practice guidelines, designing and evaluating strategies for dissemination, and using re-search to support EBP (Ciliska, DiCenso, & Cullum, 1999). Some of these centers are listed in Table 8-1.

table 8.1 Selected centers for evidence-based practice

Center	Contact
Canadian Center for Evidence-Based Nursing	ciliska@mcmaster.ca
German Center for Evidence-Based Nursing	http://home.t-online.de/home/gero.langer/ebn-zentrum/start/htm
Joanna Briggs Institute (JBI) for Evidence-Based Nursing and Midwifery	www.joannabriggs.edu.au
Knowledge Utilization Studies in Practice	www.nursing.ualberta.ca/kusp
Sarah Cole Hirsch Institute for Best Nursing Practices Based on Evidence	http://fpb.cwru.edu/HirshInstitute/
UK Centre for Evidence-Based Nursing	www.york.ac.uk/healthsciences/centres/evidence/cebn.htm
The Center for the Advancement of Evidence-Based Practice, Arizona State University	http://nursing.asu.edu/
University of Texas at San Antonio, Academic Center for EBP (ACE)	http://nursing.uthscsa.edu/research/environment.shtml#ace

The Joanna Briggs Institute, established in 1996, has multiple sites, including Western Australia, Victoria, New South Wales, South Australia, Tasmania, Queensland, Northern Territory, New Zealand, Thailand, and Hong Kong. The Institute advances the incorporation of qualitative research in systematic reviews through the Qualitative Assessment and Review Instrument. This system ranks evidence for feasibility, appropriateness, meaningfulness, and effectiveness, and it is part of a software program (Pearson, 2002). The German Center has used a "train-the-trainer" model, educating nurse leaders from across Germany who then return to their own institutions to train people in their clinical sites in EBP. The German Center for Knowledge Utilization Studies in Practice focuses on developing knowledge and research utilization to increase the use of research by nurses in order to improve outcomes.

The challenges for EBP centers are similar around the world: funding as well as identifying effective dissemination and utilization strategies to transmit evidence-based findings. The Sarah Cole Hirsh Institute was established in 1998 at the Frances Payne Bolton School of Nursing at Case Western Reserve University. A large bequest was provided to establish the center. The Joanna Briggs Institute obtains funds through institutional membership fees in return for certain services, such as assistance with development of policies and procedures and with implementation of EBP. The CREP at the University of Rochester School of Nursing has obtained extramural funds from AHRQ and from foundations. Still other centers have no ongoing funding or raise funds by conducting workshops.

The identification and evaluation of dissemination and utilization strategies is common to all the centers as well. Ultimately, the centers must show that they can successfully disseminate products, such as systematic reviews, in a way that the consumers (e.g., practitioners, managers, policy makers, and patients/clients) can use. Factors related to the innovation, individual users, organizations, and environment must be considered in planning and evaluating the strategies (Dobbins, Ciliska, Cockerill, Barnsley & DiCenso, 2002).

Facilitating Evidence-Based Practice in Organizations

When practitioners were taught how to identify and critically appraise research literature, they responded with enthusiasm. However, they reported that they had difficulty applying these skills to their practice because of heavy patient loads and shift work (Royle et al., 1996), thereby emphasizing the critical role that organizations play in fostering EBP.

Little research has focused on evaluating effective strategies for developing and sustaining EBP. Most literature that explores changing the practice of healthcare professionals has focused on physicians (Cochrane Review Group on Effective Practice and Organization of Care, 1999). However, 44 systematic reviews focusing on the effectiveness of strategies to change the practice of healthcare professionals were located and analyzed, and the following conclusions were drawn:

- Passive dissemination of research is ineffective.
- A range of interventions has been shown to be effective in changing the behavior of healthcare professionals.
- Multifaceted interventions are more likely to be effective than a single intervention.
- Individual practitioners' beliefs, attitudes, and knowledge influence their behavior but other factors, including organizational, economic, and community environments, also are important.
- A diagnostic analysis should be conducted to identify barriers and supportive factors likely to influence the proposed change in practice.
- Successful strategies to change practice need to be adequately resourced and require people with appropriate knowledge and skills.

> 66 *Tell me and I'll forget. Show me and I'll remember. Involve me and I'll understand.* 99
>
> —*Confucius*

Any systematic approach to changing professional practice should include plans to monitor, evaluate, and maintain any change (Cochrane Review Group, 1999). This means, for example, that sending an exciting study to your colleagues (passive dissemination) stating that individuals with diabetes can safely inject insulin through their clothing (Fleming, Jacober, Vandenberg, Fitzgerald, & Grunberger, 1997) is not likely to alter the content of how they teach preparation of the skin for injection. As another example, just because opinion leaders (e.g., individuals who are highly respected in an environment and able to facilitate change) were effective in changing physician practice in Ontario (Lomas et al., 1991) does not mean that they will be effective in promoting change with other types of health professionals who practice in different settings (e.g., nurses in labor and delivery) (Hodnett et al., 1996).

Broader, more intensive strategies must involve more resources and support, as well as an organizational culture change. Strategies that have potential for promoting practice change (Dobbins et al., 2002) include:

- One-on-one sessions between health professional educators and individual staff to explain the desired practice change
- Manual and computerized reminders to prompt practitioner behavior change
- Educational meetings or inservices that require active participation of the learners
- Audits and feedback in which clinical performance is monitored through electronic database or chart review
- Direct observation and feedback

A critical question remains: What else can organizations do to support EBP? As described above, some strategies have been tried and evaluated in some organizations but need further testing. Other strategies have been implemented by clinical leaders and researchers but have not been formally evaluated.

Offer Incentives

One strategy that an organization can implement to improve the inquiring approach to clinical practice is to have a clinical question contest (J. Rush, personal communication, 1998). This strategy can be used on a particular unit or within an entire institution. It begins with the use of inservice promotions, such as self-learning packages and electronic communication to teach the staff how to pose a searchable clinical question (Flemming, 1998). Individuals are then encouraged to submit questions related to their clinical practices. After a defined number of weeks, the "best" formulated and relevant question is chosen (e.g., by the unit manager or a nursing research associate), and the question writer receives a prize (e.g., a book, registration at a local research conference).

This strategy has several potential benefits. First, it can create an environment or culture of reflective inquiry into practice. Second, the questions can be submitted to the librarian to search for evidence to answer the questions. It is likely there will be some relevant, quality evidence that can then be critiqued and brought forward for decision making related to practice. Third, where there are no quality studies, the questions can be prioritized and proposals written for outcome management protocols, pilot studies, and full studies to answer the questions.

Enhance Job Description

Another strategy that managers can implement to facilitate environmental change is explicitly including EBP in performance appraisals and requiring evidence to support proposed changes in practice and policy decisions (Titler et al., 1994). When the evidence exists, supporting the change with resources is required. If no evidence exists, a consensus process similar to that described under practice guidelines is suggested.

Allot Time, Funds, and Other Resources

Administrators can further support the development of EBP by allowing practitioners time to learn skills related to EBP, such as searching bibliographic databases, searching for preappraised studies through resources that incorporate methodological filters, and learning how to critically appraise research studies. Time is needed also for computer access or going to the library, conducting searches, and holding team meetings to consider clinical questions, relevant research, and application to clinical practice and institutional policy development.

Administrators must commit to providing expertise and funds so that agency library holdings will include research relevant to clinical practice, including subscriptions to research journals. Electronic access to databases, full-text journal articles where they exist, and resources such as the *Cochrane Library* and *Clinical Evidence* are necessary.

Clinical research can become an institutional commitment, either by establishing formal research committees and appointments for clinical researchers or by collaborations with other healthcare agencies and educational institutions. Mitchell and colleagues found that healthcare institutions that reported change based on research were more likely to have a research committee and access to individuals with expertise in clinical research (Mitchell et al., 1995). Sharing arrangements such as cross-appointments can be made. Educational institutions can gain by such partnerships through provision of a "real-world" laboratory for the development of research questions and proposals, as well as the actual conduct of the research.

The concept of the "knowledge broker"—of having a person who is familiar with clinical practice and the language of research—is untested except for two pilot studies by the CREP at the University of Rochester School of Nursing that are currently testing the effects of an EBP mentor on nurse and patient outcomes in acute and community health settings. (B. Melnyk, personal communication, 2003). This is usually a role for clinical specialists, nurse educators, or nurse researchers within a clinical agency. Nurses in these roles know the organization, the culture, the environment, the dynamics of the healthcare team, and the staff's skill level in EBP. They have knowledge of how to access and critically appraise the research, as well as the ability to communicate the relevance and applicability of a study in a way that is usable by the practitioners. Organizations might consider how individuals in these roles can be used to transfer research-based messages for practice and information for clinical decision making (Thompson et al., 2001a; Thompson et al., 2001b).

In conclusion, EBP is a relatively new paradigm for nurses and other healthcare practitioners. Models have evolved from those focused specifically on research utilization to those that set research utilization within the evidence-based decision-making process, both at individual and organizational levels. Because of the relative newness of the paradigm, little evaluation exists to guide identification of the "best" strategies for implementing EBP. Some strategies are successful in some settings and with some health professional groups but do not transfer successfully to other settings and other health professional groups (Cochrane Review Group, 1999). Recent innovations need to be evaluated and creative strategies remain to be discovered.

references

Agency for Healthcare Research and Quality (AHRQ). (2002). Systems to rate the strength of scientific evidence. Fact Sheet. (AHRQ Publication No. 02-P0022). Rockville, MD: AHRQ. www.ahrq.gov/clinic/epcsums/strenfact.htm.

AHRQ. (2002). Retrieved November 10, 2002,from http://www.ahrq.gov/clinic/epcix.htm

Bhuta, T., Henderson-Smart, D. J. (2002). Elective high frequency jet ventilation versus conventional ventilation for respiratory distress syndrome in preterm infants. In *Cochrane Library, 4.* Oxford: Update Software.

Bostrum, J., & Suter, W. N. (1993). Research utilization: Making the link to practice. *Journal of Nursing Staff Development, 9,* 28–34.

Bustillo, J. R., Lauriello, J., Horan, W. P., & Keith, S. (2001). The psychosocial treatment of schizophrenia: An update. *American Journal of Psychiatry, 158,* 163–175.

Champion, V. L., & Leach, A. (1989). Variables related to research utilization in nursing: An empirical investigation. *Journal of Advanced Nursing, 14*(9), 705–710.

Ciliska, D., DiCenso, A., & Cullum, N. (1999). Centres of evidence-based nursing: Directions and challenges. *Evidence-Based Nursing; 2,* 102–103.

Ciliska, D., Mastrilli, P., Ploeg, J., Hayward, S., Brunton, G., & Underwood, J. (2001). The effectiveness of home visiting as a delivery strategy for public health nursing interventions to clients in the prenatal and postnatal periods. *Primary Health Care, 2,* 41–54.

Clinical Evidence (2002). Retrieved November 10, 2002, from www.clinicalevidenceonline.org Cochrane Collaboration. Retrieved November 10, 2002, from www.update-software.com.

Cochrane Review Group on Effective Practice and Organization of Care (1999). Getting evidence into practice. *Effective Health Care Bulletin, 5.*

Cronenwett, C. (1994). Using research in the care of patients. In G. LoBiondo-Wood & J. Haber (Eds.), *Nursing research: Methods, critical appraisal, and utilization* (pp. 89–90). St. Louis: Mosby.

DiCenso, A., Cullum, N., Ciliska, D., & Guyatt, G. Introduction to evidence-based nursing. In A. DiCenso, N. Cullum, D. Ciliska, & G. Guyatt (Eds.) (2004) *Evidence-based nursing. A guide to clinical practice.* Philadelphia: Elsevier.

DiCenso, A., Virani, T., Bajnok, I., Borycki, E., et al. (2002). A toolkit to facilitate the implementation of clinical practice guidelines in healthcare settings. *Hospital Quarterly, 5*(3), 55–60.

Dobbins, M., Ciliska, D., Cockerill, R., Barnsley, J., & DiCenso, A. (2002). A framework for the dissemination and utilization of research for health care policy and practice. *Online Journal of Knowledge Synthesis for Nursing, 9,* 7.

Drakulovic, M. B., Torres, A., Bauer, T. T, Nicolas, J. M., Nogues, S., & Ferrer, M. (1999). Supine body position as a risk factor for nosocomial pneumonia in mechanically ventilated patients: A randomized trial. *Lancet, 354,* 1851–1858.

Early Supported Discharge Trialists. (2002). Services for reducing duration of hospital care for acute stroke patients. *Cochrane Library, 4.* Oxford: Update Software.

Estabrooks, C.A. (1998). Will evidence-based nursing practice make practice perfect? *Canadian Journal of Nursing Research, 30,* 15–36.

Fleming, D. R., Jacober, S. J., Vandenberg M. A., Fitzgerald, J. T., & Grunberger, G. (1997). The safety of injecting insulin through clothing. *Diabetes Care, 20,* 244–247.

Flemming, K. (1998). Asking answerable questions. *Evidence-Based Nursing, 1,* 68–70.

Funk, S. G., Tornquist, E. M., & Champagne, M. T. (1989). A model for improving the dissemination of nursing research. *Western Journal of Nursing Research, 11*(3), 361–367.

Geyman, J. (1998) Evidence-based medicine in primary care: An overview. *Journal of the American Board of Family Practice, 11,* 46–56.

Goode, C. & Piedalue, F. (1999). Evidence-based clinical practice. *Journal of Nursing Administration, 29,* 15–21.

Grol, R. (1997). Beliefs and evidence in changing clinical practice. *British Medical Journal, 315,* 418–421.

Guyatt, G., Cook, D., Devereaux, P. J., Meade, M., & Strauss, S. (2002). Therapy. In G. Guyatt & D. Rennie (Eds.), *Users' guides to the medical literature.* Chicago: AMA Press.

Guyatt, G., & Rennie, D. (Eds.) (2002). *Users' guides to the medical literature.* Chicago: AMA Press.

Hallas, D., & Melnyk, B. M. (2003). Evidence-based practice: The paradigm shift. *Journal of Pediatric Health Care, 17* (1), 46–49.

Haynes, R., Sackett, D., Gray, J., Cook, D. & Guyatt, G. (1996.) EBM Notebook: Transferring evidence from research into practice: 1. The role of clinical care research evidence in clinical decisions. *Evidence Based Medicine, 1,* 196–198.

Haynes, R. (2002). What kind of evidence is it that evidence-based medicine advocates want health care providers and consumers to pay attention to? *BMC Health Services Research, 2,* 3.

Haynes, R. B., Devereaux, P. J., & Guyatt, G. H.(2002). Clinical expertise in the era of evidence-based medicine and patient choice. *ACP Journal Club, 136*(2), A11–A14.

Hodnett, E. D. (2002). Caregiver support for women during childbirth. *Cochrane Library, 4*. Oxford: Update Software.

Jerum, A., & Melnyk, B. M. (2001). Effectiveness of interventions to prevent obesity and obesity-related complications in children and adolescents. *Pediatric Nursing, 27*(6), 606–610.

Kajermo, K. N., Nordstrom, G., Krusebrant, A., & Bjorvell, H. (1998). Barriers and facilitators of research utilization, as perceived by a group of registered nurses in Sweden. *Journal of Advanced Nursing, 27*, 798–807.

Kim, S. (1999). *Models of theory-practice linkage in nursing.* International Nursing Research Conference: Research to Practice. University of Alberta, Edmonton, Canada.

Kitson, A. (1999). Research utilization: current issues, questions and debates. *Canadian Journal of Nursing Research, 31*(1), 13–22.

Kitson, A., Harvey, G., & McCormack, B. (1989). Enabling the implementation of evidence based practice: A conceptual framework. *Quality in Health Care, 7*(3), 149–158.

Lomas, J., Enkin, M., Anderson, G. M., Hannah, W. J., Vayda, E., & Singer, J. (1991). Opinion leaders vs. audit and feedback to implement practice guidelines. Delivery after previous cesarean section. *JAMA, 265*(17), 2202–2207.

Luker, K. A., & Kenrick, M. (1992). An exploratory study of the sources of influence on the clinical decisions of community nurses. *Journal of Advanced Nursing, 17*, 457–466.

Melnyk, B. M. (2002). Strategies for overcoming barriers in implementing evidence-based practice. *Pediatric Nursing, 28*(2), 159–161.

Melnyk, B. M., Fairbanks, E., & Feinstein, N. F. (2002). Informational/behavioral interventions with parents of LBW premature infants: An evidence-base to guide practice. *Pediatric Nursing, 28*(5), 511–516.

Melnyk, B. M., Alpert-Gillis, L., Feinstein, N. F., Fairbanks, E., Schultz-Czarniak, J., Hust, D., Sherman, L., LeMoine, C., Moldenhauer, Z., Small, L., Bender, N., & Sinkin, R. A. (2001). Improving cognitive development of LBW premature infants with the COPE program: A pilot study of the benefit of early NICU intervention with mothers. *Research in Nursing and Health, 24*, 373–389.

Melnyk, B. M., & Fineout-Overholt, E. (2002a). Putting research into practice. Rochester ARCC. *Reflections on Nursing Leadership, 28*(2), 22–25.

Melnyk, B. M., & Fineout-Overholt, E. (2002b). Key steps in evidence based practice: Asking compelling clinical questions and searching for the best evidence. *Pediatric Nursing, 28*(3), 262 263, 266.

Melnyk, B. M., Fineout-Overholt, E., Stone, P., & Ackerman, M. (2000). Evidence-based practice: The past, the present, and recommendations for the millennium. *Pediatric Nursing, 26*(1), 77–80.

Mitchell, A., Janzen, K., Pask, E., & Southwell, D. (1995). Assessment of nursing research utilization needs in Ontario health agencies. *Canadian Journal of Nursing Administration, 8*(1), 77–91.

National Association of Neonatal Nurses (2002). Retrieved November 10, 2002, from http://www.nann.org/public/articles/index.cfm?cat=9.

Olds, D. L., Robinson, J., O'Brien, R., Luckey, D. W., Pettitt, L. M., Henderson, C. R. Jr., et al. (2002). Home visiting by paraprofessionals and by nurses: A randomized, controlled trial. *Pediatrics, 110*(3), 486–496.

Parahoo, K. (2000). Barriers to, and facilitators of, research utilization among nurses in Northern Ireland. *Journal of Advanced Nursing, 31*(1), 89–98.

Pearson, A. (2002). Nursing takes the lead. *Reflections on Nursing Leadership, 28*(4), 18–21.

Ploeg, J., Ciliska, D., Dobbins, M., Hayward, S. & Thomas, H. (1996). A systematic overview of adolescent suicide prevention programs. *Canadian Journal of Public Health, 87*, 319–324.

Registered Nurses Association of Ontario (RNAO; 2002). Retrieved November 10, 2002, from http://www.rnao.org/bestpractices.

Retsas, A., & Nolan, M. (1999). Barriers to nurses' use of research. An Australian hospital study. *International Journal of Nursing Studies, 36*, 335–343.

Rice, V. H., & Stead, L. F. (2002). Nursing interventions for smoking cessation. *Cochrane Library*. Oxford: Update Software.

Rogers, E. M. (1995). *Diffusion of Innovations* (4th ed.). New York: The Free Press.

Rosswurm, M. A., & Larrabee, J. (1999). A model for change to evidence-based practice. Image: *Journal of Nursing Scholarship, 31*(4), 317–322.

Royle, J., Blythe, J., Ingram, C., DiCenso, A., Bhatnager, N., & Potvin, C. (1996). The research utilization process: The use of guided imagery to reduce anxiety. *Canadian Oncology Nursing Journal, 6,* 20–25.

Rycroft-Malone, J., Kitson, A., Harvey, G., McCormack, B., Seers, K., Titchen, A., & Estabrooks, C. (2002). Ingredients for change: Revisiting a conceptual framework. *Quality & Safety in Health Care, 11,* 174–180.

Small, L. (2002). Early predictors of poor coping outcomes in children following intensive care hospitalization and stressful medical encounters. *Pediatric Nursing, 28*(4), 393–398.

Stetler, C. B., & Marram, G. (1976). Evaluating research findings for applicability in practice. *Nursing Outlook, 24,* 559–63.

Stetler, C. B. (1994a). Refinement of the Stetler/Marram model for application of research findings to practice. *Nursing Outlook, 42,* 15–25.

Stetler, C. B. (1994b). Using research to improve patient care. In G. LoBiondo-Wood & J. Haber (Eds.), *Nursing research: methods, critical appraisal, and utilization* (pp. 1–2). St. Louis: Mosby.

Stetler, C. B., Brunell, M., Giuliano, K., Morsi, D., Prince, L., & Newell-Stokes, G. (1998). Evidence based practice and the role of nursing leadership. *Journal of Nursing Administration, 8,* 45–53.

Stetler, C. B. (2001a). Updating the Stetler model of research utilization to facilitate evidence-based practice. *Nursing Outlook, 49,* 272–278.

Stetler, C. B. (2001b). *Evidence-based practice and the use of research: A synopsis of basic strategies and concepts to improve care.* DC: Nova Foundation.

Stetler, C. B. (2002). *Evidence-based practice: A fad or the future of professional practice?* Fourth Annual Evidence Based Practice Conference: Creating Momentum! Improving Care! Ann Arbor, Michigan.

Teaching Learning Resources for Evidence-Based Practice (2002). Retrieved November 10, 2002 from www.mdx.ac.uk/www/rctsh/ebp/main.htm.

Thomas, L., Cullum, N., McColl, E., Rousseau, N., Soutter, J., & Steen, N. (2000). Guidelines in professions allied to medicine. *Cochrane Database of Systematic Reviews, 2*: CD000349. Review.

Thompson, C., McCaughan, D., Cullum, N., Sheldon, T. A., Mulhall, A., & Thompson, D. R. (2001a). The accessibility of research-based knowledge for nurses in United Kingdom acute care settings. *Journal of Advanced Nursing, 36,* 11–22.

Thompson, C., McCaughan, D., Cullum, N., Sheldon, T. A., Mulhall, A., & Thompson, D. R. (2001b). Research information in nurses' clinical decision-making: What is useful? *Journal of Advanced Nursing, 36,* 376–388.

Titler, M. G., Klieber, C., Steelman, V., Goode, C., Rakel, B., Barry-Walker, J., Small, S., & Buckwalter, K. (1994). Infusing research into practice to promote quality care. *Nursing Research, 43*(5), 307–313.

Titler, M. G. (2002). Use of research in practice. In G. LoBiondo & J. Haber (Eds.), *Nursing research: Methods, critical appraisal and utilization* (5th ed.). St. Louis, MO: Mosby.

Trepepi-Bova, K. A., Woods, K. D., & Loach, M. C. (1997). A comparison of transparent polyurethane and dry gauze dressings for peripheral IV catheter sites: Rates of phlebitis, infiltration, and dislodgment by patients. *American Journal of Critical Care, 6,* 377–381.

Weiss, C. (1980). Knowledge creep and decision accretion. *Knowledge: Creation, Diffusion, Utilization, 1,* 381–404.

Zaroukian, M. H. (2001). PubMed clinical queries. *Evidence-Based Medicine, 6,* 8.

chapter 8

219

Using Evidence-Based Practice Guidelines: Tools for Improving Practice

Jean Slutsky

chapter 9

> **"***Whatever you can do or dream you can, begin it. Boldness has genius, power, and magic in it.***"**
>
> —*Johann Wolfgang von Goethe*

Variation in clinical practices is a well-recognized phenomenon. It has been over 30 years since Wennberg and Gittelsohn (1973, 1982) first described the variation in treatment patterns in New England and other parts of the country. A remarkable variety of practices in the diagnosis, treatment, and management of patients exists in the United States and elsewhere. The Dartmouth Atlas of Health Care graphically demonstrates the variability of health care services in the United States (Dartmouth Medical School Center for the Evaluative Clinical Sciences, 1999). These regional variations in care are troubling reminders that patient care is still as much an art as a science.

   Evidence-based practice (EBP), "integrating individual clinical expertise with the best available external clinical evidence from systematic research"(Sackett et al., 1997) requires the clinician to determine which clinical options are supported by high-quality scientific evidence. Gaining access to up-to-date scientific clinical information can be very difficult, particularly where access to medical journals is limited, and synthesizing the information can be even harder. The U. S. National Library of Medicine (NLM) estimates that approximately 2,000 new citations are added to MEDLINE daily, making it impossible for the individual clinician to master the body of emerging evidence (NLM, 1998).

Guidelines as Tools

In reaction to these compelling findings, synthesis of published research studies and the development of clinical practice guidelines have become increasingly popular ways of addressing the variation in clinical practice and difficulty in interpreting large volumes of scientific studies. Guidelines, which cover a broad array of clinical diagnostic and therapeutic services, are used to define a minimum set of services appropriate to each clinical condition. They are also designed to allow some flexibility in their application to individual patients who fall outside the scope of the guideline or who possess significant comorbidities not adequately addressed in a particular guideline.

Rigorously and explicitly developed clinical practice guidelines can be tools to help bridge the gap between published scientific evidence and clinical decision making (Haynes, Hayward & Bridges, 1995). For both the guideline user and developer, it is critical to keep in mind the role evidence plays in developing recommendations. Most experimental studies do not take into account the characteristics of individual patients, including comorbidities and clinical settings (Berg, 1998; Cook et al., 1997; Haynes, 1993). Variations in the composition of guideline development panels, developing organization, and interpretation of the evidence are often the source of differing recommendations on the same clinical topic (Berg et al., 1997; Lohr, 1995).

The dramatic growth in guideline development is not without unintended consequences. The rigor of guidelines varies significantly, as does the reporting on how a particular guideline is formulated. There are often guidelines with conflicting recommendations, posing dilemmas for users and those trying to assess the quality of patient care. Finally, guidelines are often developed and written in ways that clinicians and organizations find difficult to implement, which limits their effectiveness in improving patient outcomes. Nevertheless, the current emphasis on evidence-based guideline development, implementation, and evaluation activities is a positive step toward evidence-based decision making at the bedside. This chapter will explore how the clinician can access, interpret, and use clinical practice guidelines to improve the care and health outcomes of their patients.

Where to Find Guidelines

Finding guidelines can be a formidable challenge. The large number of guideline developers and topics, coupled with the various forms of guideline publication and distribution, make identification of guidelines difficult and unpredictable. The term *practice guideline* can be used to define a publication type when searching NLM's PubMed database.

Access the database at **http://www.ncbi.nih.gov/entrez/query.fcgi.**

Using the keywords *practice guideline* alone, without any qualifiers, yields over 27,000 citations; most of these are not guidelines but studies, commentaries, editorials, or letters to the editor about guidelines. The search can be further refined by adding clinical areas or interventions but the result is still an overwhelming mixture of publications. Searching citation databases for clinical practice guidelines can be problematic for other reasons. Frequently, guidelines are not published in indexed journals or books, which makes them difficult to locate in traditional literature databases.

Prior to 1997, few comprehensive collections of guidelines existed. Since then, individual collections that distribute international, regional, organizational, or specialty-specific guidelines have matured (see Box 9-1). The list of individual guideline developers is long, and the distribution venues for guidelines can be as plentiful as the number of developers.

In Canada, the Canadian Medical Association (CMA) maintains the CMA InfoBase of clinical practice guidelines. Guidelines are included in the CMA InfoBase only if they are produced or endorsed in Canada by a national, provincial/territorial, or regional medical or health organization, professional society, government agency, or expert panel (**http://mdm.ca/cpgsnew/cpgs/index.asp**).

There are other country-specific guideline collections, such as the Scottish Intercollegiate Guideline Network (SIGN) sponsored by the Royal College of Physicians (**http://www.sign.ac.uk/**).

The National Institute for Clinical Excellence (NICE) in England also maintains a collection of guidelines to advise the National Health Service (**http://www.nice.org.uk/**). In New Zealand, the New Zealand Guidelines Group (NZGG) maintains a collection of guidelines developed under its sponsorship (**http://www.nzgg.org.nz/**).

Individual professional societies in the United States also maintain collections of guidelines specific to a particular practice or professional specialty. These collections vary in depth and collaboration. The American College of Cardiology and the American Heart Association have joint guideline panels and publish their guidelines in a variety of formats (**http://www.acc.org/clinical/statements.htm**; also **http://www.americanheart.org/presenter.jhtml? identifier=3004542**). The American Cancer Society also convenes multidisciplinary panels to develop cancer-related guidelines and to make the guidelines available on the Internet (**http://www.cancer.org**).

box 9.1

Selected Guideline Databases

GENERAL
- National Guideline Clearinghouse (NGC): http://www.guideline.gov
- Primary Care Clinical Practice Guidelines: http://medicine.ucsf.edu/resources/guidelines
- CMA InfoBase: http://mdm.ca/cpgsnew/cpgs/index.asp
- Health Services/Technology Assessment Text (HSTAT): http://hstat.nlm.nih.gov
- Guidelines Advisory Committee: http://www.gacguidelines.ca
- Scottish Intercollegiate Guideline Network (SIGN): http://www.sign.ac.uk/guidelines/index.html
- National Institute for Clinical Excellence (NICE): http://www.nice.org.uk/catcg2.asp?c=20034
- New Zealand Guidelines Group (NGZZ): http://www.nzgg.org.nz/library.cfm
- Guidelines International Network: http://www.G-I-N.net

SPECIFIC
- American College of Physicians: http://www.acponline.org/sci-policy/guidelines
- American Cancer Society: http://www.cancer.org/docroot/ped/content/ped_2_3x_acs_cancer_detection_guidelines_36.asp?sitearea=ped
- American College of Cardiology: http://www.acc.org/clinical/statements.htm
- American Association of Clinical Endocrinologists: http://www.aace.com/clin/guidelines
- American Association of Respiratory Care: http://www.rcjournal.com/online_resources/cpgs/cpg_index.asp
- American Academy of Pediatrics: http://www.aap.org/policy/paramtoc.html
- American Psychiatric Association: http://www.psych.org/clin_res/prac_guide.cfm
- Ministry of Health Services, British Columbia, Canada: http://www.healthservices.gov.bc.ca/msp/protoguides
- New York Academy of Medicine: http://www.ebmny.org/cpg.html
- Veterans Administration: http://www.oqp.med.va.gov/cpg/cpg.htm
- National Kidney Foundation: https://www.kidney.org/professionals/doqi/guidelineindex.cfm
- American Medical Directors Association: http://www.amda.com/info/cpg
- Registered Nurses Association of Ontario: http://www.rnao.org/bestpractices
- Association of Women's Health, Obstetric, and Neonatal Nurses: http://awhonn.org
- National Association of Neonatal Nurses: http://www.nann.org
- Oncology Nursing Society – http://www.ons.org
- University of Iowa Gerontological Nursing Interventions Research Center: http://www.nursing.uiowa.edu/centers/gnirc/protocols.htm

Although it is useful to have collections of guidelines that are specific to a disease or specialty, this makes finding guidelines in more than one clinical area difficult. In 1998, the U.S. Agency for Health Care Policy and Research, now the Agency for Healthcare Research and Quality (AHRQ, 1998), released the National Guideline Clearinghouse (NGC).

Access the National Guideline Clearinghouse (NGC) at **http://www.guideline.gov.**

The NGC was developed in partnership with the American Medical Association and the American Association of Health Plans. In developing NGC, AHRQ intended to create a comprehensive database of up-to-date English language evidence-based clinical practice guidelines (see Box 9-2). Five years later, NGC contains over 1,100 guidelines from developers all over the world. NGC also contains an archive of guideline titles that are out of date. The archived guidelines do not get circulated on the site. The database is updated at least weekly with new content and provides guideline comparison features so users can explore differences between guidelines. Users can register to receive weekly e-mails listing the guideline changes on the site. NGC receives over 70,000 visits per week.

Of the various guideline collections and databases, NGC contains the most descriptive information about guidelines. It also is the most selective about the guidelines that are included in its database; inclusion criteria are applied to each guideline before they are incorporated in the database. Furthermore, guidelines in the database reflect the most current version. In 2002, more than one third of the guidelines submitted to NGC were updates of guidelines already in the database.

The Primary Care Clinical Practice Guidelines Web site is a comprehensive collection of indexed links to full-text guidelines and other sources of guideline-related information. The site is not annotated and does not provide details about individual guidelines. Although the Web site provides a broad array of helpful links, the user is compelled to go to each link to determine information about each guideline. This can be time-consuming and confusing when there are multiple guideline links for the same topic area. Despite these limitations, it provides a very useful portal for guideline-related Web sites.

One other Web site that is very helpful is NLM Gateway. The Gateway allows users to put in a search term, which is then sent out to eight different NLM databases. One of these, Health Services/Health Technology Assessment Text (HSTAT) is especially practical. HSTAT is unique because it takes large guidelines, systematic reviews, and technology assessments and enables their text to be searchable on the Web, making them much easier to navigate electronically.

Access the NLM Gateway at **http://gateway.nlm.nih.gov/gw/Cmd**.

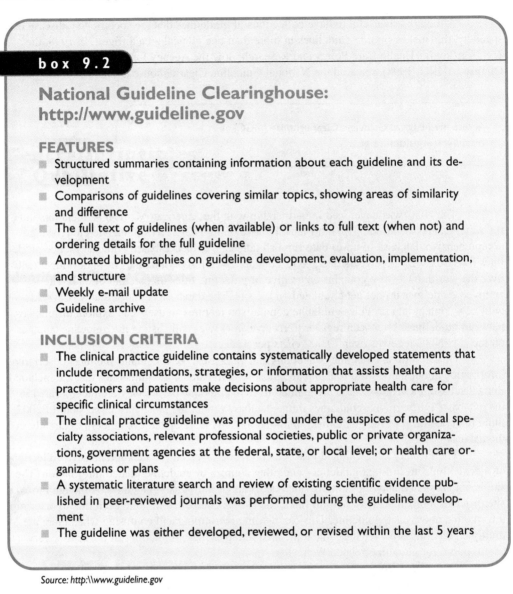

box 9.2

National Guideline Clearinghouse: http://www.guideline.gov

FEATURES

- Structured summaries containing information about each guideline and its development
- Comparisons of guidelines covering similar topics, showing areas of similarity and difference
- The full text of guidelines (when available) or links to full text (when not) and ordering details for the full guideline
- Annotated bibliographies on guideline development, evaluation, implementation, and structure
- Weekly e-mail update
- Guideline archive

INCLUSION CRITERIA

- The clinical practice guideline contains systematically developed statements that include recommendations, strategies, or information that assists health care practitioners and patients make decisions about appropriate health care for specific clinical circumstances
- The clinical practice guideline was produced under the auspices of medical specialty associations, relevant professional societies, public or private organizations, government agencies at the federal, state, or local level; or health care organizations or plans
- A systematic literature search and review of existing scientific evidence published in peer-reviewed journals was performed during the guideline development
- The guideline was either developed, reviewed, or revised within the last 5 years

Source: http:\\www.guideline.gov

There is no shortage of guideline-related sites on the Internet. The challenge is finding the source of guidelines that is easiest to use and provides the best mechanisms for making sure the contents are up to date. Because so many of guideline resources are now on the Internet, it is wise to consider the quality of the Web site when choosing a source. The European Union has developed standards that are valuable to keep in mind. The six standards are (Commission of the European Communities, Brussels, 2002):

- Transparency of health-related content
- Authority of health-related content providers

- Privacy and data protection of health data
- Updating of health-related information
- Accountability for health-related content
- Accessibility of health-related content

Extremely useful databases of clinical practice guidelines exist. Many of these resources provide guideline users with not only good information about clinical practice guidelines but also additional information on how guidelines are used and developed. Critical appraisal of guideline databases is necessary to ensure that the information is current and reliable.

Finding the Right Guideline

Locating and reviewing current guidelines on a particular subject can be overwhelming. Even after a guideline has been identified, it is often difficult to determine critical attributes of the guideline, such as how the guideline was developed, who developed and funded it, what dates the literature review covered or who was on the panel, and so on. Guidelines should be explicit in their discussion of the evidence supporting recommendations and in identifying the benefits and harms of interventions (Barrett et al., 1999). Guidelines developed using evidence of established benefit of treatments or interventions have the potential to improve health outcomes and decrease morbidity and mortality (Woolf et al., 1999). Users of guidelines need to keep in mind that "one size *does not* fit all."

Hayes describes the "three Rs" of clinical practice guideline application as their application to the *right person* at the *right time* and in the *right way* (Haynes, 1993). Davis and Taylor-Vaisey (1997) suggest that the effect of clinical guidelines on improved health care outcomes is dependent on taking into account their nature, the nature and beliefs of the target clinicians, and environmental factors when trying to implement them. Hayward and colleagues for the Evidence-based Medicine Working Group identified three main questions to consider (Hayward et al., 1995; Wilson et al., 1995). These questions concern the *validity of the recommendations*, the *identification of the recommendations,* and *the usefulness of the recommendations.*

Are the Recommendations Valid?

It is important to know whether the developers used outcomes meaningful to the patient and whether they were inclusive in considering all reasonable treatment options. The user should consider whether the developers assigned different values to the outcomes they evaluated. For example, did the developer seek patient preferences or use a multidisciplinary panel in their deliberations?

The developers should demonstrate that they have used an explicit and sensible process to systematically search and review the evidence on which the guideline recommendations are based. When combining the evidence, did the developer use a rating scheme or similar method to determine the quality and strength of the individual studies and the combined studies? Developers often use letter grades or words such as *strongly recommend* to demonstrate their assessment of the strength of the evidence for a given recommendation. In 2002, the Research Training Institute at University of North Carolina at Chapel Hill (RTI-UNC) Evidence-Based Practice Center completed a systematic review of schemes used to rate the quality of a body of evidence. The review evaluated three domains. There is no universal consensus on grading evidence or the strength of the body of evidence for a recommendation, although there are well-established norms (see Box 9-3), most notably the U.S. Preventive Services Task Force (Harris et al., 2001).

Because guidelines reflect "snapshots" of the evidence at a given point in time, they often are overtaken by new evidence. Developers can alert guideline users to ongoing research studies that may have an impact on the recommendations in the future. Guidelines should also undergo peer review and sometimes pilot testing in actual practice before being released. This allows a broader group of people to identify inconsistencies or relevant evidence that might have been overlooked. Pilot testing the guideline in actual practice allows organizational or functional problems with implementing the guideline to be identified. These can then be corrected or accommodated to enhance the chances of the guideline being implemented.

box 9.3

U.S. Preventive Services Task Force Recommendations

A—The United States Preventive Services Task Force (USPSTF) strongly recommends that clinicians routinely provide [the service] to eligible patients. (The USPSTF found good evidence that [the service] improves important health outcomes and concludes that benefits substantially outweigh harms.)

B—The USPSTF recommends that clinicians routinely provide [the service] to eligible patients. (The USPSTF found at least fair evidence that [the service] improves important health outcomes and concludes that benefits outweigh harms.)

C—The USPSTF makes no recommendation for or against routine provision of [the service]. (The USPSTF found at least fair evidence that [the service] can improve health outcomes but concludes that the balance of the benefits and harms is too close to justify a general recommendation.)

D—The USPSTF recommends against routinely providing [the service] to asymptomatic patients. (The USPSTF found at least fair evidence that [the service] is ineffective or that harms outweigh benefits.)

I—The USPSTF concludes that the evidence is insufficient to recommend for or against routinely providing [the service]. (Evidence that [the service] is effective is lacking, of poor quality, or conflicting and the balance of benefits and harms cannot be determined.)

What Are the Recommendations?

The usefulness of a guideline is dependent on how meaningful and practical are the actual recommendations. Practicality relates to the ease with which a recommendation is implemented. The recommendations should be as unambiguous as possible. They should address periodicity of screening and other interventions, and they should be explicit about areas where there are trade-offs that require informed choice by the patient. Furthermore, recommendations should address clinically relevant actions. The recommendation should be justified based on the developer's assessment of the benefits of the intervention against the harms of action. If an intervention has a significant chance of introducing harm and is based on poor evidence, the guideline should explicitly justify the basis for the recommendation.

Will the Recommendations Help Patient Care?

Applying a guideline on management of heart failure in the ambulatory setting is not the same as using a guideline on management of heart failure in the hospital. Similarly, a guideline on management of heart failure in children is not comparable with a guideline on management of heart failure in adults. The guideline should fit the setting of care, the age and gender of the patient, the presence of any comorbidities, and the type of clinician providing the care. This last point is important to consider. Patients do not generally present with only one disease or condition. Often, clinicians are faced with a patient who has multiple morbidities. Guidelines do not always take into account multiple conditions so the clinician must individualize treatment in many circumstances. Even so, guidelines can help point the clinician in the right direction when looking for the right care for their patients.

Tools for Evaluating Guidelines

Finding the right guideline to use is contingent on being able to critically evaluate the reliability of a guideline. There is ample evidence that guideline developers do not always adhere to best practices in guideline development. Two studies of guidelines developed by medical specialty societies found that a significant percentage did not adhere to accepted methodological practices in their development (Grilli et al., 2000; Shaneyfelt, Mayo-Smith, & Rothwangl, 1999). The Institute of Medicine in 1990 identified eight attributes of good guideline development, including:

- Validity
- Reliability and reproducibility
- Clinical applicability
- Clinical flexibility
- Clarity
- Documentation
- Development by a multidisciplinary process
- Plans for review (Field & Lohr, 1992)

Guidelines are complex and heterogeneous documents; therefore, evaluating them is often difficult.

Provisional Instrument for Assessing Guidelines

Lohr and Field (1992) developed a provisional instrument for assessing clinical practice guidelines. The instrument was developed because it was recognized that there was a need for an explicit mechanism to assess the soundness of individual clinical practice guidelines. The instrument was a first step in trying to identify a way to assess important attributes of guidelines. Nonetheless, it was long and difficult to complete. It was not intended to be used by practicing clinicians but by groups or organizations wanting to adopt a guideline. The instrument was also appropriate for self-assessment by guideline developers.

AGREE Instrument for Assessing Guidelines

In 1992, the United Kingdom National Health Services Management Executive set in motion the development of an appraisal instrument for the National Health Services (Cluzeau et al., 1999). This was the first attempt to formally assess the usefulness of a guideline appraisal instrument. Subsequently, the European Union provided funding for the development of the Appraisal of Guidelines for Research and Evaluation (AGREE) Instrument.

The Appraisal of Guidelines for Research and Evaluation (AGREE) Instrument can be found at **http://www.agreecollaboration.org.**

The AGREE Instrument was developed and evaluated by an international group of guideline developers and researchers. Since its release in final form in 2001, the AGREE Instrument has been translated into many languages and is gaining appeal as the standard guideline appraisal tool. The Agree Instrument contains 6 quality domains and 23 items (AGREE Collaboration, 2001) (see Box 9-4).

It is recommended that there be more than one appraiser for each guideline—preferably four—to increase the reliability of the instrument. The instrument is scored using a four-point Likert scale, with one being "strongly disagree" and four being "strongly agree." The domain scores are not meant to be aggregated into one overall score for the guideline. Thus, the instrument will produce individual domain scores but will not produce an overall rating for a guideline. The instrument allows the appraiser to give a subjective assessment of the guideline based on review of the individual domain scores.

National Guideline Clearinghouse and Others

The NGC produces structured summaries of each guideline in its database to aid the user in assessing the quality and appropriateness of a guideline. The summaries describe guideline attributes similar to those contained in the Lohr and Field (1992) provisional instrument and the AGREE (2001) Instrument. In addition, the Conference on Guideline Standardization (COGS) Statement recommends standardizing attributes that guideline developers should describe to help assess guidelines and make their implementation easier (Shiffman et al., 2003).

box 9.4

AGREE Instrument

SCOPE AND PURPOSE

Item 1. The overall objective(s) of the guideline is (are) specifically described.

Item 2. The clinical question(s) covered by the guideline is (are) specifically described.

Item 3. The patients to whom the guideline(s) are meant to apply are specifically described.

STAKEHOLDER INVOLVEMENT

Item 4. The guideline development group includes individuals from all relevant professional groups.

Item 5. The patients' views and preferences have been sought.

Item 6. The target users of the guideline are clearly defined.

Item 7. The guideline has been piloted among target users.

RIGOUR OF DEVELOPMENT

Item 8. Systematic methods were used to search for evidence.

Item 9. The criteria for selecting the evidence are clearly described.

Item 10. The methods used for formulating the recommendations are clearly described.

Item 11. The health benefits, side effects, and risks have been considered in formulating the recommendations.

Item 12. There is an explicit link between the recommendations and the supporting evidence.

Item 13. The guideline has been externally reviewed by experts prior to its publication.

Item 14. A procedure for updating the guideline is provided.

CLARITY AND PRESENTATION

Item 15. The recommendations are specific and unambiguous.

Item 16. The different options for management of the condition are clearly presented.

Item 17. The key recommendations are easily identifiable.

Item 18. The guideline is supported with tools for application.

APPLICATION

Item 19. The potential organizational barriers in applying the recommendations have been discussed.

Item 20. The possible cost implications of applying the recommendations have been considered.

Item 21. The guideline presents key review criteria for monitoring and/or audit purposes.

EDITORIAL INDEPENDENCE

Item 22. The guideline is editorially independent from the funding body.

Item 23. Conflicts of interest of guideline development members have been recorded.

Guideline Development

Determining when to develop guidelines should be systematically approached due to the amount of resources, skill, and time needed to accomplish these activities. In 1995, the Institute of Medicine issued guidance on setting priorities for clinical practice guidelines (Field, 1995). The report emphasized the importance of considering whether the guideline had the potential to change health outcomes or costs and the availability of scientific evidence on which to develop the recommendations (Field, 1995). Other criteria used by organizations include:

- The topic is clinically important, affecting large numbers of people with substantial morbidity or mortality (the burden of illness).
- The topic is complex enough to initiate debate about the recommendations.
- There is evidence of variation between actual and appropriate care.
- There are no existing valid or relevant guidelines available to use.
- There is evidence available to support evidence-based guideline development.
- The recommendations will be acceptable to the potential users.
- Implementation of the guideline is feasible.

When it is determined that there is uncertainty about how to treat or when gaps between optimal practice and actual practice have been identified, an organization may decide to develop a clinical practice guideline. Because it is difficult and expensive to develop guidelines, many organizations would be better served by adopting or adapting guidelines that have already been developed. Critically appraising already developed guidelines will allow an organization to screen for the best developed and suited guidelines for their organization. The AGREE (2001) Instrument is well suited for this purpose.

Processes and Panels

When the decision is made that a guideline will be developed, several important steps must take place. Guidelines can be developed using informal consensus, formal consensus, evidence-based methodologies, and explicit methodologies, either alone or in any combination (Woolf, 1992). Development should focus on more formal and explicit processes so that another developer using similar techniques would likely come to the same conclusions. Next, the guideline panel must be identified. The process for development should be multidisciplinary, reflecting the major stakeholders for the guideline, including users and patients (Field & Lohr, 1990; Shekelle et al., 1999; SIGN 50, 2002). Guideline panels should be composed of members who can adequately address the relevant interventions and meaningful outcomes and can weigh benefits and harms.

Review Questions

The next step in guideline development is the formal assessment of the clinical questions to be reviewed. This can be aided by the development of an "analytic framework" or "causal pathway" (Harris et al., 2001). These diagrams provide a roadmap for the precise description of the target patient, setting of care, interventions, and intermediate and final health outcomes. They also help focus the most meaningful questions that will guide the literature review and subsequent recommendations. Figure 9-1 shows an analytic framework for prevention screening used by the U.S. Preventive Services Task Force (Harris et al., 2001).

The numbers in the diagram relate to the key questions that will be considered. For example, one (1) relates to whether the screening test actually reduces morbidity and/or mortality. Five (5) asks the important question of whether treatment of clinically diagnosed patients results in reduced morbidity and/or mortality.

Literature Search and Review

After the key questions have been identified, a formal search and review of the literature takes place. It is easiest if a systematic review is already is identified by searching databases such as the *Cochrane Library*, MEDLINE, EMBASE, or Database of Abstracts of Reviews of Effects (DARE). If an already completed systematic review is not found, it is necessary to develop one. The first step is to determine what types of evidence will be considered, including study design, dates of publication, and language. A search strategy of relevant citation databases should be developed, preferably with the assistance of a medical librarian familiar with electronic searches. Once the search is completed, a process for screening titles and abstracts for relevance is done. The remaining titles are retrieved for evaluation. These articles are then screened, and data is extracted. The individual articles are reviewed for internal and external biases, and their quality

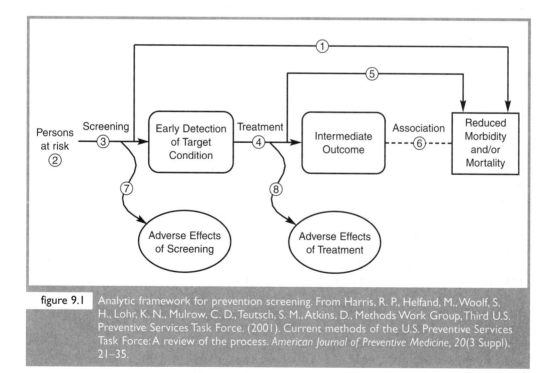

figure 9.1 Analytic framework for prevention screening. From Harris, R. P., Helfand, M., Woolf, S. H., Lohr, K. N., Mulrow, C. D., Teutsch, S. M., Atkins, D., Methods Work Group, Third U.S. Preventive Services Task Force. (2001). Current methods of the U.S. Preventive Services Task Force: A review of the process. *American Journal of Preventive Medicine, 20*(3 Suppl), 21–35.

is often rated. Once data are abstracted from the individual studies, the results are summarized, sometimes using meta-analysis to combine results from similar studies.

Recommendations

The next step is to develop recommendations based on the strength of the evidence for each of the questions that were identified in the analytic framework. Some guideline panels chose to make recommendations based solely on evidence, whereas others will use expert opinion when the evidence is poor or lacking. When expert opinion is used, it should be identified as such and be gathered using formal, explicit methods.

Peer Review

After the guideline recommendations are formulated, the guideline should be subjected to peer review to uncover any omissions or misinterpretations. In some cases, it may be wise to pilot test the guideline to determine whether it is feasible to implement and does not contain recommendations that are illogical.

Dissemination

After peer review and pilot testing, the guideline is revised accordingly and disseminated and publicized. Implementing guidelines into actual practice is difficult and will generally require multifaceted and sustained interventions. Quality measurement and feedback mechanisms can help determine whether the guideline is actually being used in practice.

Implications for Patient Care

Evidence-based clinical practice guidelines have always had the potential to dramatically improve patient care and health outcomes. When developed rigorously and implemented correctly, they can achieve their purpose. Guidelines can be an important vehicle for translating complex research findings into recommendations that can be acted on. Because organizations still struggle about the best mechanisms to implement research into practice, guideline developers should strive toward collaboration and avoidance of duplication. They should also work closely with implementers to develop guideline statements that are more easily used in computerized medical records and decision tools.

In 2002, a new international organization, the Guidelines International Network (GIN) (http://www.G-I-N.net), was formed. The organization is made up of guideline developers from throughout the world; its mission is to improve the quality of health care by promoting systematic development of clinical practice guidelines and their application into practice through supporting international collaboration. The presence of this new organization may signal a move toward globalizing evidence while still promoting localized decision making. Given the complexity and expense of developing clinical practice guidelines, the collaboration makes sense. Even more important, it signifies a universal awareness that clinical decisions can no longer be made without being informed by the best available evidence.

66 *To think is easy. To act is hard. But the hardest thing in the world is to act in accordance with your thinking.* **99**

—*J o h a n n W o l f g a n g v o n G o e t h e*

references

Agency for Healthcare Research and Quality (AHRQ), 2002. *Systems to Rate the Strength of Scientific Evidence.* Summary, Evidence Report/Technology Assessment: Number 47. AHRQ Pub. No. 02-E015, March 2002. Rockville, MD: AHRQ. Retrieved from http://www.ahrq.gov/clinic/epcsums/strengthsum.htm on November 1, 2003.

Barratt, A., Irwig, L., Glasziou, P., Cumming, R. G., Raffle, A., Hicks, N., Gray, J. A., & Guyatt, G. H. (1999). Users' guides to the medical literature: XVII. How to use guidelines and recommendations about screening. *Evidence-Based Medicine Working Group. JAMA, 281,* 2029–2034.

Berg, A. O. (1998). Dimensions of evidence. *Journal of the American Board of Family Practice; 11,* 216–223.

Berg, A. O., Atkins, D. J., & Tierney, W. (1997). Clinical practice guidelines in practice and education. *Journal of General Internal Medicine, 12*(Suppl 2), S25–S33.

Cluzeau, F. A., Littlejohns, P., Grimshaw, J. M., Feder, G., & Moran, S. E. (1999). Development and application of a generic methodology to assess the quality of clinical guidelines. *International Journal of Quality Health Care, 11*(1), 21–28.

Commission of the European Communities, Brussels (2002). eEurope: Quality Criteria for Health Related Websites. *Journal Medical Internet Resources, 4*(3), E15

Cook, D. J., Greengold, N. L., Ellrodt, G., & Weingarten, S. R. (1997). The relation between systematic reviews and practice guidelines. *Annals of Internal Medicine, 127,* 210–216.

Davis, D. A., & Taylor-Vaisey, A. (1997). Translating guidelines into practice. A systematic review of theoretic concepts, practical experience and research evidence in the adoption of clinical practice guidelines. *Canadian Medical Association Journal, 157*(4), 408–416.

Field, M. J., & Lohr, K. N. (Eds.) (1992). *Guidelines for clinical practice. From development to use.* Washington DC: National Academy Press.

Field, M. J. (Ed.) (1995). *Setting priorities for clinical practice guidelines.* Washington DC: National Academy Press.

Field, M. J., & Lohr, K. N. (Eds.) (1990). *Clinical practice guidelines: Directions for a new program.* Committee to Advise the Public Health Service on Clinical Practice Guidelines, Institute of Medicine. Washington, DC: National Academy Press.

Grilli, R., Magrini, N., Penna, A., Mura, G., & Liberati (2000). Practice guidelines developed by specialty societies: The need for a critical appraisal. *Lancet, 355,* 103–105.

Harris, R. P., Helfand, M., Woolf, S. H., Lohr, K. N., Mulrow, C. D., Teutsch, S. M., & Atkins, D.; Methods Work Group, Third U.S. Preventive Services Task Force (2001). Current methods of the U.S. Preventive Services Task Force: A review of the process. *American Journal of Preventive Medicine, 20*(3 Suppl), 21–35.

Haynes, R. B. (1993). Some problems in applying evidence in clinical practice. *Annals of the New York Academy of Sciences, 703,* 210–224.

Haynes, R. B., Hayward, R. S. A., & Lomas, J. (1995). Bridges between health care research evidence and clinical practice. *Journal of the American Medical Informatics Association, 2*(6), 342–350.

Hayward, R. S., Wilson, M. C., Tunis, S. R., Bass, E. B., & Guyatt, G. (1995). Users' guides to the medical literature. VIII. How to use clinical practice guidelines. A. Are the recommendations valid? *The Evidence-Based Medicine Working Group. JAMA, 274,* 570–574.

Lohr, K. N. (1995). Guidelines for clinical practice: What they are and why they count. *J Law Med Ethics, 23*(1), 49–56.

Lohr, K. N., & Field, M. J. (1992). A provisional instrument for assessing clinical practice guidelines. In M.J. Field & K. N. Lohr (Eds.), *Guidelines for clinical practice: From development to use.* Washington DC: National Academy Press.

Sackett, D. L., Richardson, W. S., Rosenberg, W., & Haynes, R. B. (1997). *Evidence-based medicine: How to practice and teach EBM*. New York: Churchill Livingstone.

Scottish Intercollegiate Guideline Network (SIGN) 50: A guideline developers' handbook. An introduction to SIGN methodology for the development of evidence-based clinical guidelines. Edinburgh (Scotland): SIGN; 2001 Feb. (updated 2002 Oct.).

Shaneyfelt, T. M., Mayo-Smith, M. F., & Rothwangl (1999). Are guidelines following guidelines? The methodological quality of clinical practice guidelines in the peer-reviewed medical literature. *JAMA; 281*, 1900–1905.

Shekelle, P. G., Woolf, S. H., Eccles, M., & Grimshaw, J. (1999). Clinical guidelines: developing guidelines. *British Medical Journal, 318*(7183), 593–596.

Shiffman, R. N., Shekelle, P., Overhage, J. M., Slutsky, J., Grimshaw, J., & Deshpande, A. M. (2003). A proposal for standardized reporting of clinical practice guidelines: The COGS statement. *Annals 139*(6), 493–500.

The AGREE Collaboration (Sept. 2001). Appraisal of Guidelines for Research & Evaluation (AGREE) Instrument. www.agreecollaboration.org.

U.S. National Library of Medicine (NLM) (1998). http://www.nlm.nih.gov/. Accessed October 4, 1998.

Wennberg, J., & Gittelsohn, A. (1973). Small area variations in health care delivery. *Science, 182*(117), 1102–1108.

Wennberg, J., & Gittelsohn, A. (1982). Variations in medical care among small areas. *Scientific American, 246*(4), 120–134.

Wilson, M. C., Hayward, R. S., Tunis, S. R., Bass, E. B., & Guyatt, G. (1995). Users' guides to the medical literature. VIII. How to use clinical practice guidelines. B. What are the recommendations and will they help you in caring for your patients? *The Evidence-Based Medicine Working Group. JAMA, 274*(20), 1630–1632.

Woolf, S. H. (1992). Practice guidelines, a new reality in medicine. II. Methods of developing guidelines. *Archives of Internal Medicine, 152*(5), 946–952.

Woolf, S. H., Grol, R., Hutchinson, A., Eccles, M., & Grimshaw, J. (1999). Clinical guidelines: Potential benefits, limitations, and harms of clinical guidelines. *British Medical Journal, 318*(7182), 527–530.

Acknowledgment

The views expressed in this chapter are those of the author, and no official endorsement by the AHRQ or the U.S. Department of Health and Human Services is intended or should be inferred.

Next Steps: Generating and Disseminating Evidence

Start by doing what is necessary,

then do what is possible,

and suddenly you are

doing the impossible.

St. Francis of Assisi

Generating Evidence Through Quantitative Research

Bernadette Mazurek Melnyk and Robert Cole

chapter 10

> " *Man's mind, stretched to a new idea, never goes back to its original dimensions.* "
>
> *Oliver Wendell Holmes*

When there is a lack of research reported in the literature to guide clinical practice, it becomes necessary to design and conduct studies to generate evidence. There are many areas in clinical practice that do not have an established evidence base (e.g., care for dying children, primary care interventions to improve mental health outcomes in high-risk individuals). As a result, there is an urgent need to conduct studies so that healthcare providers can base their treatment decisions on sound evidence from well-designed studies instead of continuing to make decisions that are steeped solely in tradition or opinion.

The Importance of Generating Evidence

This chapter provides a general overview and practical guide for formulating clinical research questions and designing studies to answer the questions. The chapter includes suggestions on when a quantitative approach would be more appropriate to answer a specific question. A variety of quantitative research designs are discussed, from **descriptive studies** to **randomized controlled trials** (RCTs) that are conducted to answer questions about the effectiveness of interventions or treatments. Techniques to enhance the rigor of quantitative research designs are highlighted, including strategies to strengthen **internal validity** (i.e., the ability to say that it was the independent variable or intervention that caused a change in the dependent variable or outcome, not other extraneous variables), as well as **external validity** (i.e., generalizability, which is the ability to generalize findings from a study's sample to the larger population). Specific principles of conducting *qualitative studies* are detailed in Chapter 11.

Getting Started: From Idea to Reality

> 66 *We are told never to cross a bridge until we come to it, but the world is owned by men who have 'crossed bridges' in their imagination far ahead of the crowd.* 99
>
> —*Speakers Library*

Many ideas for studies come from clinical practice situations in which questions arise regarding best practices or evolve from a search for evidence on a particular topic (e.g., Is music or relaxation therapy more effective in reducing the stress of patients after surgery? What are the major variables that predict the development of posttraumatic stress disorder in adults after motor vehicle accidents?). However, these ideas are often cast aside as competing demands for patient care or overwhelming job responsibilities prevent the transformation of ideas into study projects. Additionally, some practitioners may hesitate to conduct a study for fear they do not have adequate knowledge, skills, or resources to complete the project successfully.

Because of the nature of current clinical practice in today's healthcare environment, it is worthwhile to develop a "creative ideas" file when thoughts for studies are generated. A creative ideas file may spark practitioners to act on previous ideas at a later time. In addition, these ideas or research questions can be shared with doctorally prepared clinicians or researchers who can partner with the practitioner to launch a study. Thus, the person who had the idea or question can assume an active role on the study team but need not take on the role of the lead person, or **principal investigator (PI),** who is responsible and accountable for overseeing all elements of the research project.

> 66 *The greatest successful people of the world have used their imagination. . . . They think ahead and create their mental picture, and then go to work materializing that picture in all its details, filling in here, adding a little there, altering this a bit and that a bit, but steadily building—steadily building.* 99
>
> —*Robert Collier*

Once an idea for a study is generated, it is exceedingly important to first conduct an extensive search of the literature and critically appraise all **systematic reviews** or related studies in the area. The purpose of this search and critical appraisal is to evaluate the strengths and limitations of prior work, which is critical before another study in the same area is designed.

This process prevents unknowing replication of prior work, which typically does not enhance science or clinical practice. In contrast, deliberate replication of a prior study can be a real strength of a project because it is considered good science and it creates a solid foundation of accumulating evidence on which to base practice changes.

After an idea is generated for a study and a search for and critical appraisal of the literature has been conducted, a collaborative team can be established to be part of the planning process from the outset. Because clinicians often have a host of burning clinical questions but typically need assistance with intricate details of study design, methods, and analysis, formulating a team comprising seasoned clinicians and research experts (e.g., doctorally prepared clinical researchers) will usually lead to the best outcomes. In addition, a team of interdisciplinary professionals will add value to the project, especially in the study design and interpretation of findings. Many funding agencies now expect interdisciplinary collaboration on research projects. Convening this collaborative team for a **research design meeting** at the outset of a project is exceedingly beneficial in developing the study's design and methods, as well as establishing enthusiasm and team spirit for the project.

Research design meetings are an excellent mechanism for moving an idea into the reality of a clinical study. Approximately 1–2 weeks before the meeting is conducted, a concise, two-page study draft should be prepared and disseminated. This draft acts as an outline or overview of the clinical problem and includes the research question and a brief description of the proposed methods (see Box 10-1 for an example of a study outline, as well as Boxes 10-2 and 10-3 for completed examples of study outlines for different types of clinical studies). As the study outline develops, a list of questions related to the project should be answered:

- Is this idea feasible and clinically important?
- What is the aim of the study, along with the research question(s) or hypotheses?
- What is the best design to answer the study question(s) or test the hypotheses?
- What are the potential sources of data? Are there valid and reliable instruments to measure the desired outcomes?
- What should be the **inclusion** and **exclusion criteria** for the potential study participants?
- What are the essential elements of the intervention, if applicable?

By distributing these questions along with a concise draft of the study outline that has been developed, team members will have time to reflect on these issues and be better prepared to discuss them at the research design conference.

The research design planning session needs to foster an environment in which constructive critique and candid discussion will promote a finely tuned study design. It is important to discuss the roles for each of the study team members (e.g., percentage of effort on the study, specific functions, availability, order of authorship once the study is published). In addition, potential funding sources for the study should be discussed, as well as who will assume specific responsibilities in writing a grant proposal if funding is necessary to conduct the project (see Chapter 13 for specific steps in writing a successful grant proposal and Box 10-4 for a summary of initial steps in designing a clinical study).

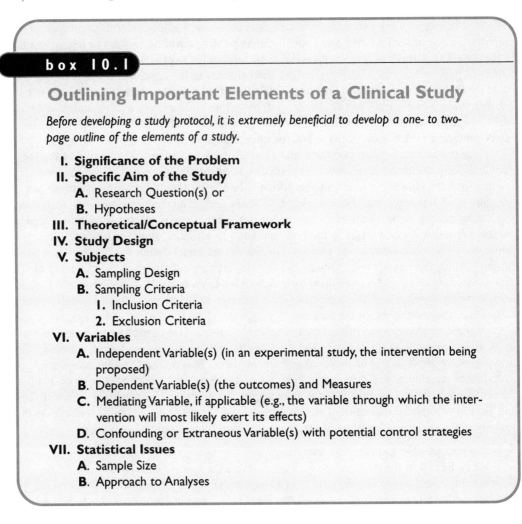

box 10.1

Outlining Important Elements of a Clinical Study

Before developing a study protocol, it is extremely beneficial to develop a one- to two-page outline of the elements of a study.

I. Significance of the Problem
II. Specific Aim of the Study
    A. Research Question(s) or
    B. Hypotheses
III. Theoretical/Conceptual Framework
IV. Study Design
V. Subjects
    A. Sampling Design
    B. Sampling Criteria
        1. Inclusion Criteria
        2. Exclusion Criteria
VI. Variables
    A. Independent Variable(s) (in an experimental study, the intervention being proposed)
    B. Dependent Variable(s) (the outcomes) and Measures
    C. Mediating Variable, if applicable (e.g., the variable through which the intervention will most likely exert its effects)
    D. Confounding or Extraneous Variable(s) with potential control strategies
VII. Statistical Issues
    A. Sample Size
    B. Approach to Analyses

Designing a Clinical Quantitative Study

Box 10-5 cites several factors to consider in developing a quantitative study. The most important of these factors is a critical analysis and synthesis of prior work conducted in the clinical area.

Critical Analysis and Synthesis of Prior Data

If this critical analysis reveals numerous studies that describe a particular construct or phenomenon, such as stressors of family caregivers of hospitalized elders, as well as studies that identify the major predictors of caregiver stress during hospitalization (e.g., uncertainty regarding the caregiving role in the hospital, lack of knowledge regarding how best to enhance outcomes in the hospitalized elder), another descriptive study in the field may not be needed. Instead, the next logical step in this example (based on the descriptive and predictive evidence already generated from prior studies) would be to design and test an educational intervention that informs

box 10.2

Example of a Completed Study Outline

A nonexperimental study entitled "Relationship Between Depressive Symptoms and Motivation to Lose Weight in Overweight Teens."

I. Significance of the Problem

Data from the Centers for Disease Control indicates that 14 percent of adolescents are overweight. The major negative consequences associated with obesity in adolescence include premature death, type 2 diabetes, hyperlipidemia, hypertension, and depression. It is known that motivation to lose weight is a key factor in weight loss, but the relationship between depressive symptoms and motivation to lose weight in adolescence has not been studied.

II. Specific Aim of the Study with Research Question(s) or Hypotheses

The aim of this study is to answer the following research question: What is the relationship between depressive symptoms and motivation to lose weight in overweight adolescents?

III. Theoretical/Conceptual Framework

Control theory postulates that, when there is a discrepancy between a standard or goal (e.g., perceived ideal weight), this discrepancy should motivate individuals to initiate behaviors (e.g., exercise, healthy eating) that allow them to achieve their goal. However, there are often barriers that may inhibit an individual in being motivated to initiate these behaviors. In this study, depression is viewed as a barrier to motivation and behaviors that would allow teens to achieve their ideal weight.

IV. Study Design

A descriptive correlational design will be used.

V. Subjects

  A. *Sampling Design:* A random sample of 80 overweight adolescents will be drawn from two randomly selected high schools in Rochester, New York; one from the city school district and one from the suburban area.

  B. *Sampling Criteria*

    1. *Inclusion Criteria:* adolescents with a body mass index of 25 or greater enrolled in the two high schools.

    2. *Exclusion Criteria:* adolescents with a current diagnosis of major depression and/or suicidal ideations.

VI. Variables

  A. *Independent variable(s):* Not applicable.

  B. *Dependent variable(s):*

  Depressive symptoms will be measured with the well-known, valid, and reliable Beck Depression Inventory (BDI-II). Motivation to lose weight will be

(continued)

box 10.2 *(continued)*

measured with a newly constructed scale that has been reviewed for content validity with experts in the field. This new scale has been pilot tested with 15 overweight teens and found to have a Cronbach's alpha of .80.

   C. Mediating variable, if applicable: Not applicable

   D. Confounding or extraneous variable(s) with potential control strategies: Gender is a potential confounding variable, because there is a higher incidence of depression in adolescent females than males documented in the literature. Therefore, stratified random sampling will be used so that an equal number of males and females will be drawn for the sample.

VII. Statistical Issues

   A. Sample size

      To obtain a power of .8 and medium effect size at the .05 level of significance, a total of 80 adolescents will be needed.

   B. Approach to analyses

      A Pearson's *r* correlation coefficient will be used to determine if a relationship exists between the number of depressive symptoms and motivation to lose weight in this sample.

family caregivers of the functions they can perform to improve their hospitalized elder's health outcomes. In contrast, if the phenomenon of caregiver stress is not well understood or adequately measured in the literature, conducting a qualitative or descriptive study *may become the beginning step in* conducting research in this area. This type of study might begin with open-ended questions to allow participants to respond in their own words to such questions as, How would you describe what it is like for you to care for your partner or parent? or How have things changed for you now, while your family member is in the hospital? Thus, research in a particular area frequently begins with qualitative work in which a phenomenon or construct is explored with heavy emphasis on interview or observation data (see Chapter 11). ^AQWhen more is known about the nature of the phenomenon through qualitative work, quantitative research is usually undertaken in which the construct of interest is described using measurement scales, test scores, and statistical approaches (see Figure 10-1).

As Figure 10-1 shows, quantitative research designs range from descriptive and correlational descriptive/predictive studies to RCTs. **Correlational descriptive** and **correlational predictive** designs examine the relationships between two or more variables (e.g., What is the relationship between smoking and lung cancer in adults? or What maternal factors in the first month of life predict infant cognitive development at 1 year old?). These designs are the study of choice when the **independent variable** cannot be manipulated experimentally because of some individual characteristic or ethical consideration (e.g., individuals cannot be assigned to smoke or not smoke). The goal in correlational descriptive or correlational predictive studies is to provide an indication of how likely it is that a cause-and-effect relationship might exist (Powers & Knapp, 1995).

box 10.3

Example of a Completed Study Outline

A Randomized Clinical Trial entitled "Improving Outcomes of Hospitalized Elders and Family Caregivers" (Li, H., Melnyk, B. M., & McCann, R., funded by the National Institutes of Health/National Institute of Nursing Research, R01 #008455-01, 4/1/03–12/31/06.

I. Significance of the Problem

There are more than 12 million elderly people hospitalized each year in the United States, many of whom experience functional decline. Family care of hospitalized elders is important, given the increasing numbers of hospitalized elders, needs for elder care in the home after hospital discharge, and responsibilities of family caregivers for providing this care. Involving family caregivers in the hospital care of their loved ones may result in positive outcomes for both the elderly patients and their family caregivers. However, there is a paucity of empirical studies that have been conducted to evaluate the effectiveness of interventions to enhance family participation in caring for hospitalized elders.

II. Specific Aim with Research Question /Hypothesis

The aim of this study is to evaluate the effects of a theoretically driven, reproducible intervention (CARE: Creating Avenues for Relative Empowerment) on the process and outcomes of hospitalized elders and their family caregivers. It is hypothesized that the family caregivers and elders who receive the CARE program will have better outcomes (e.g., less depression and functional decline) than those who receive the control program.

III. Theoretical/Conceptual Framework

The theoretical framework for this study is derived from self-regulation theory and interactional role theory. According to self-regulation theory, it is postulated that providing information to family caregivers about the potential emotions and behaviors that they can expect in their hospitalized relatives as well as signs and complications during hospitalization will facilitate the formation of a clear cognitive schema that will strengthen their beliefs about these changes as well as how to interpret them. Subsequently, stronger beliefs should lead to less worry, anxiety, and depression in the family caregivers as well as a greater participation in their loved one's care. In addition, according to role theory, it is postulated that by discussing family roles in a mutually agreed-upon family preference contract, family caregivers' beliefs about their role will be strengthened, and they will participate more in the care of their elderly relatives as well as have less role strain and more role reward and improved family-patient relationships. As a result of improved family caregivers' emotional and functional outcomes as well as role outcomes, patient outcomes also should be improved.

(continued)

box 10.3 *(continued)*

IV. Study Design

A randomized controlled trial will be used with random assignment of subjects to either the experimental CARE group or the comparison group.

V. Subjects

A. Sampling Criteria

Family members who meet the following criteria will be eligible for study participation:

1. Age 21 years or above
2. Have an elderly relative (65 years or above) admitted to the three study units within the past 24–48 hours
3. Are related to the patient by blood, marriage, adoption, or affinity as a significant other (e.g., life partner, close friend)
4. Are primary caregivers
5. Can read and speak English
6. Live within a 1-hour drive of the facility (60 miles)
7. Ineligible for participation are family members who are paid care providers, whose elderly relative is hospitalized for longer than 30 days, who are unable to complete the questionnaires or provide care because of their own mental or physical impairment, or whose relative dies during the hospital stay or within 2 months after discharge.

B. Sampling Design

A convenience sample of family caregivers who meet the inclusion criteria will participate in the study.

VI. Variables

A. Independent Variable(s)

The family caregivers in the experimental group will receive the CARE program that includes both audiotaped and written materials containing information on:

1. Emotional responses, behavioral characteristics, and possible complications of elderly patients during hospitalization
2. How family caregivers can participate in their relative's care and prevent or care for dysfunctional syndromes. In addition, family caregivers will be assisted with the development of a specific plan for their elderly relative's hospital care, based on their abilities and preferences. Family caregivers in the control group will receive audiotaped and written materials containing information on the hospital's services and policies.

(continued)

box 10.3 *(continued)*

B. Dependent Variable(s)

Measures of both process and outcome variables include family care-givers' outcomes (beliefs, anxiety, worry, depression, role performance, role strain, role adaptation, and role rewards); outcomes of quality of re-lationship between family caregiver and patient (mutuality); as well as eld-erly patients' outcomes (dysfunctional syndrome, length of hospital stay, readmission, depression, and cognitive status) during hospitalization and after hospital discharge.

C. Mediating Variable, if applicable

It is proposed that the CARE intervention will be mediated through fam-ily beliefs about their role to improve the outcomes of family caregivers.

D. Confounding or Extraneous Variable(s) with potential control strategies

The type of relationship between the family caregiver and the hospital-ized elder (e.g., spouse, daughter/son) may confound the outcomes; therefore, a randomized block design will be used that will randomly as-sign equal numbers of caregivers who are spouses and children to the CARE and control groups.

VII. Statistical Issues

A. Sample Size

To detect a medium effect with a power of 0.8 at a 0.05 level of signifi-cance, a total of 140 family caregivers and their elders will be needed. Be-cause this is a longitudinal study that will follow subjects for 2 months following discharge, 40 additional family caregivers and their elders will be recruited into the study in the event of attrition in order to assure a sample size of 140 caregivers at the end of the study.

B. Approach to Analyses

Cronbach's alpha will be used to determine internal consistency reliability for the study instruments. Analysis of covariance tests will be used to test the hypotheses if preliminary analysis reveals that the two groups are sig-nificantly different on certain demographic and clinical variables. With in-tercorrelated dependent variables, MANOVA is the first step in testing the hypotheses so that chance results will not be attributable to the ex-perimental intervention. If the MANOVA is significant, univariate ANOVAs will be used to isolate group differences on each of the de-pendent variables. If differences exist between the pooled experimental and pooled comparison groups on certain demographic or clinical vari-ables at preintervention, those differences will be controlled for statisti-cally by the use of multivariate analysis of covariance.

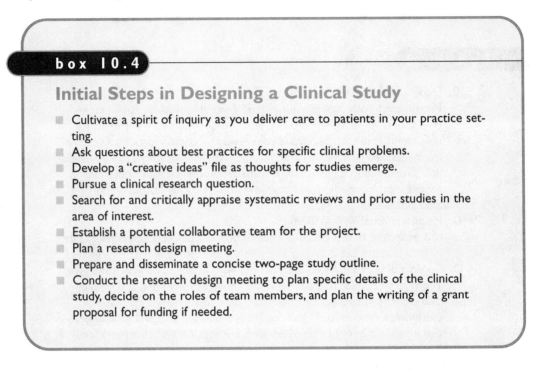

Although RCTs, or *experiments*, are the strongest designs for testing cause-and-effects relationships (i.e., testing the effects of certain clinical practices or interventions on patient outcomes), only a small percentage of studies conducted in many of the health professions are experimental studies or clinical trials. Additionally, of those intervention studies reported in the literature, many have limitations that weaken the evidence that is generated from them, including:

box 10.5

Major Factors to Consider When Designing a Quantitative Study

- Prior studies in the area
- Significance of the problem
- Feasibility
- Setting for the study and access to potential subjects
- The study team
- Ethics of the study

- Lack of random assignment to study groups
- Lack of or underdeveloped theoretical frameworks to guide the interventions
- Small sample sizes that lead to inadequate **power** to detect significant differences in outcomes between the experimental and control groups
- Omission of **manipulation checks**, assessments verifying that subjects have actually processed the experimental information that they have received or followed through with prescribed intervention activities
- Failure to limit **confounding** or **extraneous variables** (i.e., those factors that interfere with the relationship between the independent and dependent variables)
- Lack of more long-term follow-up to assess the sustainability of the treatment or intervention

Therefore, because a **true experiment** is the strongest design for the testing of cause-and-effect relationships and provides strong, or **Level II evidence** (i.e., evidence generated from an RCT, the next strongest evidence behind systematic reviews of RCTs; see Chapter 1) on which to change or improve practice, there is an urgent need for health professionals to conduct RCTs in order to inform best practices.

Descriptive Research ⟶	Predictive Research ⟶	Experimental Research

figure 10.1	Progression of quantitative research.

Significance of the Question

A second major factor to consider when designing studies is the significance of the problem or research question. There may be research questions that are very interesting (e.g., Do pink or blue scrubs worn by intensive care unit nurses impact the mood of unit secretaries?) but answering them will not significantly *improve* care or patient outcomes. Therefore, a funding agency is not likely to rate the significance of the problem as important. Problems that are significant for study are usually those that affect a large percentage of the population or those that frequently affect the process or outcomes of patient care.

Feasibility

The third factor to consider when designing a study is feasibility. Before embarking on a study, important questions to ask regarding feasibility are:

- Can the study be conducted in a reasonable amount of time?
- Are there adequate resources available to conduct the study? If the answer is no, what is the potential for obtaining funding?
- Is there an adequate number of potential subjects to recruit into the study?
- Does the lead person (PI) have sufficient time and expertise to spearhead the effort?

If the answer to any of these questions is no, further consideration should be given to the feasibility of the project.

As a general rule, it typically takes more time to carry out a clinical study than is originally projected. Even when subject numbers are projected to be sufficient for the time allotted for data collection when planning a study, it is wise to incorporate a buffer period (i.e., extra time) in case subject recruitment takes longer than anticipated. Also, certain times of the year are more conducive for data collection than others (e.g., in conducting a study with elementary school students, data collection will be possible only when school is in session, not during the summer months).

Setting

The fourth major factor to consider when designing a study is the setting(s) in which it will be implemented. Certain settings are more conducive to the conduct of clinical research than others. Settings that tend to facilitate research are those in which there is administrative approval and staff "buy-in" regarding clinical studies. Settings in which staff members perceive research as burdensome to them or their patients may confound study results as well as hamper a study's progress. Obtaining administrative approval to conduct a study and getting a sense of staff support for a project is an early and critical preparatory step for a clinical research project.

Research Team

> "*Alone we can do so little; together we can do so much.*"
>
> —*Helen Keller*

The fifth major factor to consider when designing a clinical study is the research team. Specifically, it is important to consider the experience, skills, interest, and commitment of each member of the team. It is typical for there to be much enthusiasm about a project at its beginning, but sustained interest and participation by each member of the study team will be important for its successful completion. Study team members should possess the skills needed to plan, implement, analyze, and interpret the research data. For a novice researcher, the addition of seasoned researchers to the project will be important for its success, especially as challenges are encountered in the course of the initiative.

> "*It is literally true that you can succeed best and quickest by helping others to succeed.*"
>
> —*Napoleon Hill*

Ethics, Benefits, and Risks

The final major factor to consider in planning a study is whether it is ethical in terms of subject burden as well as whether the benefits of participation in the study will exceed the risks. Serious consideration also must be given to the gender, age, and racial/ethnic composition of the sample. For federal grant applications, strong rationale must be provided if women, children, and minority subjects will be excluded from the research project. In addition, study team members need to be knowledgeable regarding the ethics of conducting a study and the rights of participant subjects. Further discussion about obtaining research subjects' review approval for a clinical study appears later in this chapter.

Specific Steps in Designing a Quantitative Study

When designing a quantitative clinical research study, there is a specific series of orderly steps that are typically followed (see Box 10-6). This is referred to as the *scientific approach to inquiry.*

Step 1: Formulate the Study Question

The first step in the design of a study is developing an innovative, answerable study question. Cummings, Browner, & Hulley (2001) use the acronym FINER (feasible, interesting, novel, ethical, relevant) to determine the quality of the research question. Feasibility is an important issue when formulating a research question. Although a research question may be very interesting (e.g., What is the effect of a therapeutic intervention program on depression in women whose spouses have been murdered?), it could take years to collect an adequate number of subjects to conduct the statistical analysis to answer the question.

On the other hand, if a research question is not interesting to the investigator, there is a chance that the project may never reach completion, especially when challenges arise that

---

box 10.6

Specific Steps in Designing a Quantitative Clinical Study

1. Formulate the study question.
2. Establish the significance of the problem.
3. Search for and critically appraise available evidence.
4. Develop the theoretical/conceptual framework.
5. Generate hypotheses when appropriate.
6. Select the appropriate research design.
7. Identify the population/sampling plan and implement strategies to enhance external validity.
8. Determine the measures that will be used.
9. Outline the data collection plan.
10. Apply for human subjects approval.
11. Implement the study.
12. Prepare and analyze the data.
13. Interpret the results.
14. Disseminate the findings.
15. Incorporate the findings in EBP and evaluate the outcomes.

make data collection difficult. Other feasibility issues include the amount of time and funding that it will take to conduct the project, as well as the scope of the study. Studies that are very broad and that contain too many goals are often not feasible or manageable.

Research questions should be novel, meaning that obtaining the answer to them should add to, confirm, or refute what is already known or they should extend prior research findings. Replication studies are important, especially if they address major limitations of prior work.

Good research questions should be ethical in that they do not present unacceptable physical or psychological risks to the subjects in the study. The institution of strict federal regulations surrounding research with human subjects has curtailed studies in which the risks exceed the benefits of participation in a study. As such, before a research study is conducted, review of the entire protocol by a **research subjects review board** (RSRB), sometimes referred to as an *institutional review board* (IRB), is necessary.

Many universities, such as the University of Rochester, have Web sites that provide comprehensive information on: (a) how to submit studies for review, (b) guidelines for writing a research proposal, and (c) information about regulations regarding research, including specific details related to HIPAA (Health Insurance Portability and Accountability Act; (see **http://www.urmc.rochester.edu/rsrb**).

In institutions where a formal RSRB is not in existence, there should be some type of ethics committee that reviews and approves research proposals.

Finally, research questions should be relevant to science and/or clinical practice.-They should also have the potential to impact health policy and guide further research (Cummings, Browner, & Hulley, 2001) (see Box 10-7).

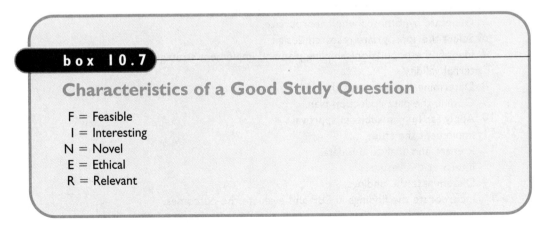

box 10.7

Characteristics of a Good Study Question

F = Feasible
I = Interesting
N = Novel
E = Ethical
R = Relevant

Source: Cummings, Browner, & Hulley, 2001

Step 2: Establish Significance of the Problem

The problem of interest should be one that is clinically important or that will extend the science in an area. When embarking on a study, it is imperative to ask questions about why the clinical problem is important, including:

- What is the incidence of this particular problem?
- How many individuals are affected by this problem?
- Will studying this problem potentially improve the care that is delivered to patients?
- Will studying this problem potentially influence health policy?
- Will studying this intervention lead to better health outcomes in patients?
- Will studying this problem assist clinicians in gaining a better understanding of the area so that more sensitive clinical care can be delivered?

Step 3: Search and Appraise Evidence

A thorough search for and critical appraisal of all relevant studies in the area is essential (see Chapters 3–6) before the study design is planned. It is first advantageous to begin searching for **systematic reviews** on the topic. A systematic review is a summary of evidence in a particular topic area that attempts to answer a specific clinical question using methods that reduce bias, usually conducted by an expert or expert panel on a particular topic (Melnyk, 2003). When it is conducted properly, a systematic review uses a rigorous process for identifying, critically appraising, and synthesizing studies for the purpose of answering a specific clinical question and drawing conclusions about the evidence gathered (e.g., How effective are educational interventions in reducing sexual risk-taking behaviors in teenagers? What factors predict osteoporosis in women?). In using a rigorous process to determine which types of studies will be included in a systematic review, author bias is usually eliminated, and greater credibility can be placed in the findings from the review. In systematic reviews, methodological strengths and limitations of each study included in the review are discussed, and recommendations for clinical practice as well as further research are presented (Guyatt & Rennie, 2002). As such, the availability of a systematic review in a particular topic area can provide an individual with quick access to the status of interventions or clinical studies in a particular area as well as recommendations for further study.

If a systematic review in the area of interest is not available, the search for and critical appraisal of individual studies should commence. In reading prior studies, the following information should be tabled so that a critical analysis of the body of prior work can be conducted:

- Demographics of the sample
- Research design employed, including the type of intervention(s), if applicable
- Variables measured with accompanying instruments
- Major findings
- Strengths and limitations

Once a table such as this is developed, it will be easier to identify strengths as well as gaps in prior work that could possibly be addressed by the proposed study.

Step 4: Develop a Theoretical/Conceptual Framework

A **theoretical** or **conceptual framework** is made up of a number of interrelated statements that attempt to describe, explain, and/or predict a phenomenon. Developing a conceptual or theoretical framework is an important step in designing a clinical study. Its purpose is to provide a framework for selecting the study's variables, including how they relate to one another, as well as to guide the development of the intervention(s) in experimental studies. Without a well-developed theoretical framework, explanations for the findings from a study may be weak and speculative (Melnyk & Feinstein, 2001).

As an example, self-regulation theory (Johnson et al., 1997; Leventhal & Johnson, 1983) has provided an excellent theoretical framework for providing educational interventions to patients undergoing intrusive procedures (e.g., endoscopy) and chemotherapy/radiation.

The basic premise of this theory is that the provision of concrete objective information to an individual who is confronting a stressful situation or procedure will facilitate a cognitive schema or representation of what will happen that is similar to the real life event. As a result of an individual knowing what he or she is likely to experience, there is an increase in understanding, predictability, and confidence in dealing with the situation as it unfolds (Johnson et al., 1997), which leads to improved coping outcomes.

Through a series of experimental studies, Melnyk and colleagues extended the use of self-regulation theory to guide interventions with parents of hospitalized and critically ill children (Melnyk, 1994; Melnyk et al., 1997), parents of low-birth-weight premature infants (Melnyk et al., 2001), and parents with young children experiencing marital separation and divorce (Melnyk & Alpert-Gillis, 1996). Extensive evidence in the literature from descriptive studies indicated that a major source of stress for parents of hospitalized and critically ill children is their children's emotional and behavioral responses to hospitalization. Thus, it was hypothesized that parents who receive the COPE (Creating Opportunities for Parent Empowerment) intervention program, which contains educational information about children's likely behavioral and emotional changes during and following hospitalization, would have stronger beliefs about their children's responses to the stressful event. It also was hypothesized that the COPE program would work through parental beliefs about their children and their role—the proposed **mediating variable** (i.e., the variable or mechanism through which the intervention works)—to positively impact parent and child outcomes. As a result of them knowing what to expect of their children's emotions and behaviors during and following hospitalization, it was predicted that parents who receive the COPE program would have better emotional and functional coping outcomes (i.e., less negative mood state and increased participation in their children's care) than would parents who did not receive this information. Ultimately, because the emotional contagion hypothesis (VanderVeer, 1949; Jimmerson, 1982) states that heightened parental anxiety leads to heightened child anxiety, it was expected that the children of parents who received the COPE program would have better coping outcomes than would those whose parents did not receive this educational information. Thus, through this series of clinical trials, empirical support for the effectiveness of the COPE program was generated in addition to data that explain how the intervention actually impacts patient and family outcomes (Figure 10-2).

Step 5: Generate Hypotheses When Appropriate

Hypotheses are predictions about the relationships between study variables. For example, when using self-regulation theory, a hypothesis that would logically emerge from the theory would be

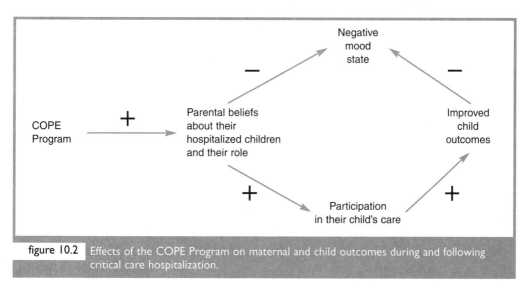

figure 10.2 Effects of the COPE Program on maternal and child outcomes during and following critical care hospitalization.

that parents who receive concrete objective information about their children's likely responses to hospitalization (i.e., the independent variable) would report less anxiety (i.e., the **dependent or outcome variable**) than would parents who do not receive this information. To include hypotheses in a clinical study, there should be either a theory to guide the formulation of these predictions or enough evidence from prior work to provide a sufficient foundation on which to make predictive statements. In situations where the evidence on which to base predictive statements is insufficient or where an investigator chooses not to use a theoretical or conceptual framework to guide his or her work (which is not advised), research questions should be developed instead of hypotheses (e.g., What is the effect of an educational intervention on coping outcomes of parents of critically ill children?).

Step 6: Select the Appropriate Research Design

The **design** of a clinical study is its foundation. It is the overall plan (i.e., the study protocol for testing the study hypotheses or questions) that includes the following:

- Strategies for controlling confounding or extraneous variables
- Strategies for when the intervention will be delivered (in experimental studies)
- How often and when the data will be collected

      A good quantitative design is one that:

- Appropriately tests the hypotheses or answers the research questions
- Lacks bias
- Controls extraneous or confounding variables
- Has sufficient **power** (i.e., the ability to detect statistically significant findings)

      If the research question or hypothesis concerns itself with testing the effects of an intervention or treatment on patient outcomes, the study calls for an **experimental design.** In contrast, if the hypothesis/research question is interested in quantitatively describing a selected variable or is interested in the relationship between two or more variables (e.g., What is the relationship between the average amount of sleep and test performance in college students? What presurgery demographic variables predict successful recovery from open heart surgery?), a **nonexperimental study design** would be the most appropriate. The next section of this chapter reviews the most common designs for nonexperimental as well as experimental studies.

Nonexperimental Study Designs

Typically, nonexperimental designs are used to describe, explain, or predict a phenomenon. These types of designs also are undertaken when it is undesirable or unethical to manipulate the independent variable or, in other words, to impose a treatment. For example, it would be unethical to assign teenagers randomly to receive an illegal drug (e.g., ecstasy) in order to study its effects on sexual risk-taking behaviors. Therefore, an alternative design would be a prospective descriptive study in which sexual risk-taking behaviors are measured over time in a group of adolescents who use ecstasy, compared with a group who has never used any drugs.

Descriptive Studies. The purpose of descriptive studies is to describe, observe, or document a phenomenon that can serve as a foundation for developing hypotheses or testing theory. For example, a descriptive study design would be appropriate to answer each of the following clinical questions:

- What is the incidence of complications in women who are on bedrest with preterm labor?
- What is the average number of depressive symptoms experienced by teenagers after a critical care hospitalization?
- In adults with type 2 diabetes, what are the most common physical comorbidities?

Survey Research Surveys are a type of descriptive study in which self-report data are typically collected to assess a certain condition or status. Most survey research is **cross-sectional** (i.e., all measurements are collected at the same point in time) versus research that is conducted over time (e.g., **cohort studies,** which follow the same sample longitudinally).

Survey data can be collected via multiple strategies (e.g., personal or telephone interviews, mailed or in-person questionnaires). For example, a group of healthcare providers might be surveyed with a questionnaire designed to measure their knowledge and attitudes about evidence-based practice (EBP). Data gained from this survey might then be used to design inservice education workshops to enhance the providers' knowledge and skills in this area.

Major advantages of survey research include rapid data collection and flexibility. Disadvantages of survey research include low response rates—especially if the surveys are mailed—and gathering information that is fairly superficial.

Correlational Studies Correlational research designs are used when there is an interest in describing the relationship between or among two or more variables. In this type of design, even when there is a strong relationship that is discovered between the variables under consideration, it is not substantiated to say that one variable caused the other to happen. For example, if a study found a positive relationship between adolescent smoking and drug use (e.g., as smoking increases, drug use increases), it would not be appropriate to state that smoking causes drug use. The only conclusion that could be drawn from these data is that these variables **co-vary** (i.e., as one changes, the other variable changes as well).

Correlational Descriptive Research   When there is interest in describing the relationship between two variables, a correlational descriptive study design would be most appropriate. For example, the following two research questions would be best answered with correlational designs:

1. What is the relationship between number of days that a person is on bedrest after a severe motor vehicle accident (the independent variable) and the incidence of decubiti ulcers (the dependent variable)?
2. What is the relationship between watching violent television shows (the independent variable) and the number of anger outbursts in adult males (the dependent variable)?

Correlational Predictive Research   When an investigator is interested in whether one variable that occurs earlier in time predicts another variable that occurs later in time, a correlational predictive study should be undertaken. For example, the following research questions would best lend themselves to this type of study (see Figure 10-3):

- Does maternal anxiety shortly after a child's admission to the intensive care unit (the independent variable) predict posttraumatic stress symptoms 6 months after hospitalization (the dependent variable)?
- Does level of stress during the first three months after starting a new job (the independent variable) predict performance one year later?

Establishment of a strong relationship in correlational predictive studies often lends support for attempting to influence the independent variable in a future intervention study. For example, if findings from research indicated that job stress in the initial months after starting a new position as a practitioner predicted later job performance, a future study might evaluate the effects of a training program on reducing early job stress with the expectation that a successful intervention program would improve later job performance. Although it should never be definitively stated that a cause-and-effect relationship is supported with a correlational study, a predictive correlational design is stronger than a descriptive one with regard to making a causal inference because the independent variable occurs before the dependent variable in time sequence (Polit & Hungler, 1999).

Case-Control Studies.   Case control studies are those in which one group of individuals (i.e., cases) with a certain condition (e.g., migraine headaches) is studied at the same time as another group of individuals who do not have the condition (i.e., controls) to determine an association between one or more predictor variables (e.g., family history of migraine headaches, consumption of red wine) and the condition (i.e., migraine headaches). Case control studies are usually

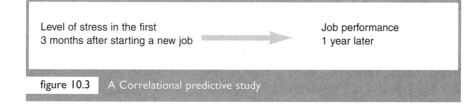

| Level of stress in the first 3 months after starting a new job | Job performance 1 year later |

figure 10.3   A Correlational predictive study

retrospective, or ex post facto (i.e., they look back in time to reveal predictor variables that might explain why the cases contracted the disease or problem and the controls did not).

Advantages of this type of research design include an ability to determine associations with a small number of subjects, which is especially useful in the study of rare types of diseases, and an ability to generate hypotheses for future studies (Newman, Browner, Cummings, & Hulley, 2001). One of the major limitations to using this study design is **bias** (i.e., an inability to control confounding variables that may influence the outcome). For example, the two groups of individuals previously presented (i.e., those with migraines and those without migraines) may be different on certain variables (e.g., amount of sleep, stress) that also may influence the development of migraine headaches.

Cohort Studies.   A cohort study follows a group of subjects longitudinally over a period of time to describe the incidence of a problem or to determine the relationship between a predictor variable and an outcome. For example, if an investigator were interested in whether daughters of mothers who had breast cancer have a higher incidence of the disease versus those whose mothers did not have breast cancer, this type of design would be appropriate. Two groups of daughters (i.e., those with and without a mother with breast cancer) would be studied over time to determine the incidence of breast cancer in each group. A major strength of prospective cohort studies includes being able to determine the incidence of a problem and its possible cause(s). A major limitation is the lengthy nature of this type of study, the costs of which often become prohibitive.

Experimental Designs

A true experiment, or RCT, is the strongest design for testing cause-and-effect relationships (e.g., whether an intervention or treatment impacts patient outcomes) and provides strong evidence on which to change and improve clinical practice. For evidence to support causality (i.e., cause-and-effect relationships), three criteria must be met:

1. The independent variable (i.e., the intervention or treatment) must precede the dependent variable (i.e., the outcome) in terms of time sequence.
2. There must be a strong relationship between the independent and dependent variables.
3. The relationship between the independent and dependent variables cannot be explained as being due to the influence of other variables (i.e., all possible alternate explanations of the relationship must be eliminated).

Although true experiments are the best designs to control for the influence of confounding variables, it must be recognized that control of potential confounding or extraneous variables is very challenging when conducting studies in the "real" world—not in the laboratory. Other limitations of experiments include the fact that they are usually time-consuming and expensive.

Intervention studies or clinical trials typically follow a five-phase development sequence:

Phase I: Basic research that is exploratory and descriptive in nature and that establishes the variables that may be amenable to intervention or in which the content, strength, and timing of the intervention are developed, along with the outcome measures for the study

Phase II: Pilot research (i.e., a small-scale study in which the intervention is tested with a small number of subjects so that feasibility of a large-scale study is determined and alternative strategies are developed for potential problems)

Phase III: Efficacy trials in which evaluation of the intervention takes place in an ideal setting and clinical efficacy is determined (in this stage, much emphasis is placed on internal validity of the study and preliminary *cost-effectiveness* of the intervention)

Phase IV: Effectiveness of clinical trials in which analysis of the intervention effect is conducted in clinical practice and clinical effectiveness is determined, as is cost-effectiveness (in this stage, much emphasis is placed on external validity or generalizability of the study)

Phase V: Effects on public health in which wide-scale implementation of the intervention is conducted to determine its effects on public health (Whittemore & Grey, 2002)

Many practitioners assume a leadership role in Phases I and II of this sequence and more of a participative role as a member of a research team in Phases III through V

Randomized Controlled Trial or True Experiment. The best type of study design or "gold standard" for evaluating the effects of a treatment or intervention is an RCT, or true experiment, in that it is the strongest design for testing cause-and-effect relationships. True experiments or RCTs possess three characteristics:

1. An experimental group that receives the treatment or intervention
2. A control or comparison group that receives standard care or a comparison intervention that is different from the experimental intervention
3. **Randomization** or **random assignment,** which is the use of a strategy to randomly assign subjects to the experimental or control groups (e.g., tossing a coin)

Random assignment is the strongest method to help ensure that the study groups are similar on demographic or clinical variables at baseline (i.e., before the treatment is delivered).

Similarity between groups at the beginning of an experiment is very important in that if findings reveal a positive effect on the dependent variable, it can be concluded that the treatment, not other extraneous variables, is what affected the outcome. For example, results from an RCT might reveal that a cognitive behavioral intervention reduced depressive symptoms in adults. However, if the adults in the experimental and control groups were not similar on certain characteristics prior to the start of the intervention (e.g., level of social support, number of current stressful life events), it could be that differences between the groups on these variables accounted for the change in depressive symptoms at the end of the study, instead of the change being due to the positive impact of the cognitive behavioral intervention itself.

Examples of true experimental designs along with advantages and disadvantages of each are presented in Figures 10-4 through 10-9. *R* in these figures indicates random assignment; *X* represents an intervention or treatment (*X1* indicates the experimental intervention, and *X2* and *X3* indicate study groups who received an intervention different from the experimental intervention); and *O* indicates the time at which an observation or outcome measurement occurs (*O1* indicates the first time that an observation or measure is gathered, and *O2* and *O3* indicate the second and third times a measure is collected). These designations have been used for years in the literature since the publishing of a landmark book on experimental designs by Campbell and Stanley (1963). Note that time moves from left to right, and subscripts can be used to designate different groups if necessary.

The major advantage of the design illustrated in Figure 10-4 is that it is a true experiment, the strongest design for testing cause-and-effect relationships. As seen in Figure 10-4, the inclusion of a comparison group in the design that receives a different/comparison or "control"

R	O_1	X_1	O_2
R	O_1	X_2	O_2

figure 10.4 Two group randomized controlled trial with pretest/ posttest design and structurally equivalent comparison group. R = random assignment; X = intervention/treatment, with X_1 being the experimental intervention and X_2 being the comparison/control intervention; O = observation/measurement, with O_1 being the first time the variable is measured (at baseline) and O_2 being the second time that it is measured (after the intervention).

intervention similar in length to the experimental intervention is important, especially in psychosocial research, because it helps to support that any positive effects of the experimental intervention are not just the result of giving participants something instead of nothing but are due to experimental intervention itself. However, at the same time, it must be realized that including a comparison intervention may dilute some of the positive effects of the experimental intervention, especially if an outcome being measured in a study is tapping a psychosocial variable, such as anxiety (e.g., giving participants something instead of nothing, as would be the case with a pure control group, might reduce anxiety simply because someone spent time and provided some type of intervention). The benefits of this design (i.e., including a control or comparison intervention) outweigh the risk of diluting the positive effects of the experimental intervention. Although pretesting the subjects on the same measure that is being used as the outcome for the study (e.g., state anxiety) may in itself sensitize them to respond differently when answering questions on the anxiety measure the second time, this approach allows one to determine whether subjects are similar on anxiety at the commencement of the study. A disadvantage of this design, as with all experiments, is that it typically is expensive and time-consuming.

The advantage of conducting a two-group RCT with a posttest only design is that there is no pretesting effect, which may confound the outcome in a study (Figure 10-5). For example, if you were interested in evaluating the effects of a fire safety educational program on school-aged children's knowledge of fire safety procedures, you may not want to pretest the experimental and control groups on their knowledge by asking them questions such as, What do you do if fire gets on your clothes? or What do you do if you find matches? The administration of a

R	X_1	O_1
R	X_2	O_1

figure 10.5 Two-group randomized controlled trial with posttest design only. R = random assignment; X = intervention/treatment, with X_1 being the experimental intervention and X_2 being the comparison/control intervention; O = observation/ measurement.

pretest in itself may lead the control children, who were not receiving the educational information, to ask their parents or teachers for the answers to these questions. As a result, findings may reveal no difference in knowledge between the two study groups at the end of the study—not because the intervention did not work but due to the strong influence of pretesting effects on the outcome.

The main disadvantage of a posttest only design is that baseline data on the study groups are unknown. Even though random assignment in the design illustrated in Figure 10-5 was used, which is the strongest strategy for controlling extraneous or confounding variables in an experimental study, there is still a chance that the two groups may be unequal or different at the start of the study. Differences in important baseline study measures between experimental groups may then negatively impact a study's outcomes or interfere with the ability to say that it was the intervention itself that caused a change in the dependent variable(s).

If an investigator is interested in whether an intervention produces both short- and long-term effects on an outcome, it is important for a study to build into its design repeated measurements of the outcome variable of interest (Figure 10-6).

The advantage of this type of design is that repeated assessments of an outcome variable over time allow an investigator to determine the sustainability of an intervention's effects. A disadvantage of this type of design is that *study attrition* (i.e., loss of subjects) may be a problem that may threaten the internal validity of the study. Another disadvantage of this design is that it is costly to follow subjects for longer periods of time. In addition, repeated follow-up on the same measures also may have the disadvantage of introducing testing effects that influence the outcome. For example, individuals may think about their answers and change their beliefs as part of the repeated follow-up sessions, not as the result of the intervention. Also, subjects may learn how repeated follow-up sessions work and, if the study entails extensive questioning when individuals admit to certain things (e.g., being depressed or taking drugs), they may learn to respond negatively to avoid lengthy follow-up testing or interviews.

The real disadvantage to conducting an RCT with a true control group, as illustrated in Figure 10-7, is that any positive intervention effects that are found may be solely related to giving the intervention group "something" versus nothing or the typical standard of care. This is especially true in studies that are measuring psychosocial/mental health variables, such as depression and anxiety. For example, if a healthcare provider were studying the effects of a stress reduction program on college students with test anxiety, someone simply spending extra time with them could reduce their anxiety, regardless of whether the intervention itself was helpful.

| R | X_1 | O_1 | O_2 | O_3 |
| R | X_2 | O_1 | O_2 | O_3 |

figure 10.6 Two-group randomized controlled trial with long-term repeated measures follow-up. R = random assignment; X = intervention/treatment, with X_1 being the experimental intervention and X_2 being the comparison intervention; O = observation/measurement, which will occur at 3 different time points (i.e., O_1, O_2, and O_3) after the intervention/treatment is delivered.

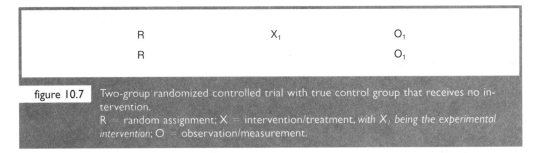

R	X_1	O_1
R		O_1

figure 10.7 Two-group randomized controlled trial with true control group that receives no intervention.
R = random assignment; X = intervention/treatment, with X_1 being the experimental intervention; O = observation/measurement.

The inclusion of a third group, as shown in Figure 10-8, allows an investigator to separate the effects of giving something (i.e., a comparison intervention) from a pure control group—a very strong experimental design. Disadvantages typically include the need to recruit additional subjects and costs to conduct the study.

The main advantage to conducting an experimental study that employs a **Solomon four-group design** (i.e., an experiment that uses a before-after design for the first experimental and control groups and an after-only design for the second experimental and control groups; Polit & Beck, 2003) is that it can separate the effects of pretesting the subjects (i.e., gathering baseline measures) on the outcome measure(s) (see Figure 10-9). Disadvantages include the addition of subjects as well as costs for increasing the size of the sample.

A factorial design (Figure 10-10) is an experiment that has two or more interventions or treatments. A major advantage of this type of design is that it allows an investigator to study the separate and combined effects of different types of interventions. For example, if a health-care provider were interested in the separate and combined effects of two different interventions (i.e., educational information and an exercise program) on blood pressure in adults with hypertension, this type of design would result in four groups:

1. A group of subjects who would receive educational information only
2. A group of subjects who would receive an exercise program only
3. A group of subjects who would receive both educational information and an exercise program
4. A group of subjects who would receive neither information nor exercise

R	X_1	O_1
R	X_2	O_1
R		O_1

figure 10.8 Three-group randomized controlled trial (i.e., one group who receives one type of experimental intervention; one group who receives a different or comparison intervention; and a pure control group who receives no intervention or standard care.
R = random assignment; X = intervention/treatment, with X_1 being the experimental intervention and X_2 being the comparison intervention; O = observation/measurement, which only occurs once (i.e., postintervention).

R	O_1	X_1	O_2
R		X_1	O_2
R	O_1	X_2	O_2
R		X_2	O_2

figure 10.9 Solomon four-group design in which a pair of experimental and control groups receive pretesting as depicted by O_1 and a pair who do not receive pretesting. R = random assignment; X = intervention/treatment, *with X_1 being the experimental intervention and X_2 being the comparison/control intervention*; O = observation/measurement, *with O_1 being the pretest (i.e., measured at baseline) and O_2 being the posttest (i.e., measured after the intervention is delivered).*

A major strength of this design is that it could be determined whether education or exercise alone positively impacts blood pressure or whether a combination of the two treatments is more effective than either intervention alone. Disadvantages to this design typically include additional subjects and costs.

      Quasi-Experimental Studies. Designs in which the independent variable (i.e., a treatment) is manipulated or introduced but where there is a lack of random assignment or a control group are called **quasi-experimental designs.**

      Although **quasi-experiments** may be more practical and feasible, they are weaker than true experimental designs in the ability to establish cause-and-effect inferences (i.e., to say that the independent variable or treatment was responsible for a change in the dependent variable and that the change was not due to other extraneous factors).

      There are times when quasi-experiments need to be conducted because random assignment is not always possible. For example, individuals cannot be assigned to smoking and non-

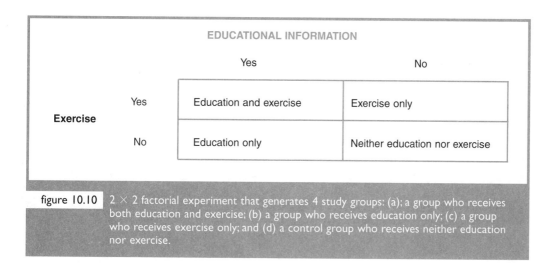

figure 10.10 2 × 2 factorial experiment that generates 4 study groups: (a); a group who receives both education and exercise; (b) a group who receives education only; (c) a group who receives exercise only; and (d) a control group who receives neither education nor exercise.

smoking conditions. Even when it is ethically feasible to use random assignment, the study setting might preclude it. For example, school principals frequently resist assigning children to programs based on random assignment. In addition, random assignment can be disruptive in schools (e.g., taking children out of their regular classrooms for special programs). Quasi-experiments, that is, designs that compare groups created by some method other than random assignment, provide an alternative to true experiments. Despite their limitations, some of these designs can be quite powerful in their ability to eliminate alternative explanations for the relationship between an intervention and the outcomes in a study.

Two examples of quasi-experimental designs are shown in Figures 10-11 and 10-12. In Figure 10-11, there is an experimental and control group who both receive a treatment, but the subjects have not been randomly assigned to the two study groups. As a result, the probability of equal study groups cannot be assured. Therefore, a pretest is administered so that it can be determined whether the two study groups are equal at baseline, before the intervention is delivered. In quasi-experiments, pretesting is especially important in order to assess whether the subjects are similar at baseline on the variable(s) that will be used as the outcome(s) in the study. If only posttesting is conducted in a quasi-experimental design in which random assignment was not used, it would be very difficult to have confidence in the findings because it could not be known whether the study groups were similar on key variables at the commencement of the study. In contrast, when random assignment is used in true experimental designs, it is very likely that the study groups will be equivalent on pretest measures.

Another example of a quasi-experimental study is the time series design (Figure 10-12). In this study, there is no random assignment or comparison/control group. This design incorporates a long series of pretest observations, an intervention, and a long series of posttest observations.

The time series design is used most frequently in communities or agencies that maintain careful archival records. It also can be used with community survey data if the survey questions and sample remain constant over time. An intervention effect is evidenced if a stable pattern of observations over a long period of time is found, followed by a marked change at the point of the intervention, then a stable pattern again over a long time after the intervention. For example, adolescent truancy rates might be tracked over several years, followed by an intervention with tracking of truancy rates for several additional years. If there is a marked drop in truancy rates at the point of the intervention, there is reasonable evidence for a program's effect. Even though this is a one-group design, there is ample evidence to rule out a variety of alternative explanations.

$$O_1 \qquad X_1 \qquad O_2$$
$$O_1 \qquad X_2 \qquad O_2$$

figure 10.11 A quasi-experiment with pretest and posttest design and a comparison/control group but lacking random assignment.
X = Intervention, with X_1 being the experimental intervention and X_2 being the comparison/control intervention; O = Observation, with O_1 indicating measurement at baseline and O_2 indicating measurement after the intervention is delivered.

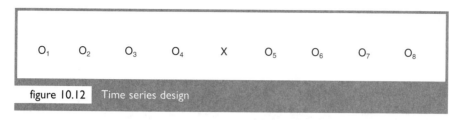

$$O_1 \quad O_2 \quad O_3 \quad O_4 \quad X \quad O_5 \quad O_6 \quad O_7 \quad O_8$$

figure 10.12   Time series design

One frequent challenge to single group designs is the threat of **history**, which involves the occurrence of some event or program unrelated to the intervention that might account for the change observed. History remains a viable alternate explanation for a change in the dependent variable only if the event happens at the same time point as the intervention. If the event occurs earlier or later than the experimental intervention, it cannot explain a change in outcome that occurs at or around the time of the intervention.

Another possible alternate explanation for observed changes in a one-group design is the **maturation** threat. Maturation is a developmental change that occurs even in the absence of the intervention. A true maturation effect will occur gradually throughout the pretest and posttest periods and thus could not account for sharp changes that occur at the point of the intervention.

Observed changes also might occur because of repeated testing or changes in instrumentation. Repeat testing of individuals typically influences their subsequent scores. In addition, performance on skills-based tests should increase over time simply due to practice. Finally, mortality as well as attrition or movement into and out of a community also could influence the outcome data but they offer an alternate explanation only if it started at the point of treatment.

Tamburro and colleagues (2002) employed an interrupted time series design in their evaluation of the impact of the Mid-South Safe Kids Coalition on rates of serious unintentional injuries (i.e., those leading to hospitalization or death). Consistent data were available for 1990 and 1991, the two years prior to the implementation of the coalition, and for 1993 through 1997, about six years following the implementation. All children in the county under 10 years old who were treated in a single hospital were included in the sample. Analyses showed a statistically significant drop in the rates of targeted injuries from 3.5 to 2.0 per 1,000 children, beginning precisely at the point the coalition was formed.

Pre-experimental Studies.   Pre-experiments lack both random assignment and a comparison/control group (Figure 10-13). As such, they are very weak in internal validity and allow too many competing explanations for a study's findings.

Other Important Experimental Design Factors.   Methods to ensure quality and consistency in the delivery of the intervention (i.e., maintenance of integrity) are crucial for being able to determine whether and how well an intervention works.

Integrity and Reproducibility   Frequently, investigators spend inordinate amounts of time paying particular attention to the dependent variable(s) or measure(s) to be used in a study and do not give sufficient time and attention to how an intervention is delivered. In addition, at the outset of an intervention study, it is critical to give thought to whether the intervention will be able to be reproduced by others in different settings. Reproducibility is critical if translation

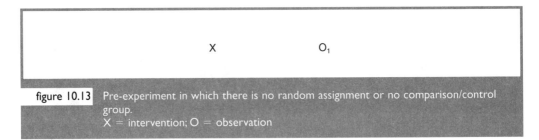

figure 10.13 Pre-experiment in which there is no random assignment or no comparison/control group.
X = intervention; O = observation

of the intervention into real-life practice settings is going to occur. As such, it is important to manualize or create standardized materials that specifically outline the content of the intervention so that others can replicate it and expect the same results in their practice settings. Use of videotapes, audiotapes, DVDs, or other types of reproducible materials to deliver an intervention is helpful in that this strategy ensures that each subject will receive all of the intervention content in exactly the same manner. However, not always is this type of delivery best suited to a particular clinical population. For example, groups may be the best strategy to deliver interventions to teens at high risk for sexually transmitted diseases because they allow for the teaching of refusal skills through role-playing.

In a study conducted by Morrison-Beedy and colleagues (2002a; 2002b), several healthcare providers were used to deliver an information/motivation/behavioral skills training program in four 2-hour group sessions to urban minority female adolescents. The content of the program and necessary skills to be taught for each of the sessions were detailed in a written manual. However, before the actual study commenced, intensive training of the interventionists occurred (e.g., practice groups, role-playing) to ensure that each of them would deliver the content of the program and the teaching of behavioral skills in the same manner. Once the study started, sessions were audiotaped and reviewed by the investigators to ensure quality and completeness in the delivery of the educational information and behavioral skills.

If rigorous standards to ensure integrity of an intervention do not occur in a study, it would be difficult to know whether the findings generated were the result of the intervention itself or other extraneous variables. When integrity of an intervention is maintained, greater confidence can be placed in a study's findings.

Pilot Study   Before conducting a large experimental study, it is extremely beneficial to first conduct a pilot study, which is a preliminary study that is conducted with a small number of subjects (e.g., 30–40) versus a full-scale clinical trial with large numbers of subjects. A pilot study is critical in determining the feasibility of subject enrollment, the intervention, the protocol or data collection plan for the study, and the likelihood that subjects will complete follow-up measures. With the development and implementation of new study measures, it also is essential to pilot them before use in a full-scale study to determine their validity and reliability. Pilot work enables investigators to identify weaknesses in their study design so that they can be corrected for the full-scale study. Subjects used for the pilot study should match those individuals who will be participating in the full-scale clinical trial.

Pilot studies are frequently conducted by advanced practice nurses and other master's-prepared clinicians and often lead the way to full-scale clinical trials. Working through the details for a large-scale intervention trial with a pilot study saves much time, energy, and frustration, as well as provides convincing evidence that a large-scale clinical trial is feasible and well worth the effort.

Manipulation Checks   Manipulation checks are important assessments to determine whether the intervention was successfully conducted. For example, if an investigator were delivering an educational intervention intended to teach healthcare providers about a disease and its treatment in order to improve patient outcomes, a manipulation check might be a test with a number of multiple-choice questions about the content of the intervention to which the subjects would respond. Answering a certain percentage of these questions correctly would indicate that the subjects successfully processed the educational information. As another example, an investigator may be interested in the effects of a new aerobic exercise program on weight loss in young adults. Therefore, subjects in the experimental group would be taught this program and instructed to complete the prescribed activities three times per week. A manipulation check to ensure that subjects actually complied with the prescribed exercise activities may involve keeping a log that lists the dates and number of minutes spent adhering to the program. These types of assessments are critical in order to verify that manipulation of the independent variable or completion of the treatment was achieved. If manipulation checks are not included in an experimental study and results indicate no differences between the experimental and control/comparison groups, it would be very difficult to explain whether it was a lack of intervention potency or the fact that subjects did not attend to or adhere to the intervention that was responsible for a lack of intervention effects.

Intervention Processes   When preparing to conduct an intervention study, it is important to think not only about the dependent variables or outcomes that the intervention might impact, but also about the process through which the intervention will exert its effects. The explanations about how an intervention works are important in facilitating its implementation into practice settings (Melnyk, 1995; Melnyk & Feinstein, 2001).

For example, an investigator proposes that a cognitive behavioral intervention (the independent variable) will reduce depressive symptoms (the dependent variable) in adults with low self-esteem. At the same time, however, the investigator proposes the mechanism of action (i.e., the mediating variable) through which the intervention will work. Therefore, it is hypothesized that the experimental intervention will enhance cognitive beliefs about one's ability to engage in positive coping strategies, which in turn will result in a decrease in depressive symptoms (see Figure 10-14). Conceptualization of a well-defined theoretical framework at the outset of designing an intervention study will facilitate explanations of how an intervention program may impact a study's outcomes.

Control Strategies   When conducting experimental studies, it is critical to strategize about how to control for extraneous factors that may influence the outcome(s) so that the effects of the intervention itself can be determined. These extraneous factors include those internal or intrinsic to the individuals who participate in a study (e.g., fatigue, level of maturity) and those external to the participants (e.g., the environment in which the study is conducted).

The best strategy to control for extraneous variables is randomization or random assignment. By randomly assigning subjects to study groups, there is a good probability that the subjects in the groups will be similar on important characteristics at the beginning of a study. When random assignment is not possible, other methods may be used to control extraneous or confounding variables. One of these strategies is **homogeneity,** or using subjects who are simi-

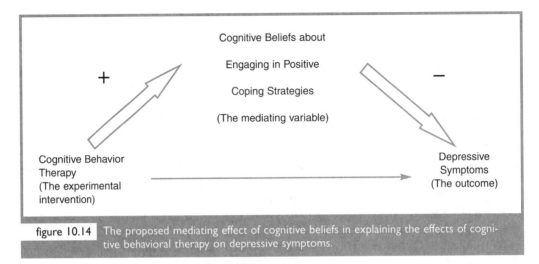

figure 10.14   The proposed mediating effect of cognitive beliefs in explaining the effects of cognitive behavioral therapy on depressive symptoms.

lar on the characteristics that may affect the outcome variable(s). For example, if a study were evaluating the effects of an intervention on parental stress during the critical care hospitalization of children, it may include only parents from intact marriages because divorced parents may have higher stress levels than nondivorced parents. In addition, very young mothers may have high stress levels. Therefore, this study's inclusion criteria may include only those parents who are from intact marriages as well as those who are older than 21 years. A weakness of this strategy is that at the end of the study, findings can be generalized only to married parents older than 21 years.

Another strategy to control intrinsic factors in a study is **blocking.** Blocking entails deliberately including a potential extraneous intrinsic or confounding variable in a study's design. For example, if there were a concern that level of motivation would affect the results of a study to determine the effects of aerobic exercise (i.e., the treatment) on weight loss in young adults, an investigator may choose to include motivation as another independent variable in the study, aside from the exercise program itself. In doing so, the effects of both motivation and exercise on weight loss could be studied in a 2 x 2 **randomized block design** (see Figure 10-15) involving two independent variables with two levels: (a) exercise and no exercise; and (b) high motivation and low motivation. The benefit of this type of design is that the interaction between motivation and exercise on weight loss also could be determined (i.e., Do individuals with high levels of motivation have greater weight loss than those with low motivation?).

Threats to Internal Validity   **Internal validity** is the extent to which it can be said that the independent variable (i.e., the intervention) causes a change in the dependent variable (i.e., outcome), and that the results are not due to other factors or alternative explanations. There are a number of major threats to the internal validity of a study that should be addressed in the planning process.

Attrition   The first threat to internal validity is **attrition,** or dropout of study participants, which may result in nonequivalent study groups (i.e., more individuals lost from the study in the control group than from the experimental group or more individuals with a certain

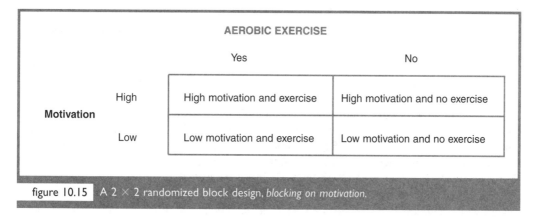

figure 10.15   A 2 × 2 randomized block design, *blocking on motivation.*

characteristic withdrawing from participation). As a result of losing more subjects from the control group than from the experimental group or more subjects with a certain characteristic (e.g., high anxiety), the study findings may be different than if those individuals had remained in the study. For example, if individuals with the poorest outcomes felt that they were not gaining any benefit from the study, which led them to drop from a study, differences between the two study groups may not surface during statistical analyses.

One strategy for preventing differential attrition is not to overly persuade potential subjects to participate in a study. There is a fine line between encouraging a potential subject to participate in a study and overly persuading him or her to participate. If someone decides to participate with much hesitation, there is an increased probability that he or she may drop from the study.

Another strategy for preventing attrition is to offer research subjects a small honorarium for participating in a study. Some studies provide an honorarium during each time point that a subject completes a specific phase of a study protocol (e.g., completing a set of questionnaires or receiving an intervention), whereas others provide an honorarium when the subjects complete the entire study protocol. Providing an honorarium sends the message that an individual's time for participating in a study is valued.

If there will be substantial time between contacts in a study, it is important to maintain communication through periodic cards or telephone calls. Lengthy lapses in communication with subjects makes it easier for them not to return phone calls and questionnaires as well as to miss follow-up appointments. To prevent attrition, another helpful strategy is to maintain consistency in who provides follow-up with the participants. One consistent person on the research team who follows a subject longitudinally over time will enhance the chances of successfully obtaining repeated follow-up data.

Finally, it is important to reduce subject burden to prevent attrition from a study. Participants can become easily overwhelmed if each contact involves the completion of several questionnaires that require a lot of time. An important question to ask for each proposed dependent variable is, How key is the measurement of this outcome or is it just a nice additional piece of data to include in the study? As a general rule of thumb, the easier and less time-consuming it is to participate in a study, the greater will be the probability of completion.

Confounding Variables/Selection   The best strategy to minimize the influence of confounding variables is to randomly assign subjects to study groups. In addition to establishing thoughtful inclusion and exclusion criteria, it also is important to maintain consistent study conditions for all participants. One way to ensure consistency is to establish clearly written study protocols so that every individual on the team understands the intricacies of when and how the interventions will be delivered, as well as the specific steps of data collection.

Nonadherence and Failure to Complete Protocol   Designing a realistic intervention is important so that it will eventually be transportable to the real world. There is a delicate balance in designing an intervention that will produce sustainable effects versus one that will be easy to implement in practice. As such, much thoughtful consideration must be given to the logistics of the intervention (e.g., feasibility, user-friendliness).

If there are multiple sessions with ongoing phases of the intervention, it is important to record which and how many sessions are attended and completed by study participants because this will facilitate evaluation of whether a dose response exists (i.e., the greater the number of sessions one attends, the larger the effect of the intervention).

Measurement of Change in Outcome Variables   In intervention studies where it is important to demonstrate a change in key dependent variables that the treatment will impact, it is critical to use measures that are sensitive to change over time. For example, if a certain measure has high **test–retest reliability** (i.e., it is stable over time), there will be little opportunity to affect a change in that measure. This is in contrast to other types of studies in which high test–retest reliabilities on certain measures are desirable (e.g., cohort studies that do not employ interventions in which you are following certain variables over time). For example, an individual's trait anxiety is the general predisposition to anxiety over time, which has been empirically shown to be a stable construct. In contrast, an individual's state anxiety fluctuates, depending on the situation. Therefore, an intervention would most likely affect state, not trait anxiety. Therefore, state anxiety would be a better outcome measure in an intervention study than would trait anxiety.

In conducting intervention studies, it is important to use the same measures longitudinally so that intervention effects over time can be determined. Carefully planning the timing of assessments is critical, especially if there is interest in both the short- and long-term effects of an intervention. It also is important to use measures that have good variability and that have been tested in the population of interest to avoid **"ceiling"** and **"floor"** effects (i.e., participant scores that cluster toward the low end or high end score of a measure).

In addition to measuring the outcomes of interventions with quantitative scales, it is important to administer an evaluation questionnaire at the end of a study so that subjects can provide open-ended responses to whether and how they believed the intervention was helpful. These types of responses are especially important if, by chance, the quantitative measures in the study reveal no statistically significant differences between study groups on key outcome variables.

It also is important to assess both clinical meaningfulness and statistical significance when determining whether an intervention has been successful. For example, the greater number of subjects that are included in a study, the more statistical *power* there will be to detect statistically significant differences between groups. In contrast, the smaller the sample size, the lower the power and the more difficult it will be to detect statistically significant findings. For example, in one hypothetical study with 1,000 subjects, an investigator found that teens who were enrolled in an expensive smoking cessation program smoked two cigarettes less per day than did teens who did not receive the program. This finding was statistically significant at the 0.05 level. As a result of this significant finding, the costly smoking cessation program was widely implemented. Although the finding was statistically significant, the clinical meaningfulness of this finding is weak. In contrast, another investigator conducted the same study with 50 adolescents and found that the experimental group teens smoked 10 cigarettes less per day than did teens who did not receive the smoking cessation program. This difference, however, was not statistically significant due to a small number of subjects and low statistical power. Therefore, a decision was made not to implement the program routinely because there was not a statistically significant difference between the study groups. However, a 10-cigarette difference between groups is more clinically meaningful than a 2-cigarette difference. This is a good example of how faulty decisions can be made if only statistically significant findings are considered important and their clinical meaningfulness is ignored.

History   History is another major threat to the internal validity of a study. This condition happens when external events take place concurrently with the treatment that may influence the outcome variables. For example, if a study were being conducted to determine the effects of a violence prevention intervention on anxiety in school-aged children and a school shooting occurred that received extensive media attention during the course of the trial, children's anxiety levels at the end of the study could be high, despite any positive effects of the intervention. The best way to minimize the threat of history is random assignment because at least both groups then should be equally affected by the external event.

Maturation   The passage of time alone can impact the outcomes of a study. For example, when studying infants who are growing rapidly, an acceleration in cognitive development may occur, regardless of the effects of an intervention that is aimed at enhancing cognition. The best way to deal with the threat of maturation is to use random assignment to allocate subjects to experimental and control groups as well as to recognize it as a potential alternative explanation for a study's findings.

Testing   Completing measures repeatedly could influence an individual's responses the next time a measure is completed. For example, answering the same depression scale three or four times could program someone to respond in the same way on subsequent administrations of the scale.

On the other hand, lengthy lapses in the administration of an instrument may result in a failure to detect important changes over time. Therefore, the best way to deal with this threat to internal validity is to think very carefully about how many times subjects are being asked to complete study measures and provide a strong rationale for these decisions.

Step 7: Identify the Sample and Enhance External Validity

External validity addresses the **generalizability** of research results (i.e., our ability to apply what we learn from a study sample to the larger population from which the sample was drawn). Clearly, a great deal is learned from the samples we study. However, there is always interest in applying that knowledge to a broader population (e.g., to the next 1,000 patients, not just the 100 in a particular study).

The key to external validity is the degree to which the sample that is being studied is representative of the population from which it was drawn. Creating a representative sample is a complex and challenging task. Samples are rarely if ever perfectly representative of the populations of interest, but there can be reasonable approximations.

There are four steps to consider when building a sample (Trochim, 2001):

1. Carefully define the theoretical population. The theoretical population is the population to which you wish to generalize your results (e.g., all 3-year-old children).

2. Describe the population to which you have access (i.e., the study population). Continuing with our example, this might include all 3-year-old children in the county in which you work, or perhaps in all of the counties in which your collaborators work. At this point, it is necessary to consider how similar the study population is to the target population. Typically, if the county is large and diverse, it is reasonable to assume that the study population is an acceptable substitute for the theoretical population. However, if the focus of your work is strongly influenced by regional factors, such as climate, culture, or access to services, the choice of a study population could severely limit generalizability to the theoretical population.

3. Describe the method you will use to access the population; in other words, define the sampling frame. It is highly unlikely that there will be a single comprehensive list of all 3-year-old children living in any one region at a particular time. You must find some practical method of identifying eligible children; then assess how the available methods might introduce bias or nonrepresentativeness. One strategy might be to approach the day care programs in the region. This would certainly be efficient, but not all 3-year-olds attend day care, and those who do are unlikely to be fully representative of the study population. For example, children whose mothers do not work outside the home are less likely to attend day care. Another approach might be to contact all of the pediatric offices in the region and solicit their cooperation in identifying the 3-year-olds under their care. Certainly, all young children see a pediatrician or nurse practitioner from time to time, even if they do not regularly keep their well child appointments. However, not all children in the region may receive care at the local pediatric offices. Perhaps families at one or both ends of the socioeconomic spectrum travel outside of the region for their care; perhaps others avoid care because of a lack of insurance and use only the emergency department on an "as needed" basis. Finally, the records at the pediatric offices might be out of date. A child may have come in for a 2-year visit, then moved away. Each of these possible alternatives needs to be reviewed and evaluated. The method that balances efficiency with representativeness will be the best choice. If there are more sites (day care centers, pediatric offices) than one can efficiently work with, a mechanism to choose a portion of the sites must be selected. The options will be described in the next section, along with mechanisms for selecting actual subjects from the sampling frame.

4. Typically, the sampling frame will include many more potential subjects than are required for the study. Thus, the fourth step in the process is identifying a method to select those individuals who will be invited to participate. Once again, the method chosen should balance efficiency and representativeness.

Random Sampling

Randomly sampling study sites (e.g., clinics or day care centers) and then subjects is the method most likely to avoid bias. In **random sampling,** every potential subject has an equal chance of being selected. The most straightforward way to think about random sampling is to imagine taking the list of everyone in the sampling frame, cutting it into small pieces with one name on each piece, placing all the names in a bowl, and drawing from the bowl the number of names required for the study design. This might work for selecting 6 day care programs from a list of 25 but in practice, it is an inefficient way to draw a sample of 200 children from a sampling frame of 10,000. That is quite a bit of cutting! A more efficient method is to assign everyone in the sampling frame a unique number, then, reading down the columns of a random number table or a list of random numbers generated by a computer algorithm, select those cases whose identifiers are included in the list of random numbers. If the entire sampling frame is available electronically, most computer database programs will draw random samples of cases of any specified number.

Random sampling is an efficient way in which to create a representative sample, but it does not guarantee representativeness. By definition, the process is random. However, it is possible, although quite unlikely, that a very atypical sample might emerge. In using random sampling to create a sample of 200 from 10,000 children, every possible sample of 200 has an equal chance of being drawn. It is possible, although very unlikely, that the sample drawn will contain 200 boys and no girls. More realistically, smaller (proportionately) subgroups might be underrepresented or entirely absent. If the research involves handedness or physical stature, it is possible that the selected sample will have no left-handed children or no children below or above a given height. To avoid this possibility, sampling procedures frequently incorporate **stratification.**

Stratified Sampling

Stratification involves dividing the study population into two or more subpopulations, then sampling separately from each. For example, if you would like to ensure that exactly 50% of the 200 children in the study sample are male, you would divide the study population into male and female groups and randomly sample 100 from each. This type of simple stratification works only if information about the stratification variable is included in the sampling frame data, that is, in the day care center or pediatric office records. It is unlikely that you would be able to stratify by handedness using this simple strategy. Similarly, it would be unlikely that you would be able to stratify on measures such as depression, self-esteem, or life stress because information about these variables is unlikely to be included in any accessible preexisting database.

A variation on this theme involves a second stage of information gathering and sampling. Once the initial sampling frame is identified, a brief survey is conducted with a large random sample. The survey includes questions about variables on which you would like to stratify. A second random sample can now be drawn from the sample of completed surveys. This second-stage sampling can be stratified based on this new information. Such sampling designs are somewhat more complex to analyze, but they do ensure that all of the subgroups of interest are included in adequate numbers.

Cluster (Area) Random Sampling

If the study population is spread over a wide geographical area, you can use another variation of two-stage sampling. First, you divide the large area into regions or clusters (e.g., counties or census tracts). From the full list of clusters, you can randomly sample a sufficiently manageable number of clusters. Then individual subjects from each cluster can be randomly sampled. Clearly, it is best to have the same sampling strategy and the same sampling frame within each cluster. Like the other two-stage strategies, this requires somewhat more complex approaches to data analysis, but it makes collecting data across large geographic regions economical. If, for example, your sample population is all women in a state and you randomly sample from that population (e.g., from state motor vehicle or telephone records), you then must drive all over the state to collect your data. If you divide the state into counties and randomly sample six counties, the logistics of data collection become manageable as long as you believe these six counties fairly reflect the overall state profile.

Nonprobability or Purposive Samples

There are occasions when it is not feasible to use random sampling. Nevertheless, you should make every effort to develop a representative sample and to employ a systematic approach that can be well described. This is purposive sampling (Trochim, 2001). A good description of your sampling strategy, whether random or not, permits the readers of your work to judge for themselves the representativeness of your sample and the generalizability of your results. Simply characterizing the sampling strategy as one of "convenience" with no further discussion leaves the reader with the impression that no thought whatsoever was given to external validity and no judgment can be made about generalizability. The reader is left to believe that you are assuming that your findings are invariant across all people and all places.

Modal Instance Sampling

Unlike random sampling, you sample the most frequent or modal case. This is less useful when sampling individuals than when sampling larger units, such as counties, clinics, or schools in two-stage sampling designs or where these larger units are actually the units of analysis (i.e., where the program or treatment is applied to a region or clinic rather than to a person). For example, in a primarily rural state, when selecting counties, you would select counties with a "typical" profile rather than those having very few highly urban counties. With respect to schools, you might select from the "comprehensive" high schools rather than from magnet or other schools with specialized programming.

With respect to the sampling of individuals, if we want to sample children from predominantly middle-class schools where most children are college bound, we might want to choose students who are in fact middle-class and college bound. This will not give a truly representative picture of the entire school, but it provides a reasonable reflection of the majority.

Heterogeneity Sampling

This strategy is applicable in the same situations in which modal instance sampling is applicable. However, with this approach, instead of sampling just the modal or typical case, you take care to sample heterogeneously to ensure a broad spectrum of subjects. In the example involving counties described above, rather than sampling just the modal rural counties, you would sample rural, urban, and suburban counties. With respect to schools, you might select comprehensive, magnet, and some specialized school programs. With respect to individual children, you might sample college-bound students, those in vocational programs, and perhaps even some who have dropped out or are about to drop out of school.

Snowball Sampling

Snowball sampling is helpful when assembling a sample of infrequent or hard-to-find cases. With snowball sampling, each subject is asked to recommend other potential subjects or to inform other possible subjects about the opportunity to participate in the study. For example, if one is studying older adults with relatively rare diseases or conditions, the spouses of one case will be likely to know or at least to have met other individuals whose spouses have the same condition. In snowball sampling, the investigator is less concerned with broad representation of a large study population and more concerned with finding the relatively few members of that population who exist.

Determination of Sample Size

The determination of sample size is an important step and should be done early in the process of designing a study. It is important to remember that the sample size estimate should be calculated on how many subjects need to be followed over the course of a study, not just enrolled (Browner, Newman, Cummings, & Hulley, 2001), always building into the plan at least a 20% dropout rate for longitudinal designs. Too few subjects may result in low statistical power and the inability to detect significant findings in a study when they truly do exist (i.e., making a *type 2 error*, such as when an investigator accepts a false null hypothesis, which states there is no relationship between the independent and dependent variables). Many studies conducted in the health professions result in nonsignificant findings as a result of too small of samples. On the other hand, enrolling more subjects than needed will result in greater costs to a study than necessary. When estimating sample size, it is important to obtain the statistics on the number of patients who would have met your study criteria who were available in the clinical setting during the prior year where the study will be conducted. These data will allow you to determine the feasibility of recruiting the necessary number of subjects during the course of your study.

Power analysis is a procedure used for determining the sample size needed for a study and helps to reduce type 2 errors (Polit & Beck, 2003). Readers are encouraged to refer to a good resource to assist with the process of power analysis and calculation of sample size (Cohen, 1988; Jaccard & Becker, 1990).

Refusal to Participate and Study Attrition

The actual generalizability of the results depends not on who is approached to participate in a study but on who actually completes the study. Not everyone who is approached agrees to participate, and not everyone who agrees to participate completes the study. If the number of people who refuse or who drop out is relatively small and there is no reason to believe that any subgroup of subjects was more likely to drop out than any other (i.e., the pattern of refusals and dropouts was random), the final sample will still be representative of the study population. Quite frequently, however, those who refuse to participate and those who drop out are not a random subset.

People with exhibitionist tendencies (i.e., those who like to talk about themselves), hypochondriacs (i.e., always in need of confirmation of their illness or looking for free services), people with a strong social conscience, and those generally willing to volunteer are less likely to refuse. Thus, they will be overrepresented in any sample in which there is a substantial degree of refusal or dropout (Rosenthal & Rosnow, 1990). People who volunteer also are more likely to be affluent and well educated.

The best strategy to enhance external validity is to minimize refusal and dropout rates. To assess the potential impact of these threats, it is essential to have a clear sampling frame and to keep records of who is approached, who agrees to participate, who refuses, and ultimately who completes the study. If anything is known about those who were approached and refused, the possibility of bias can be addressed by comparing those who refused with those who did not as well as those who dropped out with those who did not. Understanding the impact of refusal rates is not possible using convenience sampling in which advertisements are placed in the newspaper or signs are posted and only those who are interested are identified. Such strategies must assume that the findings of the study (e.g., the impact of the intervention or the beliefs of the participants) are invariant across people.

Strategies to Promote Participation

There are several strategies that encourage participation in a study:

Have direct, personal contacts with prospective subjects. Avoid making prospective subjects take any action or demonstrate any initiative to enroll, such as requiring them to complete enrollment forms or make telephone calls. Be persistent but respectful when contacting prospective subjects. Send letters of introduction on official stationery introducing the study and stating who and when someone will call to explain the study further. Use high-powered mailings (e.g., special delivery and/or hand-addressed envelopes) because individuals are much more likely to open such mail. Have the letters come from the PI whose credentials lend credibility to the study. Finally, communicate that volunteering is normative, not unusual behavior. You do not want to start out by saying, "You are probably quite busy . . ." This conveys an expectation that the person will refuse and actually gives them a socially acceptable reason.

Make participation as easy as possible. Do what you can to remove any barriers, such as the cost of babysitting or transportation. If possible, have babysitting available at the study site. If that is not possible, provide a sufficient honorarium to cover the cost. Cover the cost of transportation or send a cab to transport individuals to the study site. Make the study as non-threatening, stress free, and brief as possible, given the research design. Lengthy interviews covering a number of personal topics will burden subjects. Be certain each section is essential. Train the recruiters and interviewers well. Make certain that they are comfortable with the recruitment protocol, script, and interview before working with actual subjects. Interviewers must be accepting and nonjudgmental. They must not appear shocked, awkward, or unprepared during any conversation or interview.

Make participation worthwhile. Carefully and clearly explain the importance of the work and the manner in which the study results might improve care or services to patients and/or families like theirs. Make participation sound interesting. Emphasize what the subjects might learn about themselves or their families. Tell them about any activities they might actually enjoy.

Step 8: Determine Measures

Selection of measures or instruments to assess or observe a study's variables is a critical step in designing a clinical study. As a rule, it is best to choose measures that yield the highest level of data (i.e., *interval* or *ratio data*, otherwise known as *continuous variables*) because these types of measures will allow fuller assessments of the study's variables, as well as permit the use of more robust statistical tests. Examples of interval-or ratio-level data that have quantified intervals on an infinite scale of values are weight in pounds, number of glasses of beverages consumed a day, and age. **Ordinal data** are those that have ordered categories with intervals that cannot be quantified (e.g., none, a little, some, a lot, and very much so). Finally, **categorical data** have unordered categories in which one category is not considered higher or better than another (e.g., sex, gender, race).

Measures should be both **valid** (i.e., they measure what they are intended to measure) and **reliable** (i.e., they consistently and accurately measure the construct of interest). If possible, it is best to use measures that have been used with similar samples as the study being planned, as well as those that are reported to have **reliability coefficients** of at least 0.70 or better instead of measures that have not been previously tested in prior work or have been tested with samples very different from the proposed study. It is very difficult to place confidence in a study's findings if the measures used did not have established validity or the **internal consistency reliability** of the measures was less than 0.70.

It also is important to recognize that obtaining two forms of assessment on a particular variable (e.g., self-report and observation) enhances credibility of the findings when the data from these different sources converge. For example, if a parent reports that his or her child is high on externalizing behaviors (i.e., acting-out behaviors) on an instrument that measures these behaviors, and the child's teacher also completes a teacher version of the same instrument that yields high scores, the convergence of these findings produces a convincing case for the child being high on externalizing behaviors.

If observation data are being gathered, it is important to train observers on the instrument that will be used in a study so that there is an **inter-rater reliability** or agreement on the construct that is being observed (e.g., maternal-infant interaction) at least 90% of the time. In addition, for intervention studies, it is important that observers be blind to study group (i.e., unaware as to whether the subjects are in the experimental or control groups) to avoid bias in their ratings.

Step 9: Outline Data Collection Plan

The data collection plan typically specifies when and where each phase of the study (e.g., subject enrollment, intervention sessions, completion of measures) will be completed and exactly when all the measures will be obtained. Careful planning of these details is essential before the study commences. A timetable is often helpful to outline the study procedures so that each member of the team is aware of the specific plan for data collection (see Table 10-1).

table 10.1 Timetable for a study's data collection plan

9/1/2004–10/31/2004 Hire and train research assistants. Prepare study offices, study materials, and data packets.

11/1/2004–10/31/2006 Subject recruitment, completion of all hospital data collection, ongoing data collection for posthospital phases of the study, and data entry.

11/1/2005–4/30/2006 Complete data collection and data entry for posthospital phases of study.

5/1/2005–10/30/2006 Data analysis. Preparation of reports and manuscripts.

Step 10: Apply for Human Subjects Approval

Before the commencement of research, it is essential to have the study approved by an RSRB that will evaluate the study for protection of human subjects. Federal regulations (Code of Federal Regulations, 1983) now mandate that any research conducted be reviewed to ensure the following:

- Risks to subjects are minimized.
- Selection of subjects is equitable (e.g., women, children, and individuals of a certain race/ethnicity are not excluded).
- Informed consent is obtained and documented if indicated (see Appendix for an example of an approved consent form).
- A data and safety monitoring plan is implemented when indicated (e.g., for clinical trials; see Appendix for an example of a data safety and monitoring plan).

In addition, any individual involved in a study as an investigator, subinvestigator, study coordinator, or enroller of human subjects must pass a required test on the protection of human subjects, based on the Belmont Report. The Belmont Report was issued in 1978 by the National Commission of the Protection of Human Subjects of Biomedical and Behavioral Research (1978) and outlined three principles on which standards of ethical conduct in research are to be based:

1. Beneficence (i.e., no harm to subjects)
2. Respect for human dignity (e.g., the right for self-determination, as in providing voluntary consent to participate in a study)
3. Justice (e.g., fair treatment and nondiscriminatory selection of human subjects)

Guidelines for RSRB application and review should be obtained from the institution(s) in which the study will be conducted.

See the University of Rochester's RSRB Web site at **http://www.urmc.rochester.edu/rsrb** for one example of required guidelines and forms for submission of a research study for human subjects' review.

Step 11: Implement the Study

Once human subjects' approval for the study is obtained, data collection can begin. Particular detail and attention should be paid to the process of data collection for the first 5–10 subjects regarding the ease of enrollment and completion of study questionnaires. This is a good time for the research team to work through any challenges encountered and to implement strategies to overcome them. Emphasis should be placed on the review of questionnaires after completion by study participants to prevent missing data that pose challenges for data analysis, as well as to determine whether subjects meet clinical criteria on sensitive measures or those that identify them as at risk for certain conditions (e.g., major depression, suicide). Weekly or biweekly team meetings are very beneficial in order for the research team to overcome challenges in data collection and to maintain cohesiveness during the conduct of the study.

Step 12: Prepare and Analyze Data

In the preparation phase of data analysis, it is important to assess study measures for completeness and to make determinations about what strategies will be used to handle missing data. For example, if less than 30% of the data are missing on a questionnaire, it is acceptable practice to impute the mean for missing items. If, on the other hand, more than 30% of the data are missing on a questionnaire, investigators commonly eliminate it from data analysis. There is a growing body of literature on handling missing data, although the best strategy is really avoiding it in the first place (Cole, Feinstein, & Bender, 2001).

Creating a code book regarding how certain responses will be translated into numerical form is important before data can be entered into a statistical program, such as SPSS (Statistical Package for the Social Sciences). For example, marital status could be coded as "1" married, "2" not married, "3" divorced, or "4" married for the second or third time. Verifying all entered data also is a critical step in preparing to analyze the data.

Multiple statistical tests can be conducted to answer research questions and to test hypotheses generated in quantitative studies, and readers are encouraged to consult a statistical resource for detailed information on these specific tests. For example, Munro's text (2001) is a "user-friendly" book that provides excellent information and examples of common statistical analyses for quantitative studies.

Step 13: Interpret the Results

Careful interpretation of the results of a study (i.e., explaining the study results) is important and should be based on the theoretical/conceptual framework that guided the study as well as prior work in the area. Alternative explanations for the findings should always be considered in the discussion. In addition, it is important to discuss findings from prior research that relate to the current study.

Step 14: Disseminate the Findings

Once a study is completed, it is imperative to disseminate the findings to both researchers and clinicians who will use the evidence in guiding further research in the area or in making decisions about patient care. The vehicles for dissemination should include both conferences in the form of oral and/or poster presentations as well as publications (see Chapter 14 for helpful strategies on preparing oral and poster presentations, as well as writing for publication). In addition, the findings of a study also should be disseminated to the media and to the public (see Chapter 14).

Step 15: Incorporate Findings into Evidence-Based Practice and Evaluate Outcomes

Once evidence from a study is generated, it is important to factor that evidence into a decision regarding whether it should be incorporated into patient care. Studies should be critically appraised with respect to three key questions:

1. Are the findings valid (i.e., as close to the truth as possible)?
2. Are the findings important (e.g., strength and preciseness of the intervention)?
3. Are the findings applicable to your patients? (See Unit Two.)

Once a decision is made to incorporate the findings of a study into practice, an outcomes evaluation should be conducted to determine the impact of the change on the process or outcomes of clinical care (see Chapter 12).

references

Browner, W. S., Newman, T. B., Cummings, S. R., & Hulley, S. B. (2001). Estimating sample size and power: The nitty-gritty. In S. B. Hulley, S. R. Cummings, W. S. Browner, D. Grady, N. Hearst, & T. B. Newman (Eds.). *Designing clinical research. An epidemiologic approach* (2nd ed.) Philadelphia: Lippincott Williams & Wilkins.

Campbell, D. T., & Stanley, J. C. (1963). *Experimental and quasi-experimental designs for research.* Chicago: Rand McNally.

Code of Federal Regulations (1983). *Protection of human subjects*: 45CFR46 (Rev. March 8, 1983). Washington, DC: Department of Health and Human Services.

Cohen, J. (1988). *Statistical power analysis for the behavioral sciences* (2nd ed.). Mahwah, NJ: Lawrence Erlbaum.

Cole, R . E., Feinstein, N. F., & Bender, N. L. (2001). What's the big deal about missing data? *Applied Nursing Research, 14*, 225–226.

Cummings, S. R., Browner, W. S., & Hulley, S. B. (2001). Conceiving the research question. In S. B. Hulley, S. R. Cummings, W. S. Browner, D. Grady, N. Hearst, and T. B. Newman (Eds) (pp. 17–23). *Designing clinical research* (2nd ed.). Philadelphia: Lippincott, Williams & Wilkins.

Guyatt, G., & Rennie, D. (2002). *Users' guides to the medical literature. Essentials of evidence-based clinical practice.* American Medical Association.

Jaccard, J., & Becker, M. A. (1990). *Statistics for the behavioral sciences* (2nd ed.). Belmont, CA: Wadsworth.

Jimmerson, S. (1982). Anxiety. In J. Haber, A. Leach, & B. Sideleau (Eds.). *Comprehensive psychiatric nursing.* New York: McGraw-Hill.

Johnson, J. E., Fieler, V. K., Jones, L. S., Wlasowicz, G. S., & Mitchell, M. L. (1977). *Self-regulation theory: Applying theory to your practice.* Pittsburgh, PA: Oncology Nursing Press.

Leventhal, H., & Johnson, J. E. (1983). Laboratory and field experimentation: Development of a theory of self-regulation. In P. J. Woolridge, M. H. Schmitt, J. K. Skipper, Jr., & R. C. Leonard (Eds.) (pp. 189–262). *Behavioral science and nursing theory.* St. Louis, MO: Mosby.

Melnyk, B. M. (1994). Coping with unplanned childhood hospitalization: Effects of informational interventions on mothers and children. *Nursing Research, 43*, 50–55.

Melnyk, B. M. (1995). Coping with unplanned childhood hospitalization: The mediating functions of parental beliefs. *Journal of Pediatric Psychology, 20*(3), 299–312.

Melnyk, B. M., & Feinstein, N. F. (2001). Mediating functions of maternal anxiety and participation in care on young children's posthospital adjustment. *Research in Nursing & Health, 24*, 18–26.

Melnyk, B. M., & Alpert-Gillis, L. J. (1996). Enhancing coping outcomes of mothers and young children following marital separation: A pilot study. *Journal of Family Nursing, 2*(3), 266–285.

Melnyk, B. M., Alpert-Gillis, L. J., Hensel, P. B., Cable-Beiling, R. C., & Rubenstein, J. S. (1997). Helping mothers cope with a critically ill child: A pilot test of the COPE intervention. *Research in Nursing & Health, 20,* 3–14.

Melnyk, B. M., Alpert-Gillis, L., Feinstein, N. F., Fairbanks, E., Schultz-Czarniak, J. Hust, D., Sherman, L., LeMoine, C., Moldenhauer, Z., Small, L., Bender, N., & Sinkin, R. A. (2001). Improving cognitive development of LBW premature infants with the COPE program: A pilot study of the benefit of early NICU intervention with mothers. *Research in Nursing and Health, 24,* 373–389.

Melnyk, B. M. (2003). Critical appraisal of systematic reviews: A key strategy for evidence-based practice. *Pediatric Nursing, 29*(2), 147–149, 125.

Morrison-Beedy, D., Carey, M. P., Aronowitz, T., Mkandawire, L., & Dyne, J. (2002a). Adolescents' input on the development of a HIV-risk reduction intervention. *Journal of the Association of Nurses in AIDS Care, 13*, 21–27.

Morrison-Beedy, D., Carey, M. P., Aronowitz, T., Mkandawire, L., & Dyne, J. (2002b). An HIV risk reduction intervention in an adolescent correctional facility: Lessons learned. *Applied Nursing Research, 15*, 97–101.

Munro, B. H. (2001). *Statistical methods for health care research* (4th edition). Philadelphia: Lippincott, Williams & Wilkins.

National Commission for the Protection of Human Subjects of Biomedical and Behavioral Research. (1978). *Belmont report: Ethical principles and guidelines for research involving human subjects.* Washington, DC: U.S. Government Printing Office.

Newman, T. B., Browner, W. S., Cummings, S. R., & Hulley, S. B. (2001). Designing an observation study: Cross-sectional and case-control studies. In S. B. Hulley, S. R. Cummings, W. S. Browner, D. Grady, N. Hearst, & T. B. Newman (Eds.). *Designing clinical research* (2nd edition) (pp. 197–123). Philadelphia: Lippincott, Williams & Wilkins.

Polit, D. F., & Hungler, B. P. (1999). *Nursing research. Principles and methods.* Philadelphia: Lippincott, Williams & Wilkins.

Powers, B A., & Knapp, T. R., (1995). *A dictionary of nursing theory and research.* New York: Springer.

Rosenthal, R. & Rosnow, R. L. (1990) *Essential of behavioral research: Methods and data analysis.* New York: McGraw-Hill.

Tamburro, R. F. , Shorr, R. I., Bush, A. J., Kritchevsky, S. B., Stidham, G. L., & Helms, S. A. (2002). Association between the inception of s SAFE KIDS Coalition and changes in pediatric unintentional injury. *Injury Prevention, 8,* 242–245.

Trochim, W. M. (2001). *The research methods knowledge base.* Cincinnati, OH: Atomic Dog Publishing.

VanderVeer, A. H. (1949). The psychopathology of physical illness and hospital residence. *Quarterly Journal of Child Behavior, 1,* 55–79.

Whittemore, R., & Grey, M. (2002). The systematic development of nursing interventions. *Journal of Nursing Scholarship, 34* (2), 115–120.

chapter 10

281

Generating Evidence Through Qualitative Research

Bethel Ann Powers

chapter 11

" *The future depends on what we do in the present.* "

Mahatma Gandhi

Qualitative studies are helpful in answering particular kinds of research questions. For example, when a concept or phenomenon is not well understood or adequately covered in the literature (e.g., understanding the experience of being the parents of a fetus with a life-threatening or life-altering condition), conducting qualitative studies is a good way to develop knowledge in this area. The **qualitative** research question is focused on a *how* (e.g., How do persons manage the experience?) or a *what* (e.g., What is the experience like?) in contrast to **quantitative** questions that ask *why* and look for a comparison of groups or relationships between variables for the purpose of establishing association or cause and effect. Qualitative studies also are helpful when much is known about a phenomenon, but what is known in certain areas is deficient in quality, depth, or detail. Thus, qualitative studies may explore specific concepts or variables (e.g., concepts of *hope* or *suffering*), develop theories to explain the processes individuals go through when dealing with an issue (e.g., the process of learning to live with irritable bowel disease), provide a more comprehensive view of a topic in sociocultural context (e.g., primary healthcare issues as perceived by migrant farm workers), or increase sensitivity to a human experience to enhance understanding or stimulate social action (e.g., the mental health needs of incarcerated adolescents).

Basic Understandings About Qualitative Research

Before discussing specific considerations in designing a qualitative study, it is important to address some common misunderstandings, lest they impede communication (see Box 11-1). First, the terms *qualitative* and *descriptive* often are used interchangeably and applied indistinguishably, so it is important to understand that this can create confusion. For example, referring to all nonnumerical data as descriptive or qualitative data to distinguish them from numerical or quantitative data confuses the nature of the data with the research processes that produce them. Any type of study design can produce numerical and nonnumerical data, but only qualitative studies produce qualitative data. Similarly, both quantitative and qualitative research traditions have distinct types of descriptive research designs. Therefore, it is important to distinguish between the two. Qualitative and descriptive studies also are lumped together on one end of the evidence-based practice (EBP) hierarchy of evidence continuum. However, qualitative studies are not a logical component of this linear quantitative continuum for the same reasons that they are not equivalent to quantitative types of descriptive research. Their purposes and underlying assumptions are very different.

Second, a set of simple procedural steps for designing qualitative research studies often is desired or expected by persons who do not understand that this is not possible because of the diversity and complexity of the field. It is assumed that readers of this chapter will have read Chapter 6 and immersed themselves to some degree in reading and appraising different types of qualitative research reports. This will help them understand this chapter's emphasis on general

box 11.1

Basic Understandings About Qualitative Research

- Not all descriptive research is qualitative.
- Not all qualitative research is descriptive.
- There is no single set of procedural steps for designing qualitative research studies.
- Qualitative studies designed and conducted by researchers mentored in a specified approach will have best outcomes.

principles that apply to qualitative research design and its use of different types of actual studies from Appendix B as illustrative examples.

Finally, some persons believe that reading about how to do qualitative research should be enough to enable them to conduct a qualitative research study. This chapter is not written with that objective in mind. The objective is to build on the information presented in Chapter 6 on appraising qualitative research. This time, however, it is assumed that readers might be thinking about practice-based research questions that they would like to pursue in collaboration with an experienced qualitative researcher. This chapter is designed to draw interested individuals more closely into that experience.

Not All Descriptive Research Is Qualitative

Descriptive studies are typically used in a preliminary way by quantitative researchers to establish the knowledge base and hypotheses for conducting correlational, quasi-experimental, and experimental studies. Examples of quantitative descriptive research are presented in Table 11-1. Quantitative studies may use some of the same techniques used by qualitative researchers (e.g., observation, interviews, and descriptive statistics); however, the purposes and methods of the research designs are not the same. Qualitative descriptive research reflects certain features that are common among other types of traditional qualitative research designs. It differs from quantitative descriptive research in many ways (see Table 11-2).

Multiple Purposes Focus on Understanding and Meaning
Qualitative descriptive studies do not serve the unidirectional purpose of quantitative descriptive studies that are designed as preliminary steps to more controlled correlational or experimental studies. These quantitative studies are oriented toward the measurement, testing, and verification of cause-and-effect relationships. In contrast, the different purposes of qualitative studies include discovering meaning, explaining meaning in context, promoting understanding, raising awareness, and challenging misconceptions about the nature of human experiences. Looking for cause-and-effect relationships is not the purpose of qualitative descriptive studies.

Openness and Flexibility Accommodate the Unexpected
Qualitative researchers cast a wider net. They consider all that happens in "the field" (i.e., all that is observed or brought to their awareness in any way) as data. In addition, they expect, welcome, and accommodate the unexpected in the process of data collection (Sandelowski, 2000). Procedures are more flexible to allow for decision making about new directions in data gathering influenced by simultaneous collection and analysis of incoming data.

Distinctive Procedures Assure Depth, Accuracy, and Completeness
Sampling in qualitative studies is purposeful to ensure data quality and completeness (i.e., the concept of **saturation**) and to enhance theoretical generalizability (Morse, 1999). Sample size varies, and samples are often comparatively small; however, data sets are very large and dense. Use of multiple data sources (e.g., participant observation, interview, and material artifacts) is common and ongoing. Qualitative researchers also rely on the discovery of multiple means of

table 11.1 Quantitative descriptive designs

Kind of Design	Purpose	Example
Basic	Measures the characteristics of a single group of variables	Documentation of the influence of treatment rounds on sleep and awake patterns of elderly hospitalized patients
Comparative descriptive	Describes differences in variables that occur in two or more groups	Comparison of diabetic teenage boys' and girls' self-care practices
Time-dimensional	Examines sequences and patterns of change, growth, and trends across time	Cohort studies that examine the health histories of a group of individuals over time to see how they may be related to periodically measured, predetermined variables, such as diet, exercise, and smoking
Longitudinal	Studies changes in the same subjects over time with respect to particular dependent variables	Follow-up of a group of premature babies delivered at a particular hospital over a calendar year to see when they "catch up" developmentally with full-term babies delivered in that same year
Cross-sectional	Studies a sample (slice) of a population at a single point in time	Study of parental coping styles while caring for their autistic children
Survey	Gathers self-report data via mailed or personally administered questionnaires	A researcher interested in resident satisfaction with assisted living options draws a sample from a population of residents and, in interviews, asks for information about persons' use and opinions of specific services

validation in the data collection and analysis process to ensure that findings are complete and accurate.

Presentation of Findings Involves Multiple Reporting Styles

Presentation of findings in qualitative research does not follow a uniform format. It involves multiple reporting styles. It is not structured around preselected variables and is more fully elaborated from participants' points of view and in their own words. Varied writing techniques may be used to sensitize readers to the real-life complexities and feeling tones of participants' experiences. Full narrative descriptions seek to establish "descriptive validity" through accurate portrayals of events and "interpretive validity" by accounting for the meanings that participants attribute to those events (Sandelowski, 2000, citing Maxwell, 1992).

table 11.2 Differences in qualitative and quantitative descriptive studies

Qualitative Descriptive Studies	Quantitative Descriptive Studies
Designed to provide meaning and understanding	Designed to lead to studies establishing cause-and-effect relationships
Openness and flexible data-gathering strategies accommodate the unexpected	Control for undesired data Fixed data-gathering strategies
Purposeful sampling Sample sizes tend to be small	Preferred random sampling Sample sizes tend to be larger
Repetitive process of simultaneous data collection and data analysis	Linear stepwise process of data collection followed by data analysis
Long, in-depth semistructured to open-ended interviews	Interviews may be open-ended but often more structured and preplanned
Observation participant and ongoing	Observation more structured and controlled
Multiple reporting styles	Uniform reporting format
Conclusions not based on prior assumptions—temporarily suspends and ultimately treats prior assumptions as data to be subjected to analysis	Conclusions guided by and limited to a priori assumptions
Nonhierarchical. Studies are complete, although they may lead to further research (qualitative or quantitative)	Hierarchical. Studies are preliminary and are expected to lead to further inferential research

Conclusions Are Not Based on Prior Assumptions

Qualitative researchers do not limit conclusions to those based on prior assumptions about a phenomenon (e.g., in the form of predetermined measures and items on surveys and other data collection instruments) or drawn from "the results of statistical tests, which are themselves based on sets of assumptions" (Sandelowski, 2000, p. 336). The prior assumptions of qualitative researchers are temporarily suspended (bracketed) and ultimately treated as data that need to be analyzed along with study participants' accounts.

Qualitative Research is Complete and Nonhierarchical

Qualitative descriptive research may generate basic knowledge, hypotheses, and theories to be used in the design of other types of qualitative or quantitative studies. However, it is not necessarily a preliminary step to some other type of research. It is "a complete and valued end-product in itself" (Sandelowski, 2000, p. 335). This reflects the nonhierarchical nature of qualitative research. It has no fixed counterpart to quantitative researchers' linear continuum that conceptualizes knowledge development as a progression upward from preliminary descriptive research designs to experiments and clinical trials. Nor do all qualitative investigations logically lead to experiments and clinical trials. Therefore, more often it is assumed that "[n]o method is absolutely weak nor strong, but rather more or less useful or appropriate in relation to certain purposes" (Sandelowski, 2000, p. 335).

> 66 *Don't let the fear of the time it will take to accomplish something stand in the way of your doing it. The time will pass anyway, we might just as well put that passing time to the best possible use.* 99
>
> *Earl Nightingale*

Not All Qualitative Research is Descriptive

Some qualitative research studies are interpretive, involving a higher degree of analytic complexity. All research involves interpretation in the natural course of describing what the findings signify and their perceived relevance. But not all research is interpretive in intent.

Interpretive Nature of Qualitative Designs

Qualitative research designs, in varying degrees, involve the use of deliberate interpretive strategies seeking to describe a phenomenon more completely. As a result, qualitative descriptive studies are more interpretive than quantitative descriptive studies because of their purposes and the ways in which they are conceptualized, designed, and carried out. However, they are less interpretive than other qualitative approaches. Although all qualitative research studies involve description, certain types, such as "[p]henomenologic, grounded theory, and ethnographic studies are not exclusively in the descriptive domain" (Sandelowski, 2000, p. 335).

Qualitative descriptive studies differ from other qualitative studies that represent one of the interpretive traditions in several ways. First, qualitative descriptive studies do not move as far *into* the data in terms of producing "thick" descriptions. Geertz (1973) used the term **thick description** as a metaphor for the use of interpretative devices to deepen ethnographic descriptions and, specifically, to make them more eloquently revealing of taken-for-granted, hidden meanings and symbols within everyday events. Second, qualitative descriptive studies do not move as far *away from* the data in their interpretations of findings. That is, they involve "a kind of interpretation that is low-inference, or likely to result in easier consensus among . . . most observers" about how closely description captures the actual reality of a situation or human experience (Sandelowski, 2000, pp. 335–336).

Description versus Interpretation as an End Product

Finally, in qualitative descriptive studies, description is the end product. The purely descriptive study employs "a straight descriptive summary of the informational contents of data [that are] organized in a way that best fits the data" (Sandelowski, 2000, pp. 338–339). In qualitative interpretive studies, description is the means to an end. In these types of studies, researchers are expected to "put much more of their own interpretive spin on what they see and hear," re-presenting and transforming the data by "deliberately choos[ing] to describe an event in terms of a conceptual, philosophical, or other highly abstract framework or system" (Sandelowski, 2000, p. 336).

No Single Set of Procedural Steps for Designing Qualitative Research Studies

Different types of qualitative research have unique methodological approaches that determine how researchers think about a phenomenon of interest, as well as what they do to understand it better. Creswell (1998) discusses how study designs differ across qualitative traditions, focusing on a small subset, specifically *phenomenology, biography, grounded theory, ethnography*, and *case study*.

In addition to having external diversity, qualitative traditions also exhibit significant internal diversity. For example, Creswell (1998) observed that the number of schools and subtypes of ethnography "with different theoretical orientations and aims [have led to] a distinct lack of orthodoxy in ethnography as a general approach to the description and interpretation of a cultural or social group (p. 59)." In like manner, similarities and differences in various approaches to grounded theory have been described as evidence of methodological diffusion and evolution (Kendall, 1999; Melia, 1996; Robrecht, 1995; Stern, 1994). Differences across schools of phenomenological inquiry also have been noted, e.g., the descriptive Husserlian-focused Duquesne School of phenomenological psychology; the interpretive emphasis of Heideggarian hermeneutics; van Manen's (1990) humanistic pedagogical approach; and the transcendental phenomenology of Moustakas (1994). Significant differences in approaches within the same school of phenomenology have also been documented, as in Beck's (1994) comparison of methodologies of Duquesne School phenomenologists Colaizzi, Giorgi, and VanKaam.

Consequently, the diversity, complexity, and dynamic nature of the field of qualitative inquiry require that individuals be specific about the research tradition and style that they will be following. In addition, the description of procedural steps to be used needs to be consistent with standards for that particular design.

Qualitative Studies Designed and Conducted by Researchers Mentored in a Specified Approach Will Have the Best Outcomes

Rising interest in conducting qualitative studies has been fueled by increased awareness of their usefulness as well as the greater availability of textbooks and articles about the various qualitative methods. What textbooks, in particular, largely fail to communicate are:

- The extent of diversity within traditions
- The limitations of written descriptions that attempt to reconstruct the more creative, reflective, cognitive processing aspects of interpretive qualitative methodologies
- Distinctions between quantitative and qualitative descriptive research
- Distinctions between descriptive and interpretive qualitative work

Sandelowski's (2000) presentation of qualitative description is especially helpful in addressing confusion and misperceptions related to choice of direction in qualitative research design. One of the confusions discussed is when a study has "overtones" of a particular qualitative approach (e.g., phenomenology, grounded theory, ethnography) but is not a pure example of that kind of study. Discussed misperceptions include mislabeling of research and "erroneous references to or misuses of methods or techniques" (p. 337).

Articles like this can do what textbooks do not do, as well—focus on select issues in closer detail. However, there is an abundance of resources on a wide range of topics. Therefore, the best approach to designing and conducting qualitative studies of any type is in partnership with a qualified researcher who can differentiate between what information will be more or less useful, who understands the clinical question and can propose possible research directions, and who has been mentored in the specific method to be used.

General Principles of Qualitative Research Design

All researchers, qualitative or quantitative, must address certain areas when designing a research study. The general principles that guide the development of qualitative research projects can be found in Box 11-2.

Identifying a Study Question

In qualitative research, the primary study question is the one that summarizes, in its most general form, what the study is about. Accompanying subquestions lend further focus, as in the following example from the literature. The primary study question is italicized for emphasis.

> *How do the material conditions and practices of the neonatal nursery shape mother-infant and mother-nurse interactions?* How do the mothers and nurses define "good motherhood?" What is the nature of the power relations between mothers and nurses? How do all these aspects affect the mothers' construction and practice of mothering? (Lupton & Fenwick, 2001, p. 1013)

Often, identification of research questions such as these evolves from curiosity about some phenomenon in the clinical setting (e.g., what the sense of motherhood and experience of

---

box 11.2

General Principles of Qualitative Research Design

1. Identify a study question.
2. Review the literature.
3. Define the theoretical perspective.
4. Select an appropriate research design.
5. Formulate a purpose statement.
6. Establish study significance.
7. Describe the research procedures.
8. Discuss study limitations.

mothering are like for mothers of hospitalized infants), hunches based on observation and experience (e.g., dynamics of mother-nurse relationships in the intensive care unit), and knowledge of some literature (e.g., articles on parenting).

Reviewing the Literature

A systematic literature review provides information about existing evidence related to study questions. It is used as a framework to explain why the study is important, to indicate what it may contribute to knowledge about the topic, and to set the stage for presentation of results in published reports, as in the following example (Hurlock-Chorostecki, 2002, pp. 34–35):

> A search of the literature using electronic databases revealed no studies pertaining [specifically] to the management of pain during weaning from mechanical ventilation. Comments in related literature . . . indicate that patients recall having pain . . . [and] . . . express frustration with their inability to communicate the pain experience. . . . Studies conducted on critical-care nurses' management of pain illustrate a clear pattern of findings suggestive of consistent undermedication. . . . Comparison studies indicate that critical-care nurses administer less analgesia than surgical nurses and less than patients in patient-control analgesia (Carroll et al., 1999; Tittle & McMillan, 1994). . . . The fact that critical-care nurses commonly withhold analgesia during weaning and view this as acceptable practice suggested that an examination into the nature of nurse decision-making related to analgesia administration during weaning was warranted.

This example illustrates that citing an absence of literature on a topic is not enough. Exploring related literature about patients' memories of pain experiences and comparison studies of nurses' management of patients' pain provided evidence to support the need for further study.

Defining the Theoretical Perspective

Theoretical perspectives that guide qualitative research range from the basic philosophical assumptions that are implicit in methodological practices of all qualitative studies (Creswell, 1998) and social science theories associated with particular traditions (e.g., theories of culture in ethnographic research; symbolic interaction in grounded theory research) to particular ideological perspectives and theoretical frameworks. Implicit assumptions and embedded theories of a research tradition that guide methods may be demonstrated rather than explicitly discussed in the design of a study (i.e., through explanation of study procedures). Other theoretical or ideological perspectives that pertain to the research questions may be presented early in the design of some studies as orienting/sensitizing frameworks or at the end of others, as outcomes of the research.

In the following example (Wise, 2002, p. 76), a theoretical framework used to guide understanding in a phenomenological study of the lived experience of pediatric liver transplantation is introduced at the beginning of the study.

> In this study, I adopted a functionalist approach to cognitive development to understand the culture of liver transplantation from the child's perspective. Proponents of a functionalist developmental approach suggest that both children and adults learn from experience with a

specific phenomenon rather than by chronological maturity alone (Chi, 1989; Eiser, 1990; Yoos, 1994). Experiential learning and an increase in knowledge about their disease and its treatment influence children's behavior. (Eiser, 1993)

In contrast, discussion of theory occurs at the end of theory-generating studies, as in the following example (Knobf, 2002, p. 15). "The explanatory theory of Carrying On . . . describes women's behaviors in response to the experience of premature menopause in the context of breast cancer."

In some studies, theory may occur as an orienting perspective as well as an end product. The following is an example (Merritt-Gray & Wuest, 1995, p. 401) in which feminist theory is presented at the outset of a study as the ideological "lens" or "filter" through which the research will be viewed or thought about.

[Feminist theory and grounded theory] have noncontradictory intellectual roots and can be used together to direct research (Wuest, 1995). Both . . . consider the contextual aspects of social experience. This characteristic is important for studying violence against women, because it moves the search for solutions from individual pathology to the broader interplay between individuals and their social context.

At the end of the study, a middle-range theory was produced to explain the process of leaving abusive conjugal relationships for geographically isolated women.

The process of reclaiming self is a social process of reinstatement of self in the larger social context, and not exclusively an intrapsychic process. . . . In this article we focus on the processes of counteracting abuse and breaking free, the initial stages in the process of reclaiming self. (Merritt-Gray & Wuest, 1995, p. 400).

Consequently, defining the theoretical perspective of a qualitative study involves choices about how theory will be used. The result is less uniformity than in the case of theory-testing and theory-verification research designs that consistently begin with a theoretical framework.

Selecting an Appropriate Research Design

Qualitative description is the design of choice for many basic clinical questions that involve the desire to facilitate an understanding of a human experience as a whole through in-depth engagement with study participants, most usually in their natural environments (i.e., "the field"). Styles and techniques typically involve researchers in field activities that may include active participation, observation, and/or interviews.

Choosing another type of qualitative design should be contingent on the availability of a researcher who is a specialist in that particular methodology. Commonly used possible choices, described in broad strokes, include:

- *Ethnography* when the purpose is to explain human experience in cultural context, as an interpretation or in theoretical terms
- *Grounded theory* when the purpose is to generate a theory that explains the ways in which persons move through an experience (e.g., in stages or phases)

● *Phenomenology* or *hermeneutics* when the purpose is to produce an interpretation of what an experience is like (i.e., how it feels and its meaning for individuals in the context of their everyday lives)

In selecting a design, it is important to be sensitive to two important considerations. One is that a descriptive qualitative design may involve "hues, tones, and textures . . . [i.e.] the look, sound, and feel of other [qualitative] approaches." However, these studies should not be confused with or mislabeled as examples of one of these approaches (Sandelowski, 2000, p. 337). Nor should such a study be referred to as "mixed-methods" research, because these designs are explicitly constructed to maximize the use of combined qualitative and quantitative approaches (Creswell, 2003, Tashakkori & Teddlie, 2003). The second consideration is that in choosing a traditional design (e.g., ethnography, grounded theory, phenomenology, hermeneutics), one needs to consider the diversity in these fields and accurately reflect the chosen method in the study design description.

Formulating a Study Purpose

Purpose statements draw attention to the central research focus, setting, participants, and the nature and selected elements of the research design. The following example of a purpose statement identifies a style of action research involving fieldwork and focus groups.

> The purpose of this study, conducted in juvenile detention, was the discovery of the adolescents' perceptions of risk (for HIV and other health-threatening consequences of risky behavior), as well as the dangers they identified in their home neighborhoods. In order to accomplish this goal, we used participatory action research and focus groups (Anderson et al., 2001, p. 340).

Establishing the Significance of the Study

Although activities up to and including establishing a study's significance have been described as six separate steps, in reality these efforts at laying the groundwork for a study evolve simultaneously. Identification of researchable clinical issues and literature reviews, in particular, help to establish why a study is needed and how it will contribute to improving professional practice. Often, statements of significance are combined with purpose statements, as in the following example.

> The single most important component of [an] intervention plan [for FM—fibromyalgia] is a comprehensive explanation of the condition that helps create a trusting relationship . . . [and] also alleviates, for the patient, any previous misconception that the symptoms are "all in the head." Although there is an abundance of recent quantitative research literature pertaining to [clinical symptoms of] FM . . . there is a need for research which describes and interprets the core of the lived experience. Therefore, the purpose of this research is twofold: to provide nurses and other healthcare providers with a clear understanding of the meaning of living with FM from the women's perspective, and to help fill a gap left vacant by the existing FM research literature (Sturge-Jacobs, 2002, p. 21).

Describing Research Procedures

There is no single set of procedural steps in qualitative research. What to do and how to do it are dictated by the topic plus background understandings and purposes of the selected study design. Typically, multiple common techniques are combined in various ways to achieve study outcomes. Areas to address include sampling and sampling strategy, ethical considerations, data collection and management, data analysis and interpretation, and standards of quality and scientific rigor.

Sample and Sampling Strategy

The sampling plan must describe the location and characteristics of the population from which a sample will be selected, the estimated sample size, inclusion/exclusion criteria, and recruitment procedures. A variety of sampling strategies may support purposeful selection of the best sources of information about an experience. Research questions, type of study, and previous studies or similar studies in the literature suggest rationales for estimating the size of the sample. Researchers also must explain how they will know when the necessary sample size has been reached, because this cannot easily be determined a priori. Commonly, this process involves monitoring the quality of databases as the research progresses. Decisions about when optimum sample size is achieved are based on judgments about (a) usefulness of the data in various informational categories; (b) types of additional data sources needed to capture an adequate view of the phenomenon; and (c) number of interviews and/or observations needed before informational categories are full and continued data collection produces no new information (concept of redundancy or saturation).

Ethical Considerations

Researchers need to keep up to date with the most current ethical guidelines for the protection of human subjects required by the federal government, funding agencies, and local institutions. Of note for qualitative researchers is the importance of addressing how use of common techniques involving close researcher-participant interaction (e.g., participant observation and in-depth interviews) over periods of time will take into account the issues of confidentiality, privacy, and concerns about nonconsenting members of a group and undue burden. Researchers need to realize that close attachments may develop between themselves and study participants, which will need to be monitored and managed kindly and professionally. They also need to be sensitive to the emotions of study participants who may experience distress at the baring of painful memories and be prepared to describe the steps the researcher will take if such distress occurs.

Data Collection and Data Management

Qualitative researchers may use multiple data collection strategies in a single study. Most important is matching and explaining how particular strategies will meet stated study aims. Examples of what will be observed, sample interview questions, and descriptions of other kinds of data sources (e.g., documents, artifacts, audio-visual materials) serve as indicators of the kinds of data that will be collected. Who will be collecting the data and how information will be recorded need to be described in detail. If there are multiple data collectors, how they are trained and supervised, as well as checks for inter-rater reliability also require explanation.

Data management systems for record keeping, storage, organization, and retrieval of information is an important consideration in research that typically generates large volumes of data. It is wise to lay out a plan prior to data collection. The plan may be a combination of a physical filing system for raw field notes, audiotapes, documents, and hard copy transcriptions and a computer software program, of which there are many varieties. The researcher needs to keep in mind that although some software programs support data analysis through features beyond storage and retrieval that enable manipulation and various displays of data, they do not actually perform analyses. Analysis of qualitative data is an intellectual process.

Data Analysis and Interpretation

Data analysis is an ongoing activity that occurs simultaneously with data collection. Therefore, description of procedures involves outlining approaches that will be used throughout the course of the research. For instance, it might be useful to describe the process for deciding about the need to modify the direction of questions and observation in response to new insights and informational needs. This will include how decisions and analytic thoughts and questioning of the data will be recorded and used. Specific analytic steps vary with different types of qualitative designs. Some of the more generic steps of data analysis involve:

- Reading through all the data to get a general sense of what is there and reflecting on possible meanings
- Coding/labeling, categorizing, and writing reflective notes about the data to examine it from all angles
- Generating detailed written descriptions
- Searching for recurring themes and patterns

Interpretive strategies move beyond description of what is there to reflection on the possible meaning of data (e.g., what it may suggest or symbolize; what there is to be learned as a result of new insights). An explanation of procedures might project how the interpretation will appear in the final written report. For example, meaning may be expressed by re-presenting participants' perspectives within a new explanatory or sensitizing framework that reflects what the researcher has come to understand of the participants' reality. A researcher also may use reflection, intuition, and imaginative play to arrive at a creative synthesis that produces a richly textured picture of the experience. Continuous writing and rewriting is a natural part of developing strong, oriented portrayals of all the experiential aspects of a phenomenon.

Whether the end product tends more toward description or interpretation, it is important to explain how data integration and conclusions will be reached, particularly in designs where more than one data source will be used. The importance and potential usefulness of findings need to be part of this discussion.

Standards of Quality and Scientific Rigor

How quality will be monitored and scientific rigor will be maintained needs to be directly addressed. Because general criteria for evaluating qualitative studies are discussed extensively in Chapter 6, comments here are limited to identifying broad areas to consider in designing a qualitative study. Greatest emphasis usually is placed on validity relating to concerns about accuracy, credibility, and confirmability, (i.e., which is evidence in the data to support findings and interpretations). Researchers may choose the most appropriate steps for ensuring quality and rigor from among a variety of strategies.

Similarly, strategies for documenting how decisions were made throughout the course of the study (the concept of an audit trail) may be described. This is thought by some to be similar to quantitative researchers' notions of reliability. Most important is that selected criteria are consistent with study aims and chosen design because although there are common strategies, there are no hard and fast rules about what procedures must be followed in every research approach. And some quality measures that are effective for one approach may not serve well for another.

Discussing Study Limitations

All types of research are delimited/bounded and limited by their scope and degree of generalizability. Qualitative researchers engaged in theory generation most often refer to the need for quantitative theory-testing research to determine generalizability, for example:

> Further research is needed to test the efficacy of the emerging theory [of nurse decision making during weaning from mechanical ventilation] for use in critical care. The truthfulness of the theory and its generalizability within nursing have yet to be tested (Hurlock-Chorostecki, 2002, p. 45).

In this instance, theory testing might lead to an estimate of statistical generalizability (i.e., the extent to which inferences based on one set of evidence may apply to a larger population of critical care nurses). Verification, extension, or development of new theory, in turn, would need to be based on accumulated evidence of many studies.

Transferability, or **theoretical generalizability** of qualitative research refers to the extent to which the evidence, knowledge, understandings, or insights gained may be thought to be meaningful and applicable to similar cases or other situations. For example, health professionals involved in caring for children and adolescents with liver disease, on the basis of their own experience, will be able to judge the extent to which Wise's (2002) hermeneutic phenomenological interpretation of children's experiences with liver transplantation is theoretically generalizable. Clinicians can do this by asking such questions as:

- Does it fit/make sense/ring true/resonate with my own observations?
- Does it provide insights/make me think differently or reflect more deeply on my own experiences?
- Would the understandings generated about what the experience is like be helpful to neophyte practitioners or families undergoing this experience?
- Does it add new understandings to existing knowledge in this field?
- Can insights from this study (related to listening to what children say and considering how to encourage them to be active participants in their care) also be valuable when applied to situations of children with other types of chronic or life-threatening illnesses?

In other words, "The knowledge gained is not limited to demographic variables; it is the fit of the topic or the comparability of the problem that is of concern. Recall, it is the knowledge that is generalized" (Morse, 1999, p. 6).

Validation of study findings might come in the form of application of the knowledge in practice. Although the existence of multiple interpretations, such as multiple coexisting theories about the same phenomenon, may have their usefulness, researchers often will describe their interpretation of findings as a natural limitation of the research to acknowledge that other interpretations of the same data could be made.

Other research limitations include potential pitfalls in chosen methods and issues related to the nature of the study topic. For example, researchers investigating so-called sensitive topics (e.g., drug cultures, deviance, crime, and abuse) or working with vulnerable populations (e.g., children, persons who are mentally ill, cognitively impaired, institutionalized, or incarcerated) must address limitations in terms of anticipated ethical, practical, and methodological issues associated with their research plans.

In summary, this chapter has offered broad considerations for generating qualitative evidence within the context of a research world that comprises both qualitative and quantitative approaches to EBP. Because neither approach exists in a vacuum, some necessary distinctions have been drawn in the interests of promoting clearer communication. However, the primary focus has been on general principles that guide the development of qualitative research projects. This discussion does not take the place of more specific guidance that researchers planning an actual study would need to obtain through training and consultation, as appropriate. To compensate for the principles' necessary general tone, a story to lend more specificity can be found in Appendix F.

The story *Looking for Best Evidence: "...A Rose by Any Other Name..."* illustrates each of the above-discussed principles by describing activities involved in the execution and dissemination of a completed ethnographic study. Although this chapter calls attention to qualitative descriptive research as a distinct, viable design option deserving of greater appreciation, it does not discount other traditional qualitative approaches that are more thoroughly covered in Chapter 6. The use of this traditional research design example makes this clear. Furthermore, the example goes beyond the process of conducting the study to demonstrate some equally important considerations about published representations of findings. Research dissemination does not receive as much attention as it should. However, it is a key component of generating evidence, particularly in qualitative research, where so much of the responsibility for determining validity and transferability rests with the decisions researchers make about appropriate representations of their work in different text formats and readers' informed interactions with those texts.

> ❝ *Use what talent you possess: The woods would be very silent if no birds sang except those that sang best.* ❞
>
> *Henry Van Dyke*

references

Anderson, N. L. R., Nyamathi, A., McAvoy, J. A., Conde, F., & Casey, C. (2001). Perceptions about risk for HIV/AIDS among adolescents in juvenile detention. *Western Journal of Nursing Research, 23,* 336–359.

Beck, C. T. (1994). Reliability and validity issues in phenomenological research. *Western Journal of Nursing Research, 16,* 254–267.

Carroll, K., Atkins, P., Herold, G., Mlcek, C., Shively, M., Clopton, P., & Glaser, D. (1999). Pain assessment and management in critically ill post-operative and trauma patients: A multisite study. *American Journal of Critical Care, 8,* 105–117.

Chi, M. (1989). How inferences about novel domain-related concepts can be constrained by structural knowledge. *Merrill-Palmer Quarterly, 35,* 27–62.

Creswell, J. W. (1998). *Qualitative inquiry and research design: Choosing among five traditions.* Thousand Oaks, CA: Sage.

Creswell, J. W. (2003). *Research design: Qualitative, quantitative, and mixed method approaches.* Thousand Oaks, CA: Sage.

Eiser, C. (1990). *Chronic childhood disease: An introduction to psychological theory and research.* Cambridge, MA: Cambridge University Press.

Eiser, C. (1993). *Growing up with a chronic disease: The impact on children and families.* London: Jessica Kingsley.

Geertz, C. (1973). Thick description: Toward an interpretive theory of culture (pp. 3–30). In C. Geertz (Ed.), *The interpretation of cultures.* New York: Basic Books.

Hurlock-Chorostecki, C. (2002). Management of pain during weaning from mechanical ventilation: The nature of nurse decision-making. *Canadian Journal of Nursing Research, 34,* 33–47.

Kendall, J. (1999). Axial coding and the grounded theory controversy. *Western Journal of Nursing Research, 21,* 743–757.

Knobf, M. T. (2002). Carrying On: The experience of premature menopause in women with early stage breast cancer. *Nursing Research, 51,* 9–17.

Lupton, D., & Fenwick, J. (2001). 'They've forgotten that I'm the mum': constructing and practising motherhood in special care nurseries. *Social Science & Medicine, 53,* 4011–4021.

Maxwell, J. A. (1992). Understanding and validity in qualitative research. *Harvard Educational Review, 62,* 279–299.

Melia, K. M. (1996). Rediscovering Glaser. *Qualitative Health Research, 6,* 368–378.

Merritt-Gray, M., & Wuest, J. (1995). Counteracting abuse and breaking free: The process of leaving revealed through women's voices. *Health Care for Women International, 16,* 399–412.

Morse, J. M. (1999). Qualitative generalizability. *Qualitative Health Research, 9,* 5–6.

Moustakas, C. (1994). *Phenomenological research methods.* Thousand Oaks, CA: Sage.

Robrecht, L. C. (1995). Grounded theory: Evolving methods. *Qualitative Health Research, 5,* 169–177.

Sandelowski, M. (2000). Whatever happened to qualitative description? *Research in Nursing & Health, 23,* 334–340.

Stern, P. N. (1994). Eroding grounded theory. In J. Morse (Ed.), *Critical issues in qualitative research methods* (pp. 212–223). Thousand Oaks, CA: Sage.

Sturge-Jacobs, M. (2002). The experience of living with fibromyalgia: Confronting an invisible disability. *Research and Theory for Nursing Practice: An International Journal, 16,* 19–31.

Tashakkori, A. & Teddlie, C. (Eds.) (2003). *Handbook of mixed methods in the social and behavioral sciences.* Thousand Oaks, CA: Sage.

Tittle, M., & McMillan, S. (1994). Pain and pain-related side effects in an ICU and on a surgical unit: Nurses' management. *American Journal of Critical Care, 5,* 433–441.

van Manen, M. (1990). *Researching lived experience: Human science for an action sensitive pedagogy.* London, Ontario: University of Western Ontario & State University of New York Press.

Wise, B. V. (2002). In their own words: The lived experience of pediatric liver transplantation. *Qualitative Health Research, 12,* 74–90.

Wuest, J. (1995). Feminist grounded theory: An exploration of congruency and tensions between two methods of knowledge discovery in nursing. *Qualitative Health Research, 5,* 125–137.

Yoos, H. L. (1994). Children's illness concepts: Old and new paradigms. *Pediatric Nursing, 20* (2), 134–140.

Generating Evidence Through Outcomes Management

Gail L. Ingersoll

chapter 12

The management of care delivery outcomes has become a growing concern for practitioners and researchers alike. Early discussions of the importance of measuring care delivery effectiveness focused primarily on outcomes research and the need to use sufficiently large data sets to monitor the impact of controlled clinical trials on defined populations. More recently, the focus has expanded to include **outcomes management** approaches, which pay attention to individuals and smaller groups of patients. Each of these measurement actions is designed to maximize care delivery outcome by comprehensively assessing and refining individual, organizational, and policy-derived practices to produce the most desirable effect.

Over the years, the focus of outcomes assessment has been directed primarily at medical care delivery, with most of the early large-scale studies addressing physician services only (Kelly, Huber, Johnson, McCloskey, & Maas, 1994; Schwartz & Lurie, 1991) and focusing on negative consequences of care. As interest in the measurement of outcomes has grown, however, attention has shifted to outcomes assessment activities that monitor more positive indicators, many of which have been targeted by nursing for years.

The Range of Outcomes Activities

From the outset, some confusion has been evident in the terms used to describe outcomes assessment and reporting activities. For example, one publication defines clinical outcomes as "clinical variations in care that can impact the patient's ability to progress according to the clinical pathway" (Peters, Cowley, & Standiford, 1999, p. 77). This definition implies that the outcome is the care provided, which it is not. The outcome, as defined in the statement above, is progression according to the clinical pathway. This global outcome would likely include a number of intermediate outcomes, which are achieved during the course of the hospital stay (e.g., extubation within 24 hours of surgery; temperature less than 39 degrees Celsius), and one or two more long-term outcomes (e.g., discharge from hospital within four days of surgery). Clinical variations in care delivery are the processes (in this case, perhaps unintended or undesired if the outcome is negative) that produce variation in the outcome (achievement of clinical pathway goals).

Another common problem is the equating of "quality of care" with outcomes. As Huber and Oermann (1999) have noted, achievement of an outcome does not necessarily assure quality of care. Moreover, a number of factors can influence outcomes, regardless of the quality of care provided (see Table 12-1), making confirmation of the relationships between the two difficult to discern. Furthermore, quality of care is an *attribute of the action,* not the result (or outcome). It is the global gold standard against which all care delivery is compared. How that quality is defined or identified is the crux of the matter. Clearly describing what constitutes high-quality care and specifying how to measure it in observable terms is a challenge—one that must be addressed, however, before any chance of equating quality of care to care delivery outcomes can occur.

A third issue in *outcomes measurement* is the frequent mention of process indicators as measures of care delivery outcome. These "process as outcome indicators" are often identified by practicing nurses in studies of potential nurse-sensitive outcome indicators (Alexander & Kroposki, 1999; Craft-Rosenberg, Krajicek, & Shin, 2002; Ingersoll, McIntosh, & Williams, 2000). Because the focus of outcomes measurement is on *the recipient* of services, however, measures that describe care provider action (e.g., care provider awareness of resources, assessment of client situation, goal setting, patient education [Alexander & Kroposki, 1999], appropriate use of resources [Ingersoll et al., 2000]), assessment and integration of genetic influences in care (Craft-Rosenberg et al., 2002), and completion of patient teaching survey (Hodge, Asch, Olson, Kravitz, & Sauvé, 2002) are not true outcome indicators of intervention effect. At the most, they can be described as intermediate outcomes that hopefully produce actual, or long-term, outcomes in the patient.

The increased frequency of nursing documentation about some care problem or goal (e.g., pain management) is not a true outcome indicator. The issue of importance is not the nurse's documentation per se; it is what the documentation indicates—that the process of pain assessment and resultant intervention has occurred. This action on the nurse's part is expected to improve care delivery outcome in the patient—in this case, level of pain. Therefore, "increased documentation of pain assessment" is an observable measure, or confirmation, of the nursing process of care. The ultimate goal of this process, which has been demonstrated by some observable action (documentation), is symptom control (outcome) in the patient.

A fourth major concern in the measurement of outcomes is the difficulty associated with linking some care delivery intervention to some clearly observed effect. This problem is particularly evident in nursing where nursing interventions are but one element of a multidimen-

table 12.1   Evidence-based contributors to outcomes

Contributor	Outcome Affected	Source*
Illness severity	Length of stay	Whittle et al., 1998
	Functional status	Porell et al., 1998
	Mortality	Aiken et al., 1999
		Porell et al., 1998
		Blegen et al., 1998
	Satisfaction with care	Aiken et al., 1999
		Blegen et al., 1998
	Infection	Blegen et al., 1998
	Pressure ulcers	Blegen et al., 1998
	Blood glucose level	Berlowitz et al., 1998
	Blood pressure	Berlowitz et al., 1998
	Rehospitalization	Berlowitz et al., 1998
Location of services		
Medical center/rural	Cost	Whittle et al., 1998
Magnet hospital status	Mortality	Aiken et al., 1999
	Satisfaction with care	Aiken et al., 1999
Dedicated specialty unit	Mortality	Aiken et al., 1999
	Satisfaction with care	Aiken et al., 1999
RN staff concentration	Mortality	Aiken et al., 1999
	Falls	Blegen & Vaughn, 1998
	Pressure ulcers	Blegen et al., 1998
	Satisfaction with care	Blegen et al., 1998
Patient characteristics		
Age, race, gender	Readmission rates	Berlowitz et al., 1998
Gender	Satisfaction with care	Whittle et al., 1998
Sexual preference	Satisfaction with care	Aiken et al., 1999
Education	Mortality	Aiken et al., 1999
Income	Mortality	Backlund et al., 1999
		Backlund et al., 1999
Provider characteristics		
Specialty training	Cost	Whittle et al., 1998
	Mortality	Aiken et al., 1999

Representative recent (previous 5 years) studies with potentially nurse-sensitive indicators.

sional package of activities designed to improve delivery of services. The more persons involved in an intervention and the more components included, the more difficult is the determination of which action or care provider produced most or all of the effect.

Care Delivery Outcomes

Care delivery outcomes are defined as the observable or measurable effects of some intervention or action. They are focused on the recipient of the service, not the provider, and can be measured at the individual, group, organization, or community level.

The most desirable indicators of care delivery outcome are reliable, valid, measurable, suitable to the population of interest, not overly costly to collect, and sensitive to changes within and across individuals. They can be global (applicable to any population or care delivery environment) or population-specific. The more global the indicator, the more difficult is the determination of the relationship between outcome and some individual intervention or action. The more specific the indicator, the less generalizable it is to other groups or circumstances.

Ideally, outcome indicators should be nondirectional. That is, they should not be defined according to the direction of the change desired (e.g., "increased" or "decreased"). Instead, they should be identified as the behavior or observable indication of response. Examples might be systolic or diastolic blood pressure (not decreased blood pressure), weight (not increased or decreased weight), length of stay, level of satisfaction, level of pain, perceived self-efficacy, number of unplanned emergency room admissions, and so forth. The goal of the action or intervention may be stated in directional terms, but the outcome itself is identified without the directional tag. For example:

Outcome indicator: systolic blood pressure.
Intervention goal: to reduce and maintain systolic blood pressure to within acceptable range according to age and gender.

The essential characteristics of outcome measures were defined in a 1988 publication (Lohr, 1988) as:

- Dimension of health (physical, physiologic, emotional) definiteness (observable event or reliable and valid proxy measure)
- Timing (intermediate or long-term)
- Directness (relationship between action and outcome)

Lohr also identified four attributes of an outcomes measurement plan:

1. The purpose of data collection
2. The source of information
3. The mode of data collection
4. The agent responsible for data analysis and interpretation

Each of these elements contributes to the type of data collected, its accuracy, its reliability and validity, and its likelihood of influencing the actions of others.

In addition to the measurement factors essential to all outcome indicators are some practical factors that ultimately contribute to their usefulness and accuracy in the clinical setting. Among these are practicality, utility, affordability, availability, and simplicity. In recognition of these characteristics, the most effective outcomes measurement plans are those that use existing data where possible, incorporate data collection activities into everyday operating procedures, gather data that are reasonably easy and affordable to collect, and select indicators that are acceptable and important to the practitioners responsible for managing care. On occasion, this practicality aspect may conflict with the measurement attributes of an ideal outcomes assessment plan, necessitating careful consideration of how to balance the demands of both. Collecting and reporting bad data simply because it's available does nothing to aid in informed decision making or maximization of outcome effect. The most responsible approach is to start small, using reliable, valid, and sensitive indicators, then to progress to additional activities as efficiencies in data collection processes and the beneficial effects of data-based management are observed.

Components of an outcome include the outcome itself, how it is observed (the indicator), its definition, its critical characteristics (how it is measured), and its range or parameters. The need for specifying the indicator and its definition and critical characteristics is most evident when the outcome is not readily observable, which is common with attitudinal or perceptual outcomes. For example, satisfaction, perception of being well cared for, self-efficacy, anxiety, and distress are some of the outcomes regularly discussed in nursing-related **outcomes research.** Although reasonable and potentially theory- or evidence-based, none of these outcome terms are sufficient by themselves. Each must have an observable measurement component that can be monitored for evidence of change. Each also must be defined to assure that all who use it fully understand its characteristics and attributes and how it pertains specifically to the groups or individuals assessed.

The critical characteristics and the range of parameters for anticipated or desired change help inform researchers and practitioners about what is and what is not an indication of evidence of program or intervention effect. These parameters should be established prior to data collection, although they may be revised over time, based on informed assessment of contributing factors or in response to benchmark reports from other institutions.

Commonly mentioned indicators of care delivery outcome are morbidity, mortality, length of stay, cost (most often measured as charges), readmission rate, and unplanned surgical procedure or return to surgery. A number of concerns exist with these indicators, however, and recent reports recommend exploring other alternatives, particularly in nursing (Ingersoll et al., 2000; Mitchell, Ferketich, & Jennings, 1998; Moritz, 1998). Among the concerns mentioned with these indicators is their susceptibility to a variety of individual, organizational, and reimbursement-related factors, all of which interfere with the accurate assessment of the true impact of some intervention on care delivery outcome.

Table 12-2 highlights some of the more recently proposed outcome indicators that nurse authors believe may be sensitive to nursing practice. Of note, however, is that although the indicators have been proposed as a result of consensus-building studies or comprehensive reviews of the literature, most have not been tested empirically and therefore must be assessed for their potential rather than absolute usefulness.

An important dimension receiving increased attention in outcomes measurement is the relationship between individual preference or perceived need and outcomes achieved (Huber & Oermann, 1999). A common indicator used to clarify this concern is patient satisfaction, which some authors recommend be measured as satisfaction against or in comparison with perceived need (Nelson et al., 1996a). An example would be the misinterpretation of patient satisfaction if the items included for assessment were not relevant or important to the person responding. Respondents may evaluate the item favorably but still be dissatisfied with other aspects of the care delivery process. As a result, they rate the overall quality of care poorly. In addition, they may express feelings of frustration because no one was concerned about the matters of importance to them. A method for addressing this concern is to ask patients to rate both how important the care delivery aspect is to them as well as how satisfactorily the service was provided.

Outcomes Management

Outcomes management is the use of process and outcomes data to coordinate and influence actions and processes of care that contribute to patient achievement of targeted behaviors or desired effects. Management activities often are driven by "variances," or observed variation around some desired condition or standard of acceptable practice. These variances generally refer to deviations in some process or interim outcome that contribute to differences in targeted or long-term outcome indicators. Some authors recommend focusing outcomes management activities on negative variances that alter the patient's progress toward desired outcomes (Cole & Houston, 1999). They stress the importance of attending to the three principal contributors to variance—the patient, the provider, and the system. An alteration in any one of these three contributors may result in undesirable variation in the patient's expected progress toward the targeted goal or outcome. In this approach, attention is directed at identifying and eliminating negative variances and thereby improving patient outcome.

Others suggest that effective outcomes management programs examine the full array of outcomes, including those that are marginal or deficient, as well as those that are adequate or superior (Johnson & Maas, 1999). This recommendation differs from the more common approach in which a rotational process is used to assess only those indicators that reflect an actual

table 12.2   Proposed evidence-based, nurse-sensitive outcome indicators

Indicator*	Provider Focus	Location Focus	Source
Achievement of appropriate self-care	Nurses All Providers	Any Any	Mitchell et al., 1998 Moritz, 1998
Central line bacteremia rate	Nurses	Inpatient	Hodge et al., 2002
Compliance/adherence	APNs	Any	Ingersoll et al., 2000
Failure to rescue	All Providers	Any	Moritz, 1998
Fall rate	Nurses	Inpatient	ANA, 1999
Family/child partnership in care decisions	Nurses	Any	Craft-Rosenberg et al., 2002
Functional status	Nurses	Ambulatory	Mastal, 1999
Health-promoting behaviors	Nurses	Any	Mitchell et al., 1998
Health-related quality of life	Nurses All Providers	Any Any	Mitchell et al., 1998 Moritz, 1998
Knowledge of patients & families	APNs	Any	Ingersoll et al., 2000
Length of stay	Nurses	Inpatient	Hodge et al., 2002
Mortality	All Providers	Any	Moritz, 1998
Nosocomial infection rate	Nurses	Inpatient	ANA, 1999
Nosocomial pneumonia rate	Nurses	Inpatient	Hodge et al., 2002

(continued)

table 12.2 Proposed evidence-based, nurse-sensitive outcome indicators (continued)

Indicator*	Provider Focus	Location Focus	Source
Nosocomial pressure ulcer rate	Nurses Nurses	Inpatient Inpatient	ANA, 1999 Hodge et al., 2002
Perception of being well cared for	APNs Nurses All Providers	Any Any Any	Ingersoll et al., 2000 Mitchell et al., 1998 Moritz, 1998
Protective behaviors	Nurses	Ambulatory	Mastal, 1999
Quality of life	APNs	Any	Ingersoll et al., 2000
Risk reduction behaviors	Nurses	Ambulatory	Mastal, 1999
Satisfaction with care	Nurses APNs Nurses	Inpatient Any Ambulatory	ANA, 1999 Ingersoll et al., 2000 Mastal, 1999
Satisfaction with educational information	Nurses	Inpatient	ANA, 1999
Satisfaction with pain management	Nurses	Inpatient	ANA, 1999
Support systems available to assist with caregiver burden	Nurses	Any	Craft-Rosenberg et al., 2002
Symptom reduction, change, or resolution	APNs Nurses Nurses All Providers	Any Ambulatory Any Any	Ingersoll et al., 2000 Mastal, 1999 Mitchell et al., 1998 Moritz, 1998
Trust of care provider	APNs	Any	Ingersoll et al., 2000
Utilization of services	Nurses	Ambulatory	Mastal, 1999

*By alphabetical order. Location does not constitute ranking of potential sensitivity to nursing interventions. Excluded from the list are process-related indicators and indicators for specialty populations or diagnoses.

  An additional source of proposed indicators is too extensive for inclusion in this review. Interested readers should examine the Nursing Outcomes Classification (NOC) indicators identified by Johnson and Maas (1997).

or potential problem. In the rotational process, the outcomes manager moves to another problem area when a target goal for improvement is reached. The problem with this rotational method is the failure to detect subtle changes in care delivery processes or outcomes that indicate a growing concern over time. By the time attention is directed toward a problem area, a whole host of opportunities for corrective action may have been missed. This rotational process also perpetuates the use of a reactive, problem-resolution focus to outcomes management. Ideally, outcomes management programs should be directed toward introducing activities that promote ongoing reflection about and continuous improvement in the services provided.

Outcomes management activities often are institution-specific and influenced by internal and external decision makers, including those responsible for reimbursement of services (Ingersoll, 1998). These decision makers also may prescribe which outcome indicators should be measured, how the data should be reported, and how often it should be collected and summarized. Although external authorities generally have quality of care and efficiency of resources in mind, some conflict may exist across care providers, healthcare administrators, and external decision makers whose immediate interests may not be consistent with the goals of the others.

Moreover, time constraints and limited resource availability may necessitate a sole focus on externally derived indicators. This practice seriously limits the potential for clarifying which indicators are most relevant for which patients and in which situations and environments. It seriously constrains the potential expansion of the evidence related to outcomes assessment.

Outcomes Measurement

Outcomes measurement is a generic term used to describe the collection and reporting of information about an observed effect in relation to some care delivery process or health promotion action. It requires the careful identification of reliable and valid outcome indicators, the selection of appropriate measurement methods, and the assurance of timeliness of data collection and reporting.

The effectiveness and usefulness of outcomes measurement is affected by:

- The quality of the data
- The consistency and accuracy of the data collection process
- The commitment and ability of those collecting the data and making decisions based on findings
- The timing (in addition to timeliness) of data collection

The timing of outcome data collection refers to the length of time that has passed between the collection of data and when an intervention or action was undertaken. Outcomes findings can be influenced significantly by the amount of time that has elapsed since the intervention and what may have transpired during that period.

What may be considered an acceptable or desirable outcome at one point may not be considered so at the next. In addition, perception-focused outcomes may change over time. For example, patients undergoing coronary artery bypass surgery for unstable angina may report significantly different perceptions about their quality of life depending on when they are asked. Immediately after surgery, they may report excellent surgical effect because of the elimination of chest pain and its restrictions on lifestyle and usual activity. Two months later, however, if patients are unable to return to work full time or to engage in all pre-anginal activities, they may report only moderate levels or even dissatisfaction with quality of life. Each time they were asked, they used different frames of reference to assess their quality of life, resulting in conflicting findings. Collecting data only at the immediate postsurgery timeframe may result in the clinician or researcher's erroneous interpretation of intervention effect.

The quality, consistency, and accuracy of data collection procedures are influenced significantly by several factors, including the number of persons directly entering or abstracting the data and the data source. Among the more common sources for data are hospital claims records (Thomas, Guire, & Horvat, 1997), administrative data sets (Rosenheck, Fontana, & Stolar, 1999), patient surveys (Rosenheck et al., 1999), patient medical records (Berlowitz et al., 1998; Porell, Caro, Silva, & Monane, 1998), and census data (Backlund, Sorlie, & Johnson, 1999). Each of these sources has considerable potential for error and may require careful action to assure the reliability and validity of the data.

Patient survey limitations include the reliance on self-report, which may or may not reflect actual circumstances and which may be completed by a biased portion of the sample. Medical records, on the other hand, are subject to wide variations in the quality and quantity of information included. The reporting of information by multiple care providers, the inability to externally confirm the accuracy of laboratory measurements and reports, and the potential for missing data make this data source particularly problematic, even though it is used most often. Administrative data sets and census data may or may not report information in a format useful for outcomes measurement. These data sources also rarely provide the amount of detail desired for some outcomes management projects.

Selection of a data source and method for outcomes measurement requires careful consideration of the risks and benefits associated with each. No single approach is best for all situations, and some compromise is usually required. The outcomes manager or researcher should identify the rationale for the selection of any approach and attempt to minimize the risks associated with each.

Outcomes Research

Outcomes research involves the use of rigorous scientific methods to measure the effect of some intervention on some outcome or outcomes (Ingersoll, 1998). Its goal is to establish care delivery standards or to develop policy statements about best practices. As a result, it is defined as applied research and is expected to produce evidence-based decision making and action as a result of its findings.

Outcomes research is directed toward populations; consequently, its usefulness for managing individual patients may be limited (see Table 12-3). Generally, the combined evidence of multiple investigations is required before recommendations can be made at the individual or small group level. Even so, practitioners who use outcomes research data for patient decision making do so with the appreciation that individual differences may not be clearly distinguished within a large-scale, population-based study.

The usefulness of outcomes research for the management of patients may be limited by the absence of any theory to guide the intervention tested and its proposed effect on outcomes. Sidani and Braden (1998) have discussed this problem at length and have identified six essential elements of intervention- and outcomes-focused research. The first of these is the accurate identification of the problem for which the intervention is designed. This element should describe the nature of the problem, what the problem looks like, what has caused it, and how severe it currently is or potentially could become. The problem discussion also should specify which population is experiencing the problem and under what conditions the problem occurs.

The second essential element consists of the critical inputs that clarify the specifics of the intervention, how the intervention will be delivered, and the strength of the intervention required to produce an effect.

table 12.3 Characteristics of outcomes management versus outcomes research activities

	Focus	Intent	Driving Forces
Outcomes Management	Local Regional	Manage care Individual decision making	Standards of practice Organizational goals & mission Accrediting agencies State/federal regulations Existing evidence Care provider interest & motivation
Outcomes Research	National International	Generate & test theory Guide standards of practice	Existing evidence Theory development & evolution Researcher interest & motivation

The third element, the **mediating processes,** identifies the expected activities that ultimately produce the desired outcome (Sidani & Braden, 1998). Although Sidani and Braden focus solely on the intermediate changes in the patient that subsequently produce the long-range effect, mediating processes also can occur through the actions of the care provider or persons carrying out the intervention. For example, increased collaboration among care providers (and documentation of that effect) following a care delivery-focused intervention might constitute a mediating process.

The fourth required element is the identification of outcomes expected to change as a result of the intervention.

Measurement Approach	Target Group	Reporting Formats	Target Audience
Continuous Based on resources & outcomes manager's experience with data collection Variety of measurement approaches; rarely experimental Often relies on existing data & measurement tools Aims for match with benchmarked organizations	Groups of individuals Individuals within groups	Descriptive statistics Visual displays Change over time Comparison to local targets & benchmarks	Local practitioners Local decision makers Accrediting agencies State & federal agencies
Continuous for defined period or sporadic, depending on research design & funding Guided by research question Based on resources & outcomes researcher's experience Quasi-experimental & experimental designs to demonstrate cause & effect Stresses use of reliable & valid measures with generalizability Aims for replicability	Populations of individuals Subgroups within populations	Descriptive statistics for discussion of population characteristics Nonparametric & parametric statistics depending on research design Comparisons between groups Comparisons over time Discussion of comparison to previous research	Researchers Theorists Practitioners Policy makers

The fifth is the extraneous factors that might interfere with the intervention effect. These include contextual, environmental, and client characteristics that affect both intervention processes and anticipated outcome (Sidani & Braden, 1998). If the intervention proposed involves a change in the type of care provider, for example, physician to nurse practitioner, the care provider's characteristics also can be considered extraneous factors.

The final element concerns implementation issues. Included in implementation issues are resource availability (Sidani & Braden, 1998), stage of organizational or provider readiness for introducing an intervention, the time required to fully implement an intervention, and the level of ability of the persons involved in implementing and carrying out the process. Each of these factors can weaken the intervention or create a need for significant modifications to what was originally planned. A careful assessment of the factors likely to interfere with the implementation of some intervention is best done as part of the theory-generation process. An important dimension of this element is using the information known about the setting and its potential fit with the plan both to design the intervention and to monitor the extraneous and mediating factors.

A useful model for clarifying outcomes research variables has been described by Holzemer (1994), Holzemer and Reilly (1995), and others (Cohen, Saylor, Holzemer & Gorenberg, 2000), who have taken the original input-process-output quality of care model developed by Donabedian (1966) and added the three principal constituents involved in healthcare interactions. This model is particularly helpful during the planning stages of outcomes research when the clear identification of variables and possible relationships is essential to successful measurement approach.

This outcomes measurement model uses a grid format to clarify how the client, provider, and setting all interact with and contribute to the inputs, processes, and outcomes associated with delivery of care (Holzemer, 1994; Holzemer & Reilly, 1995; Cohen et al., 2000). Use of the grid clarifies where the client, provider, or setting characteristics are likely to influence quality of care and subsequent outcomes. For example, a client's knowledge of his or her health status and treatment options might directly influence both the inputs of the care delivery process and the delivery process itself. Knowledgeable clients may enter the health system earlier and may restrict treatment options based on preexisting information (inputs). They also may participate more actively in the actual care delivery process, collaborating with care providers over decisions about treatment options and assuming self-care activities earlier than less well-informed persons. These direct linkages with the inputs and the processes components of the outcomes framework may have a beneficial effect on the intended and unintended outcomes of the process. For example, the associations in the inputs and processes components may result in reduced length of hospital stay, increased level of readiness for discharge, and more favorable perceptions of overall quality of care.

The Holzemer (1994) grid (see Table 12-4) assists in the clarification of which characteristics of the client, the provider, and the setting should be monitored in an outcomes research project. Identifying these proposed interactions helps determine what aspects are likely to produce the most significant impact, a particularly important consideration when measurement resources are limited and researchers are interested in addressing the most "pressing" issues first.

table 12.4   Outcomes variables grid

	Inputs	Processes	Outcomes
Client	Client/inputs	Client/processes	Client/outcomes
Provider	Provider/inputs	Provider/processes	Provider/outcomes
Setting	Setting/inputs	Setting/processes	Setting/outcomes

Reproduced with permission by Blackwell Publishing, 2002.

Models of Outcomes Management

Several healthcare organizations have developed outcomes management models specific to their institutional needs. These models guide the identification of problem areas, specify how best to measure and monitor care delivery outcome, and provide guidelines for developing interventions likely to reduce variation within and across groups.

Doerge Model

One such model is described by Doerge (2000) and uses a systems framework to link the healthcare organization's philosophy and strategic planning initiatives to efforts to monitor and manage financial and clinical risk. In this model, the individual patient is identified as the first building block in the outcomes framework. Outcomes for individual patients are managed by an individual or small group of nurses and care providers. The second level of the model includes high-risk patients who are defined as individuals at risk of "not making a smooth transition to the next point of care" (p. 29) and are managed by a care coordinator who intervenes to prevent transition delays.

The third level in the model focuses on high-volume target groups that pose significant risk and opportunity for improvement. Case managers or advanced practice nurses (APNs) provide disease management oversight of these groups. The care providers at this level use the full range of healthcare resources and care delivery settings available to minimize the patient's potential for adverse outcome. The last level in the model includes demographic subsets of populations and reviews care delivery actions across the wellness-to-illness spectrum. Program coordinators manage the strategies designed to facilitate favorable outcomes in these groups. Although not mentioned in the article pertaining to this model, the inclusion of policy makers and community advocates might also be beneficial at this outcomes management level.

Input-Process-Output Model

A second model, described by Maljanian, Effken, and Kaerhle (2000), uses an input-process-output approach to outcomes management. In this model, attention is directed at the generic and population-specific factors that contribute to outcomes seen. Outcomes according to this model are identified as intermediate and long-term, with intermediate outcomes used to guide program planning and care delivery process changes. Long-term outcome data are used to refine predictors of outcome, to evaluate the care provided, and to reduce variations in care.

Value of Care Model

A third model, which has served as a framework for the development of several others, was designed by Nelson, Mohr, and colleagues (1996b) and focuses on the importance of value in any assessment of healthcare quality. It provides a step-by-step process for measuring the value of care for groups of patients.

The defining aspect of the Nelson, Mohr et al. (1996b) model is its use of a clinical value compass to monitor inputs, processes, and outcomes of care. This clinical value compass divides outcome indicators into four quadrants. Clinical outcomes appear on the left of the circular compass, functional health status is at the top, satisfaction against need is assigned to the right, and costs of care are located on the bottom. Specific outcome indicators are subsumed under each of these quadrants and are used to measure the impact of some care delivery process on some group of patients. In this model, care delivery processes are examined for impact on outcomes in each of the quadrants. Then alternative processes are tested and compared with the initial approach, with the expectation that revised and improved processes will result in improved outcome (Nelson et al., 1996b).

The designers of this model have provided several examples of how to collect and report outcomes data (Nelson, Bataldan, Plume, & Mohr, 1996a; Nelson, Mohr et al., 1996b; Nelson, Bataldan, Plume, Mihevc, & Swartz, 1995). Among these are instrument panels, which are intended to provide real-time information to decision makers. The authors recommend using this future-focused approach rather than report cards, which they describe as most useful for purchasers of services. According to Nelson et al. (1995), purchasers of services are more interested in assessing institutional accountability for services provided and are less concerned about understanding processes of care and how these influence care delivery outcome and cost.

Unlike report cards, which contain static reports of prescribed indicators, instrument panels are quarterly reports that summarize the outcome findings identified in each of the quadrants of the clinical value compass. The information is presented in statistical process control chart format, which is a method for displaying variation over time (Brassard & Ritter, 1994). In the control charting process, individual group data are plotted over a prescribed period of time. Using this process, within-subgroup variation can be observed, as can between-subgroup variation when multiple groups are plotted along the same line.

Variation is observed by comparing patient group data collected over time against the mean or median and upper and lower control limits for a representative sample's findings. The upper and lower control limits are determined through statistical techniques based on the average of findings, which serve as the central figures against which other data are compared. Data that fall above or below the control limits are considered "out of control" (Brassard & Ritter, 1994). Data that fall within the upper and lower limits reflect acceptable levels of normal variation.

In reviewing the charts, the actual subgroups' mean data are compared with the expected mean/median line to determine whether any overall change in subgroup outcome has occurred. In addition, individual subgroups are observed for any patterns of variation within the limits and evidence of outcome averages falling outside those same parameters. Patterns within the limits suggest that some special cause (or process) is contributing to the pattern seen. Ordinarily, the variation would be random, not patterned, reflecting normal differences in subsamples or situations. Data points outside the upper or lower limits also denote influence by some special cause, warranting attention and investigation to determine what contributed to the effect seen (Brassard & Ritter, 1994). A further explanation of what patterns constitute special causes appears later in this chapter in the discussion of data displays.

Three-Dimensional, Multidisciplinary Model

A fourth model described in the literature used a multidisciplinary team approach to define outcomes management for the organization and to guide outcomes measurement activities, regardless of patient population (Houston, Fleschler, & Luquire, 2001). This three-dimensional model incorporated outcomes measurement, analysis of healthcare practices, and development and implementation of care delivery processes based on evidence. At the top of the circular picture of this model is the inclusion of institutional values as the driving force behind all measurements, analyses, process improvement, and reevaluation activities. Clearly indicating this component of the conceptual framework helps define for others how the processes, outcomes, and measurement approaches were derived and guided during the implementation of the outcomes management approach.

Cho's Model

A final outcomes management model focuses on measuring the effect of nurse staffing on patient outcomes (Cho, 2001). Although this model is fairly restrictive in its focus on nurse resources, several of the definitions provided by the author are useful for measuring outcomes associated with a variety of nursing actions. This model uses an error-modeling and organizational accident assessment approach to outcomes management.

In Cho's (2001) model, failures of the system that result in adverse outcome are defined as either latent or active. Latent failures are delayed-action consequences of management decisions or organizational processes. Active failures, on the other hand, are unsafe acts committed by care providers interacting directly with patients. Active failures are further classified into errors and violations. Errors result when a planned sequence of activities fails to achieve the desired outcome, whereas violations occur during deviations from safe operating practices, procedures, standards, or rules. According to Cho, errors are best addressed through improvements in information exchange, whereas violations require attention to motivational or cultural factors that influence care delivery processes and outcomes.

Cho (2001) classifies errors into three types of failure: skill-based slips and lapses that occur during the performance of some routine task; rule-based mistakes that result from the misapplication of prior learning; and knowledge-based mistakes, which occur in novel situations for which prior learning has limited application. The benefit of diagnosing the type of action that resulted in the adverse event (or outcome) is the potential for designing specific, problem-directed actions for quality improvement.

A number of other models are described in the literature; the ones identified here were selected because of their potential applicability to a variety of healthcare settings. The selection of an outcomes model or some component within that model requires careful assessment of the model's potential fit for the organization or patient population of interest. Financial and resource constraints may make some models impossible to implement or execute fully. In all cases, some refinement is likely, based on the characteristics and needs of the data manager and the decision makers or recipients of data reports.

Consistent across all of these models are several key elements of an effective outcomes management program (see Box 12-1).

Designing an Outcomes Management Plan

The development, implementation, and maintenance of an outcomes management program requires an infusion of resources prior to its undertaking. Experienced program developers have identified resource needs pertaining to allocated hours for staff education, team facilitation and

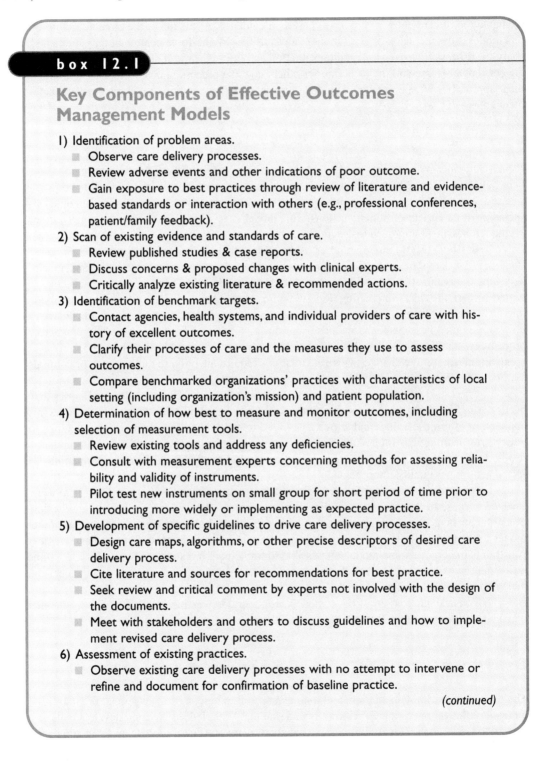

box 12.1

Key Components of Effective Outcomes Management Models

1) Identification of problem areas.
   - Observe care delivery processes.
   - Review adverse events and other indications of poor outcome.
   - Gain exposure to best practices through review of literature and evidence-based standards or interaction with others (e.g., professional conferences, patient/family feedback).
2) Scan of existing evidence and standards of care.
   - Review published studies & case reports.
   - Discuss concerns & proposed changes with clinical experts.
   - Critically analyze existing literature & recommended actions.
3) Identification of benchmark targets.
   - Contact agencies, health systems, and individual providers of care with history of excellent outcomes.
   - Clarify their processes of care and the measures they use to assess outcomes.
   - Compare benchmarked organizations' practices with characteristics of local setting (including organization's mission) and patient population.
4) Determination of how best to measure and monitor outcomes, including selection of measurement tools.
   - Review existing tools and address any deficiencies.
   - Consult with measurement experts concerning methods for assessing reliability and validity of instruments.
   - Pilot test new instruments on small group for short period of time prior to introducing more widely or implementing as expected practice.
5) Development of specific guidelines to drive care delivery processes.
   - Design care maps, algorithms, or other precise descriptors of desired care delivery process.
   - Cite literature and sources for recommendations for best practice.
   - Seek review and critical comment by experts not involved with the design of the documents.
   - Meet with stakeholders and others to discuss guidelines and how to implement revised care delivery process.
6) Assessment of existing practices.
   - Observe existing care delivery processes with no attempt to intervene or refine and document for confirmation of baseline practice.

(continued)

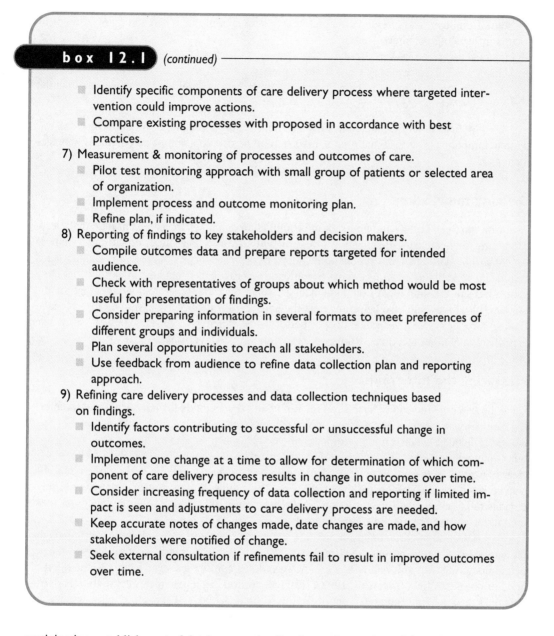

box 12.1 *(continued)*

- Identify specific components of care delivery process where targeted intervention could improve actions.
- Compare existing processes with proposed in accordance with best practices.

7) Measurement & monitoring of processes and outcomes of care.
- Pilot test monitoring approach with small group of patients or selected area of organization.
- Implement process and outcome monitoring plan.
- Refine plan, if indicated.

8) Reporting of findings to key stakeholders and decision makers.
- Compile outcomes data and prepare reports targeted for intended audience.
- Check with representatives of groups about which method would be most useful for presentation of findings.
- Consider preparing information in several formats to meet preferences of different groups and individuals.
- Plan several opportunities to reach all stakeholders.
- Use feedback from audience to refine data collection plan and reporting approach.

9) Refining care delivery processes and data collection techniques based on findings.
- Identify factors contributing to successful or unsuccessful change in outcomes.
- Implement one change at a time to allow for determination of which component of care delivery process results in change in outcomes over time.
- Consider increasing frequency of data collection and reporting if limited impact is seen and adjustments to care delivery process are needed.
- Keep accurate notes of changes made, date changes are made, and how stakeholders were notified of change.
- Seek external consultation if refinements fail to result in improved outcomes over time.

participation, establishment of databases, and collection and reporting of data. They also have stressed the importance of information systems support that relates to and manages outcomes data (Peters et al., 1999). Also described are key assumptions of an outcomes management approach:

- Clinician and administrator receptivity to information about the factors that influence care and **care delivery outcomes**

- Multidisciplinary and interdepartmental/interagency measurement and communication of factors influencing outcomes
- Informed decision making
- Management of outcomes as a nonpunitive process
- Awareness that the factors influencing care delivery and care delivery outcome are dynamic in nature (Perkins, Connerney, & Hastings, 2000).

Confirmation of the outcomes management team's appreciation for and support of these assumptions is an essential preplanning step in the development of an outcomes management plan.

Defining the Mission

According to Saks (1998), the first step in designing an outcomes management plan involves examining the healthcare organization's mission and vision for the future. Equally important is benchmarking with other institutions to identify performance targets indicative of quality care and ideal care delivery outcome. What benchmarking provides is an added assurance that the organization's or the individual's outcome data are consistent with other comparable, high-quality places. This component also helps alleviate the potential for incorrectly assuming that a local finding is reflective of a desirable level of performance, when in fact it may be well below what is happening at other locations (Rudy, Lucke, Whitman, & Davidson, 2001).

Measuring the Intervention

Once the outcome indicators have been identified and the methods for measuring and monitoring care delivery outcome are defined, the next important step is measuring the actual—as opposed to intended—intervention or process of care. This step is essential to eliminating what others have described as the "black box" of outcomes measurement (Mark, 1995). Without a clear indication of the process of care delivered, no assurance can be made about the relationship between what was done and the effect seen. This component maximizes the potential for demonstrating cause-and-effect relationships between the care provided and the outcomes measured in the patient or targeted recipient group.

A second important consideration in the measurement of care delivery processes is the measurement of intervention dose (Brooten & Naylor, 1995). Intervention dose refers to the magnitude or intensity of the intervention delivered and contributes significantly to the likelihood of program effect (Ingersoll, 1998). If only a portion of the intended intervention is delivered or if the strength of the intervention is diluted by interference from some other activity, the potential impact is reduced. The greater the magnitude of the dose and the more it contains all elements of the hypothesized intervention, the greater is the likelihood of a beneficial effect.

Accurately measuring this process component of outcomes management is difficult and fraught with potential for measurement error. Clearly defining the elements of the intervention or care delivery process is essential, as is testing the inter-rater reliability of the persons measuring the extent of intervention delivery and the components of the intervention seen. This problem was highlighted by Smith and colleagues, who reported significant differences in how care providers rated and reported the processes of care delivered to a population of frail older adults

(Smith, Atherly, Kane, & Pacala, 1997). Physicians and nurse practitioners rated the processes entirely differently on all measures assessed. These differences occurred despite acceptable levels of inter-rater reliability for the outcome measures assessed.

One method for measuring intervention dose was used in two studies of the effect of a theory-derived professional practice model on patient outcomes (Verran, Ingersoll, & Chang, 1998). In these studies, each component of the professional practice models were identified, defined, and characterized according to observable activities or processes that would indicate the component was partially or fully implemented in the practice setting.

The number of observable intervention options varied from seven at one study site to nine at the other. The minimum and maximum evidence descriptions were comparable, however, with a score of zero given for no evidence of the program's component and 7 or 9 (maximum number) for evidence that the component was fully integrated into the practice setting.

The determining characteristics of level of evidence were defined according to Rogers' (1983) theory of innovation diffusion and provided observable indicators of knowledge, persuasion, decision, implementation, confirmation, and integration stages. The lowest score (1) for evidence of any activity equated to the knowledge stage in which the concept was being discussed or explored. The next lowest level characterized the persuasion stage in which staff participated in active discussions and expressed commitment to the program component. This was followed by evidence of development of a plan (decision), evidence of some activities associated with the component (implementation), evidence of a variety of activities or elements associated with the component (confirmation), and evidence that the component was fully implemented (integration) (Milton, Verran, Gerber, & Fleury, 1995). Outcomes analyses in these studies demonstrated that the level of program implementation had a significant effect on patient outcomes (Verran et al., 1998). When the intervention score was not used, no differences were seen between experimental and comparison sites' outcomes; when it was used, significant differences appeared.

Perkins et al. (2000) have described what they believe are seven planning and action steps required for successful outcomes measurement programs. According to their process, the first step involves setting broad goals for a targeted outcome. An example of a targeted goal might be reducing the frequency of nonessential emergency room visits.

The next step involves selecting a sample of high-risk or high-likelihood patients (in the above example, emergency department patients who use the department for nonurgent needs) to monitor for current behavior (step three—describing current state) and for subsequent behavior following some planned intervention.

The third step involves carefully describing the current processes, the environment, and the group or other characteristics that are contributing to the outcomes seen (frequency of nonessential emergency department use).

During the next step, the literature is reviewed for possible best practice evidence that addresses some of the existing characteristics of emergency room use. This process can be an extensive one, particularly if the reasons for frequent use of the emergency room are multidimensional and involve both internal and external factors over which the organization or care provider have limited control. The process also can be lengthy, depending on how immediately identifiable are the contributing factors. For example, cultural norms or an individual's previous experience with healthcare services may influence how likely that person is to use the emergency room for nonessential reasons. Assessing these contributing factors may be much more difficult than identifying lack of transportation and the need to rely on ambulance transport as a reason for the nonurgent use of emergency rooms. Focused observation and assessment may be needed as a subcomponent of the overall analysis plan.

The fifth step in Perkins et al.'s (2000) process involves setting specific targets for the outcome of interest. These targets can be set using information obtained from the literature or from benchmarking with other institutions. Using a staged approach for setting outcome targets may be desirable during this process, with increasingly higher targets set over time. In keeping with the emergency department example, expected changes during the early period of a focused intervention might be an initial decline of 10% in nonessential emergency room use. Ideally, a timeframe for this initial targeted decline would be set—for example, within six months of introducing the new intervention. A greater reduction might be projected for 12 and 18 months, with additional steps taken or further strategies defined as more data are collected and early results inform subsequent action.

The sixth step in outcomes management programming involves the implementation of changes in care delivery processes or the taking of action to reduce the environmental and other factors that contribute to the outcomes seen. Of importance in this phase is the close monitoring and documentation of the change itself to assure that what was intended actually occurs. Any change in the intervention plan and any decision to alter the intended action should be documented and the rationale for the change described fully. This information will be essential to the subsequent determination of the relationship between cause (new process) and effect (outcome achieved).

The final step in this process involves reporting and disseminating the results to others (Perkins et al., 2000). The format for how the information is shared will depend on the needs of the persons receiving the information and how they will use the information for further action or decision making.

A step not included in the model by Perkins et al. (2000) is the identification of *stakeholders* interested in the outcomes measurement planning, care delivery process revision, and information dissemination components of the outcomes management approach. A stakeholder is defined as anyone who is affected in any way by the proposed changes or anticipated results of the outcomes management plan. In the case of the emergency department example, emergency department staff and administration, midlevel and senior-level hospital administration, primary care providers, patients, families, ambulatory center staff, referring hospitals, emergency medical transport personnel, and local community agencies are all examples of potential stakeholders. Careful attention to the needs of these individuals and the information they require is essential to the sustained achievement or subsequent refinement of revised care delivery processes.

Presenting Outcomes Assessment Findings

Several methods are available for presenting outcomes data to stakeholders and others. Selecting which approach to use should be guided by the overall outcomes measurement activity undertaken and the audience targeted for the presentation.

Outcomes research findings are best presented according to standard research reporting formats. The amount of information provided is dictated by the time or space available and the audience involved. In all cases, however, the discussion should include a careful description of the study's method, its sample and sample size, the setting for the investigation, the intervention tested, the predictor, outcome and extraneous variables measured, and the instruments used. This information will be needed in addition to a discussion of the study findings and their implications, which will be interpreted according to the strengths and limitations of the study design and the measurement approaches.

For decision makers and clinicians hoping to use outcomes management data to revise care delivery processes at local or site-specific samples, a more applications-focused approach may be desired. In these cases, the description of the data collection process and the specifics of the measurement plan may be of less interest than the data reports themselves.

Methods for Presenting Data

When presenting the data to decision makers, visual displays are often most effective. The components of the display should be clear, and the amount of data per frame or page should assure that the meaning of the information is not lost in the presentation. A general "artist's rule" is to place important information in the upper left-hand corner and move the reader's eye across and down. Keep descriptive information large enough for viewers to visualize at a reasonable distance (whether reviewing documents or observing presentations). Label all documents and date each to assure that the information presented is the most current. Keep track of when changes are made in the data presentation and use feedback from each audience to refine the reports as indicated.

Statistical control charts, which were mentioned previously, are useful methods for displaying subgroup comparison data. The use of control charts requires an initial data collection activity during periods when care delivery processes are considered stable. These data are then used to establish the control limits for subsequent comparisons. Generally, data from 20–30 subgroups within a stable period are used to calculate control limits (Moen, Nolan, & Provost, 1991).

Once the control limits are calculated, subgroup data are plotted according to whether they fall above or below the central line. Four types of pictorial evidence provide indication of some unusual or potentially worrisome pattern. The first of these is the location of a single point outside the upper or lower control limit (Moen et al., 1991). This pattern suggests that some specific event or characteristic is associated with that subgroup's effect.

The second pattern involves a row of eight or more points above or below the centerline (Moen et al., 1991). In this case, if the points reflect different subgroups, the pattern indicates some trend across groups. This suggests that a more widely distributed event or problem is involving several groups. If the data reflect the same subgroup over time, the pattern suggests some influence related to season or time. The assumption here is that normal variation would produce a pattern that falls randomly above and below the centerline. When an extended clustering appears that does not appear before and after the pattern, something is affecting these clustered outcomes.

The third unusual event pattern involves the clustering of six consecutive points in an upward or downward pattern (Moen et al., 1991). Again, the expectation is that the points would be randomly distributed above and below the centerline. This correlation-type patterning indicates that something is producing an observable change in the expected outcome. The fourth pattern consists of three points near either the upper or the lower control limit. Although the points remain inside the acceptable level, their clustered proximity to the cutoff points suggests this may be an early indication of some evolving event.

Other common methods for displaying outcomes data are bar graphs, pie charts, tables, and line graphs, which are particularly useful for comparing larger numbers of subgroups over time. A combination of approaches may be most effective, especially if attention is being directed at differences within and across groups at one point and at multiple times.

Clinical Example

The exemplar found in Box 12-2 highlights how outcomes management projects can lead to formal investigations of clinical issues and the development of reliable and valid measures of care delivery outcome.

---

box 12.2

Exemplar of Outcomes Management Project

The nursing staff of the Burn/Trauma Intensive Care Unit (BTICU) at Strong Memorial Hospital identified the need to better control the pain of patients treated for severe trauma or burns. Their assessment of the need for a practice change was based on feedback from patients and families, clinical experience, and discussions with other burn-trauma experts. Working with members of an interdisciplinary team, the BTICU nurses developed an evidence-based pain control protocol that they intended to introduce as standard practice on their unit. As part of this process, they recognized the importance of accurately assessing the impact of the newly designed pain control protocol on all patients, including those who were unable to respond to verbal questioning.

During the assessment planning process, the BTICU nurses identified a group of patients who were unable to rate or otherwise indicate their level of pain or pain relief. These individuals were often the most seriously injured and the most at risk for insufficient pain control; without an accurate assessment of the pain protocol's impact, the nurses would have no indication of whether the revised care delivery process was achieving the desired outcome (symptom control).

The nursing staff had been encouraged by an outside accrediting agency to use a pain assessment scale designed for children and infants (the FLACC*; Merkel, Voepel-Lewis, Shayevitz, & Malviya, 1997). This practice was not deemed acceptable to the BTICU nurses, who felt the components of the child-focused instrument did not meet the needs of nurses assessing nonverbal adult patients' level of distress or pain relief.

---

*FLACC = Face, Legs, Activity, Cry, Consolability

In this scenario, a newly designed plan for managing pain prompted the Strong Memorial Hospital Burn/Trauma Intensive Care Unit (BTICU) staff's awareness of the need to identify a reliable and valid method for measuring pain relief in patients unable to verbally express their level of discomfort. As an outgrowth of this perceived need, the nurses took the next step in the outcomes management process by examining the literature and contacting local and national experts for evidence of existing measures for assessing pain in nonverbal adults. When the nurses found nothing that met their patients' needs, they contacted a clinical researcher for assistance with developing and testing an instrument to assess symptom relief in nonverbal adults.

This action shifted the process to a more formal investigation involving the development of a psychometrically sound measurement tool that could be used in the immediate environment as well as in other settings. The focus at this point shifted from the immediate needs of the local environment to the development of a reliable and valid instrument that could benefit other researchers, practitioners, and patients.

Working with the clinical researcher, the BTICU nurses planned and conducted a pilot test of their newly proposed tool and compared assessment findings of the new tool with the existing "gold standard" for assessment of pain in nonverbal patients (the FLACC Scale, which stands for Face, Legs, Activity, Cry, and Consolability). The nurses conducted inter- and intra-rater nurse comparisons, then correlated the findings within and across scales. In contrast to findings for the FLACC scale, rarely were components of the newly devised scale labeled as not applicable or unable to assess. A physiologic-related component of the adult scale was determined to need additional refinement because of clear indication of poor inter-rater reliability. A larger study was planned to test a revised version of the scale.

During the implementation of the outcomes management program in the BTICU, nurse leaders and senior staff worked to assure that information was shared with all key stakeholders and potential users of the proposed new assessment tool. They met with physician staff, who assisted in the development of the pain management protocol. They also presented information about the protocol and the new instrument development and subsequent ongoing outcomes management process to staff at meetings and through written communications.

The nursing staff identified a timeline for completion of pain protocol, selection of symptom control measurement tool, implementation of new pain management process, and reporting of ongoing outcome assessment findings. They also identified who would be their target audiences for outcomes management reports and how frequently reports would be generated. Because the nurses also participated in a small instrument development study, they identified potential audiences and reporting formats, as well as additional research activities needed in response to that activity.

The time required to achieve this outcomes management process was considerably longer than the nurses originally envisioned. Development of a comprehensive, safe, and effective evidence-based protocol for pain management required careful review of the literature, collaboration with other healthcare disciplines, and review and comment by experts at Strong and elsewhere. The decision to develop a reliable and valid instrument to assess pain in nonverbal adults took additional time and resources to accomplish the initial and subsequent instrument development research. The nurses also had to work with others who were less enthusiastic about the idea of conducting a study at the bedside when day-to-day demands were already considerable. Nonetheless, they persevered and created an excellent, carefully thought-out and implemented outcomes management process. The steps they followed are highlighted in Figure 12-1.

		OUTCOMES MANAGEMENT (OM) PROCESS	OUTCOMES RESEARCH (OR)
STEP	OM ACTIVITY	BMTU OM ACTIONS	BMTU OR ACTIONS
Pre	Identification of problem.	Insufficient pain control in critically ill patients.	
1	Set broad goals for targeted outcome.	Ensure acceptable levels of pain control for all patients admitted to the BMTU.	
2	Identify sample of high-likelihood patients.	All patients who are unable to verbally report or otherwise make level of discomfort known to nursing and healthcare staff.	
3	Describe current state, environment, groups & other characteristics contributing to outcomes seen.	Newly injured or burned patients often are intubated. Many patients in BMTU have altered levels of consciousness. Delivery of pain medications is not standardized & varies according to physician practice & nurse assessment & responsiveness behaviors.	
4	Conduct process/outcome analysis.	Patients & families report evidence of insufficient pain control.	

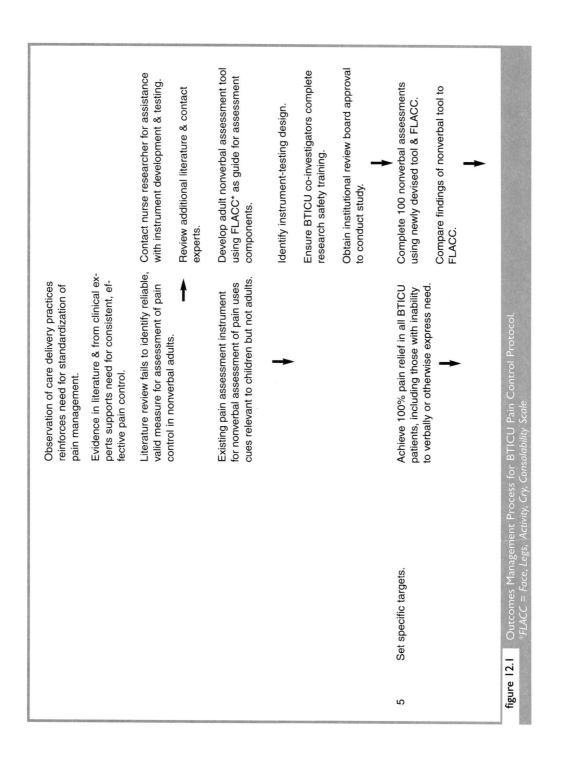

Observation of care delivery practices reinforces need for standardization of pain management.

Evidence in literature & from clinical experts supports need for consistent, effective pain control.

Literature review fails to identify reliable, valid measure for assessment of pain control in nonverbal adults.

Contact nurse researcher for assistance with instrument development & testing.

Review additional literature & contact experts.

Existing pain assessment instrument for nonverbal assessment of pain uses cues relevant to children but not adults.

Develop adult nonverbal assessment tool using FLACC* as guide for assessment components.

Identify instrument-testing design.

Ensure BTICU co-investigators complete research safety training.

Obtain institutional review board approval to conduct study.

Achieve 100% pain relief in all BTICU patients, including those with inability to verbally or otherwise express need.

Complete 100 nonverbal assessments using newly devised tool & FLACC.

Compare findings of nonverbal tool to FLACC.

5   Set specific targets.

figure 12.1   Outcomes Management Process for BTICU Pain Control Protocol.
*FLACC = Face, Legs, Activity, Cry, Consolability Scale

		OUTCOMES MANAGEMENT (OM) PROCESS	OUTCOMES RESEARCH (OR)
STEP	OM ACTIVITY	BMTU OM ACTIONS	BMTU OR ACTIONS
6	Implement changes.	Develop evidence-based pain management protocol for care of BTICU patients.	Review findings of pilot study.
		Introduce new protocol to stakeholders.	Revise new instrument based on study findings.
		Implement protocol following training of staff in use of protocol.	Design larger study using revised tool.
		Use standardized approach to assessment of symptom control outcome. →	Obtain funding to support additional research.
7	Review & report results.	Data collection ongoing.	Findings of pilot study included in application for additional funding.
		Result reporting planned for quarterly review & discussion.	Findings of pilot & other studies reported in peer-reviewed journal.
		Report format to include information related to use of symptom assessment tool and symptom relief.	Findings of pilot & other studies reported at professional conferences pertaining to care of trauma & burn patients.
		Reports to include information about change over time.	Additional studies to include other populations of adults with inability to verbally report level of pain.

figure 12.1 Outcomes Management Process for BTICU Pain Control Protocol (*continued*)

Overcoming Barriers to Outcomes Measurement

A number of factors contribute to the difficulties encountered in developing, implementing, and sustaining an outcomes measurement program. Among the most common are staff and administration resistance to the need for ongoing data collection, the difficulty associated with collecting reliable and valid data from existing sources, and the time and resources required to plan for, conduct, analyze, interpret, and report the data, then develop an appropriate intervention plan. Obstacles also include differences in how the data are defined, stored, and reported within and across institutions and the limited information available concerning the reliability, validity, and sensitivity of nurse-sensitive outcome indicators. Although these barriers may seem impossible to overcome, well-designed plans with a reasonable amount of resource support and a committed outcomes measurement team can make the process an achievable one.

Sustaining an outcomes measurement program is often the most difficult task, with competing demands interfering with the time required to measure care delivery outcomes and to design effective intervention plans. Program success also can be short-lived if patient populations shift, necessitating a revamping of program focus (Houston, Fleschler & Luquine, 2001) or if administrative support (including the provision of resources to achieve program objectives) is withdrawn or redirected. Intense pressure for early, large-scale effects also may interfere with sustained attention to groups whose outcomes are slow to change or are incremental over time.

Kite-Powell and colleagues (1999) have recommended the use of a process improvement approach to assure continued attention to outcomes measurement and management practices. They believe a focus on process improvement helps clarify which outcomes should be measured and which process refinements are most likely to produce the maximum desirable effect.

The difference between process improvement and outcomes management is the focus of the activity. In outcomes management, the initial focus is on the measurement and monitoring of outcomes. The status of these outcomes drives the actions taken to revise care delivery processes or environmental factors believed to influence the outcomes seen. With process improvement, the initial target is the process and the understanding of which components may contribute to variations in practice and ultimately differences in outcome. The overall goal of each is similar—that is, to improve the quality of care provided and the outcomes achieved. Both reinforce and inform the other, and both are required to maximize potential benefit to the organization and the individuals served.

A second important strategy for sustained attention to outcomes measurement is continued attention to the evidence generated by others. This requires a planned approach to regularly reviewing the literature for recent reports of outcomes studies, quality improvement initiatives, and recommended approaches to measuring and managing outcomes. This process can be accomplished by individuals or groups, depending on interest and need. A careful review of outcomes findings for application to practice is necessary, however, before any specific recommendations can be made.

One approach to the critical review of evidence has been proposed by Stetler (2001), who has described a model that she and colleagues use to integrate research evidence into individual or group practice. In this model, Stetler identifies six phases of evidence review that can be applied to **outcomes research.** In the first phase, the selection of studies is based on their potential usefulness to the clinical question or the care delivery problem of interest. In the second phase, the evidence is critiqued with a focus on the potential usefulness of the findings for clinical practice. In this stage, studies are reviewed both for evidence of methodologic rigor and for utilization likelihood.

The third phase of Stetler's model (2001) involves determining the fit between the study's characteristics and the clinical setting. It also includes assessing the potential feasibility of introducing the study findings into the clinical setting, determining the magnitude of the evidence, and clarifying the relationship between the evidence and current practice. In the fourth phase, specific steps for applying the findings to the clinical setting are described. The fifth phase focuses on evaluating the application process, determining the usefulness of the evidence for producing improved outcomes, and defining the need for additional refinement or revision to care delivery processes.

Selecting Resources to Assist in Outcomes Measurement

The monitoring of outcomes data can best be accomplished through the use of available resources and the careful selection of reliable and manageable measurement approaches, data storage and retrieval processes, and reporting mechanisms. With the increased availability of evidence-based data sources and the growing number of data management programs available, the outcomes researcher or manager has several options from which to choose. Selecting which instruments, programs, or formats to use should be driven by the institution or the practice providers' needs, the funds available to support the activities, and the outcomes reporting expectations required. The best approach is to start small and expand over time. If small groups of providers or organizations can link with others, additional opportunities for selection of software, equipment, or other resources may be possible.

Several authors have identified decision-making considerations for selecting outcomes management resources. The most commonly discussed are information systems, which play a critical role in determining access, ease, cost, capacity, capability, confidentiality, and reportability of outcomes management data. According to Simpson (1999), five key factors should be considered when reviewing clinical information systems for use in outcomes assessment:

1. Vendor stability and leadership
2. Functional depth and breadth of the application being reviewed
3. Integration of the software with other programs
4. Performance of the technology, especially in relation to the outcomes purposes intended
5. Vendor support, including installation and education if hardware components are purchased

Before selecting a program, it may be useful to conduct brief pilot studies to determine the data management needs and how these can best be handled. Contacting other providers or institutions that have existing programs also may be desirable, particularly if those individuals or locales will serve as benchmarks for or collaborators with the data collection plan.

Additional considerations include whether to rely on manual data entry methods or use scannable forms or hand-held data storage programs to maximize data management efficiency. Costs are associated with each of these approaches; initial and maintenance equipment costs are highest for the scannable and hand-held storage approaches (Johnson & Nolan, 2000). The costs associated with manual data entry also may be considerable, however, depending on who is entering the data and how much and how often the data are entered. Manual entry also creates additional opportunities for error, resulting in the need for data confirmation and cleaning activities, which further inflate the cost (Johnson & Nolan, 2000). Selection of which approach to use should be guided by the funding available to support the outcomes management activities, the skill of the data collectors and outcomes management personnel, and the magnitude of the data collection plan.

In addition to technology resources for outcomes measurement activities, Web site references also are available to assist with the identification of measurement strategies, the selection of data collection instruments, and the choice of data management approaches. Most of these have some costs associated with the use of materials, but many of the sites provide initial information that can be useful for decision-making purposes.

- Agency for Healthcare Research and Quality (AHRQ). Contains a variety of topics concerning the measurement of quality and outcomes of care, including several measurement approaches focused on quality of care. **http://www.ahcpr.gov.**
- Joint Commission on Accreditation of Healthcare Organizations (JCAHO). Includes descriptions of terms used in performance improvement expectations of JCAHO and updates on national safety standards. **http://www.jcaho.org.**
- Medical Outcomes Trust. Contains a list of instruments reviewed and approved by a scientific review committee. Many of these instruments pertain to the measurement of care delivery outcomes. Some are available without cost to nonprofit institutions. **http://www.outcomes-trust.org/instruments.htm.**
- University of Iowa Nursing Outcomes Classification (NOC). Contains descriptions of proposed nursing-sensitive outcome indicators and information about the classification process. **http://www.nursing.iowa.edu/noc.**
- World Health Organization (WHO). Provides handy templates for setting up outcomes monitoring programs and other reports pertaining to quality of care initiatives around the world. **http://www.who.int/health-systems-performance.**

Creating Change Through Outcomes Management and Research

Because previous outcomes measurement efforts have been directed primarily at containing healthcare costs rather than understanding the scientific basis for clinical interventions, much of the existing evidence is scattered, unfocused, and superficial. Although the control of costs is an important and essential dimension of healthcare, it is both a contributor to and an outcome of the types of care provided. Cost also is most often prescribed by external groups, such as health insurers and federal and state reimbursement programs, making manipulation of care delivery practices minimally contributory to differences seen. It does, however, provide some indication of the efficiency of care delivery processes and should be included as one component of an overall outcomes assessment plan.

Considerable research is needed to further define the effect of care delivery processes and health-related activities on care delivery outcomes. Also essential is the explicit demonstration of the ways in which outcomes management monitoring influences quality of care. Although the methods proposed in this chapter have been recommended by others and implemented in a number of healthcare organizations, few investigations have examined their usefulness for and successful achievement of improved and sustained patient outcome. The limited information to date suggests that the existing approaches may differ in the magnitude of their effect, based on the type of patient population involved and the stage of program implementation seen (Holtzman, Bjerke, & Kane, 1998).

The lack of a conceptual framework for outcomes assessment activities has contributed to the uncertainty over the effects of care provider practice or delivery process features on outcomes seen. At the very least, outcomes management programs and outcomes research projects should:

- Specify the contributing or confounding factors that may influence outcomes, regardless of intervention proposed
- Identify the process components expected to result in the outcomes achieved
- Define the outcomes anticipated
- Propose the causal relationships between intervention (including the care provider as intervention) and outcome

Figure 12-2 is a basic, simple outcomes assessment model. In this case, the intervention is the APN who provides direct care to groups of patients. The outcomes are hypothesized to change as a result of the APN's care delivery process and are based on previous research (Ingersoll et al., 2000).

Characteristics of the APN, the environment, and the client are all expected to influence the care delivery processes of the APN case manager. In addition, the characteristics of the environment and the patient are expected to have both direct and indirect effects on client outcomes through the actions of the APN case manager. Data pertaining to provider and the environmental and client characteristics should be collected in addition to information about the specific care delivery activities of the APN and the outcomes seen. In a proposed outcomes investigation, the number of outcomes measured would be reduced, with attention given to those hypothesized to be most affected by APN practice.

Future investigations of care delivery outcome should focus on the care delivery processes undertaken by nurses rather than restricting the studies to explorations of nursing resources and other structural components of care. In a comprehensive review of the literature by Lee and colleagues (1999), few investigations examined the impact of nursing processes on care delivery outcomes. The few studies available focused on the number of registered nurses providing care in comparison with the total number of nursing staff interacting with patients and other provider-type characteristics (Lee, Chang, Pearson, Kahn, & Rubenstein, 1999). Although these studies are important to the understanding of the impact of provider mix and characteris-

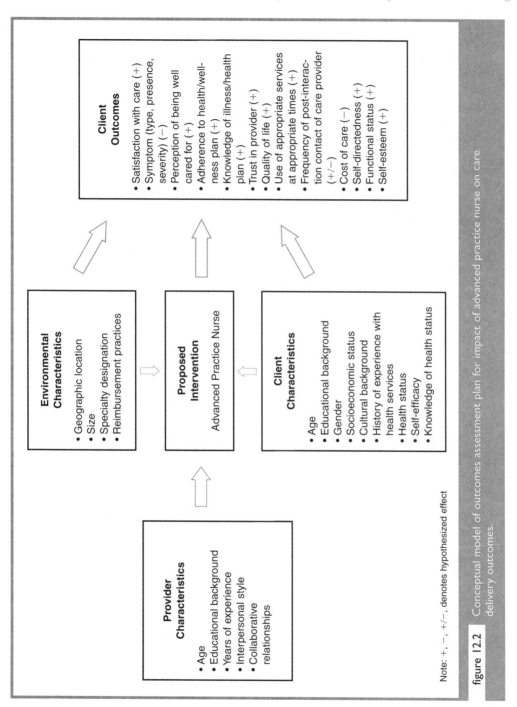

figure 12.2 Conceptual model of outcomes assessment plan for impact of advanced practice nurse on care delivery outcomes.

Note: +, −, +/−, denotes hypothesized effect

tics on care delivery outcome, they do not assist in the determination of which nursing interventions are most beneficial for patients.

Consistent, repeated testing of indicators sensitive to nursing practice is needed. This process can best be accomplished through the establishment of close collaborations between practitioners and researchers whose areas of expertise maximize the potential for applicability and usefulness of findings. These collaborative groups are much more likely to extend institution-specific findings to other locations and to maximize the potential for widespread dispersion of evidence-based results.

In addition, the process of outcomes measurement and evidence-based decision making should be seen as iterative (back and forth), with each action challenging, informing, expanding, directing, and redirecting subsequent work. This process also can proceed in several directions—internally through sideways dissemination from one area to another, outward from a local finding to another site or patient population, and inward through the use of reported evidence or linkages with other institutions interested in expanding their findings. This process serves to validate the evidence, highlight the areas needing additional attention, and refine existing theories and practice approaches over time. In each case, the discovery and reporting of evidence serves to better inform those who are delivering the care and maximize the benefits of those who are receiving it.

references

Aiken, L. J., Sloane, D. M., Lake, E. T., Sochalski, J., & Weber, A. L. (1999). Organization and outcomes of inpatient AIDS care. *Medical Care, 37,* 760–772.

Alexander, J., & Kroposki, M. (1999). Outcomes for community health nursing practice. *Journal of Nursing Administration, 29*(5), 49–56.

American Nurses Association (ANA). (1999). *Nursing-sensitive quality indicators for acute care settings and ANA's safety and quality initiative.* Available at: www.nursingworld.org/readroom/fssafe99.htm. Accessed 10/08/02.

Backlund, E., Sorlie, P. D., & Johnson, N. J. (1999). A comparison of the relationships of education and income with mortality: The national longitudinal mortality study. *Social Science & Medicine, 49,* 1373–1384.

Berlowitz, D. R., Ash, A. S., Hickey, E. C., Kader, B., Friedman, R., & Moskowitz, M. A. (1998). Profiling outcomes of ambulatory care. Casemix affects perceived performance. *Medical Care, 36,* 928–933.

Blegen, M. A., & Vaughn, T. (1998). A multisite study of nurse staffing and patient occurrences. *Nursing Economics, 16,* 196–203.

Blegen, M. A., Goode, C. J., & Reed, L. (1998). Nurse staffing and patient outcomes. *Nursing Research, 47,* 43–50.

Brassard, M., & Ritter, D. (1994). *The memory jogger.* Salem, NH: Goal/QPC.

Brooten, D., & Naylor, M. D. (1995). Nurses' effect on changing patient outcomes. *Image: Journal of Nursing Scholarship, 27,* 95–99.

Cho, S. H. (2001). Nurse staffing and adverse patient outcomes: A systems approach. *Nursing Outlook, 49,* 78–85.

Cohen, J., Saylor, C., Holzemer, W. L., & Gorenberg, B. (2000). Linking nursing care interventions with client outcomes: A community–based application of an outcomes model. *Journal of Nursing Care Quality, 15*(1), 22–31.

Cole, L., & Houston, S. (1999). Structured care methodologies: Evolution and use in patient care delivery. *Outcomes Management for Nursing Practice, 3,* 53–60.

Craft-Rosenberg, M., Krajicek, M. J., & Shin, D. (2002). Report of the American Academy of Nursing Child-Family Expert Panel: Identification of quality and outcome indicators for maternal child nursing. *Nursing Outlook, 50,* 57–60.

Doerge, J. B. (2000). Creating an outcomes framework. *Outcomes Management for Nursing Practice, 4,* 28–33.

Donabedian, A. (1966). Evaluating the quality of medical care. *Milbank Memorial Fund Quarterly, 44,* 166–206.

Hodge, M. B., Asch, S. M., Olson, V. A., Kravitz, R. L., & Sauvé, M. J. (2002). Developing indicators of nursing quality to evaluate nurse staffing ratios. *Journal of Nursing Administration, 32,* 338–345.

Holtzman, J., Bjerke, T., & Kane, R. (1998). The effects of clinical pathways for renal transplant on patient outcomes and length of stay. *Medical Care, 36,* 826–834.

Holzemer, W. L. (1994). The impact of nursing care in Latin America and the Caribbean: A focus on outcomes. *Journal of Advanced Nursing, 20,* 5–12.

Holzemer, W. L., & Reilly, C. A. (1995). Variables, variability, and variations research: Implications for medical informatics. *Journal of the American Medical Informatics Association, 2,* 183–190.

Houston, S., Fleschler, R., & Luquire, R. (2001). Reflections on a decade of outcomes management in women's services. *Journal of Gynecologic & Neonatal Nursing, 30,* 89–97.

Huber, D., & Oermann, M. (1999). Do outcomes equal quality? *Outcomes Management for Nursing Practice, 3,* 1–3.

Ingersoll, G. L. (1998). Administrative issues in the measurement and management of outcomes. *Applied Nursing Research, 11,* 93–97.

Ingersoll, G. L., McIntosh, E., & Williams, M. (2000). Nurse-sensitive outcomes of advanced practice. *Journal of Advanced Nursing, 32,* 1272–1281.

Johnson, C., & Nolan, M. T. (2000). A guide to choosing technology to support the measurement of patient outcomes. *Journal of Nursing Administration, 30,* 21–26.

Johnson, M., & Maas, M. L. (Eds.). (1997). *Nursing outcomes classification (NOC).* St. Louis. MO: Mosby-Yearbook.

Johnson, M., & Maas, M. L. (1999). Nursing-sensitive patient outcomes. Development and importance for use in assessing health care effectiveness. In E. L. Cohen & V. DeBeck (Eds.), *The outcomes mandate. Case management in health care today* (pp. 37–48). St. Louis, MO: Mosby.

Kelly, K. C., Huber, D. G., Johnson, M., McCloskey, J. C., & Maas, M. (1994). The Medical Outcomes Study: A nursing perspective. *Journal of Professional Nursing, 10,* 209–216.

Kite-Powell, D., Houston, S., Hartgraves, D., Ideno, K., Sabau, D., Deal, D., Dahlberg, C. G. W., & Luquire, R. (1999). Improving outcomes for ventilator-dependent patients: Quality enhancement to decrease mechanical ventilation time. *Outcomes Management for Nursing Practice, 3,* 95–98.

Lee, J. L., Chang, B. L., Pearson, M. L., Kahn, K. L., & Rubenstein, L. V. (1999). Does what nurses do affect clinical outcomes for hospitalized patients? A review of literature. *Health Services Research, 34,* 1011–1032.

Lohr, K. N. (1988). Outcome measurement: Concepts and questions. *Inquiry, 25,* 37–50.

Maljanian, R., Effken, J., & Kaerhle, P. (2000). Design and implementation of an outcomes management model. *Outcomes Management for Nursing Practice, 4,* 19–26.

Mark, B. A. (1995). The black box of patient outcomes research. *Image: Journal of Nursing Scholarship, 27,* 42.

Mastal, P. (1999). New signposts and directions: Indicators of quality in ambulatory nursing care. *Nursing Economics, 17,* 103–104.

Merkel, S. I., Voepel-Lewis, T., Shayevitz, J. R., & Malviya, S. (1997). The FLACC: A behavioral scale for scoring postoperative pain in young children. *Pediatric Nursing, 23,* 293–297.

Milton, D. A., Verran, J. A., Gerber, R. M., & Fleury, J. (1995). Tools to evaluate reengineering progress. In S. S. Blancett, & D. L. Flarey (Eds.), *Reengineering nursing and health care* (pp. 195–202). Gaithersburg, MD: Aspen Publishers.

Mitchell, P. H., Ferketich, S., & Jennings, B. M. (1998). Quality health outcomes model. *Image: Journal of Nursing Scholarship, 30,* 43–46.

Moen, R. D., Nolan, T. W., & Provost, L. P. (1991). *Improving quality through planned experimentation.* New York: McGraw-Hill.

Moritz, P. (1998). Demonstrating clinical impact with indicators sensitive to care and environmental context. *New Medicine, 2,* 97–102.

Nelson, E. C., Bataldan, P. B., Plume, S. K., Mihevc, N. T., & Swartz, W. G. (1995). Report cards or instrument panels: Who needs what? *Journal of Quality Improvement, 21,* 155–166.

Nelson, E. C., Bataldan, P. B., Plume, S. K., & Mohr, J. J. (1996a). Improving health care part 2: A clinical improvement worksheet and users' manual. *Journal of Quality Improvement, 22,* 531–548.

Nelson, E. C., Mohr, J. J., Bataldan, P. B., & Plume, S. K. (1996b). Improving health care, part 1: The clinical value compass. *Journal of Quality Improvement, 22,* 243–256.

Perkins, S. B., Connerney, I., & Hastings, C. E. (2000). Outcomes management: From concepts to application. *AACN Clinical Issues, 11,* 339–350.

Peters, C., Cowley, M., & Standiford, L. (1999). The process of outcomes management in an acute care facility. *Nursing Administration Quarterly, 24*(1), 75–89.

Porell, F., Caro, F. G., Silva, A., & Monane, M. (1998). A longitudinal analysis of nursing home outcomes. *Health Services Research, 33,* 835–865.

Rogers, E. M. (1983). *Diffusion of innovations* (3rd ed.). New York: Free Press.

Rosenheck, R., Fontana, A., & Stolar, M. (1999). Assessing quality of care. Administrative indicators and clinical outcomes in posttraumatic stress disorder. *Medical Care, 37,* 180–188.

Rudy, E. B., Lucke, J. F., Whitman, G. R., & Davidson, L. J. (2001). Benchmarking patient outcomes. *Journal of Nursing Scholarship, 33,* 185–189.

Saks, N. P. (1998). Developing an integrated model for outcomes management. *Advanced Practice Nursing Quarterly, 4*(1), 27–32.

Schwartz, J. S., & Lurie, N. (1991). *Outcome measurement for the assessment of hospital care* (Cooperative Agreement Report #99-c-99/69/5-0153). Springfield, VA: U. S. Department of Commerce.

Sidani, S., & Braden, C. J. (1998). *Evaluating nursing interventions. A theory-driven approach.* Thousand Oaks, CA: Sage.

Simpson, R. L. (1999). Automated outcomes management. Criteria for selection of information systems. In E. L. Cohen, & V. DeBack (Eds.), *The outcomes mandate. Case management in health care today* (pp. 226–234). St. Louis, MO: Mosby.

Smith, M. A., Atherly, A. J., Kane, R. L., & Pacala, J. T. (1997). Peer review of the quality of care. Reliability and sources of variability for outcome and process assessments. *Journal of American Medical Association, 278,* 1573–1578.

Stetler, C. B. (2001). Updating the Stetler model of research utilization to facilitate evidence—based practice. *Nursing Outlook, 49,* 272–279.

Thomas, J. W., Guire, K. E., & Horvat, G. G. (1997). Is patient length of stay related to quality care? *Hospital & Health Services Administration, 42,* 489–507.

Verran, J. A., Ingersoll, G. L., & Chang, S. (1998). *Joint analysis of innovative practice model effects. Final report* (U01 NR02153). Tucson, AZ: University of Arizona.

Whittle, J., Lin, C. J., Lave, J. R., Fine, M. J., Delaney, K. M., Joyce, D. Z., Young, W. W., & Kapoor, W. N. (1998). Relationship of provider characteristics to outcomes, process, and costs of care for community-acquired pneumonia. *Medical Care, 36,* 977–987.

Writing a Successful Grant Proposal to Fund Research and Outcomes Management Projects

Bernadette Mazurek Melnyk and Ellen Fineout-Overholt

chapter 13

> 66 *There's always a way if you are willing to pay the price of time, energy, or effort.* 99
>
> —*Robert Schuller*

Once a decision has been made to conduct a study to generate evidence that will guide clinical practice or to implement and evaluate a practice change as part of an outcomes management project, the feasibility of conducting such an initiative must be assessed. Although certain studies or outcomes management projects can be conducted with few resources, most projects (e.g., randomized controlled trials [RCTs]) typically require funding to cover items such as research assistants, staff time, instruments to measure outcomes of interest, intervention materials, and data management and analyses. This chapter will focus on strategies for developing a successful grant proposal to fund research as well as outcomes management projects. Many of these grant-writing strategies are similar, whether applying for large-scale grants from federal agencies, such as the National Institutes of Health (NIH), or more small-scale funding from professional organizations or foundations. Potential funding sources and key components of a project budget also will be highlighted.

Preliminary Strategies for Writing a Grant Proposal

A grant proposal is a written plan outlining the specific aims, background, significance, methods, and budget for a project that is requesting funding from sources such as professional organizations, federal agencies, or foundations. It is not uncommon for the process of planning, writing, and revising a rigorous detailed grant proposal for certain funding sources (e.g., NIH, the Agency for Healthcare Research and Quality [AHRQ], the Centers for Disease Control and Prevention [CDC]) to take several months. In contrast, other sources (e.g., foundations and professional organizations) may require only the submission of a concise abstract or two- to three-page summary of the project for funding consideration. When embarking on the road to writing a successful grant proposal, whether for a large or small project, there are five critical qualities that the writer must possess—the five "Ps": passion, planning, persuasion, persistence, and patience.

The Five Ps

The first quality is *passion* for the proposed initiative. Passion for the project is essential, especially because many "character-building" experiences (e.g., writing multiple drafts, resubmissions) will surface along the road to successful completion.

Second, detailed *planning* must begin. Every element of the project needs to be carefully considered, along with strategies for overcoming potential obstacles.

The third element for successful grant writing is *persuasion*. The grant application needs to be written in a manner that excites the reviewers and creates a compelling case for why the project should be funded.

Finally, *persistence* and *patience* are indispensable qualities, especially because the grant application process is very competitive across federal agencies, professional organizations, and foundations. In many cases, repeated submissions are required to secure funding. Therefore, resubmitting applications and being patient and receptive to grant reviewers' feedback are crucial ingredients for success. One tip for success is to surround yourself with uplifting motivational quotes to inspire and encourage you through the writing process (Box 13-1).

First Impressions

Remember that you never get a second chance to make a great first impression. Paying attention to details and being as meticulous as possible for the first grant submission will be well worth the effort when your grant is reviewed.

Once the idea for a study project is generated, the literature searched and critically appraised, and a planning meeting conducted to determine the design and methods (see Chapters 10–12), a search for potential funding sources should commence.

Credentials

To obtain grants from most national federal funding agencies (e.g., NIH and AHRQ), a doctoral degree is usually the minimum qualification necessary for the principal or lead investi-

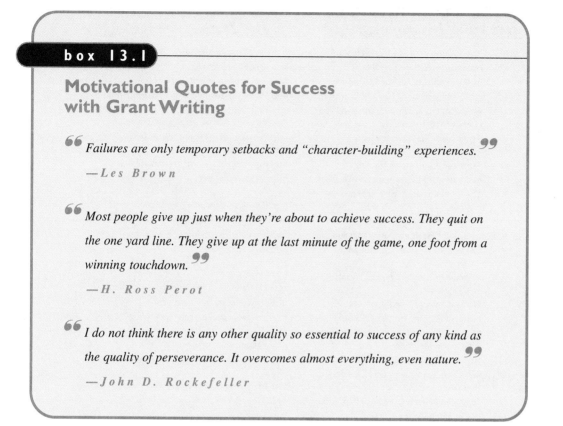

gator on the project. However, many clinicians with master's degrees make substantial contributions to federally funded studies as members of research teams that are spearheaded by doctorally prepared clinicians. For many professional organization and foundation funding sources, a master's degree is usually sufficient to obtain grant funding, although it typically fares well in the peer review of the grant proposal to have a doctorally prepared researcher as part of the team.

Potential Funding Sources

Academic medical centers, schools within university settings, and healthcare organizations frequently have internal mechanisms available to fund small research projects (e.g., pilot and feasibility studies), often through a competitive grants program. External funding agencies, such as AHRQ; foundations, such as the W.T. Grant Foundation; for-profit corporations, such as pharmaceutical companies; and professional organizations, such as the Society of Critical Care Medicine and the American Heart Association often list priorities or areas that they are interested in supporting (e.g., palliative care, pain management for critically ill patients, symptom management, and HIV risk reduction).

table 13.1   Internet links to a variety of potential funding agencies

Type	Organization	Internet Link
M	National Institute of Mental Health	http://gopher.nimh.nih.gov/grants/grants.cfm
V	National Institutes of Health	http://grants1.nih.gov/grants/funding/funding.htm
M	National Alliance for the Mentally Ill	http://www.nami.org/research/policy.html
V	National Institute of Nursing Research[1]	http://www.nih.gov/ninr/research/diversity.html
D	American Nurses Foundation (American Nurses Association)	http://www.nursingworld.org/anf/grtdev.htm
V	Sigma Theta Tau International[2]	http://www.nursingsociety.org/research/research_grants.html
D	American Academy of Nursing	http://www.nursingworld.org/aan/aafel02.htm
M	International Nurses Society on Addictions	http://www.intnsa.org/
P	The Administration for Children and Families	http://www.acf.dhhs.gov/grants.html#grants
G	Administration on Aging	http://www.aoa.dhhs.gov/
V	Agency for Healthcare Research and Quality	http://www.ahcpr.gov/fund/funding.htm
V	Centers for Disease Control and Prevention	http://www.cdc.gov/
M	Substance Abuse and Mental Health Services Administration	http://www.samhsa.gov/funding/funding.html
G	National Institute on Aging	http://www.nia.nih.gov/research/
M	National Institute on Drug Abuse	http://www.drugabuse.gov/funding.html
V	National Center for Complementary and Alternative Medicine	http://nccam.nih.gov/research/
M	Alzheimer's Association	http://www.alz.org/Researchers/overview.htm
M	American Academy of Child & Adolescent Psychiatry	http://www.aacap.org/research/index.htm
D	American Nurses Credentialing Center	http://www.ana.org/ancc/grants.htm
D	National League for Nursing	http://www.nln.org/aboutnln/grants.htm
M	American Psychiatric Association	http://www.psych.org/res_res/index.cfm
V	The Foundation Center[3]	http://www.fdncenter.org/
V	GrantsNet[4]	http://www.grantsnet.org/
V	The Robert Wood Johnson Foundation	http://www.rwjf.org/index.jsp
V	Federal Register[5]	http://www.access.gpo.gov/su_docs/aces/aces140.html
P	Annie E. Casey Foundation	http://www.aecf.org/
O	Oncology Nursing Society	http://www.ons.org/xp6/ONS/Research.xml/Funding_Opportunities.xml
O	American Cancer Society	http://www.cancer.org/eprise/main/docroot/RES/RES_5?sitearea=RES
O	American Association for Cancer Research	http://www.aacr.org/
V	University of Rochester Medical Center/Project Believe	http://www.rochester.edu

KEY: D = Nursing issues (e.g., recruitment/retention, competencies, etc.), G = Geriatric, O = Oncology, M = Mental health, P = Pediatric, V = Multitype (nonspecific, general categories)
1. Offers special programs for minority research opportunities
2. Also sponsors joint partner grants
3. Paid membership to access database of opportunities
4. Free membership to access database of opportunities
5. Official daily publication for all federal agency funding notices

Establishing a list of potential funding agencies whose priorities are matched with the type of study or project that you are interested in conducting will enhance chances for success. Internet links to a variety of potential funding agencies/organizations are listed in Table 13-1.

Additional helpful resources are databases that match a clinician's interests with federal and foundation research grant opportunities. Two databases that most universities have available to provide this type of matching include the Sponsored Programs Information Network (SPIN) and Genius Smarts. With information from more than 2,500 different sponsoring agencies, SPIN facilitates the identification of potential grants in an individual's area of interest, once specified in the database. Genius Smarts sends e-mail messages to persons who are registered in the SPIN database whenever there is a match between the identified areas of interest and potential funding opportunities. Another continuously updated database that is accessible on the Internet is GrantsNet, a resource of funding opportunities in biomedical research.

Available at **http://www.grantsnet.org** and free of charge, GrantsNet provides excellent grant-writing tools and tips.

The Foundation Center Online found at **http://fdncenter.org/** assists individuals in learning about and locating foundations that are a match with their individual interests.

The Foundation Center's mission is to support and improve institutional philanthropic efforts by promoting public understanding of the field and assisting grant applicants to succeed. Helpful online education and tutorials on grant writing also are available at this Web site. Online registration is free to the Foundation Center.

Application Criteria

Before proceeding with an application to a specific funding agency or organization, the criteria required to apply for a grant needs to be identified. For example, to be eligible for a research grant from some professional organizations, membership in the organization is required. In addition, some foundations require that the grant applicant live in a particular geographical area to apply for funding. Obtaining this type of information as well as conducting a background investigation on a particular organization or foundation will save precious time and energy in that grant applications will be submitted only to sources that match your interest area and qualifications.

Some grant writers find it helpful to contact an individual from the agency or to write a letter of inquiry that contains an abstract of the proposed project before actually writing and submitting the full proposal for funding. The names and contact information for program officers (i.e., the program development/administration contact personnel for grant applicants) are typically listed on the agency's home Web page. Although some individuals prefer to write the grant abstract after the entire proposal is completed, others find it worthwhile to develop the abstract first and seek up-front consultation about the project's compatibility with a potential funding agency's interests.

Importance of the Abstract

The proposal's abstract is key to the success of the proposal and should create a compelling case for why the project needs to be funded. Important components of the abstract should include:

- Clinical significance of the project
- Study's aims or hypotheses/study questions
- Conceptual or **theoretical framework**
- Design and methods, including sample and outcome variables to be measured, as well as the intervention if the study is a clinical trial
- Approach to analyses

Finding a Match

If the preconsultation indicates that the proposed work is not a good match for the potential funding agency, fight off discouragement. Much time and energy will be saved in developing a grant proposal for an agency that is interested in the project as opposed to one that is not. Because grant funding is very competitive, consider targeting several potential funding sources to which your proposal can be submitted simultaneously. However, first determine whether multiple submissions of essentially the same proposal to different funding agencies are allowable by carefully reading the guidelines for submission or asking the program officer from the funding source. Also, keep in mind that various agencies may be willing to fund specific parts of the overall project budget.

Once potential funding agencies are identified, it is extremely beneficial to obtain copies of successfully funded proposals if available. Review of these proposals for substantive quality as well as layout and formatting often strengthens the proposal, especially for first-time grant applicants. Federal agencies (e.g., NIH, AHRQ) will provide copies of successfully funded proposals upon request.

> A copy of a well-written NIH grant can be accessed at **http://www.niaid.nih.gov/ncn/grants/app/app.pdf.** In addition, abstracts of past and currently funded federal proposals are available at http://crisp.cit.nih.gov/.

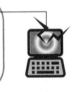

For copies of grants funded by professional organizations and foundations, requests should be made directly to the investigator(s). Abstracts of currently funded projects from professional organizations and foundations are often available on their Web sites or publicized in their newsletters.

Guidelines for Submission

Before writing the proposal, guidelines for grant submission should be obtained from each potential funding source (e.g., length of the proposal, desired font, specifications on margins), reviewed carefully, and followed meticulously. Some funding agencies will return grants if all directions are not followed, which may delay evaluation of the grant proposal until the next re-view cycle. Also, be sure that the grant proposal looks pleasing aesthetically and does not con-tain grammatical and typographical errors. A well-organized proposal that is clear and free of er-rors indicates to reviewers that the actual project will be carried out with the same meticulous detail (Cummings, Holly, & Hulley, 2001).

> Tips and answers to frequently asked questions for new applicants who are applying to the NIH for grant funding can be obtained at:
> **http://www.nigms.nih.gov/funding/tips.html**
> **http://www.niaid.nih.gov/ncn/grants/plan/plan_i3.htm**

Criteria for Rating and Reviewing

In addition to obtaining the guidelines for grant submission, ask whether the funding agency provides grant applicants with the criteria on which grants are rated and reviewed.

> The NIH publishes the review criteria on which grant applications are rated by reviewers at **http://grants1.nih.gov/grants/guide/notice-files/not97-010.html**. These criteria are fairly typical of other rating systems used by multiple funding agencies and include:
>
> - Significance of the study
> - Approach (e.g., design and methods)
> - Innovation
> - Investigator
> - Environment (e.g., whether adequate resources are available to support the project's success)

Develop the Outline

Before writing the proposal, it is helpful to develop an outline that includes each component of the grant application with a timeline and deadline for completion. If working within a team, the lead investigator can then assign specific sections of the grant proposal to various team mem-bers. Team members should be informed that before the final product is ready for submission, the document may require several revisions.

As a rule of thumb, it is important to avoid the "old and predictable." Grant reviewers look favorably on projects that are innovative.

In addition, never assume that the reviewers will know what you mean when you are writing the grant. Writing with clarity and providing rationales for the decisions that you have made about your design and methods are instrumental to receiving a positive grant review.

At the same time, avoid promising too much or too little within the context of the grant. Thinking that it is advantageous to accomplish a multitude of goals within one study is a commonly held belief, but projects that are so ambitious in scope that feasibility is in question tend to fare poorly in review.

Any time your team lacks a particular expertise related to your project, it is important to obtain expert consultants who can provide guidance in needed areas. These individuals can critique the proposal to strengthen the application before it is submitted. Of additional benefit is a mock review in which successful grant writers and others with expertise in the project area are convened to critique the grant's strengths and limitations. With this type of feedback, you can strengthen the grant application before it is ever submitted for funding consideration. Another strategy is to ask individuals with no expertise in the project area to read the grant proposal and provide feedback on its clarity.

Some individuals find it helpful to place a draft of the grant aside for a few days, then read it again. A fresh perspective a few days later is often invaluable in making final revisions. Additionally, obtaining an editorial review of the grant proposal before submitting it is important in achieving the strongest possible product. See Box 13-2 for a summary of general strategies for successful grant writing.

Specific Steps in Writing a Successful Grant Proposal

The typical components of a grant proposal are listed in Box 13-3. Although not all of these components may be required for every grant, it is helpful to consider each one when planning the project.

The Abstract

A large amount of time should be invested in developing a clear, compelling, comprehensive, and concise abstract of the project. Because it is a preview of what is to come, the abstract needs to pique the interest and excitement of the reviewers so that they will be compelled to read the rest of the grant application. A poorly written abstract will immediately set the tone for the review and may bias the reviewers to judge the full proposal negatively or dissuade them from reading the rest of the proposal, given that reviewers typically review multiple grant applications simultaneously. Please see Box 13-4 for two examples of grant abstracts from funded grants that are clear and comprehensive but concise and compelling.

Table of Contents

The table of contents containing the components of the grant and corresponding page numbers must be completed accurately so that a reviewer who wants to refer back to a section of the grant can easily identify and access it.

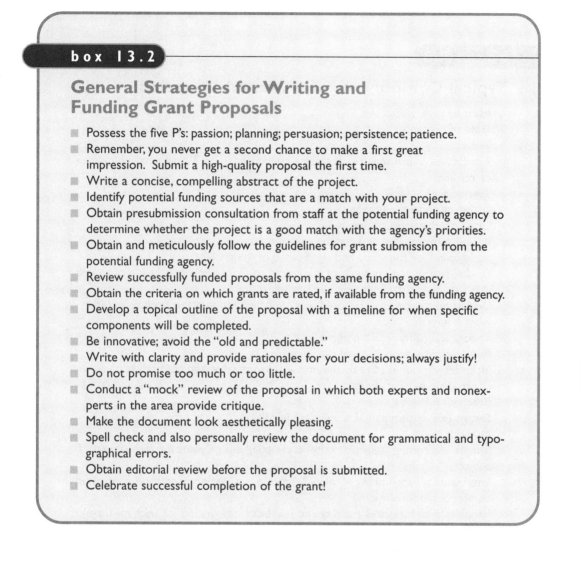

box 13.2

General Strategies for Writing and Funding Grant Proposals

- Possess the five P's: passion; planning; persuasion; persistence; patience.
- Remember, you never get a second chance to make a first great impression. Submit a high-quality proposal the first time.
- Write a concise, compelling abstract of the project.
- Identify potential funding sources that are a match with your project.
- Obtain presubmission consultation from staff at the potential funding agency to determine whether the project is a good match with the agency's priorities.
- Obtain and meticulously follow the guidelines for grant submission from the potential funding agency.
- Review successfully funded proposals from the same funding agency.
- Obtain the criteria on which grants are rated, if available from the funding agency.
- Develop a topical outline of the proposal with a timeline for when specific components will be completed.
- Be innovative; avoid the "old and predictable."
- Write with clarity and provide rationales for your decisions; always justify!
- Do not promise too much or too little.
- Conduct a "mock" review of the proposal in which both experts and nonexperts in the area provide critique.
- Make the document look aesthetically pleasing.
- Spell check and also personally review the document for grammatical and typographical errors.
- Obtain editorial review before the proposal is submitted.
- Celebrate successful completion of the grant!

Budget

Many hospitals and universities have research centers or offices with an administrator specifically skilled in developing budgets for grant proposals. It is helpful to seek the assistance of this person, if available, when developing the budget for your project to avoid over- or underestimating costs. Knowing which expenses the funding organization will and will not cover is important before developing the budget. This information is often included in the potential funder's guidelines for grant submission.

Most budgets are delineated into two categories: personnel and nonpersonnel (e.g., travel, costs associated with purchasing instruments, honoraria for the subjects). Many profes-

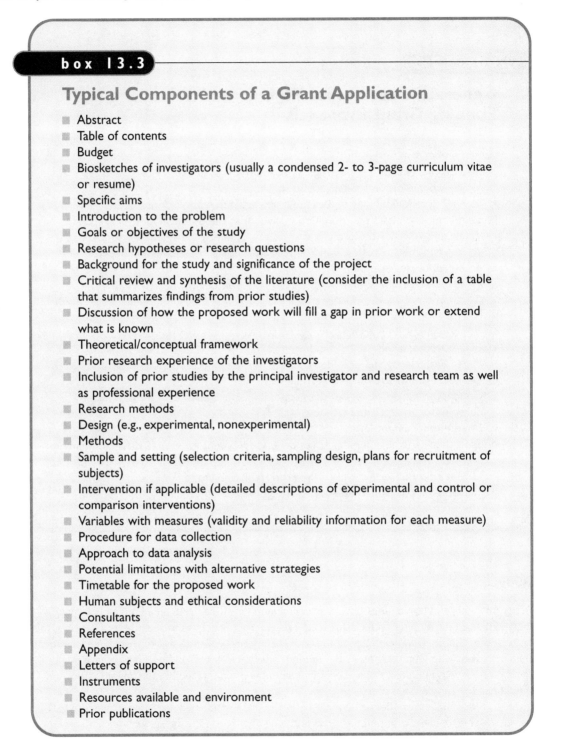

box 13.3

Typical Components of a Grant Application

- Abstract
- Table of contents
- Budget
- Biosketches of investigators (usually a condensed 2- to 3-page curriculum vitae or resume)
- Specific aims
- Introduction to the problem
- Goals or objectives of the study
- Research hypotheses or research questions
- Background for the study and significance of the project
- Critical review and synthesis of the literature (consider the inclusion of a table that summarizes findings from prior studies)
- Discussion of how the proposed work will fill a gap in prior work or extend what is known
- Theoretical/conceptual framework
- Prior research experience of the investigators
- Inclusion of prior studies by the principal investigator and research team as well as professional experience
- Research methods
- Design (e.g., experimental, nonexperimental)
- Methods
- Sample and setting (selection criteria, sampling design, plans for recruitment of subjects)
- Intervention if applicable (detailed descriptions of experimental and control or comparison interventions)
- Variables with measures (validity and reliability information for each measure)
- Procedure for data collection
- Approach to data analysis
- Potential limitations with alternative strategies
- Timetable for the proposed work
- Human subjects and ethical considerations
- Consultants
- References
- Appendix
- Letters of support
- Instruments
- Resources available and environment
- Prior publications

box 13.4

Examples of Grant Abstracts from Two Funded Studies

FUNCTIONAL OUTCOMES AFTER INTENSIVE CARE AMONG ELDERS

Funded by the American Nurses Foundation (Principal investigator: Diane Mick, PhD, RN,CCNS, GNP; Total costs = $2,700).

Objective: Both age and probability of benefit have been suggested as criteria for allocation of healthcare resources. This study will evaluate elders' functional outcomes after intensive care in an effort to discern benefit or futility of interventions.

Methods: A descriptive correlational design will be used. Subjects who are 65 years of age will be identified as "elderly" or "frail elderly" on admission to the Intensive Care Unit (ICU), using Katz's Index of Activities of Daily Living (ADL) scale. Illness severity will be quantified using the Acute Physiology and Chronic Health Evaluation II Scale (APACHE II). Functional status at admission and at discharge from the ICU, and at 1-month and 3-month post-ICU discharge intervals will be quantified with the Medical Outcomes Study 36-Item Short-Form Health Survey (SF-36). Significance of relationships among age, frailty, gender, illness severity, and functional outcomes will be determined, as well as which patient characteristics and clinical factors are predictive of high levels of physical functioning after ICU discharge.

Significance: Findings may be useful as an adjunct to clinical decision making. As the clinicians who are closest to critically ill elderly patients, nurses are positioned to facilitate dialogue about elderly patients' wishes and expectations.

IMPROVING OUTCOMES OF LOW-BIRTH-WEIGHT (LBW) PREMATURE INFANTS AND PARENTS

Funded by the National Institutes of Health/National Institute of Nursing Research; Principal investigator: Bernadette Melnyk, PhD, CPNP, NPP, FAAN; Co-investigators: Linda Alpert-Gillis, PhD, and Nancy Feinstein, PhD, RN-C (R01#05077); Total costs = $2.44 million.

Although the mortality rate of LBW premature infants has declined dramatically over the past several years, morbidity remains high as the result of negative cognitive, neurodevelopmental, and behavioral sequelae. Studies indicate that parents of LBW premature infants experience multiple ongoing stressors that result in short- and long-term negative coping outcomes, such as anxiety and depression, as well as dysfunctional parenting patterns. In the proposed study, we will build upon our prior work and previous studies that have supported the positive

(continued)

---

box 13.4 *(continued)*

benefits of educational-behavioral interventions with mothers of hospitalized young children and LBW premature infants. Among the unique contributions of this study include: (a) development of a theoretically driven, reproducible intervention that can be easily translated into clinical practice and widely disseminated, (b) evaluation of our intervention with fathers/significant others as well as mothers, (c) a prospective cost-effectiveness analysis, and (d) an intervention that begins early in the NICU stay, prior to parents developing negative perceptions of their infants and the establishment of ineffective parent-infant interactions.

The primary aim of this multisite study is to evaluate the effects of a theoretically driven, reproducible intervention (COPE = Creating Opportunities for Parent Empowerment) on the process and outcomes of mothers and fathers/significant others' coping with a LBW premature infant and infant developmental outcomes. The secondary aims are to: (a) explore how the coping process and outcomes of mothers and fathers together contribute to the outcomes of LBW premature infants, (b) determine the cost-effectiveness of the COPE program, and (c) explore what factors moderate the effects of the intervention program (e.g., temperament, family structure, SES). A two-group experiment will be used with 240 mothers and 240 fathers/significant others of LBW premature infants in the NICU. Measures of both process and outcome variables, including parental beliefs, anxiety, depression, parent-infant interaction, and infant developmental outcomes will be assessed during hospitalization and up to the infants' 2-year corrected ages. Findings from a recent pilot study with 42 mother-infant dyads support undertaking this full-scale clinical trial in that mothers who received the COPE program versus those who received a comparison program had more positive coping outcomes, and their infants scored significantly (14 points) higher on the Mental Development Index of the Bayley Scales of Infant Development at 6 months corrected age.

---

sional organizations pay only for **direct costs** (i.e., those costs directly required to conduct the study, such as personnel, travel, photocopying, instruments, and subject fees) and not for **indirect costs** (i.e., those costs that are not directly related to the actual conduct of the study but are associated with the "overhead" in an organization, such as lights, telephones, office space). Reviewers will critically analyze whether there are appropriate and adequate personnel to carry out the study and whether the costs requested are allowable and reasonable. In applying for small grants from professional organizations and foundations, which may not provide enough funds to cover a portion of the salaries for the investigators/clinicians who will implement the project, it is important to negotiate release time with administrators during the preparation of the grant so that there will be ample time to successfully complete the project if funded. Typically, subscriptions to journals, professional organization memberships, and entertainment are examples of nonallowable costs. See Table 13-2 for an example of a grant application's proposed budget.

table 13.2 Example of a grant application's proposed budget

Example of a Grant Application's Proposed Budget

Principal Investigator
Funding Agency
Submission Date

Earliest Start Date

Personnel	Role on Project	Type of Appt	% of Effort	$ Base Salary	$ Salary	Benefit Rate	$ Benefits	$ Total Sal &Ben
				First Year				
Mary Smith	Principal Investigator	12	0.05	68,000	3,400	28.50%	969	4,369
Roberta Picarazzi	Co-Investigator	12	0.05	68,000	3,400	28.50%	969	4,369
TBA (24 hours @$38)	Research Associate	12			912	28.50%	260	1,172
TBA (49 hours @$18/hr)	Research Assistant	12			882	31.00%	273	1,155
					0		0	0
					8,594		2,471	11,065

Consultant Costs			0
NA			
Equipment			0
NA			
Supplies			50
General Office Supplies		50	
Travel			0
Local			
Domestic			
Other Expenses			4,350
Lab Supplies			
Pharmacy Setup Fee		500	
Drug/material costs and labor	$15/day x 3 days	3600	Sample Size = 80
Photocopying		50	
Instrument for data collection			
Patient Satisfaction Tool			
Human Subjects Consent Form			
Presentation Materials (poster & slides)		200	
SUBTOTAL DIRECT COSTS FOR INITIAL BUDGET PERIOD			15,465
Consortium/Contractual Costs			
Direct Costs			
Indirect Costs			
TOTAL DIRECT COSTS FOR INITIAL BUDGET PERIOD			15,465
Less Equipment Costs			15,465
Indirect Costs			–

Biosketches of the Principal Investigator and Research Team Members

For the review panel to assess the qualifications of the research team so that it can make a judgment about the team's ability to conduct the proposed project, **biosketches** are typically required as part of the grant application. A biosketch is a condensed two- to three-page document, similar to a resume or brief curriculum vita, that captures the individual's educational and professional work experience, honors, prior research grants, and publications.

Introduction and Specific Aims

The significance of the problem should be immediately introduced in the grant proposal so that the reviewers can make the judgment that the project is worth funding right from the beginning of the proposal. For example, the following introduction is quickly convincing of the need for more intervention studies with teenagers who use tobacco.

> Approximately 3,000 adolescents become regular tobacco users every day. Evidence from prior studies indicates that teens who smoke are more likely to abuse other substances, such as alcohol and drugs, than teens who do not smoke. There also is accumulating evidence that morbidities associated with cigarette smoking include hypertension, hypercholesteremia, and lung and heart disease.

In the introduction to the grant, it also is important to be clear about what it is that the study will accomplish (i.e., the goals or objectives). For example, "This proposal will evaluate the effects of a conceptually driven, reproducible intervention program on smoking cessation in 15- to 18-year-old adolescents."

Background and Significance

In this section of the grant proposal, it is important to convince the reviewers that the problem being presented is worthy of study in that the findings are likely to improve the clinical practice and/or health outcomes of a specific population. How the proposal will extend the science in the area or positively impact clinical practice should be explicitly stated. In addition, a comprehensive but concise review of prior studies in the area should be presented, along with a critical analysis of their major strengths and limitations, including the gaps of prior work. It is beneficial to use a table to summarize the sample, design, measures, outcomes, and major limitations of prior studies. The literature review must clearly provide justification for the proposed study's aims, hypotheses, and/or research questions.

The inclusion of a well-defined conceptual or theoretical framework is important in guiding the study and explaining study findings. If a separate section devoted to the conceptual or theoretical framework is not specified in the guidelines for grant submission, it is typically included in the background section of the proposal. When crafted appropriately, it is clear how the theoretical/conceptual framework is driving the study hypotheses, the intervention if applicable, and/or the relationship between the proposed study variables. This section of the grant also should include definitions of the constructs being measured, along with a description of how the constructs to be studied relate to one another.

For example, if an individual is using a coping framework to study the effects of a stress-reduction intervention program with working women, it would be important in the theoretical framework to state that coping comprises two functions: emotional coping, which regulates emotional responses, such as anxiety and depression; and functional coping, which is the solving of problems, such as the ability to demonstrate high-quality work performance. Therefore, a study of working women that uses this coping framework should evaluate the effects of the stress-reduction program on the outcome measures of anxiety, depression, and work performance.

The background section should conclude with the study's **hypotheses,** which are statements about the predicted relationships between the **independent** and **dependent** or outcome variables. Hypotheses should be clear, testable, and plausible. The following is an example of a well-written hypothesis.

> Family caregivers who receive the CARE program (i.e., the independent variable) will report less depressive symptoms (i.e., the dependent variable) than family caregivers who receive the comparison program at two months following their relative's discharge from the hospital.

When there is not enough prior literature on which to formulate a hypothesis, the investigator may instead present a research question to be answered by the project. For example, if no prior intervention studies have been conducted with family caregivers of hospitalized elders, it may be more appropriate to ask the research question, What is the effect of an educational intervention on anxiety and depressive symptoms in family caregivers of hospitalized elders? than to propose a hypothesis.

Prior Research Experience

A summary of prior work conducted by the principal investigator or project coordinator as well as the research team members and/or their professional experience should be included in the grant application. Inclusion of this type of information demonstrates that a solid foundation has been laid on which to conduct the proposed study and leaves the reviewers feeling confident that the research team will be able to complete the work that it is proposing.

Study Design and Methods

The design of the study should be clearly described. For example, "This is a randomized clinical trial with repeated measures at 3 and 6 months following discharge from the neonatal intensive care unit." Another example might be, "The purpose of this 6-month project is to determine the effect of implementing interdisciplinary rounds on care delivery and patient outcomes in the burn/trauma unit of a large tertiary hospital."

In discussing the study's methods, it is important to provide rationales for the selected methods so that the reviewers will know that you have critically thought about potential options and made the best decision, based on your critical analysis. Nothing should be left to the reviewers' imagination, and all decisions should be justified.

If the proposed study is an intervention trial, it is very important to discuss the strategies that will be undertaken to strengthen the **internal validity** of the study (i.e., the ability to say that it was the independent variable or the treatment that caused a change in the dependent variable, not other extraneous factors). Please see Chapter 10 for a discussion of strategies to minimize threats to internal validity in quantitative studies.

The sample should be described in this section of the proposal, including its inclusion criteria (i.e., who will be included in the study) and exclusion criteria (i.e., who will be excluded from participation), as well as exactly how the subjects will be recruited into the study. The feasibility of recruiting the targeted number of subjects also should be discussed, and support letters confirming access to the sample should be included in the grant application's appendix. In addition, a description of how subjects from both genders as well as diverse cultural groups will be included is essential. If people younger than 21 years will not be included in the research sample, it is imperative to provide a strong rationale for their exclusion because Public Law 103-43 requires that women and children be included in studies funded by the federal government. In quantitative studies, a **power analysis** (i.e., a procedure for estimating sample size) should always be included (Cohen, 1992). This calculation is critical so that the reviewers will know that there is an adequate sample size for the statistical analysis. Remember, **power** (i.e., the ability of a study to detect existing relationships among variables and thereby reject the null hypothesis that there is no relationship [Polit & Beck, 2003]) in a study increases when sample size increases. Many clinical research studies do not obtain significant findings solely because the sample size is not large enough and the study does not have adequate power to detect significant relationships between variables.

Next, the sampling design (e.g., **random** or **convenience sampling**) should be described. When it is not possible to randomly sample subjects when conducting a research study, strategies to increase representativeness of the sample and enhance **external validity** (i.e., **generalizability**) should be discussed. For example, the investigators might choose to recruit subjects from a second study site.

For intervention studies/clinical trials, the intervention must be clearly described. Discussion about how the theoretical/conceptual framework guided the development of the intervention is beneficial in assisting the reviewers to see a clear connection between them. Issues of reproducibility and feasibility of the proposed intervention also should be discussed. In addition, it is important to include information about what the comparison or control group will receive throughout the study.

For intervention studies, it is important to provide details regarding how the integrity of the intervention will be maintained (i.e., the intervention will be delivered in the same manner to all subjects), as well as assurance that the intervention will be culturally sensitive. Additionally, it is important to include a discussion about what type of **manipulation checks** (i.e., assessments to determine whether subjects actually processed the content of the intervention or followed through with the activities prescribed in the intervention program) will be used in the study. **"Booster" interventions** (i.e., additional interventions at timed intervals after the initial intervention) are a good idea to include in the study's design if long-term benefits of an intervention are desired.

It is important to include how outcomes of the study will be measured. If using formal instruments, description of each measure must be included in the grant proposal, including **face, content,** and **construct validity** (i.e., Does the instrument measure what it is intended to measure?) and **reliability** (i.e., Does the instrument measure the construct consistently?). In addition, a description of the scoring of each of the instruments should be included, along with their cultural sensitivity. Justification for why a certain measure was selected is important, especially if there are multiple valid and reliable instruments available that tap the same construct. If collecting patient outcomes, descriptions of how, when, and by whom the data will be collected should be included in the proposal.

Internal consistency reliability (i.e., the degree to which all the subparts of an instrument are measuring the same attribute [Polit & Beck, 2003] of an instrument) should be at least 70%, whereas **inter-rater reliability** (i.e., the degree to which two different observers assign the same ratings to an attribute being measured or observed [Polit & Beck, 2003]) should be at least 90% and assessed routinely to correct for any **observer drift** (i.e., a decrease in inter-rater reliability). For intervention studies, it is important to include measures that are sensitive to change over time (i.e., those with low test–retest reliabilities) so that the intervention can demonstrate its ability to affect the study's outcome variables.

When conducting research, both self-report as well as nonbiased observation measures should be included whenever possible because convergence on both of these types of measures will increase the credibility of the study's findings. In addition, the use of valid and reliable instruments is preferred whenever possible over the use of instruments that are newly developed and lacking established validity and reliability.

The procedure or protocol for the study should be clearly described. Specific information about the timing of data collection for all measures should be discussed. Using a table helps to summarize the study protocol in a concise snapshot so that reviewers can quickly grasp when the study's measures will be collected (see Table 13-3).

The description of data analysis must include specific and clear explanations about how the data to answer each of the study hypotheses or research questions will be analyzed. Adding a statistical consultant to your study team who can assist with the writing of the statistical section and the analysis of the study's data will fare favorably in the review process.

Even if the guidelines for the proposal do not call for it, it is very advantageous to include a section in the grant that discusses potential limitations of the proposal with alternative approaches. By doing so, it demonstrates to the reviewers that potential limitations of the study have been recognized, along with plans for alternative strategies that will be employed to overcome them. For example, inclusion of strategies to guard against study attrition (i.e., loss of subjects from your study) would be important to discuss in this section.

A timetable that indicates when specific components of the study will be started and completed should be included in the grant application (see Figure 13-1). This projected timeline should be realistic and feasible.

Human Subjects

When writing a research proposal, it is essential to discuss the risks and benefits of study participation, protection against risks, and the importance of the knowledge to be gained from the study. The demographics of the sample that you intend to recruit into your study also are very important to describe in the proposal. In addition, the process through which informed consent will be obtained needs to be discussed, along with how confidentiality of the data will be maintained. Some funding agencies require the proposal to have been reviewed and approved by an

table 13.3   A summary table of a study's protocol

Example of a study protocol for a randomized controlled trial to determine the effects of an intervention program on the coping outcomes of young critically ill children and their mothers

Variables	Measures	Cronbach's Alphas	Time 1	2	3	4	5	6	7	8	9
Maternal Emotional Outcomes											
State Anxiety	State Anxiety Inventory (A-State)	.94–.96	•	•	•	•		•	•	•	•
Negative Mood State	Profile of Mood States (POMS, Short Form)	.92–.96	•	•	•	•		•	•	•	•
Depression	Depression Subscale, Profile of Mood States (POMS)	.92–.96	•	•	•	•	•	•	•		•
Stress Related to PICU	Parental Stressor Scale: PICU (PSS:PICU)	.90–.91	•	•							
Posthospitalization Stress	Posthospitalization Stress Index for Parents (PSI-P)	.83–.85	•	•	•	•					
Maternal Functional Outcomes											
Parent Participation in Care	Index of Parent Participation (IPP)	.85	•	•							
Other Key Maternal Variables											
Parental Beliefs	Parental Beliefs Scale (PBS)	.91	•								
Manipulation Checks Evaluation	Manipulation Checks Self-report	NA	•	•	•	•					
	Questionnaire	NA	•	•	•	•	•				
Child Adjustment Outcomes											
Posthospital Stress	Posthospital Stress Index for Children (PSI-C)	.78–.85	•	•	•	•					
Child Behavior	Behavioral Assessment Scale for Children (BASC)	.92–.95	•	•	•	•	•				

Time 1 = Phase I Intervention (6–16 hours after PICU admission)
Time 2 = Phase II Intervention (16–30 hours after PICU admission)
Time 3 = Phase III Intervention (2–6 hours after transfer to Pediatric Unit)
Time 4 = Observation Contact (24 – 36 hours after transfer to Pediatric Unit)
Time 5 = Phase III Intervention (2–3 days following Hospital Discharge)
Time 6 = 1 Month Postdischarge Follow-up (1 month following Hospital Discharge)
Time 7 = 3 Months Postdischarge Follow-up (3 months following Hospital Discharge)
Time 8 = 6 Months Postdischarge Follow-up (6 months following Hospital Discharge)
Time 9 = 12 Months Postdischarge Follow-up (12 months following Hospital Discharge)

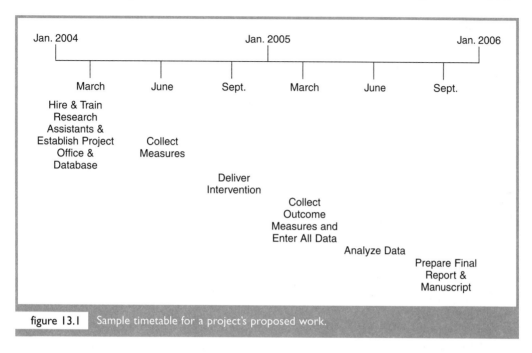

Jan. 2004   Jan. 2005   Jan. 2006

March   June   Sept.   March   June   Sept.

Hire & Train
Research
Assistants &
Establish Project
Office &
Database

Collect
Measures

Deliver
Intervention

Collect
Outcome
Measures and
Enter All Data

Analyze Data

Prepare Final
Report &
Manuscript

figure 13.1   Sample timetable for a project's proposed work.

appropriate research subjects review board, and others require proof of approval if funding is awarded before commencement of the project.

In addition, if a study is a clinical trial, federal agencies (e.g., NIH) require a **data and safety monitoring plan,** which outlines how adverse effects will be assessed and managed.

If applying to the NIH for funding, Public Law 103-43 requires that women and minorities need to be included in all studies unless there is acceptable scientific justification provided as to why their inclusion is not feasible or appropriate with regard to the health of the subjects or the purpose of the research. NIH also requires that children under the age of 21 years be included in research unless there are ethical or scientific reasons for their exclusion.

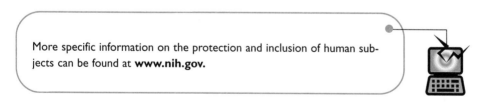

More specific information on the protection and inclusion of human subjects can be found at **www.nih.gov.**

Consultants, References, and Appendices

A section for consultants is often included in grant applications. The expertise and role of each consultant on the project should be described.

Each citation referenced in the grant proposal should be included in the reference list. All references should be accurate, complete, and formatted according to the guidelines for submission (e.g., American Psychological Association [APA] or American Medical Association [AMA] formatting).

Grant applications typically require or allow the investigator to include letters of support from consultants or study sites, copies of instruments that will be used in the study, lists of resources available, and publications of the research team that support the application. Support letters from consultants indicate to the reviewers that they are enthusiastic about the proposed study or project and that they are committed to their role on the project. Letters of support from study sites are helpful to indicate enthusiasm for the study and permission for subjects to be recruited from those sites.

Common Feedback from Grant Reviews

This section of the chapter describes feedback that is commonly provided by reviewers of federal grants and some professional organizations. It is organized according to typical categories used for rating grant applications. The purposes of feedback from a grant review should be to facilitate the professional growth of the investigator as well as to strengthen the proposed study and improve patient care (Mick & Ackerman, 1999).

Significance
Reviewers typically judge the significance of a project by whether the study addresses an important problem or extends what is known in the area. Common feedback in this category may include the following statements:

- The literature does not capture the entire body of information on the selected concepts.
- The argument for why an intervention in this particular population is needed is not strong.
- It is not clear how this study or project builds on prior work in the area.

Approach
Common feedback regarding a research study's approach (e.g., conceptual framework, design, methods, and analyses) typically includes:

- There is no, or a weak, conceptual/theoretical framework.
- The theory does not drive the intervention proposed or the selection of study variables.
- The study design is weak.
- Some of the details for the methods are unclear.
- The sample size is not adequate to test the hypotheses.
- The measures are not adequately described.
- The data analysis section needs a fuller discussion.
- The number of measures being used creates too much burden for the subjects.
- The project is too ambitious for the timetable proposed.

In addition, comments from reviewers about intervention studies typically focus on concerns about cross-contamination between the experimental and control groups (e.g., sharing of experimental information), reproducibility and feasibility of the intervention, and cultural sensitivity.

Innovation

In rating a project's innovation (i.e., whether the project employs novel approaches or methods), common feedback from reviewers includes statements such as:

- The intervention has already been tested in other populations, and the investigator is not really adding much of anything new to what has been done.
- The investigator is not convincing in the presentation of evidence that this study needs to be done.
- The use of a videotape to deliver the intervention is not necessarily innovative, given the wide array of print and media currently available.

Investigators and Institutional Support

Finally, comments about the investigator and research team frequently discuss whether the investigators are appropriately skilled and suited to conduct the work being proposed. In addition, reviewers typically comment on whether the environment is conducive to support the work being proposed (e.g., whether there is evidence of enough resources and institutional support for the project).

Major Pitfalls of Grant Proposals

There are numerous weaknesses in grant proposals that limit their ability to fare well during the review process. Box 13-5 outlines these common pitfalls.

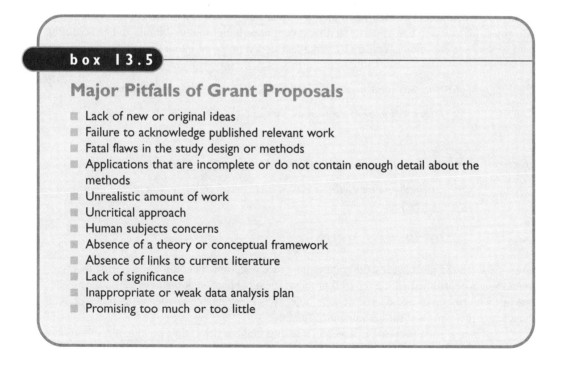

box 13.5

Major Pitfalls of Grant Proposals

- Lack of new or original ideas
- Failure to acknowledge published relevant work
- Fatal flaws in the study design or methods
- Applications that are incomplete or do not contain enough detail about the methods
- Unrealistic amount of work
- Uncritical approach
- Human subjects concerns
- Absence of a theory or conceptual framework
- Absence of links to current literature
- Lack of significance
- Inappropriate or weak data analysis plan
- Promising too much or too little

Major Characteristics of Funded Grant Proposals

Unlike proposals that are weak, strong proposals have characteristics that enhance their fundability. These characteristics include:

- Creativity
- High scientific quality
- Clarity
- Excellent technical quality (e.g., organized, easy to read, and free of grammatical and spelling errors)
- Potential to impact the clinical field
- Greater depth in thinking about conceptual issues

Successful grant proposals also include a thoughtful discussion about the limitations of the proposed work, as well as strategies for dealing with potential problems without overemphasizing these issues (Cummings, Holly, & Hulley, 2001).

> Copies of successful grant applications funded by NIH as well as a variety of professional organizations can be obtained by e-mailing Bernadette Melnyk at **Bernadette_Melnyk@urmc.rochester.edu.**

A Nonfunded Grant: Strategies for Resubmission

Many individuals feel dejected when their proposals are not successful in securing funding. However, openness to constructive feedback, continued belief in one's ability to be successful, and persistence are often necessary to turn a nonfunded proposal into a funded one.

> **"***The only limit to our realization of tomorrow will be our doubts of today.***"**
>
> *Franklin Delano Roosevelt*

> **"***If you believe you can, you probably can. If you believe you won't, you most assuredly won't. Belief is the ignition switch that gets you off the launching pad.***"**
>
> *Dr. Dennis Waitley*

Even the most successful grant writers face rejection at certain times during their careers. When confronted with a rejected proposal, being able to seek the advice of a seasoned mentor who has faced and overcome grant rejections is invaluable in addressing how you will handle the revisions and further pursuit of funding.

Once a grant proposal is rejected, it is important to determine whether a resubmission will be allowed by the funding agency. If permitted, it is important to ask whether there are specific guidelines for resubmission and, if so, to obtain them. For example, the NIH allows two resubmissions of a grant proposal. Individuals who are resubmitting are allowed a certain number of pages as an introduction to the revised proposal in which they specifically respond to how they have addressed the reviewers' concerns and suggestions.

If a resubmission is allowed, it is helpful to discuss the plans for addressing the reviewers' comments with the appropriate program officer or contact person at the funding agency. Individuals from the funding agency can often provide insights into the critique and make suggestions for revision.

After reading the reviewers' feedback, recognize that it is normal to feel sad, frustrated, and/or angry about the critique. It also is common to believe that the reviewers did not read your grant thoroughly or to feel that they did not understand your work and were overly critical of it. After reading the review comments, it is helpful to file them away for a week or two until you can come back to them with an open mind to begin the process of revising the proposal.

In the introduction to the revised application, first inform the review committee that its critique has assisted you in clarifying and strengthening your proposed work. It is critical to respond point by point to the major issues raised by the review panel, without a defensive posture. If you disagree with a recommendation from the review panel, do so gently and astutely. Be sure to include a good rationale, as in the following example.

> We agree that *cross-contamination* is always a concern in clinical intervention studies and have given it thoughtful consideration. However, we believe that this potential problem can be minimized by taking several precautions. For example, we will . . .

Finally, revise the text enough so that reviewers will note that you took their suggestions seriously, but do not completely rewrite the application as though it were new. Guidelines for resubmission will often inform applicants to use a boldface or italic font to identify the content that has been changed within the context of the grant proposal.

Unhelpful responses in the resubmission process include not taking the reviewers' critique seriously by ignoring their suggestions, as well as denigrating the review panel's criticisms. In addition, changing the research design in an attempt to please the review panel without critical thought and analysis will not fare well in the re-review of the grant proposal.

Specific Considerations in Seeking Funds for Outcomes Management or Quality Improvement Projects

Outcomes management projects and quality improvement initiatives that focus on improving practice performance, including changes in care delivery modalities (e.g., team nursing versus primary nursing), system supports for the healthcare team (e.g., computerized order entry), and evaluation of the effect of a practice change on patient outcomes within a particular environment (e.g., how, when, and by whom substance abusers are educated about drug rehabilitation and its effect on the recurrence of abuse in a small county rehabilitation program) are usually not funded by federal agencies. Internal funding sources and foundations are typically the most viable places to obtain funding for these types of endeavors. The application process for a foundation can range in rigor from a one- to two-page abstract to a full-scale NIH-style grant proposal.

For internal sources of funding within one's institution (e.g., schools of nursing, academic health centers, hospitals), guidelines are usually available upon request from the research office, if one exists, or from the department that handles professional, educational, or research affairs. As with other types of grant applications, obtaining and explicitly following the guidelines for submission are essential for success. In both cases, one of the primary tenets of securing funding is that the project reflects the mission and stated goals of the organization or foundation. Specifically, the grant application needs to be an excellent match, often between what the funding source desires and what can be provided. Generally, foundations are very clear about the specific areas in which they are willing to provide fiscal support. For example, the Kellogg Foundation limits its funding to such areas as health, food systems, rural development, youth and education, philanthropy, and volunteerism. These funding areas of interest can usually be found on the foundation's Web site.

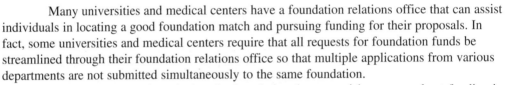

Access the Kellogg Foundation at (**http://www.wkkf.org/**).

Many universities and medical centers have a foundation relations office that can assist individuals in locating a good foundation match and pursuing funding for their proposals. In fact, some universities and medical centers require that all requests for foundation funds be streamlined through their foundation relations office so that multiple applications from various departments are not submitted simultaneously to the same foundation.

One way to determine whether the foundation that you wish to query about funding is a good match with your project is to peruse projects that were recently funded, which can typically be found on the foundation's Web site. Scanning the list of these funded projects can provide a sense of the types of projects that are currently being funded. If few to no healthcare projects are funded, realize that this may not be a good match and that more inquiry is necessary before soliciting funding from that organization. If you determine that a foundation is a good match for your project, carefully study the requirements for proposal submission. Some foundations require that the first step in the application process include only an abstract of the proposed project. If the abstract matches the organization's goals and is reviewed favorably, the applicant may be asked to provide a more detailed proposal. However, some foundations or organizations may provide funding based on the abstract alone, especially if the budget request is small (e.g., under $10,000). Other foundations require a full-scale proposal, including detailed budgets and biographical sketches for the project director and team members. By carefully following the guidelines provided by the organization, the chance of funding will increase.

Keep in mind that most foundations require that the sponsoring organization meet the regulations of the United States Internal Revenue Service as a 501c3 organization (i.e., tax exempt). When preparing to seek foundation funding, be aware that many foundations seldom provide large funding relative in size to federal grants. In perusing foundation Web sites, you may note that, on average, most foundation grants range between $500 and $50,000.

An example of an organization that funds initiatives such as outcomes management or quality improvement projects is the American Association of Critical Care Nurses (AACN).

Information about AACN's small grant opportunities can be found at **http://www.aacn.org** along with specific requirements for submission.

Funding for Performance Improvement Projects

Performance improvement projects are typically clinical projects that use research findings to improve clinical practice. They are usually conceived in response to an identified clinical problem. Unlike research studies that have a goal to generate new knowledge, performance improvement projects are usually meant to solve clinical problems through the application of existing research-based knowledge (e.g., evidence-based clinical practice guidelines).

The recent application of the pain management guidelines developed by AHRQ to healthcare settings nationwide is a good example of a performance improvement project in action. These guidelines were based on sound scientific evidence and developed by nationally known clinical experts. Managers, clinical specialists, and educators then implemented the published guidelines in their clinical settings, measuring clinical outcomes pre- and postimplementation.

Sources that fund project performance improvement projects, such as AACN's Small Project Grants, do not generally require the scientific rigor of a typical research proposal. Because the nature of this type of funding is small (i.e., usually $500–$1,500), the timeline for funding to project implementation is short (usually under 12 months), and the project usually involves the application of well-established research evidence (e.g., guidelines, procedures, protocols). Thus, the application process is modified accordingly and typically includes:

- Cover letter.
- Grant application form.
- Timetable for the project.
- Budget: Funding requested and justification for funding requested.
- Evidence of ethical review: If an institutional review board (IRB) is not available in the institution, a letter of approval from facility administration should be requested, indicating that they are aware of the project and its implications for their patients.
- Participant consent: All subjects in the project must give written consent, especially if eventual publication of project results is anticipated (exception: data abstraction from medical records with elimination of all patient-specific identifying data).
- Program questions: Specific to each grant, these questions should be answered in detail. When describing the project, use the information outlined in the methods section of this chapter as a general guide.

Remember that many organizations require membership or registration on their Web sites to be eligible to apply for funding or to gain access to funding guidelines.

If you are a member of AACN, you can obtain more information about funding at **http://www.aacn.org.**

Foundations typically restrict their focus to certain populations or service areas (e.g., rural nursing homes). For example, the Washington Square Health Foundation focuses on increasing access to healthcare among at-risk populations and expanding the community's capacity to address important healthcare needs. Its mission is to grant funds in order to promote and maintain access to adequate healthcare for all people in the Greater Chicago area. This foundation awards funding to medical and nursing educational programs, medical research institutions, and direct healthcare services (e.g., outcomes management initiatives). General guidelines for submitting a grant proposal to the Washington Square Health Foundation include:

- Collected assessment data about the healthcare needs of high-risk, underserved, and/or disadvantaged populations in service area.
- Implemented targeted activities to increase the accessibility of healthcare services to one or more high-risk, underserved, and/or disadvantaged populations.
- Designed and implemented with community involvement, new or expanded services to address the healthcare needs of one or more high-risk, underserved, and/or disadvantaged populations.
- Identified opportunities to increase assets of high-risk, underserved, and/or disadvantaged communities, such as by employing community members as staff in health programs, locating health service delivery sites in the community, negotiating purchasing contracts with local businesses for health service-related products.

The Washington Square Health Foundation can be found at **http://www.wshf.org.**

Some foundations fund demonstration and quality improvement projects as well as community initiatives versus research because of the desire to influence practice or healthcare improvements quickly. For example, the Department of Health and Human Services has announced that the Fan Fox & Leslie R. Samuels Foundation has shifted the focus of its healthcare program from applied research to patient-based and social service activities that assist older adults in New York City. According to the announcement of this change, the refocused program is designed to improve the mechanism for health and social services to be delivered through support to organizations that reflect inventive, useful, competent, and thoughtful care to their patients. Requirements for a grant application to the Fan Fox & Leslie R. Samuels Foundation include the following:

- The program will improve the overall quality of life or healthcare service delivery to New York City's elderly.
- The program has a realistic, achievable work plan and a rational, well-justified budget.
- The program staff members who will perform the work are experienced and highly qualified.
- The sponsoring organization is stable, competent, and committed.

To submit an abstract for funding to the Fan Fox & Leslie R. Samuels Foundation, applicants must compile a cover sheet with the following information: legal name, address, phone, fax, e-mail and Web site addresses (if available) of the institution or organization; the program director's name, address, phone, fax, and e-mail (if available); the name and exact title of the organization's CEO; the program title, its duration; the total dollar amount requested; and a one-paragraph summary of the proposed program. In addition, a three-page letter (1-inch margins, 12-point font) that clearly states the following must be submitted:

- The general problems and issues being addressed and their importance
- A brief description of the nature of the program and its significance, with clear goals and objectives
- The recommended approach to care or services that represents an improvement over how services are delivered now; how the proposed program makes care or service provision better
- A description of the anticipated benefit of the program to older adults, including the number of individuals who will be impacted
- The program's overall significance
- A summary of the critical activities to be performed, the timeframe for the proposed program, and a brief breakdown of the projected budget
- If successful, the likelihood that the program will be continued by the institution
- The commitment of the sponsoring institution (e.g. contribution of salaries, space, overhead, etc.) during and after the grant term

Fan Fox & Leslie R. Samuels Foundation can be found at
http://www.samuels.org/hcgdlnz.htm.

The pursuit of foundation funding is a good option to follow for a quality improvement or outcomes management initiative. Most requirements for foundation applications are readily available on the Internet, which enhances the timeliness of application submission. As with any other funding endeavor, assuring that the foundation or organization's goals are a good match for your project, carefully following the supplied guidelines, and providing the clearest and most informative presentation of the project, whether that be only an abstract or a full proposal, will increase chances for successful funding.

In conclusion, the process of writing a grant proposal is a challenging but rewarding experience. Judicious planning, careful attention to the detailed requirements of the grant application, and background homework on potential funding sources as well as prior work in the area will facilitate the writing of an innovative, compelling, clear proposal that is matched appropriately for the potential funding agency.

It is helpful to remember that the process of writing a grant proposal resembles the eating of a 2-ton chocolate elephant. If you sit on a stool in front of the elephant and look up, the whole elephant appears too large to consume. However, if you sit on the stool looking straight ahead and consume the part of the elephant that is directly in front of you, then move the stool to the next parts in sequential order and consume them one at a time, soon the whole chocolate elephant will be eaten! In addition, when writing a grant proposal, it is helpful to remember the following individuals who succeeded in their endeavors as the result of not being afraid to take risks in combination with strong belief in themselves and sheer persistence.

Babe Ruth struck out 1,330 times. In between his strikeouts, he hit 714 home runs.

R.H. Macy failed in retailing seven times before his store in New York became a success.

Abraham Lincoln failed twice in business and was defeated in six state and national elections before being elected President of the United States.

Theodor S. Geisel wrote a children's book that was rejected by 23 publishers. The twenty-fourth publisher sold six million copies of it—the first "Dr. Seuss" book—and that book and its successors are still staples of every children's library. (Kouzes & Posner, 2002, p. 214)

Remember, people often fail their way to success. This often applies to the process of grant writing. Therefore, prepare well, believe in your ability to write a great grant proposal, seek mentorship and critique, and stay persistent to resubmit until your project is funded!

references

Cohen, J. (1992). A power primer. *Psychological Bulletin, 112*(1), 155–159.

Cummings, S. R., Holly, E. A., & Hulley, S. (2001). Writing and funding a research proposal. In S. B. Hulley, S. R. Cummings, W. S. Browner, D. Grady, N. Hearst, & T. B. Newman (Eds.), *Designing clinical research. An epidemiologic approach* (2nd ed.). Philadelphia: Lippincott Williams & Wilkins.

Kouzes, J. M., & Posner, B. Z. (2002). *The leadership challenge* (3rd ed.). San Francisco: Jossey-Bass.

Mick, D., & Ackerman, M. (1999). Successful strategies for small grant funding for advanced practice nurses. *The Internet Journal of Advanced Nursing Practice*, 2N2: Retrieved from http://www.icaap.org/iuicode?88.2.2.1.

Polit, D. F., & Beck, C. T. (2003). *Nursing research. Principles and methods* (7th ed.). Philadelphia: Lippincott, Williams & Wilkins.

Disseminating Evidence

Cecily L. Betz, Kathryn Smith,
Bernadette Mazurek Melnyk, and Tom Rickey

chapter 14

This chapter focuses on ideas and pragmatic suggestions for disseminating evidence-based information. Whatever the venue (e.g., speaking before an audience, presenting a poster, publishing a paper, communicating with the media, writing a health policy brief), the key to being effective is sufficient preparation. Excellent preparation reduces performance anxiety, bolsters confidence, and enhances the success of any dissemination initiative.

Disseminating Evidence Through Podium/Oral Presentations

An effective evidence-based presentation begins with an understanding of the characteristics and needs of the audience. When asked to make a podium or oral presentation, it is important to inquire about the audience and the context of the presentation (Garity, 1999; Gross, 2002; Hadfield-Law, 2001; McConnell, 2002; Schulmeister & Vrabel, 2002; Smith, 2000; Woodring, 1995, 2000).

Preparing for the Presentation

As you begin preparing the presentation, specifically ask the following substantive questions:

- What is the educational level of the audience?
- What is the audience's current knowledge of the material to be presented?
- Is the content for an audience with limited knowledge of the evidence-based topic?
- Why is the audience interested in the presentation?
- Is the audience expected to use evidence-based approaches in providing clinical care?
- What other information, if any, will the audience be receiving?
- What previous exposure has the audience had to the content of the presentation?
- How might the members of the audience use the information from the presentation to improve their practices, teaching, or other aspects of their work?

Additional logistical questions to consider include:

- Number of participants expected to attend the presentation
- Availability of audio-visual equipment (e.g., LCD projector for Power Point presentations
- Length of the presentation
- Expectations regarding handouts
- Specific content to be addressed (Bagott & Bagott, 2001)

Once these questions are answered, formulation of the presentation can begin. The first step in this process is creating learner objectives (e.g., at the end of the presentation, the participants will be able to describe the study's major outcomes) along with a detailed outline for the presentation. For presentations with a purpose of disseminating evidence from a study, the following topical outline is suggested.

I. Introduction to the clinical problem (e.g., depression affects approximately 25% of adults in the United States)
II. The purpose/primary aim of the study (e.g., to determine the short- and long-term effects of cognitive-behavior therapy [CBT] on depressive symptoms in young adults)
III. The theoretical framework used to guide the study
IV. Hypotheses (young adults who receive CBT will have less depressive symptoms than young adults who do not receive CBT) or study questions (what are the effects of CBT on depressed adults?)
V. The design (e.g., a randomized controlled trial)
   A. A description of the interventions used if an experimental study is being presented
   B. A description of the sample with inclusion and exclusion criteria (e.g., the sample included 104 depressed adults between the ages of 21 and 30; potential subjects were excluded if they had a mental health problem with psychotic features), as well as a concise description of the demographics of the sample
   C. The dependent variables and instruments used to measure the study's outcomes, along with validity and reliability information of each instrument (e.g., the Beck Depression Inventory was used to measure depressive symptoms; construct validity of the Beck Inventory has been supported in prior work, and internal consistency reliability is reported as consistently above 0.80)
VI. Findings from the study
   A. Approach to statistical analyses (e.g., types of statistical tests used [an independent t-test was used to test the study hypothesis])
   B. Findings (it is best to represent the findings in easy-to-read graphs or tables)
VII. Discussion of the findings, along with major limitations of the study (e.g., substantial attrition rate)

VIII. Implications
    A. Implications for future research (e.g., what was learned from this study that can guide future research in the area)
    B. Implications for clinical practice (e.g., how this evidence can be used to improve practice)

Once the outline is developed, major points and the content for each section of the outline can be developed along with the time allocation for each component of the presentation. Many conferences limit research/evidence-based presentations to 20 minutes, with it being commonplace for three to four individuals to deliver their talks in the same session. For presentations with extremely limited time frames, it is critical to deliver "nuts and bolts" information only. Because many individuals, especially novices, often extend their presentation beyond the allocated time limit, it is beneficial to write out and conduct a "practice" presentation before the actual conference. Having colleagues attend and critique this practice session will strengthen the final product.

Slides to Enhance the Presentation

Once the presentation is written, slides should be developed to enhance delivery and hold the attention of the audience. Many of the currently available slide programs (e.g., Microsoft PowerPoint) are easy to use. A rule of thumb is that a minimal amount of information should be contained on each slide and that there should be no more than one or two slides per minute of presentation time. Therefore, if an oral presentation is scheduled for 20 minutes, no more than 40 slides should accompany it.

Another helpful tip in creating slides is to keep them simple in terms of the colors, graphics, and number of fonts used. A dark or medium background (e.g., navy blue) with light color lettering (e.g., yellow or white) works best. White or pale-colored backgrounds should be avoided. Individuals in the back of a room should be able to read all text. Fonts should be simple (e.g., Arial, Times New Roman). Font and background color should be consistent throughout the slide presentation. Important points should appear in boldface on slides. In addition, photographs enhance the presentation, capture the audience's interest, and assist in emphasizing important points (see Appendix G for an example of a slide presentation to accompany a 20-minute research report). Moreover, a number of Web sites contain helpful information for creating and delivering professional oral presentations.

Here are some useful Web sites for preparing a podium or oral presentation:

http://nsweb.nursingspectrum.com/ce/ce183.htm features a self-study module, "A Quick Guide to Preparing Professional Presentations," by Mary E. Greipp.

At **http://www.kodak.com/US/en/digital/av/presenters/index.shtml** can be found "The Presenter's Forum: Tips, Techniques and Lessons."

http://www.presentersonline.com/tutorials/powerpoint/slides.shtml contains excellent tutorials on creating PowerPoint slides by Epson Presenters Online, where registration is free, and templates and clip art are downloadable.

Other Types of Evidence-Based Oral Presentations

The following guidelines and tips for presenting evidence from a study also apply to delivering other types of evidence-based presentations (e.g., evidence-based implementation projects).

The format for presenting *systematic reviews* of evidence should include:

- Introduction to the clinical problem
- Purpose of the systematic review or the clinical question addressed
- Methods (e.g., search strategy)
- Results (i.e., presentation and critical appraisal of the evidence)
- Implications for future research and practice

Disseminating Evidence Through Panel Presentations

Panel presentations are effective venues for conveying divergent perspectives on evidence-based topics. This type of presentation format is especially effective in convening colleagues from various clinical settings to disseminate information on evidenced-based topics. For example, during a panel presentation, clinicians can discuss their evidenced-based approaches to promoting spiritual support services on their hematology-oncology units. Listening to a number of different views enriches the session for the audience. The style and purpose of panel presentations varies according to the roles of the moderator and panelists. The moderator may serve as the coordinator, meaning that this individual manages the agenda of the panel by first giving background or introductory information and commentary on the subject matter to be discussed. Then the moderator asks questions of the panel members to elicit their opinions on the topic. Questions from the audience are taken as a means of delving further into particular areas of interest or understanding the panelists' views better.

Another panel model features a more formalized approach in which members of the panel present prepared remarks, with the moderator serving as a discussion facilitator by offering commentary for panel response and eliciting audience questions. The panel format is dependent on a number of factors, including panelist expertise, public speaking experience, organizational practices, and the moderator's competence in the role.

Panelist Preparation

Serving as a panelist begins with knowing the expectations for participation (e.g., delivering a prepared presentation or sharing expert opinions with the audience). The panel format will dictate the type of preparation necessary for the presentation. Whatever the format, it is necessary to obtain contextual information.

First, the potential panelist must learn about the theme of and rationale for the panel, along with the session objectives. For example, is the panelist expected to provide a clinically based or theoretically oriented presentation? Coupled with this information, it is important to know information about the other panelists and their areas of expertise, and the topics that the other panelists will address along with their particular biases or perspectives. It also is necessary to know the timeframe for the entire panel, including allotment of time for audience questions, each panelist's prepared remarks, and the moderator's commentary (Garity, 1999; Gross, 2002; Hadfield-Law, 2001; McConnell, 2002; Schulmeister & Vrabel, 2002; Smith, 2000; Woodring, 2000, 1995).

If a panelist is expected to prepare remarks, it is important to inquire about the availability of audio-visual equipment. In addition, the following strategies will ensure success of the panel presentation.

- Limit the number of slides because having too many slides becomes distracting and deemphasizes the substance of the presentation. Slides should be used to highlight, not supplant what is said.
- Develop a time clock system (e.g., set a timepiece in front of the speaker or have the moderator invoke the time notification with signage or some other method).
- Use active voice that holds the audience's attention, and illustrate content with "real-life" examples.
- Identify the major theme of the presentation and add three to five major points to support the thrust of the theme.

If a panelist is expected to offer expert opinions in response to questions, the following preparatory steps are needed:

- Gather information on the projected demographics of the audience and gear responses to the needs of the group; consulting with colleagues before the panel presentation may be useful. A representative description of the projected audience will provide insight as to appropriate direction for preparation.
- Anticipate the questions that might be asked from the audience; colleagues can be asked to contribute to a potential list of questions for advance preparation.
- Paraphrase questions asked from the audience before providing a response; this allows everyone in the audience to hear the questions and allows the presenter time to organize his or her thoughts.
- Treat all questions with the same importance so as not to display a bias or preference for certain individuals in the audience.
- During the session, panelists are expected to conduct themselves professionally, with sensitivity to the fact that they are only one of several experts sharing the stage from whom the audience wants to hear new information and practice ideas. Box 14-1 lists suggestions for panelist conduct, or what some individuals refer to as "A Panelist's Do's and Don'ts."

Moderator Preparation

The moderator's main role during a panel presentation is to ensure that the session objectives are met and that the panelist presentations are "pulled together" in a cohesive fashion. The moderator will begin the session by providing introductory remarks that include an overview of the panel's purpose, a brief biographical introduction, and the evidence-based topic of each panelist. The moderator's role is to ensure the even flow of the panel discussion and questions from the audience. At the conclusion of the panel, the moderator should provide summary statements of the major themes of each evidence-based presentation; therefore, note taking dur-

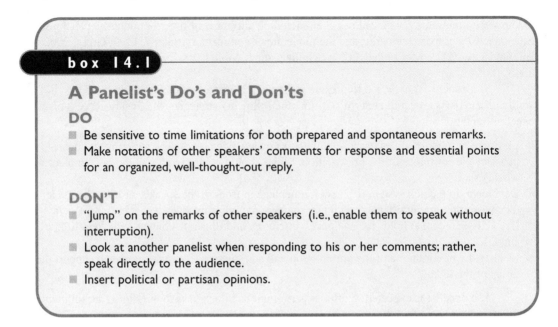

box 14.1

A Panelist's Do's and Don'ts

DO
- Be sensitive to time limitations for both prepared and spontaneous remarks.
- Make notations of other speakers' comments for response and essential points for an organized, well-thought-out reply.

DON'T
- "Jump" on the remarks of other speakers (i.e., enable them to speak without interruption).
- Look at another panelist when responding to his or her comments; rather, speak directly to the audience.
- Insert political or partisan opinions.

ing the session will be necessary while being attentive to coordinating questions from the audience and panelist responses. Box 14-2 presents specific responsibilities of the moderator during a panel presentation.

Prior to the panel session, the moderator should contact each of the panelists to obtain sufficient information about the presentation and each panelist's area of expertise. Exchange of information about the other panels also should occur, including contact information so that con-

box 14.2

Responsibilities of the Moderator During a Panel Presentation

- Provide a brief introduction of each panelist, emphasizing his or her expertise or experience with the evidence-based topic.
- Select audience members who have questions to ask of panelists.
- Repeat questions (or have panelists do it) for the audience's benefit.
- Remind the audience members or panelists of time constraints if too much time is used.
- Redirect the panelists' comments as needed to ensure that one or two panelists do not dominate the session.

tact by panel members can be established before the presentation. Additionally, the moderator can serve as a liaison for exchanging logistic information (e.g., audio-visual needs, room setup, projected number of individuals attending the presentation for distribution of handouts, and confirmation of the meeting time and place). The moderator also needs to be responsible for ensuring that the panel adheres to time constraints and clearly conveys to panelists the methods for keeping time.

Disseminating Evidence Through Roundtable Presentations

Roundtable presentations are an informal way to share information with a small group of people—literally, the number of individuals that fit around a table. Roundtable presentations offer the opportunity not only to share specific information with a group, but also to allow the group to discuss the information, experiences related to the information, and how the content will be used within their own practices.

Because the group for a roundtable is generally small (i.e., 6–12 individuals), it is appropriate to start the discussion with introductions so that the group members can get acquainted, which will allow them more easily to engage in conversation about the topic. The use of audio-visual equipment is often not possible in this setting, but PowerPoint or other types of handouts can be used to identify key points or provide supplemental information (Bergren, 2000; Cook, 1999, 1998; Evans, 2000). As in the case of a formal lecture, it is important to understand the needs of the audience and their reasons for attending the roundtable.

Preparation for a Roundtable Discussion

In planning the presentation, it is important to allow ample time for discussion. Anticipate that one half to one third of the allotted time will be spent in discussion related to the prepared evidence-based material. Preplanned discussion questions to be used by the presenter are useful to facilitate dialogue among the participants, should spontaneous conversation not occur.

Content for a roundtable is prepared in the same way as for a lecture presentation. Delivery of the material will be different, given the small group size and intimate setting in which the roundtable takes place. After appropriate introductions, the goals of the evidenced-based presentation are stated. Any handouts are distributed and described in terms of their utility and relevance to the evidence-based practice (EBP) topic. The content of the presentation is then delivered. Because the group is small, it is important to scan the group regularly, making eye contact with each person, in order to engage all present. Questions can be answered either during the presentation or at the end. If questions are taken and discussion allowed during the delivery of the content, it is important to watch the time to assure that all content will be covered (Garity, 1999; Gross, 2002; Hadfield-Law, 2001; McConnell, 2002; Schulmeister & Vrabel, 2002; Woodring, 2000, 1995).

At the end of a roundtable session, participants should be thanked for attending, and any final questions should be answered that require additional clarification. The group may wish to exchange business cards or other identification or information so that dialogue among the members may continue. The presenter should offer his/her business card to allow future follow-up and may stay in the vicinity of the roundtable for a period of time after the session to answer individual questions.

Disseminating Evidence Through Poster Presentations

Poster presentations provide an alternative option for presenting evidence-based information to a professional audience. Poster presentations are different from those given from a podium in a number of ways. Podium presentations are more formal in both style and format. The presenter typically provides more information from the podium as contrasted with the poster, wherein only the most essential aspects of information about a study or evidence-based project are given. The podium presenter adheres to a fairly standard format for providing information, with little or no time allowed to take audience questions. The poster presenter also adheres to a defined format for displaying information; however, this type of presentation allows for more interaction between colleagues in the area of clinical interest. Individuals displaying posters can explore any number of issues that are not possible with podium presentations. For example, colleagues might discuss in greater detail the clinical implications of the evidence presented, such as implementation challenges in a community-based setting compared with a tertiary care setting.

Podium presentations are confined to limited periods of time (i.e., usually 15–20 minutes in length), whereas posters are displayed for longer periods of time (e.g., several hours), which allows the presenter more time to speak directly with colleagues about their work. A poster presentation is less intimidating than a podium presentation because public speaking can be uncomfortable for professionals who are not accustomed to presenting before large numbers of people (Bagott & Bagott, 2001).

Displaying information also may be preferable to giving an oral presentation for individuals who process information better in visual rather than verbal format.

The key to developing an effective and eye-catching poster is to construct it in a way that captures the attention of the conference participants. It is useful to think about the attractive characteristics of poster presentations seen at various professional conferences (see the accompanying CD-ROM for two well-designed posters that were displayed at national/international conferences). Notable aspects of these posters include their design and symmetry, the contrast of colors used, use of key words or phrases to emphasize important content, and use of graphs/figures to present study findings. In contrast, posters that are poorly designed often present content in a disorganized format, contain too much or too little information, use colors that clash, and do not use figures/graphs to display content.

However, the display of graphics and organization of a poster are not enough. Knowing how to present information to colleagues in succinct, scholarly, and precise terms is just as important. Substance and design, when combined well in a poster, can serve as an effective vehicle for conveying information to colleagues. The poster becomes a magnet for attracting colleagues, not only to read about one's work but also to provide a venue for additional discussion with sharing of information that is the keystone of collegial discourse.

Ideally, if the resources are available, it is useful to consult with a graphic design expert when constructing a poster. Consulting with an expert certainly makes it easier, but the designer has limitations as well because this individual's area of expertise is limited to graphic design, not the poster content (Beyla & Nicoll, 1998; Taggart & Arslanian, 2000).

When a poster is accepted for presentation at a conference, authors typically receive the guidelines for construction and display of their posters (e.g., size specifications). If the guidelines are not received, it is critical to obtain them prior to beginning the poster's design so that time is not lost in preparing a product that does not meet the requirements of the poster session.

The Pragmatics of Constructing a Poster: Getting Started

The first step in developing a poster presentation is to translate ideas and images into graphic form. Sketching out or developing a "mockup" model of the poster with self-sticking notes may be useful. The professional meeting and/or association may specify poster requirements. Therefore, it will be important to obtain and carefully review poster guidelines, such as the poster size that is standard for the conference (e.g., the typical size is 4 feet × 6 feet). It also is important that the poster text and graphics be readable from a distance of 4 feet. Keeping the following principles in mind will enhance the readability of the poster.

- Remember that English-speaking participants will read the poster from left to right and from top to bottom.
- Number the order of the presentation to assist the reader in information sequencing.
- Vary the font size on the poster according to the type of information being presented, for example, 72 point (pt) or larger for the poster title (readable from 20 feet); 72 pt or larger for authors' names and affiliations; 36–48 pt or larger for poster headings and subheadings; and 14–20 pt for poster text.
- Use graphics or illustrations in lieu of text when appropriate, such as when reporting findings.
- Keep headings and subheadings brief (fewer than five words).
- Use familiar typeface (e.g., Times New Roman, Courier New, Arial) and the same font style throughout the poster.
- Keep in mind that sans serif fonts (without curlicues) are the most readable.
- Avoid using shadowing and underlines; use bold instead for areas of emphasis.
- Use active tense, e.g., "Findings reveal...."

The presentation of content should follow a logical sequence from beginning to end. This format is similar to that used for publishing research papers. The presentation of research content, although dependent on the specifications of the conference, typically includes:

- *Introduction*: The focus of the introduction section is to attract the attention of colleagues about the significance of the project by emphasizing the need, prevalence of the problem, or clinical issue.
- *Research Objectives/Hypotheses*: This section should be brief in that it states the focus of the study.
- *Methods/Design*: Brevity is the key unless there is something of interest about the methods or design that warrants emphasis (e.g., recruiting and training interviewers for culturally diverse populations).

* *Data Analysis*: This section should be concise in terms of listing analyses conducted.
* *Study Findings*: The emphasis in this section is on presenting graphs or tables with limited explanatory text to accompany them.
* *Conclusions*: Brief statements are made regarding the most significant findings as well as the clinical implications for nursing practice.
* *Acknowledgement*: When applicable, it is acceptable to recognize the names of other staff on the project and/or whether the project was funded by an extramural source.

Evidence-Based Poster Presentations

Similarly, the content of an evidence-based poster presentation would generally include the following sections:

* *Statement of the Problem*: Provide background as to the nature or status of the clinical problem (e.g., prevalence data or other statistics demonstrating the growing importance of problem).
* *Clinical Question*: Specifically identify what clinical problem or question was investigated.
* *Search for Evidence/Accepted Practice*: Identify briefly the methods and sources used to collect evidence (e.g., search strategy for the review of literature, focus groups, and surveys of institutional practices).
* *Presentation and Critical Appraisal of the Evidence*: Provide a succinct summary of the conclusions drawn from evaluating the scope of evidence available.
* *Clinical Practice Implications*: Describe clinical practice implications, based on the process of collecting and evaluating the evidence.

Expectations of Poster Presenters

Poster presenters are expected to stand beside their posters in accordance with the designated time periods for display. It is disappointing for colleagues to walk among posters without the authors or investigators because one of the primary purposes for a poster presentation is to facilitate scholarly and clinical dialogue among colleagues. Having PowerPoint handouts of the poster presentation available for distribution is helpful as well (Bergren, 2000; Cook, 1999, 1998; Evans, 2000). The handouts may contain additional information that was not possible to include in the poster display (e.g., more detail on the review of pertinent literature, the theoretical framework, research instruments, and references).

Helpful Resources for Constructing Posters

Many excellent resources are available via the Internet. These resources provide pragmatic details on aspects of constructing a poster (e.g., durable poster materials, display layout and format, logistics of color selection, photos and graphics). Some sites provide information on using PowerPoint and creating posters for online purposes. These sites are listed in Box 14-3. Listed below are some fail-safe suggestions for avoiding poster presentation disasters.

- Develop a timeline that accommodates unanticipated delays in processing over which one has no control (e.g., use of graphic designer, photo processing).
- Back up files as the poster is being developed so that no data are lost through computer malfunctioning or as a result of a virus.
- Determine the best method for transporting the poster on an airplane or by train because it may have to be carried to the passenger section and stored overhead.
- Bring a computer file of the poster, just in case it gets lost, damaged, or destroyed in transit.

---

box 14.3

Helpful Web Sites for Creating Poster Presentations

1. *Creating Posters for Humanities & Social Sciences.* This Web site provides succinct information on the construction of posters akin to listing of "helpful hints." Background information is presented on the rationale and benefits for considering poster sessions as an option for professional presentation. This background information is more appropriate for instructors or presenters who want to teach a class on poster sessions.
   http://www.lcsc.edu/ss150/poster.htm

2. *Designing Effective Posters* by Jeff Radel, Department of Occupational Therapy Education, University of Kansas Medical Center. This Web site provides the most comprehensive and detailed information about poster sessions of any Web site. Radel provides detailed information on every aspect of creating a poster, from formatting the poster title to transport and storage. This site is really a must.
   http://www.kumc.edu/SAH/OTEd/jradel/Poster_Presentations/PstrStart.html

3. *A Guide to Writing in the Biological Sciences: The Poster Session*, George Mason University, Department of Biology. This Web site contains two tutorials on creating posters, both of which have some good information on construction tips and poster format. These tutorials are worth looking at for some useful suggestions.
   http://classweb.gmu.edu/biologyresources/writingguide/Poster.htm

4. *Writing @CSU: Overview: Poster Sessions.* This Web site is produced by the Writing Center at Colorado State University and is available for use by its students, faculty, and others. This tutorial provides excellent information on all of the specifics of constructing a poster. Suggestions are offered for the novice who is unsure of how to progress in constructing a poster, such as suggesting when to call the organization to have additional questions answered.
   http://writing.colostate.edu/references/speaking/poster/index.cfm

- Ensure the security of the poster if staying in a hotel room by properly labeling it in case it is inadvertently misplaced.
- Remember to bring materials (e.g., masking tape, double-sided tape, pins) to display the poster.

Disseminating Evidence Through Small Group Presentations

Evidence-Based Grand Rounds

Grand rounds can serve as a major forum for evidence-based presentations. Very often, departments within tertiary care and academic settings will host grand rounds. Grand rounds are forums designed for clinicians to speak directly to their colleagues on topics that are innovative ("cutting edge") or that call for new approaches to care. Usually, speakers present empirically based answers to clinical practice questions, typically findings from their own or others' studies or policy updates with clinical implications for staff. Grand rounds usually consist of formal oral presentations accompanied by audio-visual slides or video presentations. Generally, a question-and-answer period follows the speaker's presentation.

Just as there are journal club Web sites (discussed in more detail later in the chapter), grand rounds presentations can be found on numerous Internet Web sites. Internet grand rounds is another setting for experts to share evidence-based information with colleagues on a particular topic. The Internet grand rounds topic may be presented or reviewed by numerous clinical experts, enabling users to e-mail questions that can later be posted on the site. The advantages of Internet usage are the widespread access that is available to users, the ability to combine the perspectives and expertise of many clinical specialists, and the convenience for the user. Additionally, users are not bound by the time constraints of real-time meetings, enabling them to participate at their own convenience.

Evidence-Based Clinical Rounds

Evidence-based clinical rounds, smaller in scope than grand rounds, are a wonderful medium through which to present evidence to guide clinical practice changes as well as intimately involve clinical staff in the process. Evidence-based clinical rounds have been used very successfully as part of the Advancing Research and Clinical Practice through Close Collaboration (ARCC) model at the University of Rochester School of Nursing, Medical Center, and community (Melnyk & Fineout-Overholt, 2002). One or a few clinicians will do the following in preparation for these rounds:

- Identify a clinical question (e.g., What is the most effective medication to decrease pain in postsurgical cardiac patients?).
- Conduct a systematic search for the evidence to answer the clinical question.
- Critically appraise the evidence found.
- Recommend guidelines for practice changes based on the evidence.

These clinicians then present the information that they gathered and make recommendations for clinical practice to their colleagues, based on the evidence, in the form of an oral presentation during a more casual session than the more formal, larger grand rounds.

Disseminating Evidence Through Community Meetings

Individuals identified as experts in a particular area may be asked to present evidence-based information in a community setting. This type of presentation can be particularly challenging because community groups may include laypersons and the media, in addition to professionals. This requires that the speaker be able to address all members of the group in a way that is understandable to everyone. Before making the presentation, it is important to collaborate with community leaders about the nature of the content to be presented as well as to be culturally sensitive to the potential participants of the meeting. Tips for presenting to a mixed audience include the following:

- Define all abbreviations and acronyms (e.g., the American College of Nurse Practitioners, rather than ACNP).
- Provide definitions as you speak (e.g., ". . . risk pool, that is, a group of individuals brought together to purchase insurance in order to spread the risk, or cost, among a larger group of people . . .").
- Avoid off-hand remarks that could be misinterpreted or misquoted by any media present. Stick with the facts as you know them or offer your professional, educated opinion when asked.
- Offer to answer individual questions after the session so that those who might be embarrassed to ask a question before a large group will have the opportunity to question the speaker privately.
- Begin the presentation with a general overview of its purpose, followed by a review of the major points or findings. When offering examples, consider the potentially mixed nature of the audience and offer exemplars that all members can understand. The use of PowerPoint slides and corresponding handouts also are useful in keeping all participants engaged and focused on the presentation (Bergren, 2000; Cook, 1999, 1998; Evans, 2000). In addition, referral to relevant Web sites and articles is always appreciated.
- Allow ample time for questions and answers as well as discussion of the topic.

Disseminating Evidence Through Hospital/Organization-Based and Professional Committee Meetings

Presenting evidence-based information to a committee of fellow professionals can be a stressful and intimidating experience. Adequate preparation is again the key for ensuring success. Anticipate questions that may reflect not only the information that is being presented but also historical information because not everyone in the group will be aware of all of the relevant history surrounding a particular issue. Consider the following:

- Why is the group interested in the topic?
- What is the history of the issue in the particular institution?
- Has there been any controversy surrounding the issue that may interfere with the presentation? If so, should it be addressed in an open manner before the presentation begins?
- Are there some members of the group who may be more resistant than others to the information presented? If it is possible to learn more about concerns ahead of time, they can be addressed more readily in the meeting.
- Is there any related information that may need to be discussed during the presentation, and does the presenter have adequate knowledge in the related area?
- Is this a group whose meetings are informal, or does the group maintain formal rules during its meeting process?

      Two of the most important pieces of information needed before beginning to prepare for a committee presentation are:

1. Who is the audience?
2. How much time will there be to share information?

      Whoever invites the presenter to the meeting or is responsible for serving as chairperson should be able to describe the anticipated number of attendees, the disciplines represented, and the relevance of the information for the group. Using the questions above as a basis for exploration should result in adequate information about the audience.

      Committee meetings are usually tightly scheduled with little opportunity to go beyond the allotted time. Therefore, it is important to be able to provide key information within the timeframe allowed. In addition, if the meeting is held in a hospital or other similar facility, staff members may come in and out of the meeting when they are answering pages or attending to patient care responsibilities. This movement in and out of the room can be distracting and unnerving for the speaker, so it is important to prepare mentally for this possibility and plan to focus on the topic and the members who remain at the meeting. In addition, anticipate that some latecomers will ask for information that has already been presented. The best approach is to provide the information in a brief manner and offer to discuss it more fully after the meeting.

      After a brief introduction as to its relevance for the group, the presentation can generally follow the format for a journal article on an EBP topic, including:

- Clinical question
- Search for evidence
- Critical appraisal
- Implications for practice
- Evaluation (if the practice change had been implemented)

      This should be followed by a period of discussion as to the utility of the information for the committee or the facility.

Disseminating Evidence Through Journal Clubs

The concept of journal clubs has evolved considerably over the years, especially with the use of the Internet as a vehicle for scholarly exchange. One only has to access the World Wide Web by using a search engine with the key words *journal club* and find a proliferation of online journal clubs, most of which are evidence-based in focus, to appreciate the widespread recognition of journal clubs as a conduit for dissemination of knowledge on clinical care. Whether journal clubs are offered on site or via the Internet, they serve as another mechanism for disseminating the best evidence on which to base nursing practice.

On-Site Journal Clubs

Journal clubs provide an opportunity for clinicians to share and learn about evidence-based approaches at their work sites. An advanced-level clinician can serve as the leader and mentor of a journal club until other colleagues achieve the knowledge and skills necessary to lead a group. The success of the journal club will depend on several factors:

- Expertise of the advanced-level clinician in selecting an appropriate review article together with other supporting articles that provide substantial sources of evidence
- Organizational resources to facilitate the activities of the journal club, such as access to online bibliographic resources that include evidence-based reviews (e.g., Cochrane Controlled Trials Register)
- Participation by motivated colleagues/staff

A journal club is typically led by an advanced-level clinician who understands research design, methods, and statistics. This clinician serves not only as the discussion facilitator, but also as an educator because it is likely that colleagues will ask additional contextual information. Questions from journal club participants typically focus on the type of research design used, sample selection criteria, instrumentation, and statistical analyses. Therefore, it is essential that the journal club leader have the knowledge to answer these types of questions adequately. Additionally, in order to be effective, the journal club leader needs facilitator skills to encourage members of the club to participate as well as to feel comfortable and supported in sharing input. The facilitation skills for an effective journal club leader include:

- Actively listening to questions asked.
- Using open-ended questions to facilitate discussion.
- Avoiding the appearance of preference or bias in responding to questions by stating that a particular question is "good" unless equivalent affirming comments are made about all questions.
- Clearly communicating messages about the purpose and expectations for the club.
- Coming to the meeting well prepared and organized to conduct the meeting smoothly. This might involve ensuring room availability and setup, as well as a sufficient number of handouts and other materials.
- Monitoring the flow of discussion to ensure that it is focused on the topic.

- Interceding when conversation "drift" occurs, redirecting the conversation back to the topic. This might include offering comments such as "getting back to our point," "as was said before," and "we were talking about . . ."
- Reinforcing responses to questions asked by members with affirming comments in order to encourage group participation.
- Summarizing major points at the end of the session before concluding the meeting.

The journal club leader will most likely have the responsibility for selecting the journal article to be discussed by the group participants. This article should meet the journal club criteria for an evidence-based presentation and should be appropriate to the clinical practice of the staff. Selected articles should be studies or evidence reviews that are current, use valid and reliable instrumentation, have an adequate number of subjects, and use a research design appropriate for the research question or purpose. Although there may be variations of the format for the journal club, the standard process for the discussion of articles is as follows:

- Study objectives/hypotheses.
- Design and methods, including the setting wherein the study was conducted (e.g., in the community, in the intensive care unit, in outpatient clinic, or in the home) as well as instruments used along with their validity and reliability for the sample studied.
- Data analyses, with rationale for the specific tests used.
- Findings, specifically in terms of the significance or nonsignificance of the findings, paying careful attention to whether the study had a large enough sample size with power to detect significant findings.
- Conclusions of the study with clinical implications, such as the clinical procedure related to aseptic management of long-term gastrostomy tubes.
- Efficient critical appraisal of the study, including its strengths and limitations as well as applicability to practice. For example, clinicians might be hesitant to change their practice based on the findings from one study that had a very small number of subjects.

Journal clubs are held at regularly scheduled times and locations, enabling participants to anticipate meetings. Articles for the journal club should be distributed to members well in advance so members can read and "digest" the material.

Online Journal Clubs

The Internet provides additional resources and opportunities for developing other types of journal clubs for healthcare professionals. There are numerous online bibliographic databases that can be accessed for obtaining evidence-based answers to questions or accessing substantive articles for a journal club.

For example, an advanced-level clinician on a pediatric unit of a major tertiary medical center wants to find a high-quality article on pediatric pain for next month's journal club. The most effective strategy for finding this article would be to access one of several online evidence-based review databases, because the most current and rigorously reviewed studies can be found there. These databases include the ACP Journal Club, Evidence-Based Medicine Reviews, Cochrane Database of Systematic Reviews, Cochrane Controlled Trials Register, and Database of Abstracts of Reviews of Effectiveness (DARE). Searching these databases for "pediatric pain" reveals the five citations listed in Box 14-4. Based on the needs of the clinical staff, the clinician selects the article published by Colwell and colleagues (1996) because it addresses specific clinical practice issues related to pediatric pain.

Finally, there are online journal clubs that incorporate the technological advantages available with the Internet. This format enables individual users to access the journal club Web site at times convenient to personal work schedules, interests, and learning style. Web site journal clubs, although highly individualized, are similar to the group meeting format in that an article is reviewed for its applicability for clinical practice. The difference with the online format is the process, which varies from site to site (e.g., a critical review of a clinical trial initiated by a contributing author and reviewed by Web site editors; individual efforts of a Web site editor with feedback from its users). A number of online evidence-based Web sites are listed in Box 14-5.

There are numerous disadvantages and advantages in using online journal clubs. The user does not have the benefit of hearing the views of colleagues, which may limit learning regarding others' own clinical areas of expertise, critical thinking, and professional attitudes and values. Having the opportunity to participate in shared discourse on professional issues is an important activity that promotes group cohesiveness and understanding, often fostering teamwork and group morale. Some learners may benefit more from the group discussion format, because it

box 14.4

Results of a Search on "Pediatric Pain" in Evidence-Based Review Databases

Greenberg, R. S., Billett, C., Zahurak, M., & Yaster, M. Videotape increases parental knowledge about pediatric pain management [Clinical Trial. Journal Article. Randomized Controlled Trial] *Anesthesia & Analgesia, 89*(4), 899–903, 1999 Oct.

Carceles, M.D., Castano, I., Carrasco, A., Santos, P., Rincon, I. S., Alonso, B., & Lopez, F. Patient controlled analgesia in postoperative pediatric pain. *Revista de la Sociedad Española del Dolor 3*(Suppl III), 69–77, 1996.

Colwell, C., Clark, L., & Perkins, R. Postoperative use of pediatric pain scales: Children's self-report versus nurse assessment of pain intensity and affect. [Clinical Trial. Journal Article. Randomized Controlled Trial]. *Journal of Pediatric Nursing, 11*(6), 375–382, 1996 Dec.

Benestad, B., Vinje, O., Veierod, M. B., & Vanvik, I. H., Quantitative and qualitative assessments of pain in children with juvenile chronic arthritis based on the Norwegian version of the Pediatric Pain Questionnaire. [Clinical Trial. Journal Article. Randomized Controlled Trial]. *Scandinavian Journal of Rheumatology, 25*(5), 293–299, 1996.

Engel, J. M. Relaxation training: A self-help approach for children with headaches. [Clinical Trial. Journal Article. Randomized Controlled Trial] *American Journal of Occupational Therapy, 46*(7), 591–596, 1992 Jul.

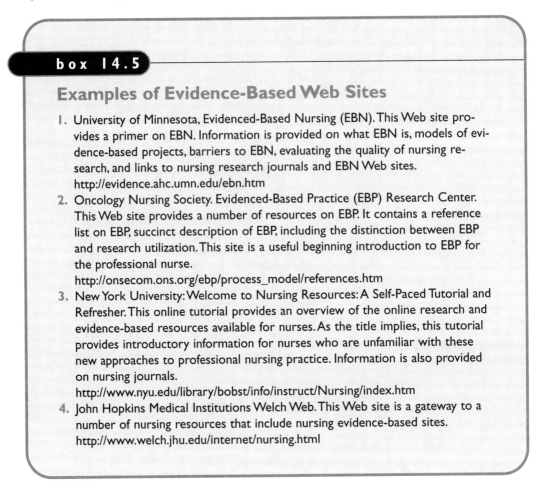

box 14.5

Examples of Evidence-Based Web Sites

1. University of Minnesota, Evidenced-Based Nursing (EBN). This Web site pro-vides a primer on EBN. Information is provided on what EBN is, models of evi-dence-based projects, barriers to EBN, evaluating the quality of nursing re-search, and links to nursing research journals and EBN Web sites.
   http://evidence.ahc.umn.edu/ebn.htm
2. Oncology Nursing Society. Evidenced-Based Practice (EBP) Research Center. This Web site provides a number of resources on EBP. It contains a reference list on EBP, succinct description of EBP, including the distinction between EBP and research utilization. This site is a useful beginning introduction to EBP for the professional nurse.
   http://onsecom.ons.org/ebp/process_model/references.htm
3. New York University: Welcome to Nursing Resources: A Self-Paced Tutorial and Refresher. This online tutorial provides an overview of the online research and evidence-based resources available for nurses. As the title implies, this tutorial provides introductory information for nurses who are unfamiliar with these new approaches to professional nursing practice. Information is also provided on nursing journals.
   http://www.nyu.edu/library/bobst/info/instruct/Nursing/index.htm
4. John Hopkins Medical Institutions Welch Web. This Web site is a gateway to a number of nursing resources that include nursing evidence-based sites.
   http://www.welch.jhu.edu/internet/nursing.html

is more suitable to their learning style. Likewise, other staff members may prefer the online for-mat, because it is more convenient and accessible.

Journal club meetings enable the moderator to model professional behavior for other staff members. Professional development is an ongoing process, and the journal club is yet an-other opportunity for leaders to model the importance of using evidence for nursing practice, to demonstrate ways of discussing practice issues in a nonthreatening venue, and to create expecta-tions for professional practice. Depending on a number of factors, such as Web site design and personnel resources, the online format may be more economical and feasible.

Disseminating Evidence Through Publishing

Many publishing options are available for individuals who are interested in sharing evidence-based information with their colleagues. Typically, writing a journal article or contributing a chapter to a book are the first ideas that come to mind when publishing is considered. Publications of this sort may appear overwhelming in terms of time, effort, and lack of prior writing experience. However, there are many other opportunities and options available for individuals who find themselves entertaining ideas about publishing.

Publishing experience can be gained by taking on less ambitious projects, such as serving on a publishing-type of committee at work or through a professional organization. Serving on these committees enables professionals to network with and learn from each other about the logistics and mechanics of publishing. Although the specific purpose of the committee may vary slightly (e.g., a newsletter committee, a publication committee), these committees are not necessarily designed for creating or fostering collective writing efforts. Publication committees may serve as panels to review publications submitted by prospective authors to an association's newsletter or journal. Other committees may provide oversight to the production of professional materials to ensure that the association or organization's affiliation is properly represented.

Regardless of the specific type of publication committee, membership enables individuals to learn through a variety of skill-enhancing efforts on how to write and professionally publish. Ideally, seasoned committee members can serve as mentors for less experienced committee members in acquiring these skills. For example, reviewing the written work of other colleagues enables one to learn through the editing process what constitutes both a well-written manuscript and one not written so well. Writing a manuscript is not only about sharing expertise concerning evidence-based approaches, it is also about learning how to present information in a manner that enhances readability for professional audiences. Reading drafts in progress is an indirect method of learning to write.

Serving on evidence-based committees provides another prospect for learning important precursor publishing skills. It is through committee participation that professionals learn the clinical framework for the organization of content and practice. Committee discussion of evidence-based issues and approaches provides an understanding of the processes involved in EBP that include:

- Posing the burning clinical question
- Searching for the best and latest evidence
- Critically appraising the evidence
- Clinically implementing a practice change
- Evaluating the change

Also, introduction to role models who have published can influence those who have not because it exposes individuals to the possibility that this new professional effort is possible.

Finding a Mentor

For individuals who have had limited publishing experience, finding a mentor is beneficial. This mentor can be found anywhere (e.g., at school or work, on the Internet, with a professional organization, and in some instances by contacting a nursing editor). A mentor can guide the novice writer through the process, starting with an idea for a topic and leading to the actual writing and submission process. It is important that the mentor selected be an individual who possesses sufficient prior publication experience.

Although experience and expertise are important, so is compatibility (e.g., writing style, temperament, and personality). A nursing colleague who has a style of interaction that is uncomfortable for the novice is a significant detriment. Those who publish must devote extra time and effort beyond their usual workloads; therefore, engaging in an effort that is unpleasant and literally painful is likely to be short lived. Persistence with a specific publishing effort is likely to be brief if these types of negative circumstances exist. Publishing should be both a professionally rewarding and a fun experience (Farella, 2002; Fetter, 1999; Fitzgerald, 2000; Sullivan, 2002).

Generating the Idea

A component of getting started with publishing an evidence-based paper is determining the topic. Generating the topic concept for publication is based on an individual's area of expertise, the clinical question that arises from clinical practice, and the availability of resources to support the initial curiosity and attention to the idea. An idea for an evidence-based publication may have been germinating for some time before it is fully acknowledged as a potential publication topic. For example, a clinician may have noticed that elderly residents in assisted living facilities have extended periods of confusion following hospital admissions. This clinical interest may lead the clinician to research the literature for information on the phenomenon and to find evidence for instituting new interventions. The experience leads the clinician to believe that other colleagues would benefit from learning about these practices. As a result, the clinician decides to write an article for a gerontology journal.

Brainstorming is another approach whereby ideas are generated through a free-association process. This process is enhanced if it can be done with other colleagues. The impetus stimulated with the rapid exchange of ideas can result in many more ideas that would otherwise not have been identified (Fitzgerald, 2000; Oermann, 1999, 2001; Pelletier et al., 2002).

Planning the Manuscript

Once an idea or a set of ideas has been "discovered," the prospective author needs to sketch out a plan on how this initial idea or concept can be developed into a manuscript (Grant, 1998). For evidence-based papers, the formats for writing articles do not vary significantly because differences are based more on style rather than substance. Although publication formats vary according to the technical specifications and editorial philosophy of the journal, the standard format for an evidence-based manuscript is as follows:

Title page: This is the first page of the manuscript and contains the article's title and all of the authors' names, job titles, affiliations, and contact information. If there are many authors, the corresponding author is indicated. The manuscript title should be succinct, and the key words in the title should be well known and accessible for content bibliographic searches. For example, if the author intends to write an evidenced-based manuscript about adolescents, having the term *children* in the title would be misleading for readers.

Abstract: An abstract contains a brief summary or synopsis of the article. Summaries indicate to the reader whether it is a research or clinical article. The abstract also identifies the major themes or findings and clinical implications.

Introduction: The introduction of the manuscript should be written in a succinct manner and should not extend beyond a few paragraphs. It contains information about the purpose of the article, the importance of the topic for the professional audience, and brief supporting evidence as to why this topic is important. Supporting evidence might include prevalence data or demonstration of need.

Manuscript narrative: This "middle section" of the manuscript will differ according to the type of evidence-based paper that is written, journal guidelines, and editorial philosophy.

Conclusions and clinical implications: The conclusions of the research evidence are presented in a summary form to emphasize the essence of the narrative discussion. For professionals who are accustomed to reading clinically oriented articles, the format of evidence-based papers may be unfamiliar and more difficult to follow. The conclusion section enables the reader to locate the information succinctly if the previous discussion is difficult to follow. The clinical implications section informs the reader about how this evidence can be applied to clinical practice. As importantly, the evidence substantiates the rationale for its use in clinical practice.

Adopting a Positive Attitude

> " *Your living is determined not so much by what life brings to you as by the attitude you bring to life; not so much by what happens to you as by the way your mind looks at what happens.* "
>
> *John Homer Miller*

Having a positive attitude toward professional publication, especially for novice prospective authors, is an absolute must. When an individual decides to write professionally, one needs to develop a resolute attitude that the publication task will be completed, no matter what problems or challenges are encountered, because there are likely to be a number of them. Typically, authors have the unusual experience of engaging in a very solitary activity that is undertaken by literally hundreds of thousands of people. Yet there are very few opportunities that enable authors to communicate with one another about the highs and lows of the writing experience. Occasionally, one will read a magazine or newspaper article about the process of writing. In 2001, Stephen King wrote a book entitled simply *On Writing* that provides insight into his life as a writer and what he has learned along the way in becoming one. However, most times authors toil at their computers, writing and deleting what they have written and rewriting until the words on the page seem to make sense of the ideas they want to convey to their readers.

> " *You measure the size of the accomplishment by the obstacles you had to overcome to reach your goals.* "
>
> *Booker T. Washington*

For many authors, uncertainty and self-doubt can interfere unduly with the process of writing, resulting in an unfinished manuscript that languishes on the computer's hard drive. For others, perhaps a harsh critique is mailed to them after the review has been completed, releasing a barrage of self-doubt and shame. For some individuals, the feedback is traumatic and demoralizing. Regrettably, these authors are unwilling to subject themselves to this harrowing experience again. However, it is important to know and appreciate that even the most successful and prominent authors have been subjected to their fair share of rejections. A major difference between those who are successful and those who are not is *persistence*. Persistence is one of the keys to getting work published.

> **66** *Criticism, like rain, should be gentle enough to nourish a man's growth without destroying his roots.* **99**
>
> *Frank A. Clark*

Another major factor that contributes to writing success is organization. That is, the process of getting an evidence-based publication submitted and accepted is dependent on creating the circumstances for it to occur, because it does not just happen. The organizational approach to getting thoughts down on paper in an acceptable professional format will require allocation of time periods for writing and achievement of the steps described in this section on publishing. Therefore, it is useful to remember the following (Wills, 2000):

- Work on eliminating negative self-talk (e.g., "I can't do this" or "This paper will never get published").
- Remember that every author at some point in his or her career had to start at the beginning.
- Negative manuscript reviews should never be personalized, because almost everyone has received at least one.
- There is a collective experience of feeling confident, unsure, hesitant, weary, excited, bored, and tired that all authors can relate to with writing for publication.
- Authors who are successful do not take no for an answer easily; they are able to brush aside criticism, look at it objectively, and revise the paper accordingly, resulting in a much improved document.
- Setting realistic goals for initiating and completing a writing task is essential to prevent the disappointment of unrealistic expectations and possibly abandoning the project entirely.
- Developing a plan that specifies a concrete course of action with attainable benchmarks of accomplishment enables an author to feel satisfaction associated with achieving a stated goal.

Deciding What to Publish

Professional publications on EBP can be found everywhere. The significance of its influence is demonstrated by the number of publications that can be found through bibliographic searches, the number of professional journals that regularly feature columns on EBP, and other publications that address the topic exclusively, such as this book and the journal *Evidence-Based Nursing*.

One of the first decisions an author makes in beginning the writing process is the choice of what to write and how it will be written. There are numerous opportunities for publishing that vary from something as straightforward as a letter to the editor to the complex writing project of editing a major nursing textbook. Here is a listing of the wide range of publishing options:

- Letters to the editor
- Books
- Chapters
- Articles
- Newsletter inserts
- Book and media reviews

- Commentaries
- Continuing education reviews
- NCLEX Questions
- Evidence-based clinical practice guidelines
- Standards of care

Authors with limited publishing experience may want to begin with manageable writing endeavors, such as a media review or contributing a chapter to a textbook. Students, under the tutelage of their instructors, may be encouraged to revamp their written class assignment into a manuscript for journal submission. Well-established authors, journal editors, and other professional leaders continually search for aspiring authors who have both the motivation and professional expertise as well as the willingness to engage in the publishing process.

Selecting a Journal

The format and content of a manuscript targeted for journal submission will be dictated by the editorial guidelines and technical specifications of the journal. The author must first target a journal that corresponds to the subject matter of the manuscript. Authors intending to submit evidence-based papers will need to apprise themselves of the following journal criteria before making the decision to submit to a particular journal (Grant, 1998; Hundley, 2002; Mason, 1999).

- Is the journal peer-reviewed?
- What is the profile of the journal's readership?
- What is the turnaround period for review?
- What is the "in press" period (i.e., from time of acceptance to publication)?
- What are the technical specifications?

Manuscripts submitted to **peer-reviewed journals** are critiqued by a team of reviewers who have expertise in the subject matter of the paper. Any identification of the manuscript's author(s) is removed and, likewise, the anonymity of the reviewers is maintained during the review process. This type of review process is known as the **blind review,** meaning that neither the authors nor the reviewers know the identities of each other. It is believed that the blind review process is the most objective and fair way of judging the significance, the technical competence, and contribution to the professional literature.

Peer-reviewed journals publish more rigorously reviewed manuscripts than those reviewed by other means. Generally, most authors prefer to have their manuscripts published in these journals for this reason. Manuscripts published in regularly featured columns of peer-reviewed journals may not be peer-reviewed. Authors need to ascertain this fact before submission. Another useful criterion to use in considering the choice for journal submission is the readership profile. Although the style and format of articles published by journals will be obvious to the author in terms of the type of article (e.g., data-based, clinical, or policy-oriented papers), having other editorial information is useful in terms of understanding the need to insert additional narrative on research methodology or clinical implications (Carroll-Johnson, 2001; De-Behnke, Kline, & Shih, 2001).

In most instances, information on the review process (e.g., the review period time frame and technical specifications) can be found in the "information for authors" section in each journal. Many authors are concerned about the timeliness in which manuscripts are published. Authors may worry that a research paper that has undergone a lengthy review process will not then be published in a timely manner. Concerns also exist regarding the delay in publishing an "in press" manuscript because a lengthy time frame will substantially slow the dissemination of research findings. Answers to these questions can be easily obtained from journal editors. There are currently numerous Web sites for nursing journals wherein technical specifications are listed, editorial philosophy is posted, and hyperlinks are available to the journal's publisher for convenient access (American Psychological Association [APA], 2002). The journal's technical specifications include the following:

- Page length
- Reference format (e.g. APA)
- Margins, font style, and size
- Use of graphics, photos, and figures
- Face page and author identifying information
- Number of hard copies
- Electronic version and software
- Inclusion of a self-addressed stamped envelope

Developing the Manuscript Concept

Developing the concept for the manuscript is contingent on the author's area of clinical expertise and the need for evidence because there is a dearth of accessible information on which to base clinical practice. A clinician may want to share information with colleagues about an innovative intervention or implementation of an exemplary program, or may report the findings of testing a new approach to providing clinical services. There is an urgent need to publish articles on the search for and critical appraisal of evidence as healthcare providers increasingly desire to base their practices on empirically tested approaches. However, the publication of evidence-based articles and reports is in the seminal stages. These types of articles have only recently begun to be published in certain healthcare professions. Unlike other areas in the healthcare literature, there has been relatively little written in any subspecialty area on the critical appraisal of accumulated evidence to guide clinical practices.

As the author proceeds with the process of refining the concept for writing an article on EBP, the perusal of the literature will assist in distillation of the topic into an organizational outline. Reviewing the literature will enable the author to gain an understanding of how to develop this publication uniquely and in a manner that contributes to the body of evidence-based nursing literature (Betz, 2001; Farella, 2002; Siwek, Gourlay, Slawson, & Shaughnessy, 2002; Webb, 2002).

Review of the Literature

Throughout the discussion on methods for disseminating evidence, such as journal clubs and public presentations, the Internet was identified as a technology resource. This also is true for publishing efforts. Use of online bibliographic databases enables writers to conduct more comprehensive and better literature searches. The following bibliographic databases will be useful when proceeding with the literature search for writing evidence-based articles and reports.

- Cochrane Database of Systematic Reviews (interdisciplinary)
- Cochrane Controlled Trials Register (interdisciplinary)
- ACP Journal Club (interdisciplinary)
- Evidence-Based Medicine Reviews (interdisciplinary)
- DARE (interdisciplinary)
- Cumulative Index of Nursing and Allied Health Literature (CINAHL, a nursing and allied health literature database that contains international journals from these disciplines)
- MEDLINE (a medical literature database of international medical, nursing, and allied health journals that contains primarily medical journals and selected nursing and allied health journals that have met the criteria for inclusion)

In conducting a literature review preliminary to writing a manuscript, a few guidelines should be followed. References cited in a manuscript should be recent, meaning those published within the past 3–5 years. In some professions, it may be difficult to find current citations from the literature, thereby necessitating accessing the interdisciplinary literature representing not only health-related disciplines but also non–health-related disciplines (e.g., education, job development, and rehabilitation, to name a few). There are classic references from any field that should be included in a publication because these are seminal works on which subsequent publications are based and cannot be ignored.

An author will have concluded his or her search for evidence when the **saturation level** of research has been reached. The saturation level is achieved once the author no longer finds any new references, but instead, is familiar and knowledgeable with the literature. Clinicians who author evidence-based articles will rely heavily on empirically based articles as they are searching for evidence. Authors will be less likely to include clinically oriented articles other than to demonstrate the relevance to clinical practice, such as the prevalence of falls in the elderly. Textbooks should be used sparingly in evidence-based publications unless the books are written on highly specialized topics and are a compilation of perspectives from experts in the field (Heinrich, 2002).

Developing a Timeline

Healthcare professionals are well acquainted with developing and adhering to a work plan that identifies benchmarks of achievement. Having a work plan specifies in a concrete fashion the necessary tasks the author must undertake to complete the writing goal. The greater the level of specificity, the better the "roadmap" the author will have for reaching his or her goal. Together with the identified tasks, *realistic* timelines should be listed along with strategies for keeping on track with accomplishing the steps of the writing project. A writing project timeline might look like the one listed below.

Operationalize the idea/select a topic—June 1
Formulate the OUTLINE—June 15
Locate journals/author guidelines—July 15
Survey the literature—September 15
Develop the first draft—November 15
Review/proofread—December 10
Formulate revisions—January 8
Submit—January 20

Writing Strategies

Content outlines for articles will vary according to the type of manuscript. The generic outline for an evidence-based article, as used in the ongoing evidence-based column in the journal *Pediatric Nursing*, follows this format:

- Introduction to the clinical problem
- The clinical question
- Search for the evidence (i.e., the search strategy used to find the evidence and the results)
- Presentation of the evidence
- Critical appraisal of the evidence with implications for future research
- Application to practice (i.e., based on the evidence reviewed, what should be implemented in clinical practice settings)
- Evaluation (includes outcomes of the practice change if they were measured).

Obviously, writing an article for publication involves much more than just following an outline. The writing process is a slow and tedious effort that is characterized by stops and starts, cutting and pasting, and the frequent use of the Delete key. However, writers use several pragmatic tips to help them complete their writing projects. Writing begins with following the manuscript outline at whatever section that can be written, even if it means first writing the simpler portions of the manuscript (e.g., the conclusion and introduction). Placing words on paper is important to "priming the pump," meaning to write anything, even if initially the words are awkward sounding and stilted. Inspiration will not necessarily happen spontaneously.

- Creativity is dependent on discipline and organizational techniques (Webb, 2002; Wong, 1999). These organizational techniques include the following:
- The manuscript outline should be followed as written. If the author discovers the narrative would be better written otherwise, the outline needs revision.
- Writing something is preferable to writing nothing. Awkward-sounding statements can always be edited and/or deleted. Initially, generating loose ideas that are difficult to couple with words can lead to more fluid thinking and word composition.
- Before completing a session of writing, leave notes within the document that can be used as prompts for the next writing activity. Leaving author notes ensures continuity with the train of thought from the last writing session and helps to facilitate recall and ease with the writing process.
- Write the paper anonymously, meaning there is no self-identification, although there may be exceptions in discussing particular programs. Use the same verb tense throughout, and avoid the use of passive voice. Note the major themes of paragraphs in the margins of the manuscript to discern the discussion sequencing, highlighting potential problems with organization.

- Avoid the use of *should*s, *must*s, and other words that sound opinionated and self-serving. Insert information that can be replicated and applied by others by avoiding the use of nonspecific terminology. For example, when discussing family support strategies, consider what more information can be shared with readers to enhance a clearer understanding of what is specifically meant.

Proofreading the Manuscript

If possible, the optimal proofreading strategy is to have colleagues or friends read the manuscript draft, including individuals who have expertise in the content area as well as those who possess no content expertise. Those without content expertise are specifically helpful in reading the manuscript for clarity, style, and grammatical errors. However, it is essential that whoever proofreads the draft be a good writer with the capacity to provide specific suggestions for editing purposes. Very often, faculty members whose students are writing for publication outside of their course assignments are willing to serve as proofreaders.

Authors can serve as their own proofreaders as well. Setting the manuscript draft aside for a week or two will create the distance needed to read it again with a set of "fresh eyes." In this manner, the author can read his or her own work more objectively and potentially single out the flaws with sentence structure, spelling, organization, and content. Once the proofreading is accomplished, the draft is revised based on collegial feedback and the author's own proofing.

Spell checking the document is an absolute must in proofing manuscripts. However, automatic spell checking is not enough in that it is not capable of detecting problems with some misspellings. The numbering of tables, graphics, and figures will need to be double-checked to ensure that they are properly matched with the sequence identified in the paper. The citation of references in the text is checked with those in the reference list for correct spelling, dates of publication, and referencing format. Other technical specifications (e.g., pagination, use of headers, margins, fonts) are reviewed to ensure conformity to those listed in the author guidelines. Permissions and transfer of copyright are included with the packet of materials that will be sent to the editorial office.

Once this process is completed, the manuscript can be submitted for review. The information for authors and/or the receipt from the editorial office will indicate the expected turnaround period for the manuscript review. If after a few weeks no feedback has been received, it is appropriate to e-mail or call the editorial office to inquire about the status of the review. As mentioned previously, it is important not to take feedback personally. An impassioned approach will serve the author well by moving beyond what might be stinging criticisms to revising the draft based on the reviewers' recommendations. It is at this juncture that the author needs to keep focused on what was and continues to be the original goal—to publish the paper and contribute to the professional literature on evidence-based practice (Ohler, 2002; Sullivan, 2002).

Disseminating Evidence to Influence Health Policy

Politically, healthcare providers are in an enviable position to advocate for change because they are highly regarded by the American public. As a leading politician recently remarked to a nursing colleague, "Political endorsements from state nursing organizations are one of the most important endorsements a politician seeks to obtain." Several public survey polls illustrate the generous views the public has of healthcare providers. A 1998 NBC News and *The Wall Street Journal* poll

table 14.1 *Wall Street Journal* **poll: Groups most responsible for making the healthcare system better**

Group	Percentage Believed to Make Healthcare System Better
Nurses	67%
Pharmacists/drug stores	63%
Physicians	55%
Hospitals	44%
Pharmaceutical companies	35%
Insurance companies	32%
Health and Human Services Departments	28%
HMOs/managed care plans	23%

NBC News and the Wall Street Journal (1998, June 18–21)

found that the public believed nurses, pharmacists, and physicians were the foremost healthcare groups responsible for making the healthcare system better (see Table 14-1). A public opinion survey conducted jointly by Harvard University, Robert Wood Johnson Foundation, and the University of Maryland found that the public rated nurses and physicians most favorably of all groups to have the best recommendations for children's healthcare (see Table 14-2). In essence, such a testimonial is *evidence* of the potential influence that healthcare providers, individually and collectively, have to effect changes in policy and to be engaged in policymaking. The key is not only recognizing this potential but also actively taking advantage of opportunities that arise to be engaged in policymaking at all levels of government and within professional organizations and service agencies.

Regrettably, opportunities to affect policy change may not be seized or recognized for their value and importance. A nursing colleague recently witnessed the unpleasant exchange of a lawmaker's stern words directed to a nursing administrator from a local nursing education department. This nursing education administrator had been invited to provide testimony on the state's nursing shortage during a legislative hearing on this workforce crisis. Unfortunately, the nursing administrator was ill prepared and had not conducted the preparatory work necessary to offer legislative testimony. The legislator was angered with her lack of preparation and her inability to answer his questions about the state's nursing shortage and statewide nursing efforts to address this issue. Not only was this an example of inadequate professional preparation but the circumstances also reflected negatively on the profession as a whole because the policy input on behalf of nurses was not heard.

These two vignettes illustrate the continuum of possibilities for healthcare professionals to influence policy. As healthcare professionals learn to become more involved in policymaking, they will be expected to integrate evidence as the basis for policy development. As policy makers, healthcare providers will be "at the table" with key stakeholders, citing evidence to improve healthcare resources and services for national and international populations. This sec-

table 14.2 Groups Americans trust for children's healthcare policies

Group	Percentage Believed to Have Best Recommendations
Nurses	77%
Physicians	72%
Church organizations	66%
Child advocacy groups	61%
Teacher's organizations	58%
Public health officials	57%
Hospital associations	50%
Health insurance companies	31%
Labor unions	22%

Blendon, et al. (1998)

tion will provide specific suggestions for integrating evidence in writing and other policymaking efforts (National Health Service Information Authority, 2001).

Developing Issues Briefs

There is a growing recognition that the most current evidence and best thinking are needed to provide policy issues to politicians (Health Resources and Services Administration, 1999). The emergence of using evidence in clinical practice throughout healthcare to improve clinical practice has now been transferred to policymaking. A legislator cannot bring forward legislation without having the necessary substantiation, based on various sources of evidence, as to the need or problem to be addressed (ESRC UK Centre for Evidence-Based Policy and Practice, 2001a, 2001b; Health Development Agency, 2002a, 2002b). One avenue for informing policy makers is by developing issues briefs (see Appendix H for a brief developed by the National Association of Pediatric Nurse Practitioners' KySS [Keep your children/yourself Safe and Secure] Campaign [Melnyk, Brown, Jones, Kreipe, & Novak, 2003] to assist policy makers in drafting a bill to improve access to children's mental health services). Issues briefs provide the current evidence, based on prevalence reports, research by scientists, and the opinion of experts.

The key to developing issues briefs is to be succinct and direct in communicating with the intended audience. A well-written issues brief summarizes and clearly communicates to the reader the scope of the policy issue. The reader should be able to scan the document quickly and be able to comprehend the major aspects of the policy issue that is featured. Tips for organizing an issues brief include the following:

- Lead with a title on the masthead that clearly conveys the purpose.
- Identify the policy issue in the first sentence so that by the end of the opening paragraph, the reader knows the policy issue.

- Include background information that highlights the major features of the issue.
- Indicate the historical pattern of response to the problem in subsequent statements.
- Identify the inherent limitations as well as the problem and why it is still a problem.

An issues brief will provide a systematic review and synthesis of literature based on the selected topic addressing the demonstrated clinical outcomes of interventions, cost-effectiveness, and applicability. As the supporting evidence is presented, the reader is led in a logical sequence through the presentation of information that enables a clear understanding of the need for policy change. The concluding remarks of this section provide the links between research, clinical practice, and policymaking. It distills for the reader what has been done and how it can be applied to policymaking, which may be difficult for the politician or stakeholders if they do not have the expertise to "point the way" (Box 14-6).

---

box 14.6

Typical Topics and Components of an Issues Brief

Issues briefs are developed to address issues of interest to policy makers:

TYPICAL TOPICS
Health care financing
Risk/benefit ratio
Ways of reducing costs
Lower rates of mortality and improved morbidity
The role of technology in health care
Human resource needs
System change to improve services

TYPICAL COMPONENTS
Title

Background of the Issue
Historical pattern of response to the problem
Inherent limitations and problems
Why it is still a problem

Review and Synthesis of the Literature
Clinical outcomes of interventions
Cost-effectiveness
Applicability
Policy Implications

System changes
Services proposed
Population outcomes

A review of the literature should be conducted differently for policy makers than for a research audience. The analysis is conducted not only with clinical knowledge in the area but also with an understanding of the practical implications for policy makers. Where the information was obtained (i.e., meaning the type of research studies reviewed and synthesized in the paper; expert opinion of researchers, clinicians, and experts) is incorporated in the brief (Huberman, 1990). Once the strength of the available evidence has been analyzed, conclusions are made about where gaps in the literature exist for which further research is needed.

The final steps of translating what is known into policy and/or practice are important (American Dental Association, 2002). The healthcare provider who is involved in constructing a policy issue brief will emphasize the application for policy and practice. That is, what is being advocated for policy change? How will the policy result in a change for services, such as treatments, assessment approaches, and evaluation of intervention outcomes (e.g., What clinical outcomes for the target population are expected, such as improved health as evidenced by better cardiovascular status and a higher level of daily functioning)?

Policy conclusions should delineate in detail the possible clinical implications. For example, implications would recommend:

- Funding priorities in the treatment of chronic conditions
- Projected effects of funding cutbacks (e.g., a decrease in access to care and treatment)
- Longitudinal studies of various treatment approaches (e.g., hormone replacement therapy)
- Identification of actual and anticipated population outcomes

In this way, issues briefs assist policy makers in understanding the evidence so they can create legislation founded on the premise that policy change is based on good science and knowledge.

Design layout is a factor in conveying the message to the audience. Obvious requirements in design layout of policy briefs are to ensure that there are graphics to highlight the major propositions, problems, facts, and recommendations. Boxes that contain bulleted, succinct statements are effective. A pullout that defines terminology may be useful if the language is unfamiliar to readers. A case example to illustrate the nature of the problem or the implications of recommendations may be helpful.

In a nutshell, policy makers are more likely to use information and evidence from a policy brief if:

- The research evidence in the brief is focused
- The document can be skimmed quickly for salient points
- It is synthesized, conclusion-oriented, and succinct (i.e., no more than 2–4 pages) (Melnyk et al., 2003)

Use of graphics and visual pointers also enables the reader to navigate through the material easily. To add depth, briefs can be accompanied by other tools, such as slides, spreadsheets, links to articles, Web sites, and a list of key contacts (Melnyk et al., 2003).

Understanding the Target Audience

Daily, consumers are bombarded with "new" or "breaking" information about healthcare that includes promising new medications and treatments, hope for medical cures, and new treatment approaches. The barrage of information can be confusing for consumers. The conflicting information on hormone replacement therapy is an excellent example of the confusion women experience in understanding what might be the long-term effects of taking hormones (National Health Service Information Authority, 2001). Policy experts have noted that the public seeks information that will enable them to better understand the disease pathophysiology and clinical application of that knowledge. In writing for a particular audience, the author needs to have an awareness of what type of information the audience is looking for and what would be looked on as most helpful.

Thoughtful and well-referenced issues briefs will be used by professional associations to assist them in the development of critical paths and practice guidelines. For example, the Agency for Healthcare Research and Quality (AHRQ) National Guidelines Clearinghouse contains over 1,000 clinical practice guidelines that clinicians can access. AHRQ is currently involved in supporting the implementation efforts of the State Child Health Insurance Program (SCHIP) by producing national performance measures for this national effort (AHRQ, 2000). Additionally, policy makers and other stakeholders can work with clinicians in suggesting topics for evidence review and development (Huberman, 1990).

Writing in Understandable Language

The content and format of a policy brief will vary depending on the characteristics of the intended audience and whether the readers are primarily consumers, policy makers, or professionals. To illustrate, if an issues brief is written for a professional audience, the summary of the research evidence can be presented using research terminology. If issues briefs are written for consumer-oriented audiences (e.g., legislators), research terminology is altered for consumer comprehension. Generally speaking, the reading level for widespread consumer distribution should be for a sixth-grade reading level (using the Flesch Kineard Reading Level found on software tools to assess reading level is most helpful). For policy makers, the format needs to emphasize practical information that is easy to read.

It is the writer's responsibility to apply or translate for the reader the synthesis of research for policy (i.e., how a particular practice can be improved and what the expected outcomes are for the targeted underserved populations). The issues brief author(s) need to keep in mind the targeted readership and the change that is being advocated. Based on these two primary criteria, the issues brief will be written in the style and format appropriate for the audience. All knowledge must have local application in order to be used. The effective issues brief will be written in a style and format enabling the policy maker to see easily the relevance for local or state application (Louis, 1996).

Lastly, information overload is a barrier to accessing and using evidence (Bryant, 2000). Having a preexisting relationship or intending to develop one with policy makers is essential to be buttressed by the evidence (Huberman, 1990). A recent study found that seeking the advice and expertise of colleagues related to medical issues was preferable to seeking information from the literature. This model would likely apply to working with policy makers, as well (Huag, 1997). Relationships and other methods of contact will strengthen the ties with policy makers, such as bulletins for decision makers that focus on a particular issue, as is done by several policy think tanks. Additionally, healthcare provider experts aware of the organizational barriers of workload, time constraints, and authority to implement change associated with projected change will be in a position to address these concerns directly through personal contacts with policy makers (Funk et al., 1991).

Policy briefs are designed to inform readers with analyses of research results that have policy relevance. Recent policy briefs of interest to healthcare providers have been published on the problems associated with needle sticks and nursing staffing. Issues briefs are effective tools for use by nursing professionals to describe, discuss, and recommend the need for policy changes.

Disseminating Evidence to the Media

Heathcare professionals need to think critically about why a reporter would want to take time to hear about their work and to listen to what they have to say. Professionals who are serious about disseminating evidence need to be prepared to answer this question (Box 14-7).

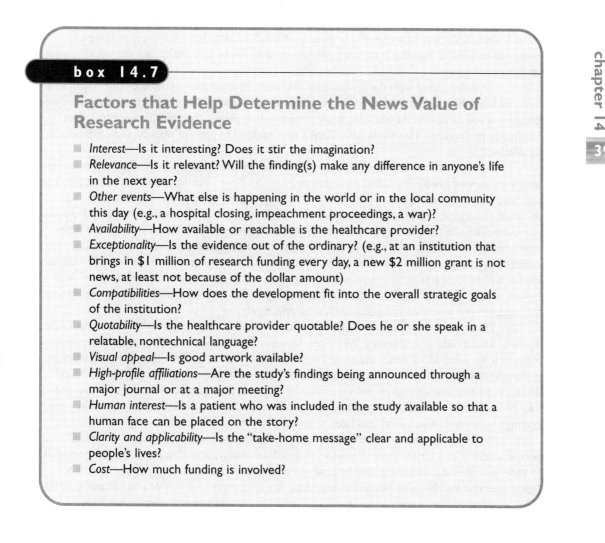

box 14.7

Factors that Help Determine the News Value of Research Evidence

- *Interest*—Is it interesting? Does it stir the imagination?
- *Relevance*—Is it relevant? Will the finding(s) make any difference in anyone's life in the next year?
- *Other events*—What else is happening in the world or in the local community this day (e.g., a hospital closing, impeachment proceedings, a war)?
- *Availability*—How available or reachable is the healthcare provider?
- *Exceptionality*—Is the evidence out of the ordinary? (e.g., at an institution that brings in $1 million of research funding every day, a new $2 million grant is not news, at least not because of the dollar amount)
- *Compatibilities*—How does the development fit into the overall strategic goals of the institution?
- *Quotability*—Is the healthcare provider quotable? Does he or she speak in a relatable, nontechnical language?
- *Visual appeal*—Is good artwork available?
- *High-profile affiliations*—Are the study's findings being announced through a major journal or at a major meeting?
- *Human interest*—Is a patient who was included in the study available so that a human face can be placed on the story?
- *Clarity and applicability*—Is the "take-home message" clear and applicable to people's lives?
- *Cost*—How much funding is involved?

This section of the chapter provides general guidance for talking to the media about findings from research and evidence-based implementation projects. Basics are covered first, and emphasis follows with regard to the dynamic nature of news, factors influencing why reporters cover certain stories, and information about how to influence the process.

The Basics

Everyone has a story to tell. A technician witnesses a miraculous patient recovery in the middle of the night; a nurse designs a study that uncovers the ineffectiveness of a tool widely used by healthcare providers; a researcher designs a novel molecule that evolves into a drug to treat the symptoms of heart disease in millions. However, these examples all deal with healthcare. What about sports, marriage, hobbies, other professions, world politics, and travel? It is a huge world out there, full of incredible stories, amazing breakthroughs, and passionate people performing great feats. Really, it is almost too much. At any instant, people can choose from hundreds of broadcast channels beamed into living rooms, select from millions of Web sites, and view news from a multitude of publications. Information is coming at everyone in a flood, making it difficult for someone to listen to a healthcare provider's story or research findings.

To make a case with the media, first you must be clear about your message. What is it that you want the world to know? Have you developed an incredible new method for identifying children at risk of abuse? Might your work inspire young people to explore research or the healthcare professions? Have you developed a new method to prevent obesity and cardiovascular disease?

Second, what is your definition of "the world"? Perhaps the only person who needs to hear your message is the president of your university because your department is slated for closure and you want him or her to be aware of your colleagues' good work. The target of your message also could be a particular company to which you hope to license a new technology that you have discovered. Your target audience could be overweight individuals who should hear your message of moderation, exercise, and weight loss. Specifically, knowing or choosing your audience is just as important as shaping your message. It may be that you need to work with the media, but perhaps you simply need to make one phone call or send a letter to one individual. Not all dissemination requires the media, particularly in this era when individuals possess more tools than ever for reaching targeted audiences effectively.

Finally, it is important to conduct a reality check in terms of assessing the competition. There is a multitude of fascinating Web sites, libraries full of books, reports to complete, and patients to be seen, all of which compete for the public's attention. Therefore, it is important to remember that just because you want someone to listen to what you have to say about the evidence on a particular topic does not mean they will listen. This may be the most common mistake of healthcare providers (i.e., making the assumption that people will be interested in your findings because so much work has been invested in a particular project).

When attempting to make contact with the media, you will often find a very intelligent person working in a virtual frenzy because of deadlines and competitive pressures. Be prepared to state your message concisely and be ready to challenge that person into paying attention. Never presume that because you have something to say, a reporter owes you the courtesy of listening. You may be one of dozens or hundreds of people who contact the reporter on that day in the midst of a multitude of demanding tasks that need to be accomplished.

To be prepared to make your case for why the media should cover what you have to say, you should place yourself and your story through scrutiny that mirrors a review from a top journal. You should know who has done or is doing work similar to yours and how your work is different. Be prepared to justify why funding was provided for your research or project. Be ready to explain the significance of your work in a way that the reporter can understand, which may result in an explanation unlike one you have ever given to other colleagues. It is important to ask yourself the question, Why should my story dominate over a typical day's smattering of "health news" (e.g., the genetic variations of malaria, cold-weather lip care, overeating as one of life's guilty pleasures, and ski-related injuries)?

News Is Dynamic

Once you have honed your message and defined the audience that you would like to reach as well as decided that the media might be a good way to communicate with that audience, you need to recognize the potential power of the media. When people turn to the Internet, the TV remote, or the radio, they simply hit a button, and a flurry of information comes sailing forth. There is a tendency in most of us simply to listen to what we hear, not quite unquestioningly but certainly passively. For example, people turn on the radio, hear "the day's top news," and make what they will of it. However, there is truthfully no central repository of events deemed to be "news" from which the media draws. Ordinary people decide what is news. If you remember nothing else from this chapter, remember this: *The news is up for grabs.*

As a news recipient, you are allowing your world view to be dictated by someone else. Whether it is an announcer in a radio booth in Albuquerque, an unseen TV editor shouting across a newsroom in Los Angeles, or a webmaster spinning tales from his living room, you are subjecting yourself to someone else's choices about what you should and should not hear. People make these choices every day (i.e., which information to pass along and which to conceal or ignore). You might inform your neighbors about the interest rate you received on refinancing your house but not tell how long you spent brushing your teeth that morning. A father might tell his young child about his first experience playing baseball but not about his first experience with a girl. We are all editors.

This also is true with the media. A ferry boat sinks and 240 people die, but it is not news because it happened halfway across the globe. The same day, a single man veers off the road and escapes without a scratch, but it is a headline news story because the driver is a politician who was driving while intoxicated.

There is no single body of events that constitutes "news" and another set of events that constitutes "non-news." Deciding the news is an incredibly dynamic process, and becoming aware of this is a huge step toward working with the media effectively. Prepare carefully first, then pursue your share of the media. It could be that the healthcare provider across town is conducting work less interesting than your own, but maybe she or he actually took the time to call a reporter. As a result, the front-page story is about the other professional's work, not yours.

In addition to the specifics of your story, there is a multitude of factors that will decide whether your "news" is the media's "news" on any given day (see Box 14-7). Being aware of these and other factors is important if your story is to make the news.

- What issues are routinely covered by the publication?
- When is the reporter's deadline, and what time of day are you contacting him or her?
- What else is going on in the world today? Has there been a big layoff locally? A major terrorism event?
- Which reporter or editor is on vacation, and who is filling in? What are his or her interests?
- What are the personal issues that the reporter is grappling with that day?
- What is the editorial approach or bias of the publication as a whole?
- From which demographics does the outlet draw the bulk of its advertising dollars?
- Who is able to provide or offer the best opportunity for artwork or a visually interesting angle?
- Which source returned the phone call most quickly?

Most of these factors cannot be controlled by you, but they mold coverage of stories. Consider for example a public relations (PR) specialist who prepared publicity about a research finding published in a top scientific journal (i.e., a fossil of a tropical beast known as a "champsosaur" that was found in the Arctic Circle) that included a global warming theme, a well-executed color sketch of an interesting beast, an animal whose name sounded like "chompasaurus," an accessible and engaging scientist, and a top-notch publication aligned to promise tremendous coverage. That same day, though, the U.S. House of Representatives voted to impeach President Clinton. As a result, the "chompasaurus" was redirected to the inside pages of newspapers everywhere by an event that the researcher had no hope to control. The story still received international attention but not as sweeping as would have occurred in the absence of a national "high-profile" event.

The point to remember is that news is a fluid medium. There are all sorts of people manipulating events to determine what you read, hear, and view. You can make the decision to sit on the sideline and receive news that is determined by others or do your best to convey your message to your audience.

You also will find that many others may attempt to manipulate your findings or story for a certain news angle. Box 14-8 provides some examples of the people who might become involved in an ordinary healthcare or research story. Your graduate student may seek to turn the findings into a job offer. The PR department may hawk the results to the media, seeking positive publicity for the institution. The fund-raising office may have in mind a meeting with a donor who is ready to give millions of dollars, based on work just like yours. Your competitors will comb through the article, seeking weak spots. The company funding your pharmaceutical research may be thrilled with the results and will promote them on Wall Street. Also, politicians may rush to claim credit for supplying the funding that resulted in such important knowledge. The list goes on and on.

Much of the competition for news space and its interpretation is invisible to the typical healthcare professional, who usually spends years immersed in his or her work, compared with time spent with an actual media representative—an exposure usually measured in minutes. Thus, many healthcare professionals approach the media with a certain bravado. Although anyone who works with the media ought to be prepared for negative fallout, healthcare providers seem to be particularly vulnerable to being caught off guard when a supposedly straightforward process of communication goes awry.

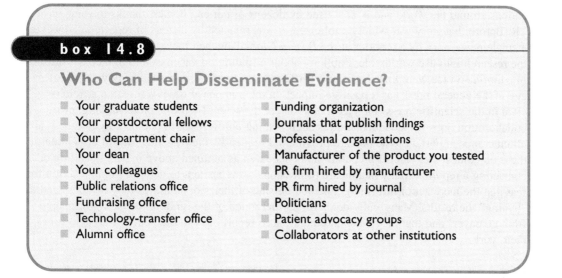

box 14.8

Who Can Help Disseminate Evidence?

- Your graduate students
- Your postdoctoral fellows
- Your department chair
- Your dean
- Your colleagues
- Public relations office
- Fundraising office
- Technology-transfer office
- Alumni office
- Funding organization
- Journals that publish findings
- Professional organizations
- Manufacturer of the product you tested
- PR firm hired by manufacturer
- PR firm hired by journal
- Politicians
- Patient advocacy groups
- Collaborators at other institutions

The Bad, the Good, and Media Exposure in General

Media scrutiny may bring with it the realization that your quote really is not true (e.g., your project is not "the first" or "the only," as you sincerely thought it was). A collaborator's name may be unintentionally omitted from an article, causing jealousy or even a rift. Your competitors (i.e., that group across the country with a huge reputation), whose work over the last 10 years will be proven completely inane if you are correct, may try and dispute your works (worse yet, they may even have better media contacts). Your colleagues down the hall may say that your work is unimportant because it was covered in the popular press when truthfully, they are jealous because prospective graduate students want to visit your team, not theirs. Or simply working with the media may consume large amounts of time that you could be spending elsewhere, and the process is no longer fun for you, but the queries keep pouring in. There are a great many pitfalls about working with the media, and the costs versus the benefits need to be weighed before deciding to pursue this avenue of dissemination.

Media attention can be extremely beneficial as well. Your student may get a great offer from an employer who was unaware of your work before it was covered in a major business magazine. You might be invited to speak at a national meeting based on an organizer's Internet search of a topic. After reading about your work, a representative from a large company may visit you, then fund your work with several hundred thousand dollars. The article may help fuel perceived momentum around an expansion of research or a healthcare topic, resulting in a spurt in donations that will fund your future initiatives. There also may be a boost in morale from the media coverage that helps your institution retain the best and brightest individuals. Publicity about the findings from a clinical trial also can speed research and fuel initiatives to better health outcomes for the public.

Publicists of research findings have witnessed all these results and more. Publicity about a nurse's study of rocking-chair therapy to treat dementia was covered by major publications around the world and is now used by dozens of nursing homes, thanks to some basic PR. Before that story was widely publicized, it was rejected by dozens of reporters. However, a single news story by a reporter at the *Boston Globe* launched the story into popularity and the research into use worldwide. Publicity about a finding on vaccines and thimerosal resulted in editorials in the *New York Times* and *Wall Street Journal*. Also, research shows that coverage in the general press has a positive impact on the number of times a research article is cited in the scientific press. Increased citations in the scientific press, more funding, greater collaboration, jobs for students, and research making a difference in people's lives—these are all outcomes important to healthcare providers. Frequently, the first step toward disseminating these outcomes after careful preparation is conducted as outlined above is simply calling or contacting a reporter. Many healthcare professionals are hesitant to take this simple action for fear that the mere act of informing a person outside of their communities may be construed as "hyping" the results. Many individuals forget that much of the funding for their work came from taxpayers and that they have an obligation to report back to the people who paid for their work.

Some Practical Advice

Even when reluctant to call the media, chances are that you will have contact with a reporter about your study's findings eventually. When this occurs, you might want to have Box 14-9 posted nearby as a starting point or simply have handy the phone number of your PR person, who should work as your advocate. Frequently, a PR representative can clarify a reporter's questions for you or provide you with the reporter's background. It is not uncommon for a local reporter to lack total understanding about research, whereas some reporters at the largest publications will have their doctorates and will relish the opportunity to grill you in detail about the methods used in your project. A PR person also can redirect a call to someone else in the organization who is more appropriate or provide you the happenings within your organization that might influence the reporter's approach. Occasionally, a PR representative will counsel you to steer clear of a certain reporter because of that reporter's poor track record.

Even as you invite a PR person into your life, you must remain aware that he or she also is altering the story to some extent and placing your work in a particular context. For instance, after a PR specialist conducts a careful interview and does some reading about the topic, he or she attempts to write a summary of the healthcare professional's work in approximately 800 words (see Appendix I for an example of a press release summary). Then the summary is provided to the professional for review. Typically a physician, nurse, or researcher will read what is written, change a couple of lowercase letters to uppercase and perhaps strike out an erroneous word or two or insert some jargon. They typically limit their comments to the words presented to them in the summary. It never occurs to many professionals that they have left the entire interpretation of their work (e.g., the context, the emphasis) up to the PR specialist. If the words are accurate, they approve the overall theme. It is great when that happens, but healthcare professionals should be encouraged to consider whether the PR person's interpretation is accurate or one that they would choose themselves.

With the input of a PR person who specializes in covering research findings, a host of other issues will arise when disseminating evidence to the media. Briefly, here are a few of those issues.

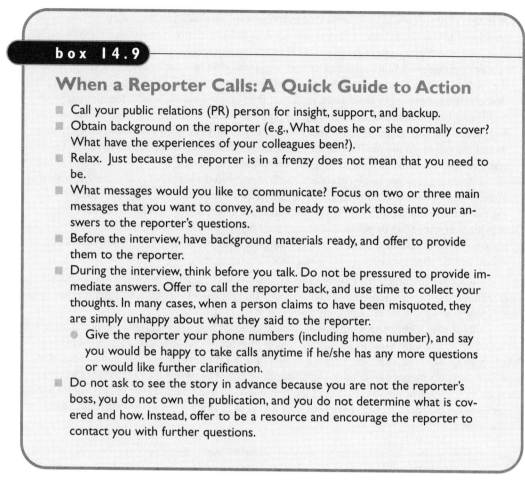

Embargoes: A news "embargo" (i.e., a restriction on the release of any media information about the findings from a study before they are published in a journal article) is oftentimes used by some journals or science organizations to give reporters time to develop a story on a complex or exciting topic. However, not all reporters agree to embargoes; many see them as authorized or misguided attempts to control the news—and not all embargoes are legitimate. To be safe, if you are part of an embargoed story, you need to clarify this up front with the reporter before you say anything of substance. That said, hundreds of research stories are embargoed every week, and rarely does anything go wrong. If you and the reporter agree on the embargo, it is fine to speak to the reporter, and the story will appear after the embargo "lifts."

Off the record: Do not go there. Anything you say is on the record, and if you talk and then say afterward, "That was off the record," the reporter has no obligation to regard those comments as off the record. You have to establish that *before* the interview. Even then, it is risky and better to avoid.

Peer review: This is crucial to veteran research reporters, as crucial to them as it is to researchers. If you are making a claim, you need to have evidence that has been reviewed by someone else. Stories claiming any type of medical or scientific progress in detail usually rely on a publication in a journal or at least a presentation at a professional meeting. Even so, the "rules" are not always clear. A journal article almost always has much more detailed evidence and has been more rigorously reviewed than an abstract for a poster presentation, so the timing can be delicate. So, too, can the publicity be around a paper or presentation. For instance, some journals will reject manuscripts if you or your institution have actively promoted the results in the media, but they will accept them even if the media covered the previously reported results, as long as you did not initiate the coverage.

Press conferences: Try not to be nervous when interviewed during a press conference. Visual elements should be available whenever possible. Keep comments short. Include speakers for the news value they contribute. If you are talking about research results, make sure you have presented at a meeting or published in a journal *before* the conference. Healthcare professionals who make claims and present study findings at a press conference without supporting evidence that has been peer-reviewed place their careers at risk.

It also is important to remember technology-transfer issues. In other words, contact your technology-transfer department and consider filing a patent on any research/program products *before* you publish or present your results.

Reporters come with a variety of interests and abilities, but all have the power to reach out to more people with your message than you will probably be able to reach without them. When dealing with a reporter on a deadline, spending 5 minutes placing an issue in perspective will save them 45 minutes of conducting research on the Web, when they really only have 5 minutes to accomplish the job. Avoiding the temptation to send them to the library, along with the other "don'ts" listed in Box 14-10, will go a long way toward building your reputation as a media source.

---

box 14.10

Some "Don'ts" When Working with Reporters

Don't use scientific jargon.
Don't assume you are a media expert.
Don't wait hours to return a call; call back immediately.
Don't expect a story to name every contributor or collaborator.
Don't assume the reporter is familiar with the details of your project or discipline—ask.
Don't dictate the "proper" questions or the story angle.
Don't talk about just the positive aspects of your research findings; also discuss the limitations.
Don't ask to see a copy of the story before it is published.

You will not want to be a source for all reporters, because some will not be very credible and/or polite. In one instance, a reporter repeatedly demanded to see a research group's "vials containing smallpox virus," no matter how many times the group tried to clarify that it had the *vaccine*, not the *virus*.

There also are reporters who have no interest in looking objectively at news and who instead are seeking a human face to place on a story already written. Additionally, there are reporters who will try to have you tell their version of a story instead of your version. In a story about why people were volunteering to be vaccinated against smallpox, a representative from a major TV network was not satisfied with the answer provided by one participant. The answer did not match the producer's preconceived notion of why people were volunteering, so he instructed the participant to use the word "patriotism" in his answer. Because the young man had been prepared for the pressure exerted by reporters, he disregarded the advice and provided an honest answer. The story was a success, in addition to being truthful.

The payoff from working effectively with the press can be enormous, but the prospect also can be daunting. It is important to prepare thoroughly, seek the assistance of an experienced PR person if one is available, build up a reservoir of patience and persistence, and give it a try. Although it would be simpler if quality work attracted attention on its own, the reality is that news is a "grab bag," and you might as well capture your share of it.

references

Agency for Healthcare Research and Quality (AHRQ). (2000). *Supporting research that improves health care for children and adolescents.* AHRQ Pub. No. 00-P017. Rockville, MD: AHRQ. Available at http://www.ahrq.gov/research/childbrf.htm. Accessed December 11, 2002.

American Dental Association (ADA). (2002). *ADA policy on evidenced-based dentistry.* Available at http://www.ada.org/prof/prac/issues/statements/evidencebased.html. Accessed December 12, 2002.

American Psychological Association (APA). (2002). *Publication manual of the American Psychological Association* (5th. ed). Washington, DC: APA.

Bagott, I., & Bagott, J. (2001). Talk the talk: Overcome your fear of public speaking. *Nursing Spectrum (Metro Edition), 2*(7), 12–13.

Bergren, M. D. (2000) Information technology. Power up your presentation with PowerPoint. *Journal of School Nursing, 16*(4), 44–47.

Betz, C. L.(2001), Frequently asked questions . . . again. *Journal of Pediatric Nursing, 16*(2), 1–2.

Beyla, S. C., & Nicoll L. H. (1998). Developing and presenting a poster presentation. *AORN Journal 67*(2), 468–469.

Blendon, R. J., Young, J. T., McCormick, M. C.,

Kropf, M., & Blair, J. (1998). Americans' views on children's health. *Journal of the American Medical Association, 280,* 2122–2127.

Bryant, A. (2000). *Information wanted? Knowledge, curiosity, uncertainty and evidence: A qualitative study of the perceived information needs of general practitioners.* Paper presented at the Qualitative Evidence-Based Practice Conference, Coventry University, 15–17 May. Available at http://www.leeds.ac.uk/educol/documents/00001417.htm. Accessed May 13, 2002.

Carroll-Johnson, R. M. (2001). Submitting a manuscript for review. *Clinical Journal of Oncology Nursing, 5*(3 Suppl), 13–16.

Cook, D. M. (1998). The power of PowerPoint. *Nurse Educator 23*(4), 5–7.

Cook, J. S. (1989). *The elements of speechwriting and public speaking.* New York: Collier Books.

DeBehnke, D. J., Kline, J. A., & Shih, R. D. (2001). Research fundamentals: Choosing an appropriate journal, manuscript preparation, and interactions with editors. *Academic Emergency Medicine, 8*(8): 844–850.

ESRC UK Centre for Evidence-Based Policy and Practice. (2001a) Working Paper 6. London: Department of Politics, University of London.

ESRC UK Centre for Evidence-Based Policy and Practice. (2001b). Working Paper 1. London: Department of Politics, University of London.

Evans, M. L. (2000). Polished, professional presentation: Unlocking the design elements. *Journal of Continuing Education in Nursing, 31*(5), 213–218

Farella, C. (2002). Read all about it! RN authors have the write stuff. *Nursing Spectrum (Greater Chicago/Ne Illinois & Nw Indiana Edition), 15*(1), 32–34.

Fetter, M. S. (1999). The privilege of publishing. *Medical-Surgical Nursing, 8*(3), 142–143.

Fitzgerald, T. (2000). 5 minutes with . . . Carolyn Zagury, PhD, RN . . . nursing and publishing. *Nurseweek (California Statewide Edition), 13*(20), 15.

Fitzpatrick, J. J. (1999). The joys of publishing. *Applied Nursing Research, 12*(2), 59.

Funk, S. G., Champagne, M. T., Wiese, R. A., & Tournquist, E. M. (1991). Barriers: The barriers to research utilization scale. *Applied Nursing Research, 4*(1), 39–45.

Garity, J. (1999). Creating a professional presentation: A template for success. *Journal of Intravenous Nursing, 22*(2), 81–86.

Grant, J. S. (1998). Writing manuscripts for clinical journals. *Home Health Nurse, 16*, 813–822.

Gross, B. (2002). Preparing to teach the large lecture course. *Tools for teaching.* Berkeley, CA: University of California, Berkeley. Available at http://teaching.berkeley.edu/bgd/largelecture.html. Accessed November 10, 2002.

Hadfield-Law, L. (2001). Presentation skills. Presentation skills for nurses: How to prepare more effectively. *British Journal of Nursing, 10*(18), 1208–1211.

Health Development Agency (2002a). Systematic or unsystematic, is that the question? Available at http://194.83.94.80/hda/docs/evidence/eb2000/corehtml/sys_unsys_phesg_hammersley.html. Accessed December 09, 2002.

Health Development Agency (2002b). Putting public health evidence into practice. Available at http://194.83.94.80/hda/docs/evidence/eb2000/corehtml/news.html. Accessed December 11, 2002.

Health Resources and Services Administration. (1999). Prepared Remarks of Claude Earl Fox, Health Resources and Services Administration, Center for Healthcare Policy and Research Initial Development Meeting, University of West Virginia Health Policy Center, Charleston, West Virginia, October 12, 1999. Available at http://newsroom.hrsa.gov/speeches/uwvhealth-center.htm. Accessed December 11, 2002.

Heinrich, K. T. (2002). Manuscript development. Slant, style, and synthesis: 3 keys to a strong literature review. *Nurse Author and Editor, 12*(1), 1–3.

Huberman, M. (1990). Linkage between researchers and practitioners: A qualitative study. *American Educational Research Journal, 27*(2), 363–391.

Hundley, V. (2002). Research notes. How do you decide where to send an article for publication? *Nursing Standard, 16*(36), 21.

Hunt, A. H. (2000). Taking the mystery out of research: Publishing your research results. *Orthopaedic Nursing, 19*(6). 55.

Johnson, S. H. (2001). Manuscript development. A memorable ending: Writing the summary or conclusion. *Nurse Author and Editor, 11*(4), 7–9.

King, S. (2001). *On writing.* New York: Pocket Books.

Louis, K. (1996). Reconnecting knowledge utilization and school improvement: Two steps forward, one step back. In A. Hargreaves, M. Fullan, & D. Hopkins (Eds.) *International handbook on school improvement.* London: Cassell.

Mason, D. J. (1999). Journalistic rights, and wrongs. *American Journal of Nursing, 99*(9), 7.

McConnell E. A. (2002). Making outstandingly good presentations. *DCCN—Dimensions of Critical Care Nursing, 21*(1), 28–30.

Melnyk, B. M., & Fineout-Overholt, E. (2002). Putting research into practice. Rochester ARCC. *Reflections on Nursing Leadership, 28*(2), 22–25.

Melnyk, B. M., Brown, H., Jones, D., Kreipe, R., & Novak, J. (2003). Improving the mental/psychosocial health of U.S. children and adolescents: Outcomes and implementation strategies from the National KySS Summit (Supplement). *Journal of Pediatric Health Care, 17*(6), S1–S28.

National Health Service Information Authority (2001). *About the "hitting the headlines" service.* National Electronic Library for Health. Available at http://www.nehl.nhs.uk/hth/about.asp. Accessed December 11, 2002.

NBC News and The Wall Street Journal (1998, June 18–21). *NBC News/Wall Street Journal Poll: Health Care/Politics.* USA: Hart-Teeter Research Companies.

Oermann, M. H. (2001). *Writing for publication in nursing*. Philadelphia: Lippincott Williams & Wilkins.

Oermann, M. (1999). Extensive writing projects: Tips for completing them on time. *Nurse Author and Editor, 9*(1), 8–10.

Ohler, L. (2002). Manuscript development. Manuscript revisions: The team approach. *Nurse Author and Editor, 12*(2), 1–3.

Pelletier, L. R. Miracle, V. A., Thom, C., Parse, R. R., & Hauger, J. (2002). The insider's view: Timely topics. *Nurse Author and Editor, 12*(3), 5–6,

Phillips, D. P., Kanter, E. J., Bednarczyk, B., & Tastad, P. L. (1991). Importance of the lay press in the transmission of medical knowledge to the scientific community. *New England Journal of Medicine, 325*(16), 1180–1183.

Schulmeister, L., & Vrabel, M. (2002). Searching for information for presentations and publications. *Clinical Nurse Specialist, 16*(2), 79–84.

Siwek, J., Gourlay, M. L., Slawson, D. C., & Shaughnessy, A. F. (2002). How to write an evidence-based clinical review article. *American Family Physician, 65*(2), 251–258.

Smith, M. F. (2000). Nurse educator. Public speaking survival strategies. *Journal of Emergency Nursing, 26*(2), 166–168.

Sullivan, E. J. (2002). Top 10 reasons a manuscript is rejected. *Journal of Professional Nursing, 18*(1), 1–2.

Taggart, H. M., & Arslanian C. (2000). Creating an effective poster presentation. *Orthopaedic Nursing, 19*(3), 47–52.

Webb, C. (2002). How to make your article more readable. *Journal of Advanced Nursing,38*(1), 1–2.

Wills, C. E. (2000). Strategies for managing barriers to the writing process. *Nursing Forum, 25*(4), 5–13.

Wong, D. L. (1999). Manuscript review. Publishing "cutting-edge" information. *Nurse Author and Editor, 9*(3), 8–9.

Woodring, B. C. (1995). Lecture is not a four letter word! In B. Fuszard (Ed.). *Innovative teaching strategies in nursing* (2nd ed., pp. 356–371). Gaithersburg, MD: Aspen Publishers.

Woodring, B. C. (2000). Professional development. Preparing presentations that produce peace of mind. *Journal of Child & Family Nursing, 3*(1), 63–64.

chapter 14

403

Creating a Culture for Evidence-Based Practice

> 66 *Without change there is no innovation, creativity, or incentive for improvement. Those who initiate change will have a better opportunity to manage the change that is inevitable.* 99
>
> *William Pollard*

tions that offer a two-week focused experience in learning EBP have been quite successful in imparting the necessary information, sharpening skills, and imbuing enthusiasm in the learners.

On a larger scale, grand rounds, usually attended by clinicians from all corners of a department, offer the chance to speak to many people at the same time. Sound advice is to keep the presentation simple (to avoid scaring off the audience) and clinically grounded (to keep them interested).

Teaching Formats: Grazing or Hunting

In small groups such as journal clubs, determining which teaching format will work best for your participants is crucial. Consider first whether a "grazing" format or a "hunting" format would best meet learners' needs. Grazing formats have been the most common to this point and typically begin with a group of individuals dividing the relevant journals in their field among themselves. Each individual is then responsible for perusing—or grazing on—one to three journals for recent publications of interest to the group. At the small group meeting, members of the group take their turns in presenting the information they have found to the rest of the group members.

The grazing process has its inherent inefficiencies. First, in this format, the number of journals reviewed tends to be a function of the number of individuals in the group. Thus, the group is likely to leave several journals unreviewed. The group effect is further complicated by members' abilities to make it to the meetings. Third, there are many citations in given journals that are of poor quality. Wading through several journals looking for quality research evidence can be quite tedious. Fourth, the time required by the group members to accomplish the given goal tends to be quite high. Due to these inefficiencies of grazing, many members may relegate the small group meeting to just another thing on their already full "to do" lists.

Despite the inherent inefficiencies, grazing is still an essential activity in keeping up with the latest information. Fortunately, there are now secondary publications that do the grazing, cutting down the time it takes to find quality research evidence. The editorial boards of these resources systematically survey the existing literature. Any relevant studies that meet certain methodologic criteria are abstracted in a quickly readable format. Examples of sources for predigested evidence are the American College of Physicians Journal Club (ACP Journal Club), Clinical Evidence, InfoPoems, American Academy of Pediatrics Grand Rounds, Evidence-Based Nursing Journal, and Worldviews on Evidence-Based Nursing. Thus, grazing is very helpful in keeping current, especially when grazing in these greener pastures.

An alternative to grazing is a hunting format. This format begins with a clinical issue and the question of interest to the individual or group. A question is posed from a concern about a clinical issue. The question is then converted into an answerable and searchable question. A literature search to find relevant research evidence is performed. Finally, any relevant studies are brought back to the group for critical appraisal and application.

The hunting format has two distinct advantages. First, it is by definition relevant to the group because its own members posed the original question, rather than relying on whatever happened to be published since the last meeting. Second, it includes the question and search components of the EBP process, which are left out of the grazing format.

It is important to make a distinct link between the applicable clinical scenario; the searchable, answerable search question; the search findings; and the subsequent critical appraisal and application of research evidence to allow the group to see the process as a coherent whole. Otherwise, because so much time is spent in learning critical appraisal, learners can quickly equate EBP with only critical appraisal instead of seeing it as a comprehensive process. It is easy to use this format. Simply assign group members the task of presenting the results of their question, search, and critical appraisal at the various meetings on a rotating basis.

Suggestions for Teaching Evidence-Based Practice Using Evidence-Based Methods

Although the evidence on the effectiveness of teaching methods for EBP is lacking in quality, there are two conclusions that can be helpful. First, research evidence supports that seminars targeting specific EBP skills can increase those skills to a moderate degree, at least in the short term (Bennett et al., 1987; Green & Ellis, 1997; Linzer et al., 1988; Norman & Shannon, 1998; Seeling, 1991).

Skills Seminars

Skills seminars typically focus on isolated individual skills in the EBP process, such as how to ask answerable, searchable questions; how to search the healthcare literature; and how to critically appraise a study on therapy or diagnosis (Guyatt & Rennie, 2002). Practical suggestions on designing these seminars include making them relevant to your participants, orienting the group to the greater context of the whole five-step EBP process, and providing hands-on practice with each skill.

It is much easier to keep learners engaged if the examples and exercises used are drawn from topics that are relevant to them. For example, if you are teaching a group of surgical nurses, it is important to use a surgical nursing example, such as comparisons of the variety of dressing changes available for open wounds. By keeping the example relevant, the group is learning the EBP process as well as something useful to their practice. If you are in doubt on what sort of topic would be of interest, ask for suggestions from the participants. Suggestions can be offered either before the seminar so that predigested examples can be used or at the time of the seminar in more of an "on-the-fly" setup.

These more spontaneous sessions tend to be risky, because if the example is too difficult, the learners quickly can become lost and disheartened, potentially viewing EBP as a tedious and difficult process. A skillful teacher who is able to craft or frame the issue in such a way that easily guides the learner to an answer that is either searchable, answerable, available, or easily critically appraised, depending on the goals of the session, can expect a handsome payoff. The group will feel that the process is not only learnable but also useful and doable, because they see it done right before them.

When establishing focused seminars in EBP skills, remember to orient your group of learners as to where the skill you are teaching fits into the greater context of the EBP process. For example, if you are teaching a seminar on how to search the healthcare literature, it is important to stress that searching is simply a tool to be used to find the most relevant, valid research evidence and not the only—or even the most important—skill that needs to be learned in the EBP process. Whetting their appetites about the focus of the article and prompting them on to the next steps of critical appraisal and application of evidence to the clinical problem can help learners to see the broader scope of the EBP process rather than focusing on a single skill in isolation.

Another practical suggestion when establishing small, focused workshops on EBP concepts is to provide a means of hands-on practice during the workshop. For example, when teaching a session on composing and formatting answerable, searchable questions, ask the participants to individually think of clinical questions from their own experience. Members would have an opportunity to share their questions with the group, then to determine whether they are foreground or background questions (see Chapter 2). If the question were foreground, the group would decide what type of question it was (e.g., treatment, diagnosis, harm, meaning) and construct it in the PICO format. Then the group would access computers to search for relevant scientific evidence to answer their questions.

Alternatively, the leader could present a case to the group members, asking them to write down questions they generate during the presentation. Then the leader asks the group, by individual, to share their questions and phrase them in the PICO format. This sort of individual practice and skill building as a group is quite powerful as a teaching and learning method. All participants are working actively, not passively, to learn the concepts, and the other group members provide immediate feedback and "reality testing" for each individual.

Another very practical suggestion is to have the group learn searching skills in a workshop led by a medical librarian knowledgeable in EBP, in which the learners obtain hands-on practice in searching for evidence to answer their own questions. This combines the principle of relevance to the learner with the evidence-based method of skill-building workshops and thereby fosters more active participation and learning.

For teaching critical appraisal skills, it is useful to break the group into three smaller groups. Each group focuses on ascertaining whether the study met or did not meet a single methodologic or validity criterion. All the criteria are divided across the small groups. (Chapters 4–7 have more information on critical appraisal of evidence.) For example, one small group would report back to the larger group on the results of the study. Another group would discuss the validity of the study results, and the third group would discuss applicability of the study findings to the given patient scenario. This process assists the learners to view the critical appraisal process as a coherent whole.

Variety: Multiple Settings, Methods, and Formats

The second recommendation for teaching EBP that can be gleaned from the literature is that the success of a curriculum in EBP is directly proportional to the number of settings, formats, and products devoted to it. In other words, the more settings in which EBP is taught, the more formats used, and the more products required, the more successful learners will be in the long run (Norman & Shannon, 1998; Sackett & Parkes, 1998). Teaching EBP should not be restricted to one instructor or to one teaching episode (e.g., inservice, orientation class, academic course). Rather, it should be woven into the fabric of units' and departments' educational objectives or academic programs' overall curricula in such a fashion that it becomes part of the culture. The learners need to see EBP used and learned in nearly every setting to which they are exposed. This ever-present implementation and learning of EBP concepts serves to model for the learners that EBP is not only an academic exercise but also is actively used in clinical practice.

Examples of application of teaching EBP are the University of Rochester School of Nursing graduate programs and the University of Rochester Internal Medicine, Pediatrics, and Medicine-Pediatrics. Students in the nursing programs receive the foundation EBP knowledge in two core courses. These courses incorporate multiple learning opportunities, settings, and formats for learning, including computer labs for students to learn searching strategies, generating internal evidence to help answer clinical questions from their own experiences through outcomes management (see Box 15-8), and small group discussions about critical appraisal of evidence. The students also see the EBP process in practice throughout their specialty education in their clinical and didactic courses. Box 15-9 provides an example of a learning opportunity in the pediatric nurse practitioner program that originates in the clinical experience and promotes the use of the EBP process.

A combination of clinical and academic settings (e.g., morning report, journal club, ambulatory conferences, skills blocks, and an EBP elective) are part of residents' learning experiences. During morning report, participants are required to present an EP once every month

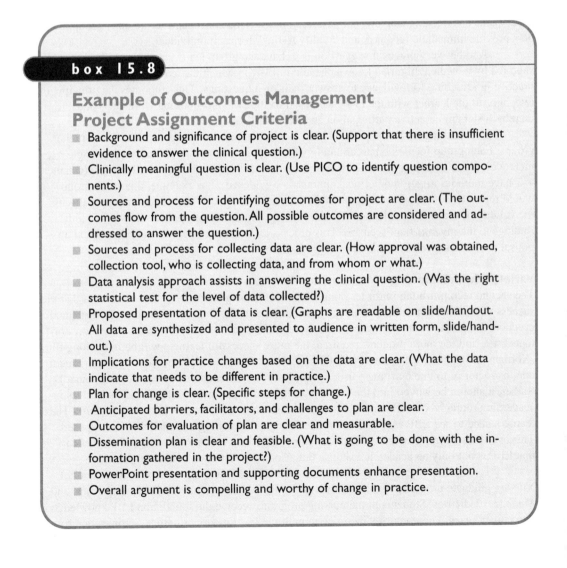

box 15.8

Example of Outcomes Management Project Assignment Criteria

- Background and significance of project is clear. (Support that there is insufficient evidence to answer the clinical question.)
- Clinically meaningful question is clear. (Use PICO to identify question components.)
- Sources and process for identifying outcomes for project are clear. (The outcomes flow from the question. All possible outcomes are considered and addressed to answer the question.)
- Sources and process for collecting data are clear. (How approval was obtained, collection tool, who is collecting data, and from whom or what.)
- Data analysis approach assists in answering the clinical question. (Was the right statistical test for the level of data collected?)
- Proposed presentation of data is clear. (Graphs are readable on slide/handout. All data are synthesized and presented to audience in written form, slide/handout.)
- Implications for practice changes based on the data are clear. (What the data indicate that needs to be different in practice.)
- Plan for change is clear. (Specific steps for change.)
- Anticipated barriers, facilitators, and challenges to plan are clear.
- Outcomes for evaluation of plan are clear and measurable.
- Dissemination plan is clear and feasible. (What is going to be done with the information gathered in the project?)
- PowerPoint presentation and supporting documents enhance presentation.
- Overall argument is compelling and worthy of change in practice.

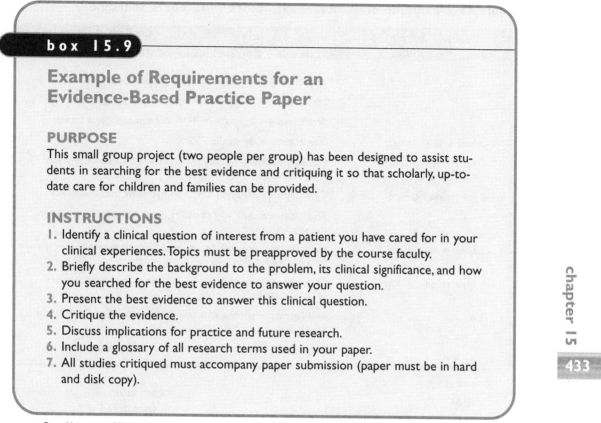

box 15.9

Example of Requirements for an Evidence-Based Practice Paper

PURPOSE
This small group project (two people per group) has been designed to assist students in searching for the best evidence and critiquing it so that scholarly, up-to-date care for children and families can be provided.

INSTRUCTIONS
1. Identify a clinical question of interest from a patient you have cared for in your clinical experiences. Topics must be preapproved by the course faculty.
2. Briefly describe the background to the problem, its clinical significance, and how you searched for the best evidence to answer your question.
3. Present the best evidence to answer this clinical question.
4. Critique the evidence.
5. Discuss implications for practice and future research.
6. Include a glossary of all research terms used in your paper.
7. All studies critiqued must accompany paper submission (paper must be in hard and disk copy).

From University of Rochester School of Nursing, Pediatric Nurse Practitioner Program, 2003.

chapter 15

433

as they rotate to different patient units. The clinical questions are to be drawn from their practice experiences, with the search, critical appraisal, and application discussed among the group. This 1-hour teaching conference usually consists of two cases being presented and discussed, each for half of an hour. Once per week, an EP is presented and discussed instead of a case. The group in attendance (including a seasoned mentor) gives immediate feedback to the resident.

Journal club meets once per week. During this noon conference, a "hunting format" is used, and the group is divided into smaller groups, each with the task of analyzing one aspect of a systematic review or study and presenting back to the large group. Skills blocks are specific two-week rotations set aside for nonclinical, classroom learning of clinical concepts, with a large portion of these sessions being devoted to the teaching of EBP concepts. These skill block minicourses are quite successful in bringing beginners to a common place of facility with EBP. Table 15-2 exemplifies a workable skill block minicourse schedule.

For the more advanced learner, an EBP elective is offered. This is a two-week course that consists of two 2-hour sessions daily. Attendance is limited to 8–10 participants for optimizing individual participation. In an introductory session where individual and group goals are set,

table 15-2 Example of workable skill block minicourse schedule

Session	Topic
1–3 hours	Introduction of principles of EBP (large group)
	Session on asking answerable questions (large group)
	Break into small groups of 8–10 and select project topics
2–2 hours (large group)	Search tutorial by medical librarian
3–1 hour (small groups)	Critically appraise and discuss an article on therapy—preselected article
4–1 hour (small groups)	Critically appraise and discuss an overview (meta-analysis)
	This overview optimally contains the article on therapy from the previous session
5–1 hour (small groups)	Critically appraise and discuss an article on diagnostic testing—preselected article
6–1 hour (small groups)	Critically appraise and discuss an article on prognosis—preselected article
7–2 hours	Small groups—participants present their project (educational prescription)
	Large group—wrap up and answer any overall questions

learning needs are identified. A session on asking an answerable and searchable question, a search tutorial with a medical librarian, and sessions on the critical appraisal and application of articles of therapy, diagnosis, prognosis, overview, and harm using preselected articles follow the introductory session. The remainder of the elective is left open for the group to decide what to present and discuss. Individuals are required to take turns in leading these open sessions, teaching the group something they did not know beforehand. This program is designed to address the three ingredients of optimal adult learning:

1. A pretest that reveals a knowledge deficit
2. A learning phase to fill the knowledge deficit
3. A posttest where the learner presents what she/he has learned

To conclude the elective, group members individually present a project of their choosing, ranging from an appraisal of related single studies to formulating a complete EP.

Lessons Learned

Among lessons learned about the structure and content of an EBP curriculum from experience at the University of Rochester, four are worth noting.

First Lesson: Deadlines

First, deadlines for any product of learning are crucial. Clinicians, both teachers and learners, are very busy in a complex clinical setting. Because there are many distractions, it is important to be explicit about the goals and timeline of any assigned learning experience. Examples of this are a two-day return on search results for a question generated by both teacher and learner, assigning an EP on a question to be presented the next day on rounds or in report, and breaking up a large project into smaller ones with shorter deadlines (e.g., divide an EBP paper assignment into three stages due one month apart: question and search strategy, critical appraisal, and application of evidence). In short, it is important to keep the learning experience on the learner's radar screen.

Second Lesson: Assess Skill Levels

The second lesson learned is that learners begin a training program with widely varied skills in EBP. Determining learners' skills prior to starting the teaching program is essential. Because becoming an evidence-based provider is a complex task, much like becoming a licensed practitioner, the program should be broken down into reasonable parts that learners can accomplish. It is important to meet learners where they are and to foster growth in knowledge and skills from that point. Any bar to reflect learner growth should be flexible enough to be angled upward or downward for a specific learner. This avoids the frustration that sets in when learners are overwhelmed with the material or process. Setting realistic expectations for each experience and providing formative feedback along the way in addition to summative information at the end of the experience will encourage learners' growth.

Third Lesson: Assure Meaning

The third lesson learned is to make the content, settings, formats, and methods meaningful to learners. This shows learners first hand that EBP is applicable and useful to them in their particular practice setting. Use relevant examples and scenarios. This is best accomplished by beginning the process with an item or question generated by the learner. It is incredibly powerful to learn the EBP process by working through an example that the learner actually cares about and that the learner can imagine her/himself using in the future. In addition, when conducting lectures or minicourses, be sure to adjust the content to the realm of the audience (e.g., surgical examples for surgical nurses and surgeons).

> **"** *To teach is to learn twice.* **"**
>
> *Joseph Joubert*

Fourth Lesson: Foster Growth

The fourth lesson learned is to foster growth in your learners with the goal that they can become teachers of EBP to their colleagues. Learners who do not readily understand intention-to-treat will improve their knowledge and comfort with the subject matter if they are provided proper mentorship and asked to teach it to someone else in a few days. It is quite satisfying for a teacher to see learners teaching what they have learned. This also is a good way of building a cadre of practitioners who are skilled at EBP, increasing the number of mentors and teachers to work with you.

Evaluation of Evidence-Based Practice Teaching Programs

The final step in the EBP process is evaluation of outcomes that are based on evidence. This also is the final step in teaching EBP. The use of scientific evidence, clinical expertise, and patient preferences and values is increasingly becoming recognized as the standard for clinical care. Haynes and Haines (1998) indicated that a barrier to implementing EBP was ineffective initiatives and programs to educate the practitioner about EBP concepts. Hatala and Guyatt (2002) further state that the evidence to support effective teaching strategies for EBP are less than desirable. Effective outcome evaluation of EBP teaching programs is as imperative as their existence. Evaluation of outcomes for learning may be conducted at different levels: the learner, the educators teaching EBP, and the overall program for teaching EBP. Each level has different aspects of evaluation that need to be addressed for the evaluation plan to be comprehensive and complete.

Learner Evaluation

Evaluating learners' integration of EBP concepts into their thinking, problem solving, and practice is not an easy task. Studies do not demonstrate that there is a "sure-fire" method of evaluating learners' grasp of EBP (Sackett & Parkes, 1998). Given this understanding, several mechanisms are discussed that can assist in determining how well learners have integrated EBP concepts into their practices.

Classroom Learning

There are many options for evaluating classroom learning of EBP concepts. Formal testing can assist the learners to identify areas in the process that need remedial work. However, synthesis papers seem to be a common option that educators use to determine whether learners have gained EBP knowledge. The foundational and other clinical courses in EBP in the graduate program at the University of Rochester School of Nursing require syntheses papers for evaluation of knowledge of EBP concepts (see Box 15-10).

An outcomes management project is required of all graduate students at the University of Rochester School of Nursing as a measure of preparation for generating internal evidence to answer clinical questions when valid scientific evidence is not available (see Box 15-8). Learners use the EBP process to accomplish this assignment. Other creative ways of evaluating learners' grasp of EBP concepts can be EBP projects, such as students working with clinical researchers or advanced clinicians on EBP initiatives. For example, in a study implementing an EBP initiative, students developed a workbook to teach other nurses and students about EBP. The students devised the text to communicate the concepts as well as examples and exercises to make the concepts come alive for the learner. This assignment assisted the instructor in evaluating how well the learners knew the EBP content. In addition to learning in the classroom, these same concepts can be integrated in the clinical area.

box 15.10

Description of an Evidence-Based Practice Synthesis Paper

The purpose of these assignments is to familiarize students with the independent identification and synthesis of existing evidence to answer a clinical question. Each student will select a clinically meaningful question and conduct an in-depth search for the best scientific evidence regarding that question. There will be components of this assignment due throughout the semester. Students will be provided feedback on those sections. The final paper should clearly describe the methods used to identify and retrieve the evidence and the rationale for exploring the clinical issue chosen. A discussion of these theories used to guide the research included in the review is expected. Clearly articulated recommendations for practice based on research evidence are essential to a successful paper. A summary table of included studies should be placed at the end of the paper, before references.

(From University of Rochester, Core Course in EBP, 2004)

Clinical Programs

Traditionally, clinical programs in nursing used care plans, care maps, and logs to evaluate clinical knowledge and application. Clinical evaluation of the application of EBP knowledge can use these tools as well; however, educators must carefully develop the instructions and requirements for these exercises. It is easy to fall back on the traditional research critique methodology that serves the learner only in gaining knowledge, not application skills. For example, a clinical course may require the learner to provide a research critique of the supporting evidence for an intervention chosen for a clinical issue encountered in the practice setting. This method does not require application of research or EBP knowledge. A better exercise may be to have the learner find and critically appraise the scientific evidence to support a chosen intervention, then to describe how this evidence influenced decision making, taking into consideration the clinical team's expertise and the patient's preferences and values.

In addition, having the learner prepare an EP can assist in evaluating EBP knowledge. The learner who applies EBP principles and processes needs time to reflect on the process and realize how application occurred and the difference the chosen evidence-based intervention made in the outcome. This processing can be in verbal or written form, in a single session with a mentor or in a group. Gaining experience in how to turn a clinical issue into a searchable, answerable question; finding relevant, valid evidence to answer the question; and coming to the point of application of evidence with confidence is not easily achieved. Evaluation of this process is equally challenging.

> 66 *What is experienced and seen in the clinical area is what will likely predict future behavior.* 99
>
> *Bob Berenson*

Preparing preceptors for teaching EBP to learners is imperative. It is known that learners emulate what they see modeled in their preceptors and educators. Berenson (2002) made that point very clear when he articulated, in a discussion about health professionals' education, that even if the benefits of EBP are clearly presented in a didactic venue, what is experienced and seen in the clinical area is what will likely predict future behavior.

During clinical discussions with learners, EBP principles need to be central. Questions about why a particular treatment option was chosen or a care trajectory was decided on are great opportunities for demonstrating operation of the EBP process. For example, during the clinical experience of one of the students at the University of Rochester School of Nursing, the healthcare team was discussing the appropriateness of the common practice of prescribing multiple assays for the diagnosis of *Clostridium difficile*. One of the preceptors indicated that current evidence does not support the use of more than one assay within a 7-day period (Renshaw, Stelling, & Doolittle, 1996) and that overall, the negative predictive value of the first stool specimen for *C. difficile* was 97% (Manabe et al., 1995). Further discussion focused on the cost savings, timing of initiation of treatment, and patient comfort by implementing current evidence. Another clinician in the group presented a patient for whom he had cared whose first two assays were negative and whose third assay was positive, indicating that the diagnosis could have been missed and at best delayed if only one assay had been collected. This clinician's experience conflicted with the current evidence. A discussion ensued, reflecting on the use of science, expertise, and patient concerns and choices together to make the best clinical decision. The role of uncertainty in clinical practice and the benefits of clinical inquiry also were discussed. Subsequently, the student was asked to design a project that would apply EBP principles to this clinical situation and evaluate the plan, including measurement of practice outcomes. This kind of application of EBP principles in the clinical area is invaluable to the learner.

Program Evaluation

Evaluating learners' ongoing absorption of EBP concepts throughout a teaching program is integral to knowing the success of the program. However, there are other outcomes of the overall program that need to be examined. Some of these outcomes may be evaluated on a continual basis, and some may be a one-time assessment.

Ongoing Quality Improvement Assessment

Continual monitoring of the environment and outcomes is necessary for either teaching or implementing EBP. Periodically, the champions of EBP need to determine where they are in reaching the goals of the EBP teaching program. This first requires a commitment to setting measurable program goals that can be monitored on an ongoing basis. Evaluation of the program's foundation can be obtained by examining the questions raised in the first part of this chapter. If there are insufficient answers (e.g., educators' knowledge of up-to-date EBP concepts is lacking), the program has not been completely successful in that area. Steps would then be taken to address the areas that lack support (e.g., send the educators to an EBP conference or hold an EBP conference on the program site).

Goals for evaluation of a teaching program should address whether the learners can formulate a searchable, answerable clinical question; efficiently find relevant evidence; discern what is best scientific evidence; and apply the best scientific evidence with clinical expertise and patient input to clinical decision making. Part of the Summit on Health Professions Education (Greiner & Knebel, 2003) competency regarding practicing using evidence states that across and within disciplines, efforts must be focused on development of a scientific evidence base. The final goal for a teaching program must be for learners to actively evaluate outcomes based on evidence.

In addition, the Summit (Greiner & Knebel, 2003) recommended that funding sources such as the Agency for Healthcare Research and Quality (AHRQ) support ongoing clinical and education research that evaluates care based on the five specified competencies. An example of this type of research could be a study to evaluate educational outcomes for an EBP teaching program across two or more disciplines (e.g., nursing and medicine).

Final Assessment

There is usually some type of cumulative assessment for learners completing a degree program, such as comprehensive exams. However, not every discipline uses this form of outcome evaluation. National licensure and certifying exams may provide outcome evaluation for some disciplines and some levels of education. Whatever form of final assessment a teaching program in EBP employs, it must address the steps of the EBP process, particularly application and evaluation. These are the most nebulous of the EBP steps. Without evaluating these steps in a final evaluation, educators cannot know whether learners are prepared to apply principles they have learned in their daily practices.

Program Effectiveness

The overall EBP program is effective if the learners are successful in integrating EBP concepts into their thinking and practice. This is very difficult to measure; however, there are several ways that offer some indication of success. Initially, a program's overall effectiveness in infusing EBP knowledge in their learners can be assessed by how many of its graduates succeed at national standardized exams, whether that is through licensure or credentialing.

National standardized licensure exams, as well as credentialing exams, are based on evidence. These are objective tests that encompass knowledge, skills, and abilities of practice. Experts provide exam questions, and the questions undergo a rigorous review process before being used in an exam. How graduates of an EBP program perform on such exams could be an indirect measure of whether a program was effective in teaching EBP knowledge to its students. Integration of EBP concepts into daily practice can be discerned by periodic follow-up with graduates to ask them about the integration of EBP in their practices. Although self-report has its drawbacks, querying what EBP initiatives learners have been involved in during the past 12 months can assist the educator in obtaining more objective information on how they have applied EBP knowledge to practice. Currently, instruments are being piloted that will provide a measure of the importance of EBP principles to a clinician's daily practice (B. M. Melnyk, personal communication, June 10, 2003).

> 66 *Words can never adequately convey the incredible impact of attitude toward life. The longer I live the more convinced I become that life is 10% what happens to us and 90% how we respond to it.*
>
> *I believe the single most significant decision I can make on a day-to-day basis is my choice of attitude. It is more than my past, my education, my bankroll, my successes or failures, fame or pain, what other people think of me or say about me, my circumstances, or my position. Attitude keeps me going or cripples my progress. It alone fuels my fire or assaults my hope. When my attitudes are right, there's no barrier too high, no valley too deep, no dream too extreme, no challenge too great for me.* 99
>
> *Charles S. Swindoll*

references

Alguire, P. C., DeWitt, D. E., Pinsky, L. E., & Ferenchick G. S. (2001). *Teaching in your office: A guide to instructing medical students and residents.* Philadelphia: American College of Physicians.

Bakken, S. (2001). An informatics infrastructure is essential for evidence-based practice. *Journal of American Medical Informatics Association. 8,* 199–201.

Berenson, B. (2002). *Crossing the quality chasm: Next steps for health professions education. Major stakeholders comment on key strategies and action plans*: June 18, 2002: Washington, DC: http://www.kaisernetwork.org/health_cast/uploaded_files/Transcript_6.18.02_IOM_Major-Stakeholders.pdf. Accessed May 17, 2003.

Bennett, K., Sackett, D., Haynes, B., Nuefeld, V., Tugwell, P., & Roberts, R. (1987). A controlled trial of teaching critical appraisal of the clinical literature to medical students. *JAMA, 257,* 2451–2454.

Breivik, B., & Gee, E. (1989). *Information literacy: Revolution in the library.* New York: American Council on Education.

Cooke, L., & Grant, M. (2002). Support for evidence-based practice. *Seminars in Oncology Nursing, 18* (1). 71–78.

Duck, J. D. (2002). *The change monster. The human forces that fuel or foil corporate transformation and change.* New York: Crown Business.

Englebardt, S., & Nelson, R. (2002*). Health care informatics: An interdisciplinary approach.* St. Louis, MO: Mosby.

French, B. (1998). Developing the skills required for evidence-based practice. *Nursing Education Today, 18,* 46–51.

Graves, K. (2000). Electronic reserves: Copyright and permissions. *Bulletin of the Medical Library Association, 88,* 18–25.

Green, M., & Ellis, P. (1997). Impact of evidence-based medicine curriculum based on adult learning theory. *Journal General Internal Medicine, 12,* 742–750.

Greiner, A., & Knebel, E. (Eds.) (2003). *Health professions education: A bridge to quality.* Washington, DC: National Academy Press.

Grimes, D. (1995). Introducing evidence-based medicine into a department of obstetrics and gynecology. *Graduate Education, 86,* 451–457.

Guyatt, G. H., & Rennie, D. (Eds.). (2002). *Users' guides to the medical literature: A manual for evidence-based health care.* Chicago. AMA Press.

Hatala, R., & Guyatt, G. (2002). Evaluating the teaching of evidence-based medicine. *JAMA, 288,* 1110–1112.

Haynes, B., & Haines, A. (1998). Getting research findings into practice: Barriers and bridges to evidence-based clinical practice. *British Medical Journal, 317,* 273–276.

Institute of Medicine (IOM). (2001). *Crossing the quality chasm: A new health system for the 21st century.* Washington, DC: National Academy Press.

IOM. (2002). *Educating health professional to use informatics.* Washington, DC: National Academy Press.

Morrison-Beedy, D., Aronowitz, T., Dyne, J., & Mkandawire, L. (2001). Mentoring students and junior faculty in faculty research: A win-win scenario. *Journal of Professional Nursing, 17,* 291–296.

Norman, G., & Shannon, S. (1998). Effectiveness of instruction in critical appraisal: A critical appraisal. *Canadian Medical Association Journal, 158,* 177–181.

Linzer, M., Brown, J., Frazier, L., DeLong, E., & Siegal, W. (1988). Impact of a medical journal club on house staff reading habits, knowledge, and critical appraisal: A randomized controlled trial. *JAMA, 260,* 2537–2541.

Manabe, Y., Vinetz, J., Moore, R., Merz, C., Charache, P., & Bartlett , J. (1995). *Clostridium difficile* colitis: An efficient clinical approach to diagnosis. *Annals of Internal Medicine, 123,* 835–840.

National Forum for Information Literacy. Retrieved October 30, 2003, from http://www.infolit.org.

Renshaw, A., Stelling, J., & Doolittle, M. (1996). The lack of value of repeated *Clostridium difficile* cytotoxicity assays. *Archives of Pathology & Laboratory Medicine. 120*(1), 49–52.

Richardson, W., Wilson, M., Nishikawa, J., & Hayward, R. (1995). The well-built clinical question: A key to evidence-based decisions. *ACP Journal Club, 123,* A12–A13.

Saba, V., & McCormick, K. (2001). *Essentials of computers for nurses: Informatics for the new millennium* (3rd ed.). New York: McGraw-Hill.

Sackett, D., Straus, S, Richardson, S., Rosenberg, W., & Haynes, B. (2000). *Evidence-based medicine: How to practice and teach EBM.* London: Churchill Livingstone.

Sackett, D. L., Haynes, R. B., Guyatt, G. H., Tugwell, P. (1991) *Clinical epidemiology: A basic science for clinical medicine* (pp. 410–414). Boston: Little, Brown and Company.

Sackett, D., & Parkes, J. (1998). Teaching critical appraisal: No quick fixes. *Canadian Medical Association Journal, 158,* 203–204.

Seeling, C. (1991). Affecting residents' literature reading attitudes, behaviors, and knowledge through a journal club intervention. *Journal of General Internal Medicine, 6,* 330–334.

Shortliffe, E., & Blois, M. (2001). The computer meets medicine and biology: Emergence of a discipline. In *Medical informatics: Computer applications in health care and biomedicine* (2nd ed.). New York: Springer.

chapter 15

441

Creating a Vision: Motivating a Change to Evidence-Based Practice in Individuals and Organizations

Bernadette Mazurek Melnyk

chapter 16

In today's rapidly changing healthcare environment in which health professionals are often confronted with short staffing, cost reductions, and heavy patient loads, the implementation of a change to evidence-based practice (EBP) can be a daunting process. Individual as well as organizational change is often a complex and lengthy process. However, there are general principles at the individual and organizational levels that will expedite the process of change when thoughtfully planned and carefully implemented.

Nearly all organizational change theories are conceptual rather than evidence-based, which limits the science base to guide decisions about implementation strategies (Prochaska, Prochaska, & Levesque, 2001). In addition, most organizational change initiatives fail because knowledge and principles of the psychology of change are not taken into consideration (Winum, Ryterband, & Stephensen, 1997).

This chapter discusses critical principles and steps for implementing change in individuals and organizations, with an emphasis on two unique non–health-care models of organizational change that may be useful in guiding successful change efforts in healthcare institutions. Strategies to enhance team functioning as well as the cooperation of individuals with various personality styles are highlighted. A major purpose of this chapter is to stimulate "out-of-the-box," or nontraditional thinking in motivating a change to best practice within individuals and organizations.

Although it is imperative to consider the structure, culture, and strategy for change within a system, it also is critical that the individual(s) implementing the change have a clear vision, belief in that vision, and persistence to overcome the many difficult or "character-building" experiences along the journey to bringing that project to fruition (Melnyk, 2001).

Essential Elements for Successful Organizational Change

Among the important elements that must be present for change to be accomplished successfully are vision, belief, strategic planning, action, persistence, and patience.

First Element: Vision and Goals

The first essential element for implementing change, whether it is at the **macro** (i.e., large-scale) or **micro** (i.e., small-scale) level, is a crystal-clear vision of what is to be accomplished. A vision of the desired outcome is needed in order to outline a plan for implementing success strategies. In numerous biographies of highly successful people, a recurrent theme is that those individuals had "big dreams" and a clear vision of the projects that they wanted to accomplish in their lives.

For example, Dr. William DeVries, the chief surgeon who inserted the first artificial heart in a human patient, commented about how he had the vision of performing this procedure for years. Dr. DeVries repeatedly rehearsed that procedure in his mind in terms of what and how he was going to accomplish it so that when the opportunity finally presented itself, he was ready to perform.

Walt Disney visualized a dream of an amusement park where families could spend quality time together long before that dream became a reality. Mr. Disney's strong visualization prompted him to take action and persist in his efforts, despite many "character-building" experiences.

Most individuals do not realize that Walt Disney was bankrupt when he traveled across the country, showing his drawing of a mouse to bankers, investors, and friends. He faced countless rejections and tremendous mockery for his ideas for years before his dream started to become a reality. However, Disney stayed focused on his dream and thought about it on a daily basis. This intense daily focus on his dream facilitated a cognitive plan of a series of events that led him to act on that dream. Walt Disney believed that once you dream or visualize what it is that you want to accomplish, the things you need to accomplish it will be attracted to you, especially if you think about *how you can do it* instead of *why you will not be able to accomplish it*. Walt Disney died before Disney World was completed and, in the opening park ceremony, a reporter commented to his brother that it was too bad that Walt never had the opportunity to see the wonderful idea come to fruition. His brother, however, commented emphatically that the reporter was incorrect and, in fact, that Walt had seen his dream for many years.

Dr. Robert Jarvik, the man who designed the world's first artificial heart, was rejected at least three times by every medical school in the United States. However, he also had a large dream that was not going to be denied. He was finally accepted into the University of Utah

School of Medicine in 1972 and, a decade later, he achieved a medical breakthrough that has gone down in history. Jarvik had none of the conventional assets (e.g., superior grades, a high score on the medical entrance exam), but he possessed important intangibles (e.g., a big dream, passion, and persistence to achieve his dream).

If you knew it were impossible to fail, what would be the vision that you have for a change to EBP in your organization?

Both within yourself and in your organization, how you think is everything. It is important to *think success* at the outset of any new individual or organizational initiative and to keep your vision larger than the fears of and obstacles associated with implementation.

Once the vision for change in your organization is established, it is imperative to create written goals for how that vision will be accomplished. Individuals with written goals are usually more successful in attaining them than those without written goals. For example, findings from a Harvard Business School study indicated that: 83% of the population do not have clearly defined goals; 14% have goals that are not written; and 3% have written goals. The study also found that the 3% of individuals with written goals were earning 10 times that of the individuals who did not have written goals (Rusnak, 2003).

Second Element: Belief

Belief in one's ability to accomplish the vision is a key element for success (Melnyk, 2001). Too often, individuals have excellent ideas, but they lack the belief and confidence necessary to successfully spearhead and achieve their initiatives. Thus, many wonderful initiatives do not come to fruition. Research indicates that cognitive beliefs affect emotions as well as the ability to successfully function or attain goals (Carver & Scheier, 1998; Melnyk, 1995). For example, if an individual does not believe or have confidence in the ability to achieve an important goal, he or she is likely to feel emotionally discouraged and not take any action toward accomplishing that goal.

> **"***Anything that the mind can conceive and believe, it can achieve.***"**
>
> *John Heywood*

Third Element: A Strategic Plan

Once an initiative is conceptualized and goals are established with deadline dates, the next essential element required for successful change is a well-defined and written strategic plan. Many initiatives fail because individuals do not carefully outline implementation strategies for each established goal. As part of the strategic planning process, it is important to accomplish a SWOT (strengths, weaknesses, opportunities, and threats) analysis. This analysis will:

- Identify the current strengths in the system that will facilitate the success of a new project.
- Identify the weaknesses in the system that may hinder the initiative.
- Outline the opportunities for success.
- Delineate the threats or barriers to the project's completion, with strategies to overcome them.

Other Elements: Action, Persistence, Patience

Other elements for the success of any organizational change project are action, persistence, and patience. All too often, projects are terminated early because of the lack of persistence and patience, especially when challenges are encountered or the results of action are not yet seen.

An analogy to this scenario may be seen in an Asian tree, the giant bamboo. The tree has a particularly hard seed. The seed is so difficult to grow that it must be watered and fertilized every day for four years before any portion of it breaks the soil. In the fifth year, the tree shows itself. Once the plant breaks the surface, it is capable of growing as fast as 4 feet a day to a height of 90 feet in less than a month. The question that is often asked is, Did the tree grow 90 feet in under a month or did it grow to its height over the five years? Of course, the answer is that it took five years to grow.

> 66 *Nurse your dreams and protect them through the bad times and tough times to the sunshine and light which always comes.* 99
>
> *Woodrow Wilson*

Thomas Edison tried 9,000 different ways to invent a new type of storage battery before he found the right combination. His associate used to laugh at him, saying that he had failed 9,000 times. However, Edison kept his dream in front of him and persisted, commenting that at least he found 9,000 ways that it would not work. What would have happened if Edison had stopped his efforts to invent a storage battery on his 8,999th attempt?

The bottom line is that, no matter how outstanding a strategic plan is conceptualized and written, action, persistence, and patience are key elements for success in accomplishing any new initiative.

Three Models of Organizational Change

Chapter 8 outlined four different models that have been used to stimulate EBP in the health professions. However, three organizational change models will now be presented because they take different elements into consideration. These models were selected because they are based either on hundreds of interviews and real-life experiences by highly qualified change experts who have worked to facilitate change in business organizations for a number of years (Duck, 2002; Kotter & Cohen, 2002) or on a behavior change model that has been empirically supported for a number of years as effective in producing behavior change in high-risk patient populations (e.g., smoking, risky sexual behavior). The principles of these models add unique perspectives and could easily be applied to healthcare organizations interested in motivating a change to EBP. Empirical testing of these models could move the field of organizational change in healthcare organizations forward.

The Change Curve Model

Duck's Change Curve model (2002) emphasizes basic assumptions for change in an organization (see Box 16-1). In addition, it emphasizes the stages of organizational change with potential areas for failure.

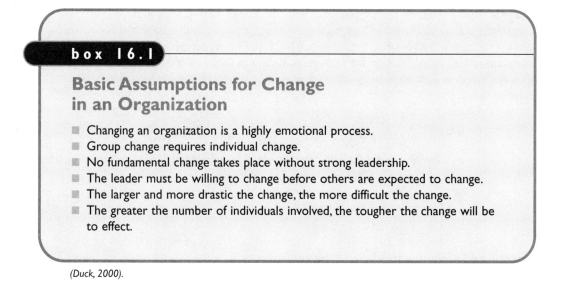

box 16.1

Basic Assumptions for Change in an Organization

- Changing an organization is a highly emotional process.
- Group change requires individual change.
- No fundamental change takes place without strong leadership.
- The leader must be willing to change before others are expected to change.
- The larger and more drastic the change, the more difficult the change.
- The greater the number of individuals involved, the tougher the change will be to effect.

(Duck, 2000).

Stage I

The first stage of organizational change in the Change Curve model (Duck, 2002) is *stagnation*. The causes of stagnation are typically a lack of effective leadership, failed initiatives, and too few resources. The emotional climate in the stage of stagnation is one in which individuals feel comfortable, there is no sense of threat, depression occurs, and/or hyperactivity exists and individuals become stressed and exhausted. Stagnation ends when action is finally taken.

Stage II

Stage II of the Change Curve model is *preparation*. In this phase, the emotional climate of the organization is one of anxiety, hopefulness, and/or reduced productivity. Buy-in of individuals is essential at this stage in which people must ask themselves, What am I willing to do? The opportunity that exists at this stage is getting people excited about the vision. The danger at this stage of change is the length of preparation: The project may fail if it is too short or too long.

Stage III

Stage III of the Change Curve model is *implementation*. In this phase, it is essential to assess individuals' readiness for the change as well as to increase their confidence in their ability to help make the change happen.

In the implementation stage, Duck (2002) emphasizes that individuals must see "what is in it for them" if they are going to commit to making a change. In addition, she asserts that when emotion is attached to the reason, individuals are more likely to change.

Stage IV

The fourth stage in Duck's model is *determination*. If results are not being experienced by now, individuals begin to experience change fatigue. The opportunity in this stage of organizational change is to create small successes along the way to change. The danger is that this is the phase in which the initiative has the highest chance of failure.

Stage V

The fifth and final stage in the Change Curve model is *fruition*. In this stage, the efforts are coming to fruition, and positive outcomes can be seen. The opportunity in this stage is to celebrate and reward individuals for their efforts as well as to seek new ways to change and grow. This stage is in danger when individuals revert back to a level of complacency and begin to stagnate again.

> **"** *I have learned that success is to be measured not so much by the position that one has reached in life as by the obstacles which one has overcome while trying to succeed.* **"**
>
> *B o o k e r   T .   W a s h i n g t o n*

Kotter and Cohen's Model of Change

Based on evidence gathered during interviews from more than 100 organizations in the process of large-scale change, Kotter and Cohen (2002) proposed that the key to organizational change lies in helping people to feel differently (i.e., appealing to their emotions). They assert that individuals change their behavior less because they are given facts or analyses that change their thinking than because they are shown truths that influence their feelings. In other words, there is a seeing, feeling, and changing pattern if successful behavioral change is going to occur. In their book *The Heart of Change* (2002), Kotter and Cohen outline eight steps for successful change in an organization (see Table 16-1).

Urgency

According to Kotter and Cohen, the first step in changing an organization is creating a *sense of urgency*. This is especially important when individuals in an organization have been in a rut or a period of complacency for some time.

Team Selection

The second step is carefully selecting a team of individuals who can guide change. Members of the team should possess the needed knowledge, skills, respect, and trust with other individuals in the organization as well as a commitment to the project. In some prior studies that have implemented interventions to facilitate a change to EBP, **opinion leaders** (e.g., individuals who have the ability to influence others) have been a critical element in change to EBP (Oxman, Thomson, Davis, & Hayes, 1995).

Vision and Strategy

In step three, the team guiding the project creates a clear vision with realistic implementation strategies for accomplishing that vision. In this step, it is important that the strategies are implemented in a reasonable timeframe because implementation that is too slow may lead to the initiative's failure.

table 16.1 Eight steps for successful change

Action	New Behavior
Step 1: Increase a sense of urgency.	"Let's go." "We need to change."
Step 2: Build the guiding team.	A group forms to guide the change and work together.
Step 3: Get the vision right.	The team develops the right vision and strategy for the change effort.
Step 4: Communicate for "buy-in."	People begin to see and accept the change as worthwhile.
Step 5: Empower action and remove barriers.	People begin to change and behave differently.
Step 6: Create short-term wins.	Momentum builds. Fewer people resist the change.
Step 7: Don't let up.	The vision is fulfilled.
Step 8: Make the change stick.	New and winning behavior continues.

From Kotter and Cohen (2002).

Communicating the Vision

Step four of Kotter and Cohen's organizational change model emphasizes the importance of communicating the vision and strategies with "heartfelt messages" that appeal to people's emotions. For example, instead of telling individuals that EBP results in better patient outcomes, stories need to be shared with them of real-life examples where EBP really made a difference (e.g., thousands of low-birth-weight infants were saved from dying as a result of a systematic review of randomized controlled trials, which indicated that dexamethasone injections to women in premature labor enhanced lung surfactant production in the fetus; mortality rates in ICUs dropped as a result of a change in endotracheal suctioning procedures). Repetition also is key so that everyone is clear on the strategies that need to be implemented.

Empowerment

In step five, individuals need to be empowered to change their behaviors. Barriers that inhibit successful change (e.g., inadequate resources or skills) should be removed. If not, individuals will become frustrated, and change will be undermined.

Interim Successes

Step six in Kotter and Cohen's model consists of establishing short-term successes. If individuals do not experience some degree of early success in their attempts to change, they will soon become frustrated, and the initiative will falter.

Ongoing Persistence

In step seven, continued persistence is essential in order to make the vision a reality. Organizational change efforts often fail because individuals try to accomplish too much in a short time or they give up too early, especially when the going gets tough.

Nourishment

In step eight, it is important to nourish the new culture to make the change last, even if the leadership team experiences transitions. This nourishment is essential if the new culture and behaviors are to be sustained.

In summary, evidence from Kotter and Cohen's work with organizations to change the behavior of professionals have indicated that change agents must communicate their vision and make their points in ways that are compelling and emotionally engaging. It is this type of communication that enables individuals to identify a problem or the solution to a problem, prompts them to experience different feelings (e.g., passion, urgency, hope), and changes behavior (i.e., they see, feel, and change).

The Transtheoretical Model of Behavior Change

For the past two decades, the transtheoretical model of health behavior change with its five stages (i.e., precontemplation, contemplation, preparation, action, and maintenance) has been empirically supported as being useful in precipitating and explaining behavior change in patients (Prochaska & Velicer, 1997).

In the stage of precontemplation, the individual is not intending to take action in the next 6 months. In contemplation, the individual is intending to take action in the next 6 months. In preparation, the individual plans to take action in the next 30 days. The stage of action is when overt changes were made less than 6 months ago. Finally, the stage of maintenance is when overt changes were made more then 6 months ago (Prochaska, Prochaska, & Levesque, 2001).

Research indicates that approximately 40% of individuals in a specific population (e.g., smokers) are in the precontemplation stage, 40% are in the contemplative stage, and 20% are in the preparation phase (e.g., Laforge, Velicer, Richmond, & Owen, 1999).

In applying these statistics, if only approximately 20% of the staff in an organization are preparing (preparation stage) to take action in implementing EBP, it will be challenging for the initiative to succeed because many of these individuals will likely view a change to EBP as imposed and become resistant to the idea (Prochaska, Prochaska, & Levesque, 2001).

The transtheoretical model is now beginning to be applied in the field of organizational change (Prochaska, Prochaska, & Levesque, 2001). The extension of this model to healthcare providers when a change to EBP is desired could continue to extend the theory's pragmatic efficacy. For example, when attempting to stimulate a change to EBP in individuals who are in the precontemplative and contemplative stages, the focus should be on making a connection with them and assisting them to progress to the next stage of readiness (e.g., from precontemplative to contemplative), rather than working with them on actual behavior change strategies.

Strategies to assist individuals to move from the precontemplative or contemplative stages to a stage of readiness to change might include:

- Strengthening their belief that EBP results in the best patient outcomes and highest quality of care
- Supporting their self-efficacy (i.e., they can indeed make the shift to EBP)

For individuals who are planning to implement EBP (i.e., in the preparation stage) or who are actively changing their practices to EBP (i.e., in the action stage), assisting them with EBP strategies (e.g., how to search for the best evidence, how to conduct efficient critical appraisal) would be an appropriate course of action. By matching the intervention strategies to the stage in which individuals are currently engaged, the model proposes that resistance, stress, and the time needed to implement the change will diminish (Prochaska, Prochaska, & Levesque, 2001). Matching the intervention to the stages of change also will allow individuals to participate in the initiative, even if they are not ready to take action.

Overcoming Major Barriers

In a systematic review of 102 trials of interventions to improve professional practice, Oxman, Thomson, Davis, and Hayes (1995) concluded that there are no "magic bullets" for improving the quality of healthcare. Dissemination-only strategies (e.g., didactic conferences or the sharing of information or evidence-based guidelines among colleagues) do not tend to produce much change in behavior or improve patient outcomes when used alone. However, multifaceted interventions consisting of a variety of strategies (e.g., use of opinion leaders, outreach visits, reminders) are moderately effective in changing behavior.

Even the best written strategic plans can go awry because of a number of barriers to implementation. As a result, it is critical to conduct an organizational analysis prior to starting the change effort to identify these barriers as well as strategies for their removal (Melnyk, 2002). Some of these barriers and recommended strategies for removing them are now discussed.

Overcoming Skepticism and Misperceptions about Evidence-Based Practice

Any time that suggested change is introduced in a system, there will be some degree of skepticism about it. Individuals tend to be skeptical about a change if they do not clearly understand the reason for it, if they are fearful about it, or if they have misperceptions about why change is needed. The best strategy for overcoming this barrier is to allow individuals to express their skepticism, fears, and anxieties about the change as well as to clarify any misperceptions that they may have about EBP (e.g., that it takes too much time). Educating them about EBP in a way that appeals to their emotions and enhances their beliefs about their ability to implement it will enhance the change process.

Individual Personality Styles

Any time that change is introduced in a system, it is important to be sensitive to the personality styles of individuals. Knowing the four major personality styles will assist in the change effort by facilitating strategies to work successfully with each of them.

Robert Rohm (1997), a seasoned psychologist who has written books on the different personality styles, uses a "DISC" model for working with individuals who possess different personality styles. Although a particular style tends to predominate, individuals often are combinations of two or more styles.

D Personality Styles: Drivers

Individuals with "D" personality styles like to take charge of projects and are highly task oriented. They are dominant, driving, and determined. An excellent strategy for working with individuals who have this type of personality style is to create excitement by giving them opportunities to lead the way by spearheading specific tasks or initiatives.

I Personality Styles: Inspired

Individuals who possess predominantly "I" personalities are typically people who are socially oriented and like to have fun. They are inspirational, influencing, impressive, and interactive. As such, they usually get excited about a new initiative by being shown that it can be a fun and exciting process.

S Personality Styles: Supportive and Steady

Individuals with predominantly "S" personalities are typically reserved and like to be led. They tend to be supportive, steady, submissive, and shy. The best strategy for working with individuals who have this personality style is to lead the way, telling them that they will be important in helping the project to succeed but that they themselves do not need to spearhead the effort.

C personality styles: Contemplators

Individuals with predominantly "C" personality styles are very analytical and detail oriented. They tend to be competent, cautious, careful, and contemplative. At one extreme, they can experience "analysis by paralysis ," to a point at which initiatives never get launched. These individuals, although they mean well, may prolong the planning stage of a new initiative so long that others lose enthusiasm for embarking in the change process. The best way to deal with these individuals is to show them all of the details of the specific action plan that will be used to accomplish the change to EBP.

Written Strategic Plan with Set Goals

Again, it is essential to have a written strategic plan with clearly established goals for a change to EBP to occur. Lack of a detailed plan is a major barrier to implementing a change to EBP within a system. The goals established should be SMART (i.e., specific, measurable, attainable, relevant, and time bound; Torres & Fairbanks, 1996). The established goals also should be high enough to facilitate growth in individuals and the organization but not so high that people will get easily frustrated by their inability to reach them.

Communicate the Vision and Strategic Plan

Communication is key to any successful organizational change plan. Individuals in the system need to be very clear about the vision and their role in the strategic planning efforts. Repetition and visual reminders of the vision and plan are important for the project's success. Involving people in creating the vision and plan will facilitate their buy-in and commitment to the project.

> **“***Change is stressful enough even when people are well prepared for its demands. Action imposed on people who are not adequately prepared can become intolerable.***”**
>
> *Prochaska, Prochaska, & Levesque, 2001, p. 258*

Teamwork

Team building is essential for a successful organizational change to EBP. Torres and Fairbanks (1996) outline six reasons for team building:

1. To establish team purpose
2. To understand the stages of team development
3. To analyze how the team works based on member role
4. To develop effective team communication
5. To examine team processes
6. To understand team leadership

It is important to understand that the team-building process is dynamic and that it requires creativity and flexibility. In addition, knowing the typical stages of team development (i.e., forming, storming, norming, and performing) will promote successful development of the team and prevent the early termination of a project due to typical team struggles, especially in the storming phase (see Table 16-2).

Resources and Administrative Support

A large number of resources are not necessary to begin a change to EBP, although there is no doubt that having ample resources will expedite the process. Systems can begin to introduce

table 16.2 Stages of team development with associated characteristics

Stage	Characteristics
Forming	Anxiety, excitement, testing, dependence, exploration, and trust
Storming	Resistance to different approaches; attitude changes; competitiveness and defensiveness; tension and disunity
Norming	Satisfaction increases; trust and respect develops; feedback is provided to others; responsibilities are shared; decisions are made
Performing	Level of interaction is high; performance increases; team members are comfortable with one another; there is optimism and confidence

From Torres and Fairbanks (1996).

small initiatives to implement a change to EBP, such as journal clubs or EBP rounds. These have been used successfully as part of the ARCC (Advancing Research and Clinical Practice through Close Collaboration model; Melnyk & Fineout-Overholt, 2002).

In these rounds, staff generate an important practice question. Then, they are assisted with searching for and critically appraising the evidence, followed by a presentation to other staff, where findings and implications for practice are discussed.

In systems that lack administrative support for a change to EBP, it is challenging but not impossible to ignite change. Assisting administrators to understand how a change to EBP can improve the quality and cost-effectiveness of patient care will facilitate their support. Sharing of important documents that herald EBP as the standard for quality care and health professional education (e.g., Institute of Medicine, 2001; Greiner & Knebel, 2003) will support the position of implementing a change to EBP in the organization.

Overcoming Resistance

Resistance in an organization is frequently the result of poorly planned implementation and is the major reason that organizational change initiatives fail (Prochaska, Prochaska, & Levesque, 2001; Winum, Ryterband, & Stephensen, 1997). Individuals who display resistance to change are often not clear about the benefits of change and/or they have fears and anxiety about their role in implementing change or how it will impact them.

When confronted with individuals who are resisting a change to EBP, it is essential to facilitate conversations that will help them express their thoughts, hesitations, and misperceptions. Listening to these individuals' perspectives on change with respect and acceptance is essential to overcoming resistance (Corey & Corey, 2002; Prochaska, Prochaska, & Levesque, 2001). Once concerns are expressed, strategies to overcome them can be implemented.

Preventing Fatigue

The barrier of fatigue typically presents itself when the implementation phase of a project is exceedingly long. An excellent strategy for preventing and/or decreasing fatigue in a system is to create small successes along the course of the change project and to recognize (reward) individuals for their efforts. Recognition and appreciation are very important in demonstrating the value of individuals' efforts and sustaining enthusiasm along the course of a project.

The road to implementing a change to EBP will be challenging but extremely rewarding. Essential elements for success include a clear vision and a well-defined written strategic plan, as well as knowledge and skills regarding the process of organizational change, team building, and working with individuals who possess different personality styles. Lastly, an ability to persist through the multiple challenges that will be confronted along the course of an organization's change will be essential for success.

> " *Never, never, never, never, never, never, never quit!* "
> *Winston Churchill*

references

Carver, S., & Scheier, M. F. (1998). *On the self-regulation of behavior.* Cambridge, England: Cambridge University Press.

Corey, M. S., & Corey, G. (2002). *Groups. Process and practice* (6th ed.). Pacific Grove, CA: Brooks/Cole.

Duck, J. D. (2002). *The change monster. The human forces that fuel or foil corporate transformation and change.* New York: Crown Business.

Greiner, A., & Knebel, E. (2003). *Health professions education: A bridge to quality.* Washington, DC: National Academy Press.

Institute of Medicine (2001). *Crossing the quality chasm: A new health system for the 21st century.* Washington, DC: National Academy Press.

Kotter, J. P., & Cohen, D. S. (2002). *The heart of change. Real-life stories of how people change their organizations.* Boston: Harvard Business School Press.

LaForge, R. G., Velicer, W. F., Richmond, R. L., & Owen, N. (1999). Stage distributions for five health behaviors in the USA and Australia. *Preventive Medicine, 28,* 61–74.

Levesque, D. A., Prochaska, J. M., & Prochaska, J. O. (1999). Stages of change and integrated service delivery. *Consulting Psychology Journal: Practice and Research, 51*(4), 226–241.

Melnyk, B. M. (2002). Strategies for overcoming barriers in implementing evidence-based practice. *Pediatric Nursing, 28*(2), 159–161.

Melnyk, B. M. (2001). Big dreams, belief and persistence: Essential elements for achieving career success. *Advance for Nurse Practitioners, 9*(3), 85–86.

Melnyk, B. M. (1995). Coping with unplanned childhood hospitalization: The mediating functions of parental beliefs. *Journal of Pediatric Psychology, 20*(3), 299–312.

Melnyk, B. M., & Fineout-Overholt, E. (2002). Putting research into practice, Rochester ARCC. *Reflections on Nursing Leadership, 28*(2), 22–25.

Oxman, A., Thomson, M. A., Davis, D., & Hayes, R. B. (1995). No magic bullets: A systematic review of 102 trials of interventions to improve professional practice. *Canadian Medical Association Journal, 15*(10), 1423–1431.

Prochaska, J. M., Prochaska, J. O., & Levesque, D. A. (2001). A transtheoretical approach to changing organizations. *Administration and Policy in Mental Health, 28*(4), 247–261.

Prochaska, J. O., & Velicer, W. F. (1997). The transtheoretical model of health behavior change. *American Journal of Health Promotion, 12*(1), 38–48.

Rohm, R. A., & Carey, E. C. (1997). *Who do you think you are . . . anyway? How your personality style acts . . . reacts . . . and interacts with others.* Atlanta: Personality Insights.

Torres, C., & Fairbanks, D. (1996). *Teambuilding: The ASTD trainer's sourcebook.* New York: McGraw-Hill.

Winum, P., Ryterband, E., & Stephensen, P. (1997). Helping organizations change: A model for guiding consultation. *Consulting Psychology Journal: Practice and Research, 49,* 6–16.

Reviewing Evidence to Guide Best Practice

Bernadette Mazurek Melnyk and Ellen Fineout-Overholt

chapter 17

The first 16 chapters of this book have emphasized how to:

- Formulate a clinical issue into a searchable, answerable question.
- Find and critically appraise relevant evidence.
- Convert that evidence into action or choose other options to generate evidence (e.g., outcomes management, quantitative or qualitative studies).
- Evaluate those initiatives (e.g., either evidence in action).

This portion of the book is a unique compilation of evidence that can assist clinicians in making the best clinical decisions to guide practice and improve patient outcomes. The chapters on the accompanying CD-ROM include 40 best evidence reviews to answer burning clinical questions in six specialty areas:

- Adults in Acute and Critical Care
- Adults in Primary Care
- Aging Adults
- Emergency and Trauma Care
- High-Risk Children and Youth
- Psychiatric Mental Health

As you find the evidence that is of interest to you in your practice area, our hope is that you will gain knowledge and be motivated to implement best practices, based on these excellent reviews. The content that follows is a brief synopsis of the evidence reviews in each of the specialty chapters. The reviews in their entirety can be found on the accompanying CD-ROM.

Best Evidence to Guide Clinical Practice with Adults in Acute and Critical Care

The pace of change is accelerating, bombarding nurses in acute and critical care with new technology and medications, evolving care delivery models, expanded nursing roles, integrated computerized systems, and a variety of ethical issues and challenges. Amidst all this change is a growing international nursing shortage. Coupled with a heavy physical workload, an emotionally draining environment, and the need to maintain unrelenting, vigilant watch over their patients, today's acute and critical care nurses often fail to question their practices, holding tightly to traditions. Yet it is through research generation that improved practice paradigms will be conceived in the future. The research process enables generation of knowledge pertaining to phenomena of interest, and within the context of critical care, phenomena are many. Crookes and Davies (1998) identified four "As" pertinent to research: awareness, appreciation, application, and ability (Daley, Elliott & Chang, 2000).

Acute and critical care nurses must possess an insatiable appetite for learning, questioning, and changing how they conduct their work. Tradition-bound practices (e.g., saline instillation during suctioning, routine lead II monitoring, and exclusion of families from access to loved ones in step-down and critical care units) must come to an end.

The focus of Chapter 18 is primarily critical care with a lesser emphasis on acute care. Anne W. Wojner, president of Health Outcomes Institute in Houston, Texas and Assistant Professor of Neurology and Neuroscience Critical Care Medicine, along with Jill Jesurum, a cardiovascular nurse practitioner and consultant with Health Outcomes Institute, considered the research priorities set by the American Association of Critical Care Nurses (AACN, 2003) as a starting point for this work. The National Quality Forum's (2003) Safe Practices compendium was reviewed as it pertains to critical care, and the Joint Commission on Accreditation of Healthcare Organizations (JCAHO, 2003) Core Measures for Critical Care also was considered. In addition, current literature was reviewed to ensure identification of phenomena of interest to acute and critical care nurses practicing in a variety of specialty areas.

Using Air Insufflation Technique and pH-Sensored Tubes to Insert Feeding Tubes
Joya D. Pickett and Lisa Tedeschi

The importance of good nutrition in critically ill patients is well documented (Babineau & Blackburn, 1994). Early adequate nutrition improves wound healing, nitrogen balance, and immunocompetence; demonstrates decreases in infection and intensive care unit (ICU) length of stay; and improves outcomes (Alexander, 1993; Braga et. al., 1996; Moore et al., 1992; Zaloga & Roberts, 1977). Enteral feeding in the patient with a functioning gut is the preferred route of food administration in the patient who cannot tolerate oral feedings (Salasidis, Fleiszer, & Johnson, 1998; Schulz, Santanello, Monk, & Falcone, 1993). Obtaining postpyloric placement of feeding tubes (FTs) can be problematic. Some methods are costly and cumbersome, causing delay and indecisiveness with regard to initiation of feedings. Recently, new pH-sensored FTs have been developed to assist in positioning of enteral tubes at the bedside by giving the user a constant digital pH reading. As the tube travels from the esophagus to the stomach and ultimately the small bowel, pH readings change. Pickett and Tedeschi reviewed six study reports to answer the clinical question, How effective are the air insufflation technique and pH-sensing feeding tubes in achieving postpyloric placement of small-bore feeding tubes in adults?

Readiness for Weaning from Mechanical Ventilation
Sandra K. Hanneman and Dorothy M. Kite-Powell

On a daily basis, approximately 41% of critically ill patients receive mechanical ventilation in the United States and Canada (Esteban et al., 2000), which translates to nearly 273,000 individuals annually. Patients who require mechanical ventilation for only a short time (e.g., $\geq$ 72 hours) generally may be weaned rapidly without untoward effects (Knebel et al., 1994; Hanneman et al., 1994). In contrast, patients who require long-term mechanical ventilation ($>$ 72 hours) may need weeks or months of weaning that is marked by setbacks and complications, interspersed with bursts of progress (Knebel et al., 1998). Hanneman and Kite-Powell reviewed guidelines, protocols, and systematic reviews to answer the clinical question, What are the most effective predictors of readiness to wean from mechanical ventilation in adult critically ill patients?

In conjunction with weaning from mechanical ventilation, Houston and colleagues focused on critically appraising the Center for Disease Control and Prevention (CDC)'s *Guideline for Prevention of Hospital-Associated Pneumonia* (2002) in answering the clinical question, What is the most effective means of preventing ventilator-associated pneumonia in adults?

chapter 17

459

The Best Methods for Assessing Sedation, Analgesia, Delirium, and Neuromuscular Blockage
Jan Foster

Appropriate sedation to minimize agitation is necessary to achieve therapeutic goals and recovery from illness and injury. Undersedation and analgesia lead to unnecessary suffering (especially during procedures), ventilator dysynchrony, agitation, delirium, and recall of events. These responses exacerbate the stress response, contribute to oxygen debt, and compromise the recovery process. Excess sedation, analgesia, and neuromuscular blockade, in contrast, contribute to prolonged and severe weakness, unrecognized cerebral insult, delayed ventilator weaning, and increased length of intensive care unit (ICU) and hospital stay, and contribute to unnecessary costs. Foster reviewed 10 instruments to measure sedation to help answer the clinical question, What are the most valid and reliable instruments supporting clinical assessment of sedation, analgesia, and delirium in adults?

Effect of Routine Nursing Procedures on Tissue Oxygenation
Susan L. Reed and Jill Jesurum

Over a span of 30 years, nursing research within the area of tissue oxygenation has largely focused on issues pertaining to the effects of routine care procedures on tissue oxygenation variables. Patient positioning, bathing, back massage, endotracheal suctioning, chest physiotherapy, ventilator weaning, and range-of-motion exercises are standard nursing care procedures that are routinely performed in the management of critically ill patients (Kozier & Erb, 1983; Luckmann & Sorensen, 1987; Potter & Perry, 2001). These routine nursing procedures are associated with an increase in oxygen demand and consequently may be poorly tolerated by critically ill patients who are susceptible to tissue oxygen deprivation (Gawlinski, 1993; Tidwell, Ryan, Osguthorpe, Paull, & Smith, 1990; Verderber & Gallagher, 1994; Weissman & Kemper, 1991; White, Winslow, Clark, & Tyler, 1990). Iatrogenic complications associated with routine nursing procedures may include hypoxemia, hypotension, cardiac dysrhythmias, and cardiac arrest (Clark, Winslow, Tyler, & White, 1990; Gawlinski & Dracup, 1998; Kinloch, 1999; Pena, 1989; Schweiss, 1987; Walsh, Vanderwarf, Hoscheit, & Fahey, 1989). Knowledge of the effects of nursing procedures on tissue oxygenation in critically ill patients can assist critical care nurses in determining when it is safe to proceed with care activities or whether activities should be postponed to avoid creating an oxygen imbalance (Jesurum, 1997). In this review, Reed and Jesurum examined three existing protocols and critically appraised 15 studies to answer the clinical question, What are the most effective nursing procedures in maximizing tissue oxygenation as measured by SVO_2 in critical care adult patients?

Effectiveness of Health Professionals' Education on Smoking Cessation
Janie Heath

Deaths in the United States related to tobacco use and dependence are greater than those combined for AIDS, alcohol, motor vehicle accidents, suicides, homicides, fire-related incidents, and illicit drugs (American Cancer Society [ACS], 2002; CDC, 1999). Due to escalating illnesses and deaths related to smoking and the significant cost to society, health care providers need to take a more aggressive approach to decrease tobacco use and dependence. However, health care providers commonly report lack of knowledge of management and treatment of tobacco dependence as a major barrier to successfully treating their patients (Cabana et al., 1999; Jaen et al., 1998; McBride et al., 1997; Secker-Walker et al., 1994; Solberg et al., 1997; Thorndike et al., 1998). Another concern is the increasing evidence that health care providers are not adequately educated on how to assist patients to stop smoking (CDC, 2001; Ferry, Grissino, Runfola 1999; Fiore, Epps, & Manley, 1994; Heath, Andrews, Thomas, Kelley, & Friedman, 2002; Sarna, Brown, Lillington, Rose, Wewers, & Brecht, 2000; Sprangler, George, Foley, & Crandall, 2002). Heath reviewed three studies to answer the clinical question, How effective is educating health care professionals about smoking cessation on patient outcomes?

Optimizing Intracranial Hemodynamics Through Manipulation of Head of Bed Positioning
Anne W. Wojner

Neurologic injuries resulting from trauma or stroke are commonly encountered in the acute care setting. In the United States alone, over 700,000 strokes occur each year and, of these, approximately 150,000 result in death (American Stroke Association, 2001). More than 500,000 moderate to severe traumatic brain injuries (TBIs) occur each year in the United States, and the majority of annual traumatic deaths are caused by a concurrent TBI (Langlois et al., 2003). Whether the result of stroke or TBI, the disability associated with neurologic impairment is both physiologically and psychologically devastating. Regardless of causative mechanism, the primary goal during acute management of stroke and TBI patients targets optimizing blood flow to ischemic brain tissue to prevent or minimize neurologic disability. One nursing measure that is routinely advocated for care of most all neurologic diagnoses, including both acute stroke and TBI patients, is elevation of the head of the bed (HOB) to 30 degrees. The goal tied with use of this intervention is reduction of ICP, thereby improving arterial blood flow to ischemic brain tissue. Wojner reviewed six studies to answer the clinical question, Should the HOB elevated to 30 degrees be used routinely to manage patients with either acute stroke or traumatic brain injury?

Effectiveness of Pneumatic and Clamp Hemostasis Devices in Prevention of Femoral Site Complications
Joya D. Pickett and Quana D. Bert

Over 2 million cardiac procedures are performed annually either to diagnose coronary artery disease (CAD) or to aid in the prevention and treatment of myocardial infarction (MI), utilizing interventional percutaneous coronary interventions (PCIs; AHA, 2002). With increasing use of PCIs, it is imperative that the incidence of procedure-related complications be minimized.

Cannulation of the femoral artery (FA) is initiated with placement of an introducer, which permits multiple diagnostic catheters and interventional devices to be exchanged (Tilkian & Daily, 1986). Puncture and manipulation of the artery predisposes the vessel to local vascular complications, such as frank bleeding, ecchymosis, and hematoma formation. More serious complications include retroperitoneal bleeding, overt hemorrhage, infection, thrombosis, pseudoaneurysm (PA), arteriovenous (AV) fistula, and limb amputation (Hessel, Adams, & Abrams, 1981; Messina et al., 1991; Pipkin, Brophy, Nesbit, & Mondy, 2000). Manual compression has been the mainstay in the postprocedural management of the femoral vascular access site. Mechanical compression devices have been proposed as an alternative to manual compression since 1974 (Semler, 1985). Pickett and Bert reviewed three studies in answering the clinical question, How effective are pneumatic and clamp hemostasis devices in the prevention of femoral site complications in patients after PCIs?

The methodical nature of these reviews made apparent the significant need for research in these areas. Acute and critical care nursing demands holistic, scientific, artful caregiving to patients at a most vulnerable and fearful time of their lives. The blend of science and art in acute and critical care nursing will continue to evolve rapidly in the coming years as the evidence supporting clinical practices grows progressively stronger.

Best Evidence to Guide Clinical Practice with Adults in Primary Care

The terrain covered by adult primary care is expansive and traverses health promotion and disease prevention, acute and chronic treatment and management, and complementary approaches to health and healing. Burning clinical questions abound and, because of the depth and breadth of adult primary care, they are diverse as clinicians seek to understand and deliver the best practice to their patients. Joanne K. Singleton, Professor at the Lienhard School of Nursing at Pace University, Carol Green-Hernandez, Associate Professor at the University of Vermont, and Edwin McMillian, a nurse practitioner, edited seven best evidence reviews that comprise Chapter ^AQ19.

Clearly, the papers in this chapter are just scratching the surface, but each of the reviews that can be found on the CD-ROM is important in its own right. The reviews are important because they were stimulated by clinicians' questions, and by following the systematic approach discussed in Chapter 1, these clinicians have found answers to the questions posed and are able to discuss implications for research and practice.

The burning questions identified by the adult primary care clinicians who contributed to this section include:

- Current physician practices and national recommendations regarding mass screening for prostate cancer, especially in men over the age of 74
- Use of wrist splints as a single first-line therapy for the relief of symptoms in adults with carpal tunnel syndrome
- Delays in seeking care of patients with acute myocardial infarction
- Zinc preparations and the symptoms of the common cold in adults
- Gabapentin for controlling diabetic neuropathic pain
- Insulin resistance and hyperinsulinemias in polycystic ovarian syndrome
- Obesity counseling in assisting adults in primary care to lose weight or reduce their body mass index (BMI)

Answers to these undoubtedly diverse questions make an important contribution to adult primary care. The following synopsis provides an overview of this contribution.

Mass Prostate Screening
Randi Z. Moskowitz

Over 220,000 new cases of prostate cancer will be found in the United States in 2003 (Jemal, Murray, Samuels et al., 2003). Prostate cancer is the most frequently diagnosed malignancy and represents the second leading cause of cancer-related deaths in America (Jemal et al., 2003; Ries, Eisner, Kosary et al., 2000). As a likely consequence of the introduction and use of the screening tool serum prostate-specific antigen (PSA) in the period between 1988 and 1992, the diagnosis of prostate cancer cases increased significantly (American Cancer Society, 2002). Since that period, the frequency of prostate cancer diagnosis has declined. This has probably occurred because the numbers diagnosed in the period from 1988 to 1992 represented new and previously existing cases of prostate cancer. Subsequent testing identifies mostly new cases (Barry, 2001).

The practice of mass screening using such tests as digital rectal exams (DREs) or serum PSA is a controversial subject. During the last 10 years, advocacy groups, an increasingly aging population, high disease frequency, and a cultural norm promoting aggressive disease intervention have contributed to an increased concern regarding screening for prostate cancer (Voss & Schectman, 2001). Evidence-based guidelines built on randomized trials that display a decrease in mortality attributable to screening do not exist. Two such trials are currently being undertaken, with only preliminary results available. The average life expectancy for men in America is now 74 years. With this statistic in mind, Moscowitz asks the question, In the United States, what are current physician practices and national recommendations regarding mass screening for prostate cancer, especially in men over the age of 74?

Carpal Tunnel Syndrome
Mary McCormack

Carpal tunnel syndrome (CTS), a predominantly idiopathic neuropathy resulting in pain and paresthesia to fingers of the affected hand, may be found in nearly 4% of all males and over 10% of all females. The incidence for females peaks near late middle age; for males, the incidence continues to increase with age (O'Connor, Marshall & Massy-Westrop, 2003). Evidence suggests that this condition is increasing in frequency (Manente, Torrieri, & Di Blasio, 2002), with some of the additional cases attributable to the ubiquitous presence and use of computer keyboards. Other occupations with repetitive-use tasks that contribute to this disease include cashiers and mechanics.

For mild to moderate symptoms, a conservative approach to treatment is probably appropriate. Recommendations from national organizations include, among other suggestions, the use of nonsteroidal antiinflammatory drugs, steroids, and wrist splints. Potential side effects of and contraindications against the use of medications suggest the consideration of wrist splints as a first-line single therapy for CTS.

McCormack investigated existing evidence-based literature to answer the clinical question, How effective is the use of wrist splints as a single first-line therapy for the relief of symptoms (e.g., pain, numbness, tingling, and burning) in adults with CTS?

Timely Care of Adults with Acute Myocardial Infarction
Jill R. Quinn

Well over a quarter of those who experience an acute myocardial infarction (AMI) experience a delay of treatment for longer than 3 hours. It has been established that heart disease is the number one cause of mortality in the United States and that each moment that passes after an AMI without appropriate treatment reduces the patient's chances of recovery. Medical interventions developed over the last 20 years have significantly improved patient survival rates but rely on application as soon as possible after the cardiac event, with a significant decrease in efficacy by 3 hours after AMI (GISSI Trial, 1986; Berger et al., 1994; Ryan et al., 1999). Observations suggest a decline in the rate of delay over the last 40 years but that delay is still significant. The range of median delay time has been reported from 2 to 6.5 hours (Dracup & Moser, 1997; React Study Group, 2000). Delay-reducing interventions, if effective, may improve survival rates for victims of heart attacks.

In her review of the evidence, Quinn attempts to answer the clinical question, In adults at risk for AMI, does distribution of information via mass media about symptoms of AMI and how to seek care reduce patient delay time in seeking care?

Zinc for the Relief of Common Cold Symptoms
Maria Claudia Escobar

The impact on human beings in the United States of the common cold can be measured in several ways. The common cold is one of the most frequent reasons for visits to ambulatory care settings (Schappert, 1998), with approximately 62 million cases annually (Fast Stats, 1996). The average adult suffers from two to four colds per year, and economic costs from lost work time alone are about $5 billion (Fact Sheet, 2001). Even with advancements in medicine and science, there exists no cure for this ubiquitous affliction.

Seeking relief from health problems such as the common cold, increasing numbers of Americans are investigating and using "alternative" treatments. It is estimated that 53% of U.S. residents use these supplements daily (Slesenski, Subar, & Kahle, 1995). One such treatment is the use of zinc in a variety of forms for the alleviation of cold symptoms. Godfrey, Godfrey, and Novick (1996) propose that the effect of zinc on cold symptoms is due to an interaction of zinc on the surface of the virus, the facial nerves, and the inflammatory process. The use of zinc for treating the common cold began more than 20 years ago and has been investigated in clinical trials since then. Several systematic reviews published before 1998 suggest it is an efficacious intervention for cold symptoms but have been criticized for design flaws. Escobar searched relevant literature for rigorously designed, recently conducted studies to answer the clinical question, Does taking oral or nasal zinc preparations effectively reduce the symptoms of the common cold in adults?

Gabapentin for Diabetic Neuropathy
Agatha A. (Tracy) Quinn

Diabetes mellitus is a disease that affects millions of people worldwide. Because of changing lifestyle habits, it is likely that the current epidemic of diabetes will get worse before it gets better. The complications of diabetes are well known to clinicians. Among the most common of these is diabetic neuropathy. Its painful sequelae have been, until recently, a source of frustration for providers who have had little or nothing to offer patients in the way of relief. Over the last several years, some patients have found that topical application of capascin provided some measure of pain control, although nothing alleviated symptoms of numbing.

More recently, some primary care providers have begun to prescribe amitriptyline in an effort to control neuropathic pain. However, neither agent has proven to be totally satisfactory in the majority of patients. Further, not everyone tolerates amitriptyline (Morello, Leckband, Stoner, Moorhouse, & Sahagian, 1999). Unfortunately, even if pain is controlled, patients who experience the numbness of diabetic neuropathy are still at risk for tissue injury. Consequently, these individuals risk tissue breakdown because they lack normal nerve conductance that would otherwise protect them from sources of physical injury, including normal bumps and bruises (National Diabetic Fact Sheet, 2003). In her review, Quinn attempts to find evidence to answer the clinical question, How effective is gabapentin in controlling diabetic neuropathic pain in adults with diabetes mellitus?

Insulin Resistance and Hyperinsulinemias in Polycystic Ovarian Syndrome
Joyce Knestrick

Polycystic ovarian syndrome (PCOS) is not a common health problem but nevertheless affects 6–10% of women in the United States (Kordella, 2002). Further, symptomatology may worsen over a woman's lifetime (Goldman & Bennett, 2000). Some of the studies reviewed by Kovarian suggested that hyperinsulinemia produces hyperandrogenism by increasing ovarian androgen production. Hyperinsulinemia itself places any patient at risk for associated comorbidities such as high blood pressure, increased clot formation, heart disease, and type 2 diabetes mellitus (Carmina et al., 1992; Dunaif, 1995).

There is evidence that suggests PCOS is a syndrome that involves insulin resistance and hyperinsulinemia. It may be that the management of PCOS will become more challenging in those women whose lifestyles make them more resistant to managing their endogenous insulin resistance syndrome. Kovarian's reviews evidence to answer the clinical question, In women with PCOS, how effective are antidiabetic agents in reducing syndrome symptoms?

Counseling and Weight Loss in Adult Obesity
Mary B. Neiheisel

Obesity has surpassed other diseases as a significant cause of morbidity and mortality in the United States (Baron, 2000). Although problems with overweight are typically seen as individuals grow older, health care providers are seeing an increasing incidence in obesity among adolescents and children (Lenfant, 2001). More worrisome is the fact that obese children become obese adults (Schmitz & Jeffery, 2000). Obesity is an outcome of excessive caloric intake in comparison with an individual's generated metabolic rate.

Clinicians use several methods to control obesity. These can include but are not limited to:

- Counseling
- Exercise programs
- Behavior change strategies
- Medications
- Several kinds of diets
- Surgical procedures

The goals of any method chosen to manage obesity should optimally include weight reduction, sustained weight reduction over time, and behavior modification needed to bring about and maintain changed eating and exercise habits in order to maintain the weight loss. Neiheisel's examination of the relevant literature dealing with counseling and weight loss in adult obesity assists in answering the clinical question, How effective is obesity counseling in assisting adults in the primary care setting with a body mass index (BMI) of greater than 25 to lose weight or reduce their BMIs?

Each of the seven areas addressed have made a contribution in assessing the nature and quality of clinical evidence on the topic and how this evidence can be used in practice. Additionally, it points to limitations or quality of the existing evidence and, in each of the areas, makes recommendations for future research.

Not only is there the need for more clinical research in each of the topics addressed, there are also numerous other areas in adult primary care that are ripe for answers to clinical questions. Some are emerging areas where little clinical research has been conducted (e.g., end-of-life issues), whereas others areas have had some research, but it is inconclusive or contradictory. Smoking cessation research has led to the development of evidence-based clinical practice guidelines, but as discussed in another chapter, patient characteristics (e.g., gender and ethnicity) have yet to be studied to help enhance clinicians' selection of first-line interventions. In the area of women's health, ongoing research in hormone replacement therapy has called into question past evidence, dramatically influencing practice. In addition, research on complementary approaches to health and healing is challenging and is still in its infancy.

This chapter illustrates the process that real-life clinicians can use to answer their burning clinical questions, helping to bridge the research-practice gap. Through evidence reviews of clinical interventions, we also are able to see areas in need of further research or more rigorous research designs. Ultimately, our efforts are aimed at best practice and improved patient outcomes.

Best Evidence to Guide Clinical Practice with Aging Adults

We often think of aging as an individual matter. However, in recent years, increased emphasis is placed on the aging of the population. This emphasis is driven by the unprecedented growth in the number of older people. Between 1990 and 2000, the number of older Americans increased by 3.7 million, a 12% increase. In 2000, there were 35 million people 65 years of age or older, approximately one in every eight Americans. The growth in the aging population is most rapid in persons over 85 years of age (Administration on Aging, 2002). By 2030, it is estimated that 20% of the population will be 65 years of age or older.

The United States is experiencing this unprecedented growth in the number of elders for a variety of reasons. First, when birth rates fell, there were fewer children in the population, so the average age increased. Second, population aging occurred because of increased life expectancy. People live longer because of improved mechanisms to control infectious diseases and improvements in health care. Third, birth cohorts influence the age of the population. For instance, the cohort born during the Depression of the 1930s was relatively small and had limited impact on the average age of the population. In contrast, the Baby Boomers born after World War II comprise a large cohort and, because of their size, they will hasten the aging of the population. All three of these events (i.e., increased life expectancy, decreased birth rates, and cohort influences) are occurring simultaneously in the United States, thereby contributing to the dramatic increase in the number of older people (Moody, 2002).

Many older people have at least one chronic condition, and many have multiple conditions. Limitations in activities of daily living because of chronic illness increase with age. In 2000, almost half of the people 75 years of age and older reported that they were limited in daily activities due to a chronic illness. This is in sharp contrast to the 2.8% of people under 65 years of age who reported limitations in activities of daily living. Limitations in activities of daily living frequently necessitate help from other people. Family members provide 85% of assistance for community-dwelling elders. Approximately 36% of family caregivers provide care 21 hours per week or more. More than half of the family caregivers reported working full time, and one third of them reported losing time from work due to caregiving responsibilities (Stone, 2000). There is an abundance of research on burdens and health risks associated with caring for an elderly family member. More recently, attention has focused on benefits and the importance of preparing family caregivers to assist older persons (Clyburn, Stone, Hadjistavropoulos, & Tuikko, 2000; Cornman-Levy, Gitlin, Corcoran, & Schinfeld, 2001; Schulz & Beach, 1999).

Often, exacerbation of chronic conditions contributes to hospital admissions in older adults. In 2000, older people had approximately four times the number of days in a hospital, compared with persons less than 65 years of age. The average length of hospital stay for elders was 6.4 days, compared with 4.6 days for all people. In addition, older people averaged more contacts with doctors than younger persons (Administration on Aging, 2002). Older persons' out-of-pocket expenditures for health care increased more than half between 1990 and 2000. On average, elders spent $3,493 in out-of-pocket costs in 2000. The cost breakdown consisted of $1,775 (51% for insurance), $884 (25%) for drugs, $693 (20%) for medical services, and $142 (4%) for medical supplies.

Given the demographics and statistics on health care utilization, health care professionals can expect to have frequent contact with older people, whether they practice in acute care hospitals, primary care, long-term care, or home health care. As a result, it is essential for health care professionals to examine the evidence to support interventions for common conditions elders experience.

Margaret J. Bull, a gerontological researcher and practitioner at Marquette University, selected the topics for Chapter 20 because they illustrate nonpharmacological interventions for common conditions or situations.

Nonpharmacological Interventions for Elders with Alzheimer's Disease
Fay L. Bower and Cyndi S. McCullough

In the first paper, Bower and McCullough present the evidence for use of nonpharmacological interventions to reduce agitation and disorientation for persons with Alzheimer's disease (AD). By 2025, approximately 22 million persons worldwide will be affected by AD. To date, there is no cure for the disease. Treatment consists of encouraging self-care and alleviating symptoms. A comprehensive review of the literature yielded 21 studies that provide promising evidence for four categories of intervention:

1. Increasing socialization
2. Reducing disorientation
3. Reducing agitation
4. Improving performance

The authors examine strengths and weaknesses of each approach and suggest that there is a variety of ways in which health care professionals can intervene effectively with older persons who have AD.

Prompted Voiding for Urinary Incontinence
Mary H. Palmer

In the second paper, Palmer examines the effectiveness of prompted voiding in alleviating the problem of urinary incontinence. This condition affects more than half of the nursing home residents in the United States, with direct annual costs estimated at $3,687 per institutionalized elder. It also is a significant problem among noninstitutionalized elders and affects their self-esteem and quality of life. Prompted voiding is a behavioral intervention that involves reminding the person to toilet, usually on two-hour intervals, and providing social reinforcement. From a total of 41 articles, three original research reports and one systematic review met the author's criteria of reporting patient outcomes, using prompted voiding for urinary incontinence, using prompted voiding as an intervention, and implementing the intervention in a long-term care facility. The strengths and weaknesses of the studies are examined, and the theoretical foundations of the intervention and implications for practice are discussed.

Stress Management Interventions with Elders
Margaret J. Bull and Ruth E. McShane

The third paper in this chapter examines the effectiveness of stress management strategies with older adults. Many illnesses are caused or exacerbated by stress. In fact, extreme levels of stress have been shown to damage health, delay recovery, and impact mortality. The severity of chronic illnesses has been associated with stress. Although much research on stress management has been focused on younger adults, less attention has been given specifically to stress management with elders. Bull and McShane uncovered 23 studies in their review; however, only three studies focused specifically on stress management with elders. The strategies used with elders were progressive muscle relaxation and reminiscence. A variety of beneficial outcomes are described. Implications for practice and future research are discussed.

End-of-Life Models of Care for Dying Residents in Nursing Homes
Sarah A. Wilson

In the fourth paper, Wilson reviews factors that have contributed to increased emphasis on end-of-life care and examines effectiveness of models for the delivery of end-of-life care in nursing homes. The majority of older adults die in institutions. Approximately 20–25% percent die in nursing homes, and it is estimated that this will increase to 40% by 2040. A comprehensive literature search yielded four studies that described delivery systems and included family member evaluations of the care delivery system. The author suggests that the application of hospice concepts in nursing homes can improve pain management and family satisfaction with care.

Depression Management Programs in Primary Care for Older Adults
Merrie J. Kaas

In the fifth paper, Kaas examines the effectiveness of depression management programs in primary care for improving outcomes for older adults. Depression is largely unrecognized and untreated in elders seen in primary care. Elders account for 20% of the suicides and 16% of the annual hospitalizations for depression. Symptoms of depression in elders are associated with decreased functional ability, increased morbidity and mortality, poorer overall quality of life, and higher health care costs. The evidence from 10 randomized clinical trials is evaluated for relevance to clinical practice.

Interventions Involving Family Caregivers to Improve Outcomes of Hospitalized Elders
Hong Li and Bernadette Mazurek Melnyk

In the final paper, Li and Melnyk examine the effectiveness of nursing interventions in involving family caregivers in the hospital care for older adults. Their comprehensive review of the literature yielded eight intervention studies. The limitations of each study are discussed. The authors suggest that clinicians can play an important role in involving family caregivers in the care of hospitalized elders. The findings of studies also suggest that family member involvement has benefits for both the elder and the family member.

Best Evidence to Guide Clinical Practice in Emergency and Trauma Care

The clinical specialties of emergency, trauma, and disaster care transcend trends in health care, from birth until death. Concerns for personal, family, and community safety in light of world events makes the need for evidence-based practice (EBP) even more crucial. In Chapter 21, Lisa Bernardo and her colleagues focus on the current issues in EBP in emergency, trauma, and disaster specialty practice.

Predictors of Survival Post-Cardiopulmonary Arrest in Adult Patients
Renee Semonin-Holleran

In the first paper, two respected emergency clinicians discuss the important issues of resuscitation in the emergency department. Semonin-Holleran outlines the predictors of survival after cardiopulmonary arrest in adult patients. Despite advances in cardiopulmonary care, such as early defibrillation, endotracheal intubation, and medication administration, outcomes from unwitnessed cardiopulmonary arrest continue to be dismal. Emergency nurses and physicians are confronted with the question, When should resuscitation efforts cease? Ethically, emergency nurses are required to do no harm. However, is prolonged resuscitation unethical when EBP indicates that life cannot be restored? Evidence-based research reports indicate that, despite best efforts of bystanders and prehospital care providers, death in the emergency department is likely following sudden cardiopulmonary arrest in the out-of-hospital setting. Semonin-Holleran concludes with the American Heart Association's recommendations (Cummins, 2002) for when cardiopulmonary resuscitation efforts should and should not be initiated. Emergency clinicians are faced with these difficult decisions in their daily practices. As such, using evidence-based findings to guide the development of emergency department guidelines for adults in cardiopulmonary arrest is vital.

Predictors of Outcome in Children Sustaining Out-of-Hospital Cardiopulmonary Arrest
Bonnie J. Clemence

Although the resuscitation of adults in cardiopulmonary arrest has dismal results, the outcomes are even more profound in children. Clemence discusses EBP related to predictors of outcome in children sustaining out-of-hospital cardiopulmonary arrest. Unlike adults, children of varying ages differ in factors leading to cardiopulmonary arrest, respond differently to medications, and have other physiologic features that affect their outcomes. Emergency clinicians are faced with the same ethical dilemma of doing no harm to children who arrive in the emergency department in cardiopulmonary arrest; resuscitation efforts continue until cardiac activity is restored. Evidence shows that very few children respond to resuscitation efforts, and those who do are left with a poor quality of life. Clemence concludes her review by citing that the best predictor of outcome in children sustaining out-of-hospital cardiopulmonary arrest is the return of spontaneous circulation in the prehospital setting (with a short interval of CPR). Prolonged resuscitation efforts in the emergency department are likely to be futile, causing more pain and suffering to families and the children. As in adults, emergency clinicians should consider developing interdisciplinary protocols or guidelines for treating children in cardiopulmonary arrest and outlining parameters for when resuscitation efforts should cease.

Despite advances in trauma care and prevention, this disease continues to be the leading cause of death and disability in individuals under the age of 45 years. Unlike the emergency area of specialty, trauma care encompasses the entire health care spectrum, from injury prevention, prehospital and emergency care, critical care (operating room, postanesthesia care unit, intensive care unit), acute care, rehabilitation, and reintroduction into the community. Similar to emergency care, there are subspecialties to this practice, such as pediatric trauma nursing, and subroles, such as trauma coordinator.

The Role of Emergency Department Thoracotomy in the Resuscitation of Injured Children
Bonnie J. Clemence

Three evidence reviews in this section reflect trauma care in the emergency department, intensive care unit, and reintroduction into the community. Clemence discusses the role of emergency department thoracotomy (EDT) in the resuscitation of injured children. Resuscitation of children and adults following cardiopulmonary arrest from traumatic events (e.g., exsanguination following a gunshot wound to the chest) continues from the prehospital setting into the emergency department. One resuscitation measure is EDT, whereby a patient's chest is opened and cardiac massage and internal cardiac defibrillation are attempted. This resuscitation measure is used as a last attempt at saving a patient's life. EDT may be most effective when patients have "signs of life" (i.e., a palpable pulse, blood pressure, spontaneous respirations, Glasgow Coma Score > 3, pupillary responses, and cardiac activity on the monitor) prior to emergency department arrival (Mazzorana, Smith, Reilly, & Brar, 1994). Because trauma is the leading cause of death in the pediatric population, EDT may be indicated in children under the aforementioned circumstances. Clemence reviews the evidence as to when EDT should be undertaken in the pediatric trauma population. Although guidelines developed for adults are extrapolated to children, the evidence is unclear for the efficacy of EDT in children sustaining trauma arrest. This conclusion is due to the retrospective nature of the research conducted in this area. Because randomized clinical trials may not be ethical to conduct in this patient population, relying on retrospective, descriptive data may be the only method for studying this problem. Clemence concludes her review with recommendations for the initiation of EDT based on the findings of the presented research but cautions that emergency nurses, physicians, and trauma surgeons may be willing to forgo the evidence if they can use EDT to save a child's life.

Predictors of Skin Breakdown in Injured Patients Receiving Treatment in the Intensive Care Unit
Lisa Bernardo and Jessica Muto

Bernardo and Muto review the evidence for predictors of skin breakdown in injured patients receiving treatment in the intensive care unit. Skin care is one aspect of patient care over which clinicians have the most influence because they are with patients 24 hours a day; are able to assess the skin during nursing procedures, such as turning, positioning and bathing; and within their scope of practice can initiate measures to relieve skin pressure or prevent skin shearing.

Based on the evidence, predictors of skin breakdown in adult trauma patients include a Braden score of ≥ 10 and ≤ 16; low body mass; hospitalization for more than 2 days but especially hospitalization for 2 weeks; head and spinal cord injuries; and cervical collar use. Health care providers can assess for these risk factors on admission and can plan their preventive care accordingly.

Although the validity and reliability of this reported literature leads to sound EBP in adults, little is written about the skin care needs of pediatric or geriatric trauma patients. Future research should include these patient populations to determine whether similar risk factors for skin breakdown are present.

The Effectiveness of Psychological Interventions to Prevent Posttraumatic Stress Disorder Following Traumatic Events

Ann M. Mitchell, Teresa J. Sakraida, and Kirstyn K. Zalace

The aftermath of trauma, as experienced by injured people, witnesses, or health care providers, can lead to negative psychological and physical outcomes. One such outcome is posttraumatic stress disorder (PTSD). Various strategies exist to prevent PTSD or to mitigate its effects. Mitchell, Sakraida, and Zalace review the evidence to determine the effectiveness of psychological interventions to prevent PTSD. Their review of published meta-analyses on this topic demonstrates a limited positive effect in preventing PTSD with acute psychological preventative interventions. Preventive psychological interventions immediately following a traumatic experience must take into consideration a number of intervening factors, such as a history of prior traumatizing events. However, acute psychological preventive interventions also may provide opportunities for working through these prior traumatic events. At present, the effectiveness of psychological debriefings in reducing the psychological distress (usually PTSD) often associated with a traumatic event remains unknown.

The Safety and Efficacy of Existing Vaccines in the Prevention of Pneumonic Plague

Tener Veenema and Catherine Vladutui

Clinical care before, during, and after disasters has occurred throughout history. Disasters, or events that overwhelm existing healthcare and community resources, occur throughout the world. Disasters can be natural (floods, earthquakes, tornadoes) or man-made (overwhelming environmental contamination with nuclear, chemical, or biological agents). Man-made disasters are further classified as unintentional, where the event was not planned or intended, or intentional, such as criminal acts or acts of terrorism. Wars, although man-made, bring about their own set of circumstances, including multiple casualties, displaced populations, and complex humanitarian emergencies.

With the increased incidence of terrorist acts throughout the world, clinicians in all healthcare settings must be prepared to care for individuals following a mass-casualty event where hundreds of people are injured or a public health emergency where hundreds of people are stricken with infectious or communicable diseases. As such, disaster care encompasses the entire healthcare spectrum—prevention, prehospital and emergency care, critical and acute care, rehabilitation, and return to the community. The disaster continuum of preparedness, mitigation, response, recovery, and evaluation includes clinical care, as well. Added features of the disaster clinical specialty area include the quarantine of patients exposed to infectious and communicable diseases, such as smallpox; the care of hundreds of injured people, whereby hospitals may need to admit many more patients (surge capacity) than what they are licensed to provide; and the surface decontamination of large numbers of people exposed to chemical agents.

World events have sparked new interest in this area of clinical practice, and the near future holds promise for new textbooks, research, and education in this specialty. Two experts in the disaster and emergency clinical specialty area outline very important and timely issues. Veenema and Vladutui review the evidence on the safety and efficacy of existing vaccines in the prevention of pneumonic plague. The anthrax-related illnesses and deaths in 2001 underscore the need for early detection and prevention of bioterrorist-related pathogens. Pneumonic plague has a high morbidity and mortality rate, making it a significant disease process and public health concern that must be controlled. As a result, scientists have developed several vaccines to prevent plague outbreaks around the world. Based on their review, Veenema and Vladutui report a negative review of evidence-based reports, because there were no human trials or well-done studies that would satisfy the requirements for safety, efficacy, and tolerability of existing plague vaccines. Such findings are disconcerting, because clinicians throughout the healthcare spectrum and the disaster continuum may unknowingly care for patients with pneumonic plague and may themselves become stricken with the disease. Future research in this and other vaccines is sorely needed.

Minimizing Errors in Children Following a Biochemical Weapons-of Mass-Destruction Incident
Susan Hoenhaus

In mass casualty situations, children, adults, and elderly are likely to be involved. Under such stressful circumstances, nurses and healthcare professionals may unintentionally make medication or treatment errors when caring for children. In patients requiring surface decontamination, nurses and healthcare professionals wear personal protective equipment that limits their dexterity in drawing up medications and in administering intramuscular and intravenous medications to children. To prevent errors from occurring, nurses need to have access to reference materials that will assist them in administering age- and weight-appropriate doses of medications and antidote, and using age-appropriate equipment under dire circumstances. Hoenhaus reviews the EBP on minimizing errors in children following a biochemical weapons-of-mass-destruction incident. Her review supports the use of the Broselow Emergency Tape and the Broselow-Luten Color Coding System to accurately and quickly determine age- and size-appropriate equipment and resuscitation medications in the pediatric population. The Broselow Emergency Tape is readily available, inexpensive, and easy to use. It will be included in the Strategic National Stockpile push packs. More research needs to be conducted in the use of the Tape and the Broselow-Luten Color Coding System to prepare for the care of children in disasters and public health emergencies.

In conclusion, the clinical specialties of emergency, trauma, and disaster overlap in their patient populations, care, and prevention. Each specialty has its own body of knowledge in which research, education, and administration opportunities are continually evolving. The papers in this chapter represent the future of these specialties. Healthcare providers are encouraged to apply evidence-based findings in their practices; to continue to ask questions; and to use research, patience, and awareness to change and improve clinical care.

Best Evidence to Guide Clinical Practice with High-Risk Children and Youth

The nature of childhood morbidity and mortality has changed considerably in the last few decades. Currently, mental health/psychosocial problems, chronic illnesses (e.g., asthma, diabetes, obesity), and preventable injuries cause more morbidity and mortality in the pediatric and adolescent population than acute physical illnesses and disorders (Hayman, Mahon, & Turner, 2002; Melnyk, Brown, Jones, Kreipe, & Novak, 2003; Melnyk et al., 2002). In addition, with currently 200 of 100,000 children experiencing a critical care hospitalization, it is expected that the number of pediatric critical care beds will continue to escalate in the new millennium with a higher severity of illness in children who occupy them (Zimmerman, 1998).

Multiple factors have contributed to this shift in morbidities, including vaccine and antimicrobial discoveries, changes in the composition of families (e.g., divorce, single parenting), recent terrorism and school violence, high levels of parental conflict and psychopathology (e.g., maternal depression), a trend toward earlier sexual activity, and the surge in technology, which has contributed to both a higher survival rate in low-birth-weight premature infants with long-term neurodevelopmental disabilities and the prolongation of life in critically ill children (Melnyk et al., 2003; Melnyk, Alpert-Gillis et al., 2001). In addition, other factors influencing current child and adolescent morbidities include demographic factors (e.g., poverty, growing minority populations with associated health disparities, adolescent parents, and low parental education), as well as service factors (e.g., lack of health insurance or adequate coverage, lack of primary care, and service systems that do not function adequately) (Weitzman, 2003).

As a result of the current pediatric and adolescent morbidities, recent initiatives at the national level have been initiated. Among these initiatives include increased opportunities for research funding in many of these focus areas by the National Institutes of Health (NIH)/National Institute of Nursing Research (NINR), and the National Institute of Mental Health (NIMH), as well as the Agency for Healthcare Research and Quality (AHRQ). In addition, new bills to improve mental health access for children are being introduced in the legislation (Melnyk et al., 2003). There also has been a recent call for proposals specifically in dissemination and implementation research from the NIMH with the intention of moving interventions that have been empirically supported as effective in research into clinical practice settings in order to improve clinical care and patient outcomes. Many of the *Healthy People 2010* objectives also target the current pediatric morbidities as a high priority (U.S. Department of Health and Human Services [U.S. DHHS], 2000).

As another example of initiatives to address some of these escalating problems, the National KySS (Keep Your Children/Yourself Safe and Secure) Campaign (an evidence-based initiative to promote the mental health and safety of children and teens) has been launched through the National Association of Pediatric Nurse Practitioners (NAPNAP) (Melnyk et al., 2003; Melnyk, Moldenhauer et al., 2001) along with NAPNAP's HEAT (Healthy Eating and Activity Together) initiative to deal with the epidemic of childhood obesity. Despite national recent and ongoing projects, there is an urgent need to make greater investments in children and adolescents, accelerate current initiatives, and launch additional collaborative efforts across multiple professional organizations, healthcare systems, and federal agencies to tackle the most pervasive problems, with an emphasis on preventive efforts as well as the early identification and evidence-based management of these most pressing child and adolescent morbidities. David Satcher, the sixteenth United States Surgeon General, so eloquently reinforced these needs as he made the following statements at the 2003 National KySS Summit: "We don't invest enough in children and there are not enough resources dedicated to them. We underestimate childhood as the foundation for the rest of adult health. What happens to children impacts the quality of life in adulthood" (Melnyk et al., 2003).

In choosing the papers for Chapter 22, Marion Broome, Associate Dean for Research and Professor at the University of Alabama at Birmingham School of Nursing, and Bernadette Melnyk, Associate Dean for Research, Professor, and Director of the Center for Research & EBP, and Pediatric Nurse Practitioner (PNP) and Dual PNP for the Psychiatric Mental Health NP Programs at the University of Rochester School of Nursing, decided to include evidence reviews that address some of the most pervasive problems in the care of children and adolescents today, many of which focus on topics where there are no systematic reviews to date that can guide clinical practice. In addition, reviews of evidence were included that would answer some of the most pressing clinical questions in the care of high-risk children and youth.

Parental Concern as a Reliable Predictor in Early Identification of Autism in Children
Michelle Beauchesne and Barbara Kelly

In the first paper, Beauchesne and Kelly tackle the tough clinical question of whether parental concern can be a reliable predictor in the early identification of autism in children. Recognizing features of autism in infancy is important for early diagnosis and treatment of this disorder but frequently poses many challenges for pediatric healthcare providers. Along with evidence to support that parental concern is a reliable predictor in the early identification of autism, this paper provides a critical review of current screening tools and practices for autism.

Effective Interventions to Reduce the Risk of HIV
Dianne Morrison-Beedy and Marilyn J. Aten

Given that HIV is now the ninth leading cause of death in adolescents and that the majority of HIV transmissions occur sexually (CDC, 2000), it was important to include a review of evidence to support the most effective interventions to reduce the risk of this disease. In a comprehensive review of the literature, Morrison-Beedy and Aten critically appraise prior studies to make recommendations about the best evidence to guide clinical practice. They conclude their review with the components that are critical in developing and implementing successful HIV prevention programs in both community and school settings. These components include information presented in combination with behavior skills that assist teens in avoiding risk behaviors as well as:

- The provision of credible, visible role models whose words and actions support participants' desires to make risk-reducing changes in behavior
- Development of skills to resist pressure from others to engage in risk behaviors
- Creation of an environment that reinforces the desired behaviors to reduce risk practices
- Development of mechanisms that foster individual pride as well as concern for one's own and others' health

Abnormal Sleep Patterns of Children in Pediatric Intensive Care Units
Margaret Carno

The purpose of the third paper by Margaret Carno is to describe abnormal sleep patterns in children hospitalized in pediatric intensive care units. Findings from this evidence review point to the urgent need to develop and test interventions to improve the sleep patterns of critically ill children.

Effective Parent-Focused Interventions for Improving Mental Health Outcomes in Critically Ill Children
Bernadette Mazurek Melnyk, Leigh Small, and Margaret Carno

The fourth review by Melnyk, Small, and Carno answered the question of what parent-focused interventions are most effective in improving mental health/coping outcomes in critically ill children. In their paper, Melnyk and colleagues highlight two reproducible interventions with positive outcomes that now need to be disseminated and implemented in pediatric intensive care units (PICUs) throughout the country to improve parental and child coping with critical illness in order to reduce long-term negative mental health outcomes.

Using Pain Assessment Measures in Children
Myra Martz Huth, Renee Ladwig, Michelle Czarecki, and Donna Harris

In the fifth paper, Huth and colleagues review studies that have examined the utility of pain assessment measures. Pain assessment and management methods, although studied systematically for the past two decades, remain a challenge in practice. Although clinicians have become more knowledgeable about and more positive in their attitudes about pain assessment over the last decade, their actual documentation of assessment is inconsistent in several studies (Broome & Huth, 2003). Huth and colleagues make a strong argument for multidimensional pain assessment, yet little systematic investigation of the value of multidimensional versus one-dimensional pain assessment has been conducted.

Feeding Methods for Premature Infants
Barbara S. Turner, Debra H. Brandon, and Mary K. Cornwell

The sixth evidence review focuses on gavage feedings in at-risk neonates by Turner and colleagues and provides a thorough review of the issues involved in deciding the best feeding method for premature infants. Although there are many dramatic procedures experienced by premature infants, few are more important to their long-term well-being than feeding. Feeding practices have varied throughout the United States for many years, with choice of feeding based on many factors other than data. The choice of feeding also is not without risk and can further challenge the well-being of these infants if not appropriate. Unfortunately, the evidence from the 11 studies reviewed in this paper is not clear. Even more unfortunate is the lack of adequate description of the intervention tested (i.e., type of feeding). Such limited description in the literature restricts the ability of others to replicate and evaluate the appropriateness of the intervention for their settings. The conclusion of Turner and colleagues is that semicontinuous feeds provide another option for clinicians to consider in their units.

Guidelines for Asthma Management in Children
Barbara Velsor-Friedrich

Because asthma is one of the most common childhood illnesses, with over 4.8 million children under 18 years of age diagnosed with this chronic illness (CDC, 1999), it was felt that this specialty chapter would not be complete without a review of evidence in this area. Although research-based guidelines for asthma management by health professionals have been available for the past decade, there remains a critical need to implement the most effective, evidence-based self-management strategies in order to improve outcomes of this disease. Based on the results of the review in this chapter by Velsor-Friedrich, clinicians should be teaching children early in their disease process to:

- Use a peak flow meter.
- Monitor their skill on a regular basis.
- Become more self-aware of their symptoms and associated outcomes.

This can be especially challenging with low-income, low-literacy children and families, especially those living in less structured environments (Slutsky & Bryant-Stephens, 2001). Yet it is these children who are most at risk for hospitalization and death.

The Influence of Family on the Health of Adolescents with Type 1 Diabetes
Robin Whittemore and Margaret Gray

In the final review entitled "The Influence of Family on Physiological and Psychosocial Health in Youth with Type 1 Diabetes," Whittemore and Gray emphasize the family demands associated with having a child with type 1 diabetes. The purpose of their synthesis is to summarize the empirical research regarding the relationships among family functioning, adherence to diabetes self-management, metabolic control, and psychosocial adjustment of youth with type 1 diabetes. Findings of this synthesis indicate that the structure and functioning of families have a critical influence on adherence to the diabetes regimen, metabolic control, and psychosocial adjustment of youth with type 1 diabetes. Implications for clinical practice are highlighted, including the need for ongoing assessment of the changing structure and functioning of families who have a child with type 1 diabetes.

Evidence to Guide Clinical Practice in Psychiatric Mental Health

Mental health and mental illness are often conceptualized as "points on a continuum" (U.S. Department of Health and Human Services [U.S. DHHS], 1999a, p. 4). At one end of the continuum is mental health, a difficult concept to define and measure because individual interpretations vary among persons (U.S. DHHS, 1999a). Moreover, although there are numerous identifiable characteristics frequently ascribed to mental health, not all of them are uniformly present in healthy individuals. Mental health can be described as a dynamic state of cognitive, affective, and behavioral equilibrium associated with successful growth and development, effective coping and adaptation, and an ability to relate to others and contribute to society (U.S. DHHS, 1999a). These qualities are generally consistent with a productive and satisfying life.

At the other end of the continuum is mental illness, the subject of Chapter 23. Mental illness is a collective term used to describe all mental disorders that are diagnosable (U.S. DHHS, 1999a). In a given year, approximately 44.3 million Americans ages 18 and older have a diagnosable mental disorder (NIMH, 2001b). One of four children and adolescents (i.e., 15 million) also have a mental health disorder severe enough to interfere with their functioning at home or at school (Melnyk et al., 2003). Mental disorders are diagnosed using the criteria outlined in the *Diagnostic and Statistical Manual of Mental Disorders* (DSM-IV-TR; American Psychiatric Association [APA], 2000). These disorders cause disturbances in thought, mood, or behavior and may include schizophrenia, major depression, bipolar disorder, and various anxiety, eating, or addictive disorders. Many individuals have more than one disorder at a time. All racial, ethnic, socioeconomic, and age groups are affected.

Although many forms of mental illness are pervasive and long-standing, effective treatments have been developed and are well documented. Patricia Wilke, a doctoral student at Kent State University, recruited six experts to write reviews of the best and latest scientific evidence that will answer the most pressing clinical questions in the psych-mental health field.

Postdisaster Disorders
Rene Love

The first section of the Psychiatric Mental Health chapter describes the current research on the psychological sequelae of disasters. This topic is significant and timely because many healthcare providers, including nurses, may be the first responders to these events. In fact, healthcare providers in all clinical areas will likely treat patients who exhibit symptoms of disaster-related stress in their practices and will need to provide the appropriate physical and psychological care. In addition, persons who have survived a disaster may be at an increased risk for the development of long-term illnesses.

According to Love, there has been a heightened interest in the psychological sequelae of disasters since the tragedy of September 11, 2001 by individual healthcare providers and by communities at large. Prior to the Oklahoma bombing of 1993, research had primarily focused on the effects of natural disasters.

In this section, Love reviews the literature on two disasters of mass destruction, a natural disaster, and several mass shooting incidents. Seven studies with adults and seven with children are included. The postdisaster studies reviewed are generally descriptive in nature and identify persons most at risk for the development of posttraumatic symptoms. Various psychometric rating scales and personal interviews were used to determine outcomes. The findings from the research reviewed suggest that most adults and children exhibit some form of physiological, psychological, or behavioral symptoms after experiencing traumatic events. Several studies with adults associated female gender, ethnicity, and a preexisting mental disorder with higher levels of posttraumatic stress. Similarly, bereavement, female gender, ethnicity, and a history of predisaster anxiety increase the likelihood of posttraumatic symptom development in children. Furthermore, stress reaction was positively associated with the amount of disaster coverage viewed on television (i.e., the more television coverage viewed, the greater the stress reaction).

Because the postdisaster studies reviewed focus on the identification of persons most at risk for symptom development, there seems to be a need for further research on interventions that will enhance coping and adaptation after surviving a traumatic event. Advanced practice clinical researchers are in an excellent position to address this need through implementation and evaluation of methods designed to reduce the symptoms of posttraumatic stress.

Postpartum Depression
Doris Noel Ugarriza

In the second paper, Ugarriza reviews four studies on postpartum depression. Postpartum depression is frequently unrecognized and, therefore, untreated. Thus, there is an urgent need for healthcare providers to diagnose and treat this disorder to prevent the tragic consequences that often ensue. According to the author, the "psychosocial sequelae" of postpartum depression may affect the family and the community, as well.

The first study reviewed in this paper is a qualitative study based on the explanatory model of illness (Kleinman, 1980). Thirty women with postpartum depression were interviewed and asked about the cause, symptoms, and management of their illness. The purpose of the study was to compare the participants' explanatory model of postpartum depression with the biomedical model, based on the DSM-IV (APA, 1994) criteria. The findings of the content analysis indicated that the participants' explanatory model of postpartum depression was not consistent with the DSM-IV (APA, 1994) criteria; in general, the participants described milder symptoms and experienced sleep deprivation rather than sleep disorders. Hence, many postpartum depressed women may experience and report symptoms differently than those listed in the DSM-IV (APA, 1994). Healthcare providers should therefore be apprised that depressed postpartum women might not always report the expected symptoms.

The second study reviewed by Ugarriza was conducted to validate the Postpartum Depression Screening Scale (PDSS; Beck & Gable, 2001). Conventional instruments used to screen for depression are generally not appropriate for use with this population because of their inability to detect the symptoms specific to postpartum depression. To address this problem, Beck and Gable (2000, 2001) created the PDSS. A sample of 150 postpartum women completed the brief 35-item self-report instrument in order to determine which women were most at risk for postpartum depression. Content validity was assessed by a panel of five experts and a focus group of 15 nurses. The study validates the PDDS (Beck & Gable, 2000, 2001) for use with postpartum women, with internal consistency reliabilities ranging from 0.83 to 0.94.

Another study reviewed by Ugarriza examined the effect of interpersonal psychotherapy on a sample of 120 postpartum depressed women. Women were randomly selected for an interpersonal therapy group or a control group. The results indicated that the postpartum depressed women in the therapy group experienced a significant decrease in depressive symptoms when compared with the postpartum depressed women in the control group. This intervention may be especially useful for women who are reluctant to use medication to treat their postpartum depression.

Finally, a study on the effectiveness of fluoxetine and cognitive behavioral counseling was reviewed. Eighty-seven postpartum depressed women were randomly assigned to one of four cells, fluoxetine or placebo, and one or six sessions of counseling. The trial lasted 12 weeks; data were collected at 1, 4, and 12 weeks. The findings indicated that after 4 weeks, all four groups had improved. Specifically, (a) the fluoxetine group had greater improvement than the placebo group; (b) improvement was greater after six counseling sessions than after one; and (c) the interaction between counseling and fluoxetine was not significant. In other words, fluoxetine and counseling were effective in treating nonpsychotic postpartum depression, but there was no advantage to using both management strategies.

Continued inquiry to determine effective methods of assessment and intervention for postpartum depression is recommended. It may be beneficial to replicate the qualitative study included in this review with a more diverse sample in an effort to determine whether the "accepted" symptom pattern for postpartum depression should be altered. If the study can be replicated, a reevaluation of assessment tools and diagnostic criteria would be in order.

Late-Life Depression
Jacqueline A. Zauszniewski

In the third section, Zauszniewski describes the evidenced-based interventions for late-life depression. Although roughly 2 million Americans ages 65 or older experience late-life depression in a given year (NIMH, 2001a), this illness often goes unrecognized and untreated. For this reason, late-life depression, like postpartum depression, poses a significant public health risk.

Zauszniewski surveyed the current literature on late-life depression and identified a variety of commonly used evidenced-based treatments. In addition to antidepressant medications, electroconvulsive therapy (ECT) and psychosocial interventions have often yielded good results. However, a review of 60 studies indicated that antidepressants and ECT are the most effective treatments for late-life depression.

A majority of clinical trials have investigated tricyclic antidepressants (TCAs) and selective serotonin reuptake inhibitors (SSRIs). Nortriptyline and desipramine, both TCAs, have been widely studied. Although these drugs cause few anticholinergic and sedative effects, they can cause cardiac conduction problems and may not be the drugs of choice for the elderly. Zauszniewski reviews the results of trials that have demonstrated the efficacy of various SSRIs, including fluoxetine, fluvoxamine, sertraline, paroxetine, and citalopram, for decreasing the symptoms associated with depression. These medications produce fewer cardiac effects but may cause interactions with other medications. Recently, trials on four newer classifications of antidepressants have been undertaken:

1. Norepinephrine antagonists and serotonin antagonists (NASAs)
2. Serotonin norepinephrine reuptake inhibitors (SNRIs)
3. Norepinephrine dopamine reuptake inhibitors (DNRIs)
4. Specific noradrenalin reuptake inhibitors (NARIs)

The author reports that mirtazapine, a NASA, seems promising for use with the elderly because it produces a faster treatment response and fewer side effects than do SSRIs.

When antidepressant medications are ineffective or poorly tolerated, ECT is a useful treatment alternative. ECT also may be used in conjunction with antidepressant therapy. According to the review by Zauszniewski, ECT may be an excellent choice for elders who are suicidal, because it produces a rapid response with few medical complications.

Another mode of evidenced-based treatment for late-life depression is psychosocial intervention. Studies comparing psychodynamic psychotherapy with other forms of psychotherapy in the treatment of depression have found little difference in outcomes. Although cognitive-behavioral and reminiscence psychotherapies have been studied with mixed results, there is some evidence that supportive psychotherapy is effective and much evidence that interpersonal psychotherapy is effective for treating depressed elders. Treatment with a combination of interpersonal psychotherapy and antidepressant medications was found to be more effective than either treatment alone for recurrent depression. However, inconsistent results were noted with the use of cognitive-behavioral therapy and antidepressants.

Continued research to develop more effective means of assessing the elderly for late-life depression is critical. Recognition and diagnosis of this disorder frequently presents a challenge to healthcare providers because the symptoms of late-life depression may be manifested differently and may be compounded by coexisting cognitive and medical conditions. Failure to recognize late-life depression, however, can lead to premature death, because 20 % of all suicides in this country occur in persons ages 65 and older (U.S. DHHS, 1999b).

Chronic Mental Illness
Alice R. Kempe

In the fourth paper, Kempe surveys the research that supports collaboration among patients, families, and healthcare providers in the treatment of persons with chronic mental illness. Chronic mental illness, also known as severe mental illness, affects more than 5 million adults and 7 million children in the United States each year (National Alliance for the Mentally Ill, 1999). Because of the limited community resources available, families are often forced to assume a caregiving role for their family members with mental disorders. Thus, successful treatment outcomes cannot be accomplished unless the patient, the family, and the healthcare team work together to achieve the same goals.

The literature reviewed by Kempe suggests that advanced practice psychiatric mental health providers must be committed, caring, knowledgeable, and able to communicate effectively and advocate for the chronically mentally ill and their families. Further, expertise in navigation through the healthcare delivery system is essential to address issues of managed care and reimbursement. There is growing evidence that advanced practice nurses (APNs) with prescriptive authority provide cost-effective, quality care. In fact, when Kempe reviewed a large study of 223 patients in an outpatient clinical setting, the results indicated that advanced practice psychiatric nurses (APPNs) provided more cost-effective care with equal or better patient outcomes than either physicians or psychologists.

Research evaluating methods of rehabilitation with this population indicate that multiple strategies work best, including social and cognitive skills training, family education, behavioral interventions, vocational rehabilitation, counseling, and case management. Kempe reviewed two other studies on the effects of case management; one study reported an increase in patient treatment compliance, and another found an increase in patient hospitalization rates.

Suggestions for further inquiry include the following:

1. Investigation of a patient-family-APPN "team" approach in the care and treatment of chronic mental illness
2. Further development of EBP guidelines
3. Continued research validating the cost-effectiveness and expertise of APPNs

Psychotic Disorders
Sarah F. Farrell and Irma H. Mahone

Farrell and Mahone highlight the evidenced-based interventions for psychotic disorders in the fifth section. Psychotic disorders are a group of disorders that are considered to be the most serious and persistent of all the mental disorders. According to the DSM-IV-TR (APA, 2000), the most prevalent of these are the schizophrenias: schizophrenia, schizophreniform, and schizoaffective disorder. Because of their severe and enduring nature, these disorders were included in this chapter. The authors propose that when EBP is used, including psychopharmacological and psychosocial interventions, persons with psychotic disorders have a greater chance for improvement.

According to Farrell and Mahone, there is a great deal of evidence to suggest that the newer atypical antipsychotics (AAPs) are superior in treating both the positive and the negative symptoms of schizophrenia with minimal extrapyramidal side effects, when compared with the older drugs. Furthermore, one study reviewed in this paper concluded that adherence was improved with the use of AAPs. Commonly prescribed AAPs include clozapine, risperidone, olanzapine, quetiapine, and ziprasidone. Though clozapine is the most efficacious for reducing negative symptoms and is the drug of choice for nonresponders, it has a potentially fatal side effect of agranulocytosis, thus necessitating frequent blood tests.

Research on the psychosocial management of psychotic disorders has investigated various methods of teaching illness self-management, including social skills training (SST), psychoeducation, assertive community treatment (ACT), supported employment, and integrated substance abuse treatment. Positive outcomes have been documented with all of these interventions. The research studies surveyed in this section offer compelling evidence for the following:

- SST promotes the development of social and independent living skills.
- Family psychoeducation reduces the rate of recidivism.
- ACT promotes symptom stability and quality of life.
- Supported employment provides job placement.
- Integrated substance abuse treatment improves housing outcomes.

Continued investigation of psychopharmacological and psychosocial interventions is necessary to improve the quality of life for persons with psychotic disorders. Studies that validate the effectiveness of community-based treatment centers in reducing the rates of recidivism and improving the quality of life for these individuals are suggested.

Cognitive-Behavioral Therapy for Schizophrenia
Wanda K. Mohr

In the final section of this chapter by Mohr, the evidence-based research that supports the efficacy of cognitive-behavioral therapy (CBT) for persons with schizophrenia is reviewed. Schizophrenia, a psychotic disorder, is a debilitating psychiatric illness. It is chronic in nature and characterized by the presence of hallucinations, delusions, disorganized speech and behavior patterns, avolition, alogia, and emotional flattening (APA, 2000). In this section, Mohr examines three studies that implement the use of CBT with persons who have schizophrenia.

The first study reviewed in this section was conducted over 4 years with a sample of 40 persons with schizophrenia or a related psychotic disorder and refractory hallucinations. Participants received CBT and coping training and were tested at 2 and 4 years. The results indicated that a majority of participants reported fewer hallucinations and cognitive problems and enjoyed an improved quality of life.

The second study described by Mohr, a randomized controlled trial, compared the efficacy of CBT with a nonspecific supportive intervention. The sample consisted of 90 treatment-compliant persons with schizophrenia who received a mean of 19 individual treatment sessions over 9 months. The sessions lasted 45 minutes for the first 2 months, then declined in frequency. They were evaluated at baseline, after treatment, and again at a 9-month follow-up. The results revealed that both groups experienced a significant reduction in positive, negative, and depressive symptoms. However, at the 9-month follow-up, only the CBT group continued to improve.

The last study Mohr reviewed compared CBT and supportive counseling. A sample of 79 treatment-compliant persons with chronic schizophrenia was divided into three groups. The first group received CBT and routine care, the second group received supportive counseling and routine psychiatric care, and the control group received only routine care. At the end of 10 weeks, the CBT group showed a significant improvement in positive symptoms; the supportive therapy group showed a nonsignificant improvement.

The results of these three studies suggest that for some persons, CBT may be an effective adjunct to conventional treatment for the positive symptoms associated with schizophrenia. For this reason, continued investigation with CBT is suggested. In addition, research to discover interventions that can improve the negative symptoms of schizophrenia is warranted.

references

Administration on Aging. (2002). *A profile of older Americans: 2002.* Washington, D.C.: U.S. Department of Health and Human Services.

Alexander, J. W. (1993). Immunoenhancement via enteral nutrition. *Archives of Surgery,* 128, 1242–1245.

American Association of Critical Care Nurses. (2003). AACN Research priority areas. Available at https://www.aacn.org/AACN/research.nsf/. Aliso Viejo, CA: AACN. Accessed September 6, 2003.

American Cancer Society. (2002). *Cancer facts and figures.* Atlanta, GA: American Cancer Society.

American Psychiatric Association (APA, 1994). *Diagnostic and Statistical Manual of Mental Disorders* (4th ed.). Washington DC: APA.

APA. (2000). *Diagnostic and Statistical Manual of Mental Disorders* (text revision). Washington DC: APA.

American Stroke Association. (2001). *Acute stroke treatment guide.* Dallas, TX: American Heart Association/American Stroke Association.

Babineau, T. J., & Blackburn, G. L. (1994) Time to

consider gut feeding. *Critical Care Medicine,* 22, 191–193.

Baron, R. B. (2000). Nutrition. In L. M. Tierney, S. J. McPhee, & M. A. Papadakis (Eds.). *Current Medical Diagnosis & Treatment.* New York: Lange Medical Books.

Barry, M. J. (2001). Prostate-specific antigen testing for early diagnosis of prostate cancer. *New England Journal of Medicine, 344,* 1373–1377.

Beck, C., & Gable, R. (2000). Postpartum depression screening scale: Development and psychometric testing. *Nursing Research, 49,* 272–282.

Beck, C., & Gable, R. (2001). Further validation of the postpartum depression screening scale. *Nursing Research, 50,* 155–164.

Berger, P. B., Bell, M. R., Holmes, D. R., Gersh, B. J., Hopfenspirger, M., & Gibbons, R. (1994). Time to reperfusion with direct coronary angioplasty and thrombolytic therapy in acute myocardial infarction. *American Journal of Cardiology, 73,* 231–236.

Braga, M., Gianotti, L., Cesart, A., Vignallli, A., Pellegatta, F., et al. (1996). Gut function and immune and inflammatory response in patients perioperatively fed with supplemented enteral formulas. *Archives of Surgery, 131*, 1257–1265.

Broome, M., & Huth, M. (2003) Nursing management of the child in pain. In N. Schechter, C. Berde, & M. Yaster (Eds.). *Pain in infants, children and adolescents* (2nd ed., pp. 417–433.). Philadelphia: Lippincott, Williams and Wilkins.

Cabana, M. D., Rand, C. S., Powe, N. R., et al. (1999). Why don't physicians follow clinical practice guidelines? A framework for improvement. *JAMA, 282*, 1458–1465.

Carmina, E., Koyama, T., Chang, L., Stancyzk, F. Z., & Lobo, R. A. (1992). Does ethnicity influence the prevalence of adrenal hyperandrogenism and insulin resistance in polycystic ovary syndrome? *American Journal of Obstetrics and Gynecology, 167*, 1807–1812.

Centers for Disease Control and Prevention (CDC). (1999a) *Asthma: A public health response.* Available at www.cdc.gov.nceh.

CDC. (1999b). Cigarette smoking-attributable mortality and years of potential life lost-United States. *Morbidity and Mortality Weekly Report, 42:*, 645–649.

CDC. (2000). HIV/AIDS surveillance in adolescents L265 slide series (through 2000). Available at http://www.cdc.gov/hiv/graphics/adolesnt.htm.

CDC. (2001). Cigarette smoking among adults—United States, 1999. *Morbidity and Mortality Weekly Report, 50*, 869–873.

CDC. (2002). *2002 Draft guidelines for prevention of hospital-associated pneumonia.* Developed by the CDC's Healthcare Infection Control Practices Advisory Committee (HICPAC). Available at http://www.cdc.gov/ncidod/hip/pneumonia/pneu_mmw.htm#top.

Clark, A. P., Winslow, E. H., Tyler, D. O., & White, K. M. (1990). Effects of endotracheal suctioning on mixed venous oxygen saturation and heart rate in critically ill adults. *Heart & Lung, 19*, 552–557.

Clyburn, L., Stone, M. J., Hadjistavroupoulos, T., & Tuikko, H. (2000). Predicting caregiver burden and depression in Alzheimer's disease. *Journal of Gerontology, 55B*(1), S2–S13.

Cornman-Levy, D., Gitlin, L., Corcoran, M. A., & Schinfeld, S. (2001). Caregiver aches and pains: The role of physical therapy in helping families provide daily care. *Alzheimer's Care Quarterly, 2*(1), 47–55.

Crookes, P. A., & Davies S. (Eds.) (1998). *Research into practice: Essential skills for reading and applying research in nursing and healthcare.* Edinburgh: Baillere Tindall.

Cummins, R. (Ed.). (2001). *ACLS Provider Manual.* Dallas, TX: American Heart Association.

Daley, J., Elliott D., & Chang, E. (2000). Research in nursing: Concepts and processes. In J. Daley, S. Speedy, & D. Jackson (Eds.), *Contexts of nursing, an introduction.* (pp. 89–106) Eastgardens, New South Wales: MacLennan & Petty Pty Limited.

Dracup, K., & Moser, D. K. (1997). Beyond sociodemographics: Factors influencing the decision to seek treatment for symptoms of acute myocardial infarction. *Heart and Lung, 26*, 253–262.

Dunaif, A. (1995). Hyperandrogenic anovulation (PCOS): A unique disorder of insulin action associated with an increased risk of non–insulin-dependent diabetes mellitus. *American Journal of Medicine*, 98, 335–395.

Esteban, A., Anzueto, A., Alia, I., Gordo, F., Apezteguia, C., Palizas, F., et al. (2000). How is mechanical ventilation employed in the intensive care unit? An International Utilization Review. *American Journal of Respiratory and Critical Care Medicine, 161*, 1450–1458.

Fact sheet: *The common cold.* (2001). Available at www.nih.gov/factsheets/cold.htm. Retrieved March 2003.

Fast Stats: *The common cold.* (1996). *Vital Health and Statistics 10* (200). Available at www.cdc.gov/nchs/faststats/colds.htm. Retrieved March 2003.

Ferry, L. H., Grissino, L. M., & Runfola, P. S. (1999). Tobacco dependence curricula in U.S. undergraduate medical education. *JAMA, 290*, 825–829.

Fiore, M. C., Epps, R. P., & Manley, M. W. (1994). A missed opportunity: Teaching medical students to help their patients successfully quit smoking. *JAMA, 271*, 624–626.

Gawlinski, A. (1993). Effects of positioning on mixed venous oxygen saturation. *Journal of Cardiovascular Nursing, 7*, 71–81.

Gawlinski, A., & Dracup, K. (1998). Effect of positioning on SVO_2 in the critically ill patient with a low ejection fraction. *Nursing Research, 47*, 293–299.

GISSI Trial (Gruppo Italiano per lo Studio della Stretochinasi nell'Infarto Miocardico) (1986). Effectiveness of intravenous thrombolytic treatment in acute myocardial infarction. *Lancet, 8478,* 397–401.

Godfrey, J. C., Godfrey, N. J., & Novick, S. G. (1996). Zinc for treating the common cold: Review of all clinical trials since 1984. *Alternative Therapies in Health & Medicine, 2*(6), 63–73.

Goldman, L., & Bennett, J. C. (2000). *Cecil textbook of medicine* (21st ed.). Philadelphia: W.B. Saunders.

Hanneman S. K., Ingersoll, G., Knebel A., Shekleton, M., Burns, S., & Clochesy, J. (1994). Weaning from short-term mechanical ventilation: A review. *American Journal of Critical Care, 3,* 421–443.

Hayman, L, Mahon, M., & Turner, R. (2002). *Chronic illness in children: An evidence-based approach.* Springer Publishing.

Heath, J., Andrews, A., Thomas, S. A., Kelley, F .J., & Friedman, E. (2002). Tobacco dependence curriculum in acute care nurse practitioner education. *American Journal of Critical Care, 11,* 27–32.

Hessel, S. J., Adams, D. F., & Abrams, H. L. (1981) Complications of angiography. *Radiology, 138,* 273–281.

Jaen, C. R., Crabtree, B. F., Zyzanski, S. J., et al. (1998). Making time for tobacco cessation counseling. *Journal of Family Practice, 46,* 425–428.

Jemal, A., Murray, T., Samuels, A., et al. (2003). Cancer statistics, 2003. *CA A Cancer Journal for Clinicians, 53*(1), 5–26.

Jesurum, J. (1997). Tissue oxygenation and routine nursing procedures in critically ill patients. *Journal of Cardiovascular Nursing, 11,* 12–30.

Joint Commission on Accreditation of Healthcare Organizations (JCAHO). (2003). ICU core measures. Available at http://www.jcaho.org. Accessed September 6, 2003. Oakbrook Terrace, IL: JCAHO.

Kinloch, D. (1999). Instillation of normal saline during endotracheal suctioning: Effects on mixed venous oxygen saturation. *American Journal of Critical Care, 8*(4), 231–240.

Kleinman, A. (1980). *Patients and healers in the context of culture.* Berkeley, CA: University of California Press.

Knebel, A., Shekleton, M., Burns, S., Clochesy, J., Hanneman, S. K., & Ingersoll, G. (1994). Weaning from mechanical ventilation: Concept development. *American Journal of Critical Care, 3,* 416–420.

Knebel, A., Shekleton, M., Burns, S., Clochesy, J.,

& Hanneman, S. K. (1998). Weaning from mechanical ventilatory support: refinement of a model. *American Journal of Critical Care, 7*(2), 149–52.

Kordella, T. (2002). A tale of two conditions. *Diabetes Forecast, 55*(6), 107–110.

Kozier, B., & Erb, G. (1983). *Fundamentals of nursing* (2nd ed.). Reading, MA: Addison-Wesley.

Langlois, J. A., Kegler S. R., Butler, J. A., Gotsch E. E., Johnson, R. L., Reichard A. A., et al. (2003). Traumatic brain injury-related hospital discharges. Results from a 14-state surveillance system, 1997. *Morbidity and Mortality Weekly Report—Surveillance Summary, 52*(4), 1–20.

Lenfant, C. (2001). Physicians need practical tools to treat the complex problems of overweight and obesity. *American Family Physician, 63,* 2139, 2145.

Luckmann, J., & Sorensen, K. C. (1987). *Medical-surgical nursing: A psychophysiologic approach* (3rd ed.). Philadelphia: W.B. Saunders.

Manente, G., Torrieri, F., & Di Blasio, F. (2001). An innovative hand brace for carpal tunnel syndrome: A randomized controlled trial. *Muscle and Nerve, 24,* 1020–1025.

Mazzonrana, V., Smith, R., Reilly, P., & Brar, H. (1994). Limited utility of emergency department thoracotomy. *American Surgeon. 60,* 516–521.

McBride, P., Plane, M., Underbakke, G., Brown, R., & Solberg, L. (1997). Smoking screening and management in primary care practices. *Archive of Family Medicine, 6,* 165–172.

Messina, L. M., Brother, T. E., Wakefield, T. W., Zelenock, G. B., Lindenauer, M., Greenfield, L. J., et al. (1991). Clinical characteristics and surgical management of vascular complications in patients undergoing cardiac catheterization: Interventional versus diagnostic procedures. *Journal of Vascular Surgery, 13,* 593–600.

Melnyk, B. M., Alpert-Gillis, L., Feinstein, N. F., Fairbanks, E., Schultz-Czarniak, J., Hust, D., et al. (2001). Improving cognitive development of LBW premature infants with the COPE program: A pilot study of the benefit of early NICU intervention with mothers. *Research in Nursing and Health, 24,* 373–389.

Melnyk, B. M., Brown, H., Jones, D. Kreipe, R., & Novak, J. (2003). Improving the mental/psychosocial health of U.S. children and adolescents: Outcomes and implementation strategies from the National KySS Summit (Supplement). *Journal of Pediatric Healthcare, 17* (6), S1–S24.

Melnyk, B. M., Feinstein, N. F., Tuttle, J., Moldenhauer, Z., Herendeen, P., Veenema, et al. (2002). Mental health worries, communication, and needs of children, teens, and parents during the year of the nation's terrorist attack: Findings from the national KySS survey. *Journal of Pediatric Healthcare, 16,* 222–234.

Melnyk, B. M., Moldenhauer, Z., Tuttle, J., Veenema, T. G., Jones, D., & Novak, J. (2003). Improving child and adolescent mental health. An evidence-based approach. *Advance for Nurse Practitioners, 11*(2), 47–52.

Melnyk, B. M., Moldenhauer, Z., Veenema, T., McMurtrie, M., Gullo, S., O-Leary, E., et al. (2001). The KySS (keep your children/yourself safe and secure) campaign: A national effort to decrease psychosocial morbidities in children and adolescents. *Journal of Pediatric Healthcare, 15*(2), 31A–34A.

Moody, H. R. (2002). *Aging concepts and controversies.* Thousand Oaks, CA: Sage.

Moore, F. A., Feliciano, D. V., Andrassy, R. J., et. al. (1992). Early enteral feeding, compared with parenteral, reduces postoperative septic complications. *Annuals of Surgery, 216,* 172–183.

Morello, C., Leckband, S., Stoner, C. P., Moorhouse, D. F., & Sahagian, G. A. (1999). Randomized double-blind study comparing the efficacy of gabapentin with amitriptyline on diabetic peripheral neuropathy pain. *Archives of Internal Medicine, 159,* 1931–1937.

National Diabetic Fact Sheet (2003). Available at http://www.diabetes.org/main/inofo/facts/facts_natl.jsp. Retrieved February 7, 2003.

National Institute of Mental Health (NIMH). (2001a). *Older adults: Depression and suicide facts.* (NIMH Pub. No. 01-4593). Available at http://www.nimh.nih.gov/publicat/elderlydepsuicide.cfm. Retrieved March 8, 2003.

NIMH. (2001b). *The numbers count. Mental disorders in America.* (NIMH Pub. No. 01-4584). Available at http://www.nimh.nih.gov/publicat/numbers.cfm. Retrieved March 8, 2003.

National Quality Forum. (2003). Safe practices for better healthcare: A consensus report. Washington, D.C.: National Quality Forum.

O'Connor, D., Marshall, S., & Massey-Westrop, N. (2003). Non-surgical treatment (other than steroid injection) for carpal tunnel syndrome (Cochrane Review). *The Cochrane Library, Issue 1.*

Pipkin, W., Brophy, C., Nesbit, R., & Mondy, J. (2000). Early experience with infectious complication of percutaneous femoral artery closure devices. *Journal of Vascular Surgery, 32,* 205–208.

Potter, P. A., & Perry, A. G. (2001). *Fundamentals of nursing.* St. Louis, MO: Mosby.

REACT Study Group (2000). Effect of a community intervention on patient delay and emergency medical service use in acute coronary heart disease (REACT Trial). *Journal of American Medical Association, 284,* 60–67.

Ries, L., Eisner, M., Kosary, C., et al. (2000). *SEER cancer statistics review, 1973–1997.* Bethesda, MD: National Cancer Institute.

Ryan, T. J., Antman, E. M., Brooks, N. H., Califf, R. M., Hillis, L. D., & Hiratzka (1999). ACC/AHA Guidelines for the management of patients with acute myocardial infarction: 1999 update: A report of the American College of Cardiology/American Heart Association Task Group on Practice Guidelines (Committee on Management of Acute Myocardial Infarction). Available at http://www.acc.org/clinical/guidelines and http://www.americanheart.org. Accessed on February 17, 2003.

Salasidis, R., Fleiszer, T., & Johnston, R. (1998). Air insufflation technique of enteral tube insertion: A randomized, controlled trial. *Critical Care Medicine, 26,* 1036–1039.

Sarna, L., Brown, J., Lillington, L., Rose, M., Wewers, M., & Brecht, M. (2000). Tobacco-control attitudes, advocacy, and smoking behaviors of oncology nurses. *Oncology Nursing Forum, 27,* 1519–1528.

Schappert, S. M. (1998). Ambulatory care visits to physician offices, hospital outpatient departments and emergency room departments: United States, 1996. *Vital Health Statistics 13*(143), 12.

Schmitz, K., & Jeffery, R. (2000). Public health interventions for the prevention and treatment of obesity. *Medical Clinics of North America, 84,* 491–512.

Schulz, R., & Beach, S. R. (1999). Caregiving as a risk factor for mortality: The caregiver health effects study. *Journal of the American Medical Association, 282,* 2215–2219.

Schulz, M. A., Santanello, S. A., Monk, J., & Falcone, R. E. (1993). An improved method for transpyloric placement of nasoenteric feeding tubes. *International Surgery, 78–82.*

Schweiss, J. F. (1987). Mixed venous hemoglobin saturation: Theory and application. In K. Tremper, & S. Barker (Eds.). *Advances in oxygen monitoring* (pp. 113–136). New York: Anesthesia Clinics.

Secker-Walker, R., Chir, B., Solomon, L., et al. (1994). Comparisons of the smoking cessation counseling activities of six types of health professionals. *Preventive Medicine, 23*, 800–808.

Semler, H. J. (1985). Transfemoral catheterization: Mechanical versus manual control of bleeding. *Radiology, 154*, 234–235.

Slesinski, M. J., Subar, A. F., & Kahle, I. L. (1995). Trends I use of vitamin and mineral supplements in the United States: The 1987 and 1992 National Health Interview Surveys. *Journal of the American Dietetic Association, 95*, 921–923.

Slutsky, P., & Bryant-Stephens, T. (2001). Developing a comprehensive, community-based asthma education and training program. *Pediatric Nursing, 27*, 449–457.

Solberg, L. I, Kottke, T., Conn, S., Brekle, M., Calomeni, C., & Conboy, K. (1997). Delivering clinical preventive services is a systems problem. *Annuals of Behavioral Medicine, 19*, 271–278.

Sprangler, J., George, G., Foley, K., & Crandall, S. (2002). Tobacco intervention training: Current efforts and gaps in U.S. medical schools. *JAMA, 288*, 1102–1109.

Stone, R. I. (2000). *Long-term care for the elderly with disabilities: Current policy, emerging trends, and implications for the twenty-first century.* New York: Milbank Memorial Fund.

Thorndike, A., Rigotti, N., Stafford, R., & Singer, D. (1998). National patterns in the treatment of smokers by physicians. *JAMA, 279*, 604–608.

Tidwell, S. L., Ryan, W. J., Osguthorpe, S. G., Paull, D. L., & Smith, T. L. (1990). Effects of position changes on mixed venous oxygen saturation in patients after coronary revascularization. *Heart & Lung, 19*, 574–577.

Tilkian, A., & Daily, E. (1986). *Cardiovascular procedures: Diagnostic techniques and therapeutic procedures.* St. Louis: Mosby.

U. S. Department of Health & Human Services (U.S. DHHS). (1999a). *Mental health: A report of the surgeon general.* Rockville, MD: SAMHSA, CMHS, NIH, and NIMH.

U.S. DHHS (1999b). *The surgeon general's call to action to prevent suicide, 1999. At a glance: Suicide among the elderly.* Retrieved February 24, 2003 from http://surgeongeneral.gov/library/calltoaction/fact2.htm.

U.S. DHHS (2001). *Healthy People 2010.* Retrieved from http://www.healthypeople.gov.

Verderber, A., & Gallagher, K. (1994). Effects of bathing, passive range-of-motion exercises, and turning on oxygen consumption in healthy men and women. *American Journal of Critical Care, 3*(5), 374–381.

Voss, J. D., & Schectman, J. M. (2001). Prostate cancer screening practices and beliefs. *Journal of General Internal Medicine, 16*, 831–837.

Walsh, J. M., Vanderwarf, C., Hoscheit, D., & Fahey, P. J. (1989). Unsuspected hemodynamic alterations during endotracheal suctioning. *Chest, 95*(1), 162–165.

Weitzman, M. (2003). Who is and who isn't providing mental health services for our nation's children (featured presentation). Rochester, NY: the National KySS Summit.

Weissman, C., & Kemper, M. (1991). The oxygen uptake-oxygen delivery relationship during ICU interventions. *Chest, 99*, 430–435.

White, K. M., Winslow, E. H., Clark, A. P., & Tyler, D. O. (1990). The physiologic basis for continuous mixed venous oxygen saturation monitoring. *Heart & Lung, 19*(5), 548–551.

Zaloga, G. P., & Roberts, P. A. (1998). Bedside placement of enteral feeding tubes in the intensive care unit. *Critical Care Medicine, 26*, 987–988.

Zimmerman, J. J. (1998). The pediatric critical care patient. In B. P. Furhman, & J. J. Zimmerman (Eds.). *Pediatric critical care* (2nd edition). New York: Mosby.

Case Examples: Evidence-Based Care and Outcomes in Adult Depression and in Critically Ill Children

appendix A

Case Example A-1: Evidence-Based Care and Outcomes in Adult Depression

An evidence-based approach to changing treatment modality for depressed adults in an in-patient psychiatric unit

As a new psychiatric/mental healthcare provider on an adult in-patient unit, you observe that various therapists are using different treatment modalities (e.g., group cognitive-behavior therapy; individual cognitive-behavior therapy; relaxation therapy; interpersonal therapy) with depressed patients. When asked about the different treatment modalities, the unit director tells you that therapists should employ the treatments they have found to work the best from their own clinical experiences. However, the director is open to further discussion and learning about the empirical effectiveness of different treatment modalities for adults with depressive disorders. Therefore, you volunteer to search the literature to answer the following clinical questions: (1) How effective is group cognitive-behavioral therapy (CBT) in comparison to individual CBT in the treatment of adult depression? and (2) How effective is CBT in comparison to relaxation therapy and interpersonal therapy in the treatment of adult depression?

A search for systematic reviews of randomized controlled trials, the strongest level of evidence upon which to base practice changes, is first undertaken in the Cochrane Database of Systematic Reviews. The key words searched include group therapy, adults, depression, and cognitive-behavior therapy. Results of this search reveal that there are no systematic reviews in the Cochrane Library published specifically to answer the clinical questions. A search for evidence-based clinical guidelines is then performed at the National Guidelines Clearinghouse at www.guideline.gov. A total of 46 guidelines are uncovered when "adult depression" is searched; however, there are no guidelines that contain data regarding effectiveness of group versus individual CBT.

The search continues with MEDLINE and CINAHL using the same key words. The results include one meta-analysis of 13 clinical trials comparing CBT, mainly in group form, with other treatment modalities (e.g., relaxation therapy, interpersonal treatment therapy) and indicate an overall positive effect for CBT with 63% of patients showing clinically significant improvement at the end of treatment compared to approximately a 20% lesser improvement in patients receiving other types of treatments. Critical appraisal of this meta-analysis and five randomized controlled trials lead to the conclusion that CBT therapy is the most effective treatment for depression. Not enough evidence is available to support a definitive conclusion that individual CBT is more effective than group CBT.

This evidence is shared with the unit director. As a result, the unit director decides to implement a practice change on the unit. Therapists are now required to conduct group CBT with the depressed patients instead of using other modes of therapy, unless individual or family factors or preferences warrant another type of treatment. As a result of this practice change, positive outcomes measured and achieved include:

- A shorter length of stay, resulting in reduced costs
- More positive interactions and communication between the patients and the staff
- Higher job satisfaction among the therapists
- More time available for therapists to spend with the most complicated mental health patients

Case Example A-2: Evidence-Based Care and Outcomes in Critically Ill Children

An evidence-based approach to identifying critically ill children at highest risk for negative mental health outcomes.

As a nurse working in a pediatric intensive care unit (PICU) for the past 2 decades, you note that the characteristics of pediatric hospitalization have been drastically changing in recent years. For example, the number of general pediatric beds has been decreasing, but the numbers of pediatric intensive care unit beds are increasing. From reviewing the literature, you also note that critical care hospitalization has the potential for long-lasting negative outcomes on children and their parents, such as posttraumatic stress disorder syndrome as well as negative behavioral, emotional, and academic outcomes as many as 10 years after hospitalization (Haslum, 1988; Melnyk et al., 1997).

Because of higher nursing caseloads in the intensive care unit along with short staffing and less time available to deliver intensive psychosocial interventions to patients and their families, you believe it is critical for you to answer the following clinical question, "What demographic variables and factors during a child's critical care hospitalization predict poor outcomes 6 months after the hospital experience?" You believe that the answer to this question is critical in order to assist healthcare professionals in identifying high-risk children before their discharge from the hospital so that targeted interventions to reduce negative outcomes can be implemented.

Your search for evidence begins with the Cochrane database of systematic reviews and National Guidelines Clearinghouse ™, which reveals no systematic reviews or EBP guidelines published on predictors of outcomes following childhood critical care hospitalization. As a result, you continue your search for individual studies from the past 20 years using Medline, CINAHL, and PsycINFO databases, which reveal eight predictive studies that can assist you in answering your question (Small, 2002). Through your critical appraisal of these studies, you conclude that the following factors have accumulated enough evidence to support them as predictors of negative outcomes in critically ill children:

- Increased parental anxiety and depressive symptoms
- A high number of family life stressors
- Marital stress and divorce
- A less cohesive family environment
- Younger age
- Male gender
- First-time hospital admissions.

After presenting the results of your search and critical appraisal to your nurse manager and medical director as well as to your colleagues, a working group was formed on your unit to develop a risk scale that could be completed by each child's primary nurse within 24 to 48 hours of admission to the PICU. With the assistance of clinical researchers from the affiliated schools of nursing and psychology, the scale was then refined and tested on a full-scale level to determine the range of scores that would predict the poorest posthospital discharge outcomes.

As a result of this EBP initiative, each child in the PICU now receives a risk assessment using a valid and reliable tool. All critically ill children who score in the highest risk category and their families are now provided with an evidence-based educational/behavioral intervention program (*COPE = Creating Opportunities for Parent Empowerment*), which has been shown to result in less externalizing behavior problems (e.g., aggression, acting out) and less attention problems for children and less posttraumatic stress symptoms for parents, up to 1 year following discharge from the hospital (Melnyk et al., 1997; Melnyk et al., 2001). As a result, the number of children and their parents who suffer long-term negative outcomes as a result of critical care hospitalization at your medical center is substantially lower than when there was no risk assessment and intervention program being implemented in your PICU.

References

Haslum, M. N. (1988). Length of preschool hospitalization, multiple admissions and later educational attainment and behavior. *Child: Care, Health and Development, 14,* 275–291.

Melnyk, B. M., Alpert-Gillis, L., Feinstein, N. F., Fairbanks, E., Schultz-Czarniak, J., Hust, D., et al. (2001). Improving cognitive development of LBW premature infants with the COPE program: A pilot study of the benefit of early NICU intervention with mothers. *Research in Nursing and Health, 24,* 373–389.

Melnyk, B.M., Alpert-Gillis, L., Hensel, P. B., Cable-Beiling, R. C., & Rubenstein, J. (1997). Helping mothers cope with a critically ill child: A pilot test of the COPE intervention. *Research in Nursing & Health, 20,* 3–14.

Small, L. (2002). Early predictors of poor coping outcomes in children following intensive care hospitalization and stressful medical encounters. *Pediatric Nursing, 28* (4), 393–398, 401.

Walking the Walk and Talking the Talk: An Appraisal Guide for Qualitative Evidence

appendix B

Care in Different Practice Settings

#1 **Chase-Ziolek, M. & Iris, M. (2002). Nurses' perspectives on the distinctive aspects of providing nursing care in a congregational setting.** *Journal of Community Health Nursing, 19,* 173–186.

Question: What is distinctive about providing nursing care in a congregational setting?

Design: Qualitative descriptive study (conceptualized as naturalistic inquiry) using two research techniques (focus group and individual telephone interviews).

Sample: Parish nurses (N=17) participating in a hospital-sponsored, volunteer health ministry program in a U. S. urban area — All women with an age range of 30 to 72 years (8 Black, 6 White, 3 Asian American). The fifteen congregations active in the program at the time of the study all were represented.

Procedures: Results of a focus group exploring the general topic of what is distinctive about providing nursing care in a congregational setting were used to construct a structured set of open-ended questions to pursue in individual telephone interviews. Questions probed parish nurses' understanding of how their interventions made a difference in clients' lives and their perceptions of unique opportunities and challenges. Content analysis was used to study transcriptions of focus group and telephone interviews. Using a two-step coding process, the researchers first predetermined response categories and linked them to topics addressed in direct questions. Second, key topics and naturally occurring categories were coded as they emerged in the responses. These were organized into higher-level analytical categories along with representative statements. Initial coding, performed by the principal researcher, was reviewed by the second researcher with differences in coding resolved through discussion. (See Chase-Ziolek & Gruca, 2000, for a companion study examining clients' perspectives of parish nursing.)

Appraisal:

- *What were the results of the study?* Nurses' responses were grouped into three key topic areas within which specific categories of information represented by sample quotes provided descriptive detail. The categories were: (a) how nurses felt they were able to make a difference (with examples related to health promotion and prevention, advocacy, and education/health counseling); (b) unique opportunities (with examples related to integration of faith and health, a more relaxed psychosocial environment, the comfort of established long-term relationships, and nurse autonomy); and (c) unique challenges (with examples related to client autonomy, the impact of religious beliefs on accepting the healthcare provider's advice, the affect of a sense of being "on call" on nurses' worship experience, and the constraints of balancing multiple time demands). Conclusions were that (a) parish nurses provide a valuable adjunct to the traditional healthcare system and that (b) the congregational context for care creates a distinctive set of experiences that affect both nurses and clients in ways that have implications for ongoing development and implementation of health ministries.
- *Are the results valid?* Yes. The sampling was inclusive with representation of all 15 congregations and a high level of parish nurse participation (17 out of 20). Accuracy and completeness (credibility and dependability) were assured by means of a deliberate sequencing of two different well-described data collection techniques, a two-step coding process, and independent coding and review by the two researchers, with differences over the analysis resolved through discussion. Findings fit the data from which they were generated (confirmability) and meaningfully reflect what needs to be taken into consideration when developing and implementing health ministries. This is a good example of a qualitative descriptive study that pays attention to social contexts that influence nurses' perspectives, uses quotes and examples effectively, and provides insights about the parish nurse role that are plausible, believable, and transferable. (These latter effects would have to be experienced first-hand by reading the article.)
- *Will the results help me in caring for my patients?* Findings may increase awareness of how the synergy between parish nurses' professional values and personal faith, the spiritual and health needs of parishioners, and congregational climates shape nursing practice in these types of health ministries. The study described how nurses make a difference and provided suggestions for the support that may be needed for this emerging role.

#2 Wallace, D. C., Tuck, I., Boland, C. S., & Witucki, J. M. (2002). Client perceptions of parish nursing. *Public Health Nursing, 19,* 128–135.

Question: What are clients' knowledge of and experiences with parish nursing?

Design: Spradley's (1979) ethnographic interview approach.

Sample: 17 church members (12 female, 5 male) from two southeastern Appalachia congregations served by parish nurses — a primarily African American inner city congregation (n=8) and a primarily Caucasian suburban/rural congregation (n=9).

Procedures: A set of three types of open-ended questions (descriptive, structural, and contrast) was used in audio taped face-to-face interviews in private homes or at church facilities. Interview transcripts were coded, domains and categories emerged, and themes were identified through simultaneous data collection and analysis. (See also Tuck & Wallace, 2000, for an ethnographic study report; taxonomies of parish nurse attributes, actions, offering, roles, and entrance requirements; and discussion of cultural themes.)

Appraisal:

- *What were the results of the study?* Clients perceived having a parish nurse as beneficial for individuals, congregation, church, and community. Parish nurses also were seen as meaningful and effective healthcare providers. Quotes and examples of clients' experiences with parish nursing related to five major themes: (a) "being available" and approachable; (b) "integrating spirituality and health" by acknowledging the spiritual aspect of persons; (c) "helping us help ourselves" by empowering persons to be actively involved in maintaining or improving their health; (d) "exploring parish nursing" as a congregational program option; and (e) "evaluating parish nursing" in terms of satisfaction with the outcomes.
- *Are the results valid?* Yes. These results that focus on client perspectives provide a contrast with those of nurse perceptions reported in the previous study by Chase-Ziolek and Iris (2002). Sample composition (males, females, and fairly even representation from each of the two congregations) and size (N=17) reflects study needs. Females were over-represented; and it would be interesting to know more about the sampling strategy, i.e., how individuals were selected. Was sampling purposeful or did it rely more on convenience and persons' availability or willingness to participate? What was the congregational response? How does the sample reflect the internal make-up of each of the two congregations? Nevertheless, procedures are adequately outlined and appropriately focused on the ethnographic interview (credibility and dependability). The implication is that this report is part of a larger set of findings that include parish nurse perceptions of their roles and more about the cultural context within which parish nursing takes place. Selective use of extensive quotes to support the five themes resulting from the data analysis provides flavor and draws the reader into the described experiences (confirmability). The individual reader must judge this and the transferability of findings first-hand. It may seem trite to conclude that clients perceived parish nursing to be helpful. However, the meaningfulness of the article rests more on what clients actually said about how they perceived this service to be helpful and about their realizations of what was required of them in terms of using the nurse as a resource and accepting more responsibility for their own health-related decisions. Explicit conclusions about how insights based on this information might be used to develop future health programs and design studies and measures of an alternative nursing delivery model are not elaborated. But there is the potential for the implicit understandings derived from the findings themselves to stimulate different insights in readers' minds as they directly engage with the written text.
- *Will the results help me in caring for my patients?* Findings may promote understanding of what clients value most about the parish nurse role. They identify broad assessment areas involving perceptions of parish nurses' effectiveness and impact that could be considered when

evaluating health services within a church community. They also encourage this mode of healthcare delivery.

#3 Lupton, D., & Fenwick, J. (2001). 'They've forgotten that I'm the mum': Constructing and practising motherhood in special care nurseries. *Social Science & Medicine, 53,* 1011–1021.

Question: How does the neonatal nursery experience affect how mothers construct and practice mothering?

Design: Qualitative interpretation using concepts from a Foucauldian perspective on power relations.

Sample: 31 mothers (age range from 19 to 41) of babies in neonatal nurseries in two major New South Wales, Australia hospitals (16 from a Sydney hospital and 15 from a regional hospital) *and 20 nurses. Of the nurse participants, all but one of whom were female, 18 were registered nurses (17 were qualified midwives) with 1-20 years of neonatal nursing experience; and 2 were student midwives.*

Procedures: Data sources included individual interviews, field observation and informal chats with mothers and nursing staff, and voice-activated taped recordings of crib-side interactions between parents and nurses. In data analysis, conceptions of power, knowledge, subjectivity, and social relations consistent with those of Foucault (a postmodern historian, philosopher, and social critic) were used as the means to examine "material practices and technologies (such as the nursery rules and regulations, the practices around caring for the infants, the layout of the nurseries) and the discursive practices shaping women's experiences and their sense of self as a mother in the nursery" (p.1012). (See Lupton, 1997, for a discussion of Foucault and the medicalization critique.)

Appraisal:

● *What were the results of the study?* Although mothers' and nurses' discourses (ways of talking and thinking based on unspoken assumptions) contained similarities, there were important differences. Mothers' first few days of motherhood were described as traumatic and distressing because of enforced separation with inability to hold or breastfeed infants, distress of seeing babies connected to wires and surrounded by machines, and dealing with the possibility that their babies might not survive. They felt constantly "supervised" by the staff and spoke of being "allowed" or "not allowed" and needing to "gain permission" from staff to touch or care for their infants. Later, mothers' feelings of distance and detachment gave way to a strong urge to reclaim the role of mother by using strategies of learning about infants' medical conditions and seeking mother-infant physical interaction and breastfeeding as much and as soon as possible. As their sense of competence increased mothers began to feel they knew their babies and could observe changes in their conditions better than the nursing staff. Some acted against nurses' instructions, although many were wary of being labeled as "difficult" and realized they needed to be "nice" to facilitate good relations. As the mothers attempted to construct themselves as "real mothers," the nurses attempted to position themselves as "teachers and monitors of the parents," "protectors of the infants," and "experts" by training and experience. Differences in defining the situation resulted in resentment and anger on the part of mothers and both overt and covert disciplinary and surveillance actions on the part of many nurses. The influence of nurses' attitudes toward and treatment of mothers not only shaped mothers' relationships with their infants in the nurseries but also extended beyond infants' hospital stays.

- *Are the results valid?* Yes. This is a good example of qualitative interpretation from a perspective of postmodern critique. Sampling procedures produced participants who were representative, in terms of age, marital status, and socioeconomic background, of women with hospitalized infants in the nurseries involved. The study focused on mothers because they tended to spend far more time in the nursery than did the fathers. Nurses involved in caring for the infants of study participants were particularly sought for the purpose of eliciting views "from both sides of the mother-nurse dyad." Length of time researchers spent in the settings (nine months) and their use of multiple data sources assured accuracy and completeness (credibility). Subjection of empirical findings to analysis guided by a Foucauldian perspective on power relationships was carefully explained (dependability). And results that address how these mothers and the nurses caring for their infants constructed notions of motherhood are consistent with stated study aims. Description of the context that contributed to the development of these practices and constructions of motherhood and the systematic use of quotes infuse meaning and enrich the reading experience (confirmability and transferability).
- *Will the results help me in caring for my patients?* The title – "They've forgotten I'm the mum" – is an important reminder as well as an indicator of a source of difficulty for mothers. The article offers a possible way to understand the cultural and power relationship bases for problematic communication patterns as a step toward improving care to infants and families (i.e., an explanation of meaning in context). The social agenda of the research is one of advocating for change through increased sensitivity to the effects on mothers of having their babies in this type of environment, taken-for-granted nursery routines and practices, and the value-laden nature of mother-nurse relationships. A shared understanding of what constitutes "being a mother" under these circumstances calls for changing closed communication power struggles driven by implicit personal and professional values into open communication partnerships between mothers and nurses that enable explicit negotiations of roles and responsibilities.

#4   Powers, B. A. (2001). Ethnographic analysis of everyday ethics in the care of nursing home residents with dementia: A taxonomy. *Nursing Research, 50,* 332–339.

Question: What is the moral basis of ordinary daily issues affecting quality of life for nursing home residents with dementia?

Design: Ethnography – using combined anthropological methods of participant observation and in-depth interviewing.

Sample: 30 case examples (residents at different stages of dementia, family members and staff) and 10 ethics committee cases in a 147-bed voluntary not-for-profit nursing home in a Northeast U.S. city.

Procedures: Content analysis of fieldnotes, interview transcripts, and documents supported the construction of paradigm cases representing different kinds of everyday issues (see Powers,

2003) and creation of a classification scheme (taxonomy) to organize and interpret findings, which is the focus of this article.

Appraisal:

- *What were the results of the study?* The taxonomy of everyday ethical issues includes four domains: (a) learning the limits of intervention; (b) tempering the culture of surveillance and restraint; (c) preserving integrity of the individual; and (d) defining community norms and values. Each domain is associated with individual or social values and positive or negative moral rights. Thus, the domains of learning the limits of intervention (individual values focus) and tempering the culture of surveillance and restraint (social values focus) are oriented toward the negative moral right not to have something done to or taken from an individual (such as the right not to be forced or the right not to be restrained). And, the domains of preserving individual integrity (individual values focus) and defining community norms and values (social values focus) are oriented toward the positive moral right to have something done for or given to an individual (such as the right to follow a preferred routine or the right to attend community events). The domains are discussed in terms of: (a) cultural perspectives on the environmental contexts within which ethical issues arise; (b) study participants' concerns; and (c) ethical perspectives that reflect how ethical and clinical ways of thinking intersect (i.e., how the nature of dementia influences resident rights and values that affect those rights).

- *Are the results valid?* Yes. This is a good example of a traditional ethnographic approach using combined anthropological methods of participant observation and in-depth interviewing. Purposeful sampling was used to obtain cases that met study aims of examining the ethical content of commonly recurring issues. Personal involvement and time spent in the setting (two years) by the researcher as well as the use of multiple data sources assured accuracy and completeness (credibility). Data analysis procedures are described in detail; and the rationale and goal of the taxonomy approach are well discussed (dependability). Domains of the taxonomy are enlivened by the use of contextualized examples and quotes from the case material (confirmability). The effect of the report on perceptions of what counts as an ethical issue and practical use of the taxonomy is dependent on the backgrounds and judgments of readers as they independently relate to the article's narrative content (transferability).

- *Will the results help me in caring for my patients?* Findings discuss the cultural context within which dementia care issues in nursing homes occur and offer ways to think about them as exercises in everyday ethics. This involves identifying common concerns and reframing them as "ethical issues." Examples of commonly expressed concerns include what are thought of as "behavior issues" (e.g., refusals of care, socially disturbing behavior, or resident-resident altercations), "treatment issues" (e.g., safety concerns, appearance, hygiene, and clinical care), or "resource issues" (e.g., service-related difficulties or delays attributed to human or material shortages). These ways of thinking, framed from care provider points of view, invite logistical, value-neutral problem solving approaches to resident-centered issues that can strip them of their moral significance. Thus, the research's social agenda is one of encouraging acknowledgement of the value-laden nature of daily life experiences in caring for persons in nursing homes with dementia by redefining ordinary everyday issues in ethical terms, framed from a resident point of view.

#5 **Hurlock-Chorostecki, C. (2002). Management of pain during weaning from mechanical ventilation: The nature of nurse decision-making.** *Canadian Journal of Nursing Research, 34,* 33–47.

Question: How do beliefs about pain and sedation influence critical care nurses' decision-making during the weaning of patients from mechanical ventilation?

Design: Grounded theory

Sample: 10 ventilator-certified critical care nurses in an intensive care unit (ICU) of an urban Canadian hospital.

Procedures: Theoretical sampling was used to select participants representative of a range of levels of skill acquisition, from novice to expert as described by Benner (1984), and to determine that defined categories, in the end, were substantial and mutually exclusive. Participants were encouraged to "tell their own story" in response to the statement: "Tell me about your nursing activities when caring for your patient during weaning." Probing questions were used to clarify and expand descriptions. The topic of pain management was not explored until raised by the participant. Constant comparative analysis included careful reading and comparison of information in transcribed interviews and analytic memos of the researcher's thoughts used to build and link categories and to link the findings to existing knowledge. A qualitative data analysis software program facilitated the processing and analyzing of textual material.

Appraisal:

- *What were the results of the study?* Decision-making was found to be influenced by two powerful forces outside of the nursing process and individual skill levels. The first force was the nurse's beliefs about the existence and importance of managing pain during weaning. Despite published evidence that pain is experienced during weaning, more than half of the nurses held a strong belief that it is not and that analgesia is unnecessary (further described as differences in style between "the diagnostic nurse" vs. "the humanistic nurse"). Beliefs were well established a priori and level of skill acquisition had no bearing on a tendency to adopt either style of nursing practice. The second force was beliefs about the nurse's role. Nurses fitting the description of "the soldier nurse" took a passive role in decision-making, following orders and maintaining a position in the chain of command. In contrast, "the nurse advocate" participated actively, using the care team structure to identify patient needs and produce a plan of care. In addition, two approaches to knowing the patient were described: the technical survey (monitoring technological and behavioral indicators) and contemplating the big picture (a holistic focus on getting to know the patient as an individual and using intuition). Humanistic nurses tended toward the latter approach. However, the degree to which it was taken depended on skill level, with the more-skilled nurses placing greater value on the whole patient. The emerging belief-decision continuum theory posited that "knowing the patient" through identifying and interpreting patient cues is strongly influenced by a priori beliefs, such as beliefs about pain. And, also, in a dynamic and continuous process of knowledge gathering, knowledge interpretation, and action, role beliefs determine whether the nurse will participate passively or actively in decision-making about the weaning process. It was concluded that "while level of skill, style of nursing, a priori beliefs, and 'knowing the patient' influence the course of action, the greatest influence is the belief about the role of the nurse" (p.43).

- *Are the results valid?* Yes. This example of grounded theory analysis of a critical care intervention process uses language, concepts, and procedures consistent with traditional practice of the method developed by Glaser and Strauss, as described by Chenitz and Swanson (1986). Measures taken during data collection and analysis to assure validity and reliability included bracketing to reduce bias, member checks, and expert consultation (dependability). In order to establish truthfulness, the final draft of the theory was presented to the study participants for their comments (credibility). Diagramming of the theory and effective use of representative quotes enhances the clarity and consistency of the findings as well as demonstrates how they are grounded in the data (dependability). Discussion further situates concepts that form the basis of this emerging theory within the contexts of relevant extant literature (transferability).

- *Will the results help me in caring for my patients?* Findings raise ideas about factors (described as personal beliefs, styles, and approaches) related to use of analgesia and sedation when weaning patients from ventilators that may be helpful for practitioners to reflect upon and discuss. How well the substantive theory fits with and captures the individual reality of similar practice situations will determine its transferability (theoretic generalizability). Testing the theory quantitatively would suggest the extent to which it may more universally apply to current trends in clinical practice (statistical generalizability).

#6 Varcoe, C. (2001). Abuse obscured: An ethnographic account of emergency nursing in relation to violence against women. *Canadian Journal of Nursing Research, 32,* 95–115.

Question: How does the social context of emergency room care influence nursing practice in relation to women who have been abused?

Design: Critical ethnography informed by a feminist understanding of violence and oppression (Varcoe, 1996).

Sample: 30 healthcare providers (21 white, female nurses and 9 other providers including admitting clerks, social workers, physicians, and administrators) and 5 women who had been abused.

Procedures: In addition to interviews, data collection involved more than 200 hours of participant observation in the Emergency Departments (EDs) of 2 urban hospitals in Canada and the communities they served. Twelve nurses, an extensively observed core sample, were interviewed twice. Of the nine additional Emergency nurses interviewed, four were from the study sites and five were from various other hospitals throughout the province in which the two sites were located. Three of the women who had been abused were met in Emergency and two in the community during fieldwork. Analysis drew on critical ethnography approaches informed by feminist ideological perspectives.

Appraisal:

- *What were the results of the study?* Findings illustrate how abuse was obscured by a focus on physical problems, rapid patient processing, and stereotypical thinking. Most nurses did not think they saw much abuse, recognizing it only when there was significant physical evidence that fit the pattern of emergency practice. This pattern involved stripping down patients to "manageable problems" — usually a physiological label such as "chest pain," "laceration," "fracture," or "overdose," with known solutions. Nurses felt pressured to process patients as quickly as possible and felt unable to engage patients or attend to anything but the most blatant physical abuse. Stereotypical thinking involved the association of abuse with direct physical trauma, and anticipation of violence among poor and "racialized" people rather than among white, middle-class or wealthy groups. Perceptions of persons' deservedness influenced the care provided. When abuse was recognized, healthcare provider response fell into three overlapping patterns: (a) *Doing nothing for the undeserving victim* (judged on the basis of such things as perceived alcohol abuse, misuse of ED services, and lifestyle) involved recognizing but not pursuing cues of abuse, dealing only with obvious physical injuries, and shifting responsibility to other providers or family members. Reasons nurses gave for doing nothing were the same as those given for failing to recognize abuse – the focus on physical problems, not knowing what to do, and lack of adequate resources. (b) *Influencing choices for the deserving victim* (judged on the basis of social status and severity of injury) involved guiding women toward what was thought to be the best choices, i.e., existing solutions and resources such as leaving the relationship or disclosing the abuse and calling the police. (c) *Offering choices to women with personal agency* involved providing care that the women requested, i.e., listening, respecting choices, and encouraging them to return to Emergency. Sometimes offering choices required giving up control and ran counter to patterns of practice because of emotional and time commitments that reduced efficiency. Some nurses in this study experienced moral distress over the judgmental attitudes they observed in others and themselves. But the researcher's conclusions were that "improved practice in relation to violence against women requires more than concerned nurses. [Care that is effective] rather than merely efficient in terms of patient processing, requires political will and adequate resources" (p.111).

- *Are the results valid?* Yes. This is a good example of critical ethnography guided by a feminist understanding of violence and oppression that paid particular attention to power relations between patients and healthcare providers and among healthcare providers. Validity was assured through purposeful sampling that continually sought competing and contradictory perspectives; use of multiple data sources; intense researcher participation in the study settings; involvement of participants in the analysis; and researcher attempts to account for her own biases, particularly with respect to racism (credibility and dependability). Empirical findings are supported by relevant quotes and contextualized descriptions (confirmability). A first-hand reading of the article is the best way to judge the social action effects (transferability) of the interpretation that seeks to motivate constructive change through uncovering the complexities and social contextual constraints affecting providers of professional care to women who have been abused.

- *Will the results help me in caring for my patients?* Findings constitute a critique of emergency department cultures that serve to mask and fail to address the needs of victims of violence and abuse. Insights reveal and challenge practice patterns that obscure abuse through rapid patient processing focused on manageable physical problems and stereotypical treatment of individuals on the basis of race and social status. Thus, a format to encourage more open awareness, personal reflection, and discussion is provided. However, it is pointed out that nurses' recognition of organizational constraints on their ability to provide optimal care suggests that bringing about resolution of these issues requires not only individual awareness and education but systemic changes, as well. Therefore, this study's political agenda is one of providing evidence to motivate personal, professional, and social efforts toward corrective and constructive action.

#7   Anderson, N. L., Nyamathi, A., McAvoy, J. A., Conde, F., & Casey, C. (2001). Perceptions about risk for HIV/AIDS among adolescents in juvenile detention. *Western Journal of Nursing Research, 23,* 336–359.

Question: What sociocultural contexts and interactional dynamics shape at-risk adolescents' beliefs about risk and danger?

Design: A blend of Participant Action Research (PAR) with focus groups and individual interviews.

Sample: 42 adolescents (19 female, 23 male) arrested for a variety of alleged violations and residing in a detention facility pending outcomes of court appearances.

Procedures: Eleven small groups composed of 2 to 5 teens were formed, and adolescents worked in partnership with researchers during field study activities. The combination of sequential focus group discussions, individual interviews, and participant observation helped to fill in gaps that would have resulted with any of these techniques used alone. Data analysis was an interactive process. Through card sorts constructed from clusters of words used during their first focus group sessions, the teens prioritized information and extended, clarified and qualified their original discussions – taking advantage of the opportunity to voice their concerns. Researchers reviewed, compared and contrasted these data sets with original group and interview discussions as well as demographic data. Researchers and participants collaborated at each data analysis phase to make the final outcome an agreed upon mutual endeavor.

Appraisal:

- *What were the results of the study?* Findings clustered under two categories: (a) perceptions about HIV/AIDS and (b) teen definitions of risk and danger. These teens did not identify HIV/AIDS as a primary concern but discussed it openly once the topic was raised. It was mentioned spontaneously most often in connection with other STDs resulting from promiscuous sexual behaviors. All could identify mode of transmission and strategies for prevention; and many had been tested. But, personal concerns and characterizations of danger focused mainly on teens' relationships with people at home, at school, and in their neighborhoods. Relationships were reviewed in the context of the present ("doing time"), reliving past experiences, and planning the future. And, in the process, the partnership that developed between participants and researchers in this study produced positive outcomes for these adolescents. That is, opportunity to be recognized and respected and to talk with persons considered as trustworthy "caught their attention and inspired them to think about AIDS as an issue of relevance to themselves" (p.355). Thus, a conclusion based on these findings was that planning for future AIDS education courses might consider more empowering approaches "by making the adolescents ... equal partners in the education enterprise" (p.355). (For additional insights on resolutions and risk-taking of adolescents in juvenile detention, see Anderson 1990, 1994, 1996, 1999.)

● *Are the results valid*? Yes. This is a good example of participant action research (PAR). Its validity is supported by detailed description of the procedures used in all phases of the study [dependability] because, as the authors explain, "incarcerated teens are a particularly vulnerable and powerless population" (p.355). Use of multiple field techniques (focus groups, individual interviews and participant observation) combined with active involvement of the teens in the participatory aspects of the research assured accuracy and completeness (credibility). Quotes fit the findings they are intended to illustrate (dependability). Presentation of the overall results gives voice to the study participants and promotes an understanding of how these teens perceived risk and which risks and dangers in their communities were of greatest concern to them. But assessment of meaningfulness and transferability is dependent on individual reader judgments.

● *Will the results help me in caring for my patients*? Findings offer a perspective that may enhance understanding of what members of some vulnerable teen populations find relevant to their personal needs and compatible with the concerns that occupy their attention. Such understanding is an essential preliminary step in planning interventions that will be effective in reaching them with appropriate risk-reduction strategies. In this study, "the participants willingly shared their perceptions of risk for HIV/AIDS as they taught the researchers about how they defined adolescent risk" (p.353). They also reported that most courses that had been provided for them had not "captured their interest or motivated them to take risk-reducing precautions" (pp. 354–355). Study outcomes suggest that the research's modeling of an empowering approach that involved teens as equal partners in the educational enterprise has implications for the design of future programs.

#8 Aston, M. L. (2002). Learning to be a normal mother: Empowerment and pedagogy in postpartum classes. *Public Health Nursing, 19,* 284–293.

Question: How are concerns and aspirations of new mothers constructed and mediated by pedagogical practices experienced in postpartum classes?

Design: Qualitative interpretation using concepts from poststructuralist and feminist methodologies.

Sample: 2 public health nurses and 6 first-time mothers participating in two public health unit postpartum classes in Ontario, Canada.

Procedures: Data collection involved audio taped in-depth interviews in mothers' homes and in nurses' health units combined with participant observation in both postpartum groups. Theoretical concepts offering particular perspectives on subjectivity, the process of normalization, difference, and relations of power were used, in analysis, as ways to understand and interpret women's concerns and aspirations about baby care and mothering as influenced by social constructions and pedagogical practices.

Appraisal:

● *What were the results of the study*? Isolation was a common theme for all of the mothers. They described feeling unprepared, being physically isolated, not feeling like a "mother" yet, and believing that there was much information on baby care and mothering that they needed to obtain to be "a normal mother." Each, at times, wanted medical advice on baby care, sometimes viewing this "expert advice" as more legitimate than advice of other mothers and friends. This was found to interfere with public health nurses' attempts to challenge the notion of "expert knowledge" by encouraging mothers to focus on and share the knowledge they possessed with each other in class as a way to support and empower them. The nurses viewed their roles as facilitators of conversations between new mothers, checking what is already known, and offering new information to address assumed learning needs. But no matter how the class was structured, it was difficult for the mothers to see themselves as "equal partners" in a learning situation experienced as involving various relations of power. Both nurses and mothers, in different ways and at different times, acknowledged assumptions that the public health nurse was a particular kind of expert who, whether lecturing or facilitating conversation, controlled an information exchange that was invested in medical discourse. Therefore, moving away from traditional problem-based, teacher-directed learning toward supportive client-centered practices of education was difficult. Different ideas about how sharing knowledge and comparing parenting styles should be done also posed difficulties. Although the public health nurses commented on the acceptability of having one's own style, opportunity to discuss differences was not provided. Therefore, mothers' sense of isolation and lack of confidence continued, with any explicit or implicit sharing or comparing that occurred raising concerns about normalcy and deviance.

- *Are the results valid?* Yes. This is a good example of qualitative interpretation from a post-structuralist feminist perspective. Sampling strategies assured an equal number of participants from each postpartum class; and sample size was appropriate for the intensive in-depth nature of the interviews and subsequent analysis. Accuracy and completeness were enhanced by use of combined field techniques that included participant observation (credibility). The analysis was supported by a detailed presentation of the theoretical concepts used to understand the conversations with participants and to interpret the women's concerns and aspirations about baby care and mothering practices (dependability and confirmability). A stated limitation of the study was that participants were predominantly white, middle class, heterosexual women in their thirties. The researcher recognizes that although "the study raises many interesting points.... Further research is necessary that would incorporate more diverse experiences of mothering that might include, for example, other races, age groups, or sexual orientations" (p.288). Transferability must be judged by reflective first-hand reading of the article.

- *Will the results help me in caring for my patients?* Findings offer insights on the nature of postpartum class experiences that go beyond analysis of different teaching-learning styles. The result is an interpretation of how social structures construct individuals' experiences and mothering practices, which, in turn, influence the postpartum class experience. "Based on the findings in this study, the learning needs of new mothers clearly need to be reconceptualized so that they incorporate an understanding of the social structures of isolation, investment in medical discourse, and processes of normalization" (p. 292). The study provides evidence that explains some of the acknowledged tensions and struggles of both mothers and nurses with regard to support and sharing, as follows. "Although the public health nurses were using concepts from nursing systems theory that focuses on equality of all participants, each woman's experiences of learning encompassed various relations of power that resisted an ideal experience of 'equal partners'" (p. 290). Therefore, this study's social action agenda advocates change in pedagogical practices based on new understanding of issues of empowerment, language, support, and knowledge exchange.

Family Issues and
Personal Relationships

#1   Young, H. M., McCormick, W. M., & Vitaliano, P. P. (2002a). Attitudes toward community-based services among Japanese American families. *The Gerontologist, 42,* 814–825.

Question: What shapes preferences and attitudes influencing utilization of community-based long-term care services by Japanese American families?

Design: Qualitative descriptive study using in-depth interviews and grounded theory approaches involving theoretical sampling, constant comparative analysis, and development of a coding scheme to account for the data.

Sample: Japanese Americans living in Washington State — 26 family caregivers, 4 care recipients, and 14 professional care providers (N=44) — selected from a larger long term care project for the purpose of augmenting already obtained quantitative data. The focus is on a particular set of long-term care options (including nursing home, assisted living, adult day care, and meal services) provided within the boundaries of and with volunteer support from an ethnic community.

Procedures: Theoretical sampling was used to produce a varied, representative, and theoretically relevant sample in terms of gender, age, marital status, caregiving situation, health status, functional ability, and use of long-term care services (i.e., participants were selected to represent those actually using services, those not using services, and those involved in decision making about services). Audio taped, semi-structured interviews were conducted in private and in the primary language of the participant. As themes, relationships and contributing factors were identified through a constant comparative method of concurrent data collection and analysis, the interview guide was modified to explore these in more detail. A qualitative data analysis software program facilitated processing and analyzing of textual material. Text was broken down into single ideas, coded, categorized, and organized to determine common themes and relationships among ideas. (See Young, McCormick, & Vitaliano, 2002b, for a focus on evolution of cultural values underlying service delivery and family expectations.)

Appraisal:

- *What were the results of the study?* Attitudes toward services were identified along six dimensions: ability to meet care needs, autonomy in daily life, quality of care and staff, cost, emotional connotation, and social and physical environment. The study supported previous findings of the acceptability of services among this population but suggested that utilization rests on more than their availability. Services that supported needs for autonomy in daily life and privacy were valued. Quality of services was a concern. Many participants stated preferences for having Japanese American care providers because of their cultural understanding, and for older care receivers, ability of care providers to speak Japanese was an issue. Participants also valued traditional Japanese meals and programs. Knowledge of actual costs and eligibility for services was not widespread; and decisions sometimes were based on incomplete information. In general, participants gathered information about services being immediately considered rather than considering a full service range; and, in discussing various options, they expressed confusion about actual provided services, financial aspects, and their eligibility. Emotionally, it was hard to rely on others; and some participants found home care stressful when older homemakers saw their home helper as a guest, thus creating work for them that the service was intended to alleviate. Maintaining and creating familiar social and natural surroundings were important. And, families remained involved and played important roles in sustaining and ensuring quality of services as well as sharing responsibility for overall care. These findings illustrate the importance of communication and collaboration among families and providers. Overall, the study illuminated needs for cultural sensitivity and illustrated the dynamic nature of the interplay between families and formal services.

- *Are the results valid?* Yes. This is a good example of the use of grounded theory approaches in a qualitative descriptive study. As noted, theoretical sampling produced a varied, representative, and theoretically relevant sample. Constant comparative analysis concurrent with data collection and use of systematic coding and data management techniques assured accuracy and completeness (credibility and dependability). Findings fit the data from which they were generated with effective use of quotes to illustrate participants' attitudes toward services, perspectives about facilitating factors and barriers, and actions used to augment services (confirmability). Transferability must be judged by reflective first-hand reading of the article.

- *Will the results help me in caring for my patients?* Family members' limited exploration of options and their confusion about available services is not an unusual finding. In general, health care providers could be more proactive in helping families anticipate changing needs of elders and accept more responsibility for guiding them to appropriate services. Also, as for this sample, services that support needs for personal autonomy and privacy have been found to be very important to the elder population at large. Specifically, this study illustrates how utilization of available services is influenced by cultural and family expectations. Better understanding of this dynamic and of the active roles that families play in caregiving regardless of living situation, may increase cultural sensitivity and optimize service delivery for older and disabled populations.

#2 Anderson, D. G., & Imle, M. A. (2001). Families of origin of homeless and never-homeless women. *Western Journal of Nursing Research, 23,* 394–413.

Question: What may at-risk, never homeless women find in childhood family environments that is not available to women who eventually do become homeless?

Design: Naturalistic inquiry involving in-depth interviews.

Sample: 12 homeless and 16 never-homeless women in a northwestern U. S. city — similar in age, education, ethnicity, abuse histories, number of persons in family of origin, and percent who grew up in stepfamilies. None were homeless as children.

Procedures: An interview guide was used to ensure that key topics pertaining to family history and composition over time were explored with each participant. Lofland's (1995) conceptions of the "social units" of meanings, practices, episodes, roles, and relationships were used to organize findings.

Appraisal:

- *What were the results of the study?* Themes identified within each social unit supported the importance of family nurturance during childhood as the basis for meaningful adult relationships. A key meaning for homeless women was "being without" (love, security, acceptance, and/or age appropriate expectations) in their families of origin. In contrast, the never-home-less women were able to describe episodes in their lives of "being with" (close family gatherings, special relationships) as well as "being connected" to family (loved and accepted) into adulthood, despite childhood traumas. Never-homeless women also had fewer episodes of transience and abuse, whereas homeless women's childhood experiences of transience of residence, parental employment, and parental relationships as well as physical abuse, lack of connection, and a sense of abandonment were accepted as normal at the time. In contrast to never-homeless women, most homeless women discussed having the role of a little adult as a child with a predominance of negative relationships full of betrayal, devaluation, destructive coalitions, oppression, and coercion. Never-homeless women were able to describe positive as well as negative childhood experiences. Thus, even though all participants experienced traumatic childhoods, the outcomes were different for never-homeless women. And data suggest that this might be because some family member countered violence and abuse with unconditional love, acceptance, and a safe haven; there was family stability in times of transience; and there was someone to turn to in times of loss and need.

- *Are the results valid*? Yes. Sample composition and size were appropriate for this naturalistic study following Lofland and Lofland's (1995) approach to analyzing social settings. Effective recruitment strategies were used to obtain participants who met the study's inclusion criteria. The never-homeless women were recruited through the use of flyers posted in locations housing women's support groups. The homeless women were recruited through a local urban cafe that served meals and provided referral and support services to homeless and poor women and children. Findings fit the data from which they were generated and were illustrated appropriately by stories and quotes (confirmability). However, there was a limitation in matching the women for the study. Although women in both studies had experienced abuse, the experience of transience and losses were not as frequent or severe for the never-homeless women. Systematic approaches to interviewing (including structured questions with probes and use of genograms) and examination of narrative data (involving social units) enhanced accuracy (credibility and dependability). Transferability must be judged by reflective first-hand reading of the article.

- *Will the results help me in caring for my patients*? Findings provide support for the influence of a woman's family of origin as a precursor to homelessness. Healthcare providers can be instrumental in "identification of girls and young women who are at high risk for adjustment problems and [need assistance with] intervention[s] to help them begin building positive attachments...before homelessness becomes an issue in their lives" (p. 412). When positive family relationships are lacking, long-term interventions include, i.e., relationship building, developing support networks, violence prevention, and positive female role modeling.

#3 Wuest, J., & Merritt-Gray, M. (2001). Beyond survival: Reclaiming self after leaving an abusive male partner. *Canadian Journal of Nursing Research, 32,* 79–94.

Question: What are the experiences of women who have left abusive male partners and not gone back?

Design: Grounded theory from a feminist perspective (Wuest, 1995).

Sample: 15 Caucasian women who originated and lived in small towns and geographically isolated areas in eastern Canada (ranging in age from late teens to mid-50s). About half had accessed women's shelters at some point in the leaving process. None had access to support groups and very few had sought professional counseling.

Procedures: Data were collected through unstructured audio taped interviews. Theoretical sampling of data from repeat interviews, interviews with new participants, and focus group data from an earlier study to explore sociocultural perspectives on women's abuse (Wuest & Merritt-Gray, 1997) provided information to illuminate the theoretical properties of emerging concepts. Theoretical coding was used to clarify relationships between concepts and facilitate theory development. In repeat interviews, the emerging theory was shared with the participant for discussion and refinement.

Appraisal:

- *What were the results of the study?* Reclaiming self* was the basic social psychological process (BSPP) that involved four stages: (a) *counteracting abuse*: learning strategies for minimizing abuse and building personal strengths (Merritt-Gray & Wuest, 1995); (b)*breaking free*: testing different exits and discovering the consequences of leaving the relationship; (c) *not going back*: attempting to establish and protect physical and emotional territory separate from the abuser despite increased risk from escalating violence (Wuest & Merritt-Gray, 1999); and (d) *moving on. Moving on* is the stage that is the focus of this paper. It involves shedding the identities of victim and survivor and moving through the following process: (a) *Figuring it out* involves searching for reasons abuse happened and why women remained in the relationship as long as they did. (b) *Putting it in its rightful place* describes the process of no longer allowing the abuse experience to define their existence, incorporating the abuse as part of their past and recognizing the positive consequences of the relationships. (c) *Launching new relationships* takes place within a social environment (e.g., social or sporting events) where women are expected to have a partner. Participants expressed reluctance to trust while acknowledging that trust was essential in the kind of relationship they wanted. (d) *Taking on a new image* involves leaving behind the image of abused woman or survivor and taking pride in the person one has become. For example, women with children spoke of becoming better parents. Others saw the possibility of a future with a career, returning to school, or owning a home.
- *Are the results valid?* Yes. This is a good example of feminist grounded theory. Method-appropriate systematic procedures to assure accuracy and completeness were described (dependability). Theoretical sampling guided a simultaneous process of data collection and analysis. Information to illuminate concepts emerging from data analysis was sought from repeat interviews, interviews with new participants and focus groups. Theoretical coding (Glaser, 1978) was used to clarify relationships between concepts and support the development of a theoretical framework (credibility). Feminist perspectives on violence, as explained in terms of gender and power issues in society at-large, supported interpretation of the meanings of women's subjective accounts. This ensured that their experiences would be examined in social context. Stages of the basic social-psychological process (BSPP) of *reclaiming self* were illustrated by descriptions and quotes that demonstrated how study findings were grounded in the data (confirmability). Conclusions are plausible, believable, and transferable, as best judged by individuals' first-hand reading of the article.
- *Will the results help me in caring for my patients?* Health professionals may use this theory when screening for abuse to determine where a woman may be in the leaving process and

tailor assistance according to needs associated with that stage. Women in the process of leaving abusive relationships also may use it to frame their progress and make sense of their experience (p.90-91). Clinicians can help women by understanding their need not to define themselves in terms of being victims or survivors of abuse; using language that reflects their orientation toward the future and moving on; offering validation and anticipatory guidance when old feelings resurface; encouraging them not to accept an unreasonable amount of responsibility or assign blame; and confirming their strengths and growth "in order to foster the development of their new image" (p.92). It is particularly important for health providers to avoid revictimizing women who have *moved on*. To that end, "findings extend knowledge of the leaving process by describing how the abuse experience and survival process may be displaced as the center of women's intra-psychic, interpersonal, and social existence" (p.79).

#4 **Rose, L., Mallinson, R. K., & Walton-Moss, B. (2002). A grounded theory of families responding to mental illness. *Western Journal of Nursing Research, 24,* 516–536**.

Question: How do families manage the experience of mental illness and where in the process do they seem to need help in coping?

Design: Grounded theory methods of Strauss and Corbin (1990).

Sample: Participants were 29 family members of 17 patients with diagnoses of schizophrenia, major depression, or bipolar disorder. Most patients had a history of at least 3 hospitalizations; and time since initial diagnosis ranged from 2 to more than 10 years. Approximately half were living with their families. Family members were parents (n=13), spouses (n=4), adult siblings (n=8), or adult children (n=4) ranging in age from 18 to 73 years. Ethnicity was Caucasian (n=19), African American (n=8), and Hispanic (n=2); and 19 were female – 10 were male.

Procedures: Purposive sampling was used to achieve variation on key characteristics of caregivers and status of psychiatric patients (hospitalized and community based). Theoretical sampling was used as the study progressed to refine categories and strengthen the emerging theory (e.g., seeking contrasting cases to increase variation in family member composition and length of illness experience). Three interviews were scheduled over a 2-year period. The first explored the nature of the illness and current concerns. The second and third interviews were used to provide additional data and validate the emerging theory. Of the 17 families interviewed at Time 1, 12 also participated at Times 2 and 3. Data collection continued until categories were saturated. Constant comparative methods described by Strauss and Corbin (1990) were used. And the substantive theory was developed using the coding paradigm of contexts, conditions, strategies, and consequences.

Appraisal:

- *What are the results of the study*? The basic process that explained most of the variation in family coping with mental illness over time was a perspective of pursuing normalcy for the patient. This involved confronting the ambiguity of the diagnosis, seeking to control the impact of the illness, and adopting a stance of seeing the realities and possibilities for the future. Goals were managing crises, containing and controlling symptoms, and crafting a revised notion of normalcy that involved reaffirming hope, redefining relationships, maintaining stability while striving for growth, and reaching conclusions about priorities, decisions, and evaluations of what being normal means, e.g., including a wish that the patient be happy. Strategies included being vigilant, setting limits on patients, invoking logic, dealing with a sense of loss, seeing patients' strengths, and taking on roles (e.g., communicator, teacher, advocate). Families were most concerned about understanding the behavior they were seeing and helping others to see it as illness based. The emergence of normalcy as a central concept illustrates the complex and difficult process of accepting the social implications of mental illness. "All family members, regardless of where they were in the illness experience, acknowledged that they continued to need help to reconcile societal goals of independence and productivity with the behaviors of young adult or even middle-aged mentally ill relatives" (p.533).

- *Are the results valid?* Yes. This is a good example of grounded theory using the methods described by Strauss and Corbin (1990). Method-appropriate systematic procedures to assure accuracy and completeness were described (dependability). These included theoretical sampling, as already described, to achieve theoretical sensitivity by seeking diversity in study participants, as well as data collection and coding procedures consistent with this grounded theory approach. Trustworthiness (accuracy) of data was discussed in relation to coding procedures. Credibility was addressed by sharing emerging conceptualizations with families at the third interview. Also discussed were data management procedures used to maintain validity and establish an audit trail. *Living with ambiguity of mental illness* was identified as a basic social problem (BSP). Stages of the basic sociopsychological process (BSPP) of *pursuing normalcy* were illustrated by diagram, descriptions, and quotes that demonstrated how study findings were grounded in the data (confirmability). Conclusions are plausible and were situated within the contexts of relevant extant literature (transferability).

- *Will the results help me in caring for my patients?* Findings stress understanding the normalizing strategies families may use to cope with the impact of mental illness. In this study, families tried to make sense of mental illness, using age-based expectations and knowledge of the person prior to the illness as reference points (p. 532). Here, help was needed most in reconciling societal goals of independence and productivity with the behaviors of ill adult relatives. And despite some families' efforts to be positive about the future, "the devastation...of ruined lives and permanently altered relationships [described by others] cannot be dismissed or ignored" (p. 533). The diversity and complexity of experiences need to be considered when focusing on what families do well in trying to achieve a sense of normalcy.

#5 Butcher, H. K., Holkup, P. A., & Buckwalter, K. C. (2001). The experience of caring for a family member with Alzheimer's Disease. *Western Journal of Nursing Research, 23*, 33–55.

Question: What is the essence of the Alzheimer's Disease or related disorder (ADRD) family caregiving experience?

Design: Secondary data analysis using van Kaam's (1966) four-stage, 12-step descriptive psychophenomenological method.

Sample: Transcripts of 103 verbatim, in-depth, open-ended, unstructured interviews with ADRD caregivers living in four states (Arizona, Iowa, Indiana, and Minnesota) — 29 were male caregivers and 37 caregivers were other than spouses.

Procedures: Each description was read and reread with a focus on identifying, naming, and grouping descriptive expressions in the exact language of informants (analysis stage). Descriptive expressions were organized and synthesized into 8 essential structural elements. Qualitative data analysis software supported data management; and an expert (judge) with experience in phenomenological methods reviewed structural elements for congruence. Final wording of structural elements (translation stage) was submitted for review by two independent expert judges and was followed by the final synthetic description/structural definition (transposition stage). In the last stage (phenomenological reflection), judges' suggestions were integrated into the final synthetic description/structural definition and findings were submitted to two advanced practice nurses and shared with a family caregiver for comments.

Appraisal:

- *What were the results of the study?* Participants' verbatim descriptive expressions were presented to support and illustrate the following final structural elements that captured the essence of the lived experience: (a) enduring stress and frustration; (b) immersed in caregiving; (c) finding meaning and joy; (d) integrating ADRD into our lives; (e) moving with continuous change; (f) preserving integrity; (g) gathering support; and (h) suffering through the losses.
- *Are the results valid?* Yes. This is an interesting example of the use of a phenomenological approach to perform a secondary analysis on a large amount of in-depth interview data. Although most phenomenological studies involve small samples, van Kaam's (1966) four-stage, 12-step method is accommodating to large data sets. Another of its unique features is the reporting of frequencies and percentages that provides easier comparison and summary of the categorization of all the data (p.37). Already described rigorous method-specific procedures involving review at different stages by expert judges and comments of advanced practice nurses and a family caregiver assured accuracy and credibility (dependability). (Reading the article will provide even more step-by-step procedural details.) Selection of transcripts to include in the analysis was based on Hinds, Vogel, and Clark-Steffin's (1997) criteria for evaluating the completeness and quality of qualitative data for secondary analysis (credibility). "To assure that there was no selection bias between the 245 participants [in the original study] and the 103 selected for inclusion in the phenomenological analysis, respondents selected for the phenomenological analysis were compared to those not selected on variables that might influence the discussion of caregiving....There were no statistical differences between the selected and unselected groups across all variables" (p.39). Effective use of a data grid to report relative frequencies of preliminary essential elements and quotes to illustrate the connections between the resultant interpretation and the data illuminated common themes (confirmability). The authors conclude that "the methodological innovativeness of this study expands and deepens understanding of the experience of caring for a family member with ADRD...and the larger and more diverse sample...strengthens the transferability of findings" (p.50).
- *Will the results help me in caring for my patients?* Findings raise awareness of how family members' (78% in this study) may find meaning amidst the stress and anguish of caring for the person with ADRD by valuing positive aspects of the relationship and caregiving experience and by "creating moments of joyfulness together" (p.51). By extending knowledge based on quantitative studies of caregiving, the research addresses health professionals' needs for fuller understanding of "the shared meanings that family members attribute to their expe-

rience as caregivers p.35." Attention to the positive aspects of caregiving that accompany the pain and the loss reflects a recent focus in the literature.

#6 Norton, S. A., & Bowers, B. J. (2001). Working toward consensus: Providers' strategies to shift patients from curative to palliative treatment choices. *Research in Nursing & Health, 24,* 258–269.

Question: What strategies do professional care providers use to shift patients and families from curative to palliative treatment choices?

Design: Grounded theory

Sample: 15 participants (10 nurses, 5 physicians) from a midsize Mid-western city. These data are part of a larger study of reconciling decisions near end of life.

Procedures: Constant comparative analysis and theoretical sampling revealed many strategies used by healthcare providers to assess patients' understandings of their situations and to help them alter what were viewed as unrealistic or unreasonable perspectives. Common to all those who described such strategies was a goal of either preventing a "bad death" or hoping to achieve a "good death." (See Norton & Talerico, 2000.)

Appraisal:

- *What were the results of the study?* Provider responses to perceived unrealistic patient or proxy/family member goals included: (a) avoiding interactions with the patient and family; (b) referring the patient and family to another provider; and (c) using strategies aimed at shifting unrealistic goals and treatment decisions to more realistic ones. Strategies to shift patients and families from curative to palliative treatment choices were grouped according to the following purposes: (a) *Laying the Groundwork* involved establishing trust and rapport; *teaching* about prognosis and treatment choices; and *planting seeds* to open up the possibility that the patient might not survive. (b) *Shifting the Picture* involved creating a new context, refocusing, or reframing previous understandings; *working together* with other providers to present a united front to patient and family regarding prognosis and treatment options; *family meetings*; *creating new expectations* to help patients and families expect deterioration and anticipate changes with a clear understanding that death is inevitable; *changing the scope of choice* such as advance directives, hospice, do not resuscitate, and comfort care only; *changing the value of treatment options* to raise the value of patient comfort and quality time for patients and families together; and *changing indicators*, information used to monitor the patient's condition, to help patients and families shift their understanding of the big picture. (c) *Accepting a New Picture* involved helping patients and families make decisions that will more likely result in a good death by *involving others*, such as social workers or clergy, to help families accept a terminal prognosis; *redirecting hope* for a good death, *and repeating and reiterating information.*
- *Are the results valid?* Yes. This is a good example of grounded theory using axial coding and dimensional analysis as an adjunct data analysis tool. Systematic method-specific procedures involved theoretical sampling, in-depth interviews with ongoing member checks, constant comparative analysis, coding (dependability), and Schatzman's (1991) approach to examining the "parts, attributes, interconnections, context, processes, and implications" of a phenome-

non (p.309). Procedures to maximize credibility of the results included: verbatim transcription of interviews that were checked for accuracy and stored in a computer software program designed to assist qualitative data management; use of memos and matrices to track the evolving theory and methodological choices made by the researcher during the study; and weekly meetings of the principal researcher with a multidisciplinary grounded theory dimensional analysis group. A diagram of providers strategies to shift patients from curative to palliative treatment choices and selected quotes enhanced understanding (confirmability and transferability), best judged by a first-hand reading of the article.

● *Will the results help me in caring for my patients?* Until patients and families shift their understanding of the patient's condition to accommodate palliative treatment choices when curative choices are of no further benefit, clinicians may be hampered in their efforts to assist the person toward "a good death." Findings raise awareness of the process professional care providers use in facilitating movement from unrealistic curative goals to realistic palliative goals. The model (described in terms of laying the groundwork, shifting the picture, and reinforcing acceptance of the new picture) may serve as a useful guide for helping patients and families make this transition at end of life.

#7 McGrath, P. (2002). Qualitative findings on the experience of end-of-life care for hematological malignancies. *American Journal of Hospice & Palliative Care, 19*, 103–111.

Question: What is the experience of patients with hematological malignancies and their families during the time traditionally associated with hospice care, i.e., the last six months of the dying trajectory and twelve months into the bereavement period?

Design: Descriptive study using a phenomenologically oriented open-ended interview approach.

Sample: Bereaved carers (N=10) in Queensland, Australia who were attending a grief course and were willing to provide retrospective insights on end-of-life experiences of loved ones with hematological malignancies.

Procedures: A researcher with counseling background and experience in working with families coping with this type of malignancy conducted audio taped interviews. Participants were encouraged to tell their stories about what the illness experience was like for patient and family from the point of the prediagnostic symptomatology up to the present (time of interview). Verbatim transcripts were analyzed thematically.

Appraisal:

● *What were the results of the study?* Multiple quotes are used to partially re-create participants' accounts of experiences that are distinguished by: (a) distressing dying scenes involving increased use of high-technology, tests, and invasive procedures; (b) traumatizing and alienating intensive care unit experiences; (c) lack of referrals to palliative care; (d) evidence of posttraumatic stress symptoms in family caregivers; and (e) absence of supportive follow-up from the hospital for family members.

● *Are the results valid?* Yes. This example of a qualitative descriptive study with phenomenological overtones enlisted participants from a grief course that resulted in 100 percent enrollment (N=10). "By the time of the third or fourth interview, it became obvious that participants were reporting very similar experiences. Consequently, by the tenth interview a high level of confidence had been achieved as to the importance and relevance of the issues being reported" (p.104). A computer software program designed to assist in qualitative data management supported analysis procedures that collapsed 104 coded data bits into five major themes. The description of these (dependability and credibility) is supported by extensive verbatim quotes (confirmability). The results are plausible, believable, and transferable, as best judged by individual readers' direct engagement with the written text of the article.

- *Will the results help me in caring for my patients?* Findings raise awareness of hardships families may encounter in the dying experience within "curative" acute care hospital settings. Insights and specific suggestions are aimed at encouraging development of more holistic family-centered palliative care strategies. These include anticipatory support in the form of providing information about hospice and palliative care early in the treatment phase; appropriate referral of patients to palliative care services at sufficiently early points in the dying trajectory; supportive care to families both during and after the terminal stage; and special consideration of following up family caregivers who may be vulnerable to symptoms of post-traumatic stress.

Individual Human Experiences

#1 Samuelsson, M., Radestad, I., & Segesten, K. (2001). A waste of life: Fathers' experience of losing a child before birth. *Birth, 28,* 124–130.

Question: How do fathers experience losing a child through intrauterine death?

Design: Phenomenology

Sample: 11 fathers in Sweden (age range between 31 to 46) whose offspring died during weeks 29 to 42 of pregnancy. For five fathers, the stillborn child was their first; six already had children. Four fathers had become fathers again after the death of the child in question; and four of the men's partners were pregnant.

Procedures: Interviews were conducted 5 to 27 months after the stillbirth. Transcribed text was analyzed in several steps: (a) reading through several times to obtain a complete picture of the content; (b) highlighting experiences related by the fathers in various subject areas; and (c) identifying and analyzing meaningful central units to pinpoint the core meaning – the essence – of the phenomenon.

Appraisal:

- *What were the results of the study?* Results were presented under 18 categories of meaning within 5 timeframes: (a) *Experiencing that the baby was no longer alive* included *feelings of an impending catastrophe* (involving shock, lack of feeling and denial); *great disappointment; consolation in their adversity* (through confirmation of their misgivings, support and information); and an urgent need to *get rid of the burden*, being concerned that the dead baby could harm their partner. (b) During the *time between being told of the baby's death and induction of labor* fathers thought that *having time to adjust* to the fact that the baby was dead was essential. Taking care of practical details and *protecting their partner* was important. (c)

The delivery was characterized by *frustration and helplessness* that at times made them feel left behind, outside of it all, confused, and submerged in a totally female-dominated world. Many missed not having another man to talk to. To most fathers *it felt right that their partner should give birth vaginally*, believing that the natural procedure (as opposed to a caesarian section) conveyed more dignity. Some felt they had played an important role and given good support to their partner. (d) The final confirmation – *the stillbirth and aftercare* – was felt as a terribly sad *waste of life*. Fathers said they approached the baby with respect, dignity, and a certain *fear of seeing their child*. All of the fathers had *tokens of remembrance from the baby*, including photos, hand and footprints, a lock of hair, and mother's and baby's identification wristbands. Aftercare was administered in the maternity ward, and most fathers remained there for 24 hours. (e) *The first time at home* was experienced as pronounced emptiness and silence. They felt cheated by life, abandoned, and vulnerable. *There were three of them when they left for the hospital, but only two came back.* The room prepared for the baby now seemed like a slap in the face. Primary elements in coming to grips with their grief and *finding their way back to everyday life* were the collected tokens of remembrance of the child and the support of the obstetric staff and hospital chaplain. Fathers perceived that *receiving support* was an urgent need, the most valuable help of which was the good relationship with their partners. Most felt their partners needed to talk and could express their feelings better, whereas they felt they were more silent and brooding. The most important help was from hospital chapel personnel and the chapel's support group for those who had lost a child before and up to a year after birth. The question of why the baby had died did not go away until the fathers had been given a definitive answer and an *explanation* of the cause. However, some fathers realized, that it is not always possible to find an answer. The fathers were at different stages of grieving, but they had begun to learn to live with the loss and move on.

- *Are the results valid*? Yes. The sampling strategy is clearly described and sample size is adequate. Information about the interview process and questions is provided. And, previously described procedures are appropriate for a phenomenologically oriented analysis of the in-depth interview data (credibility and dependability). The report of the results carefully identifies the number of fathers whose experiences are most strongly represented by certain themes, accounts for their collective experiences, and uses quotes to illustrate findings (confirmability). The writing is effective, although the individual reader must assess this along with the transferability of findings.
- *Will the results help me in caring for my patients*? Although attention is more often focused on mothers' responses to perinatal loss, these findings raise awareness of fathers' experience of stillbirth and needs for understanding the ways they manage their grief. Insights on what they found to be helpful may serve as a guide to care providers to ensure that fathers are not the "forgotten mourners" (p.125).

#2 **Jain, A., Sherman, S.N., Chamberlin, L.A., et al. (2001). Why don't low-income mothers worry about their preschoolers being overweight?** *Pediatrics, 107,* **1138–1146.**

Question: What are mothers' perceptions about childhood obesity and existing barriers to its prevention and management?

Design: Three focus groups with 6 participants in each.

Sample: 18 low-income mothers of preschool children at risk for later obesity (13 black, 5 white). The setting was a clinic of the Special Supplemental Nutrition Program for Women, Infants, and Children in Cincinnati, Ohio.

Procedures: Two of the authors, one white and one black, jointly moderated the focus groups. After each of the first two focus groups, the two leaders reviewed the questions, reworded them, and added probe questions. There was strong convergence in responses across the focus groups; and no new ideas emerged in the third. The six authors coded focus group transcripts independently and then agreed on common themes. An independent reader also reviewed the transcripts and recorded a set of themes. All of these themes were among the 22 themes identified by the primary readers through group consensus (later collapsed into 10 major themes).

Appraisal:

- *What were the results of the study?* Themes were grouped under the three major target areas for discussion. *Definition*, (exploring perceptions of how mothers determine that a child is overweight), revealed disagreement with health professionals' classifications (four themes): (a) There was shared dislike and distrust of the growth charts and the claim that they were not relevant to their children. (b) Mothers described their children's sizes in terms of bone structure (big-boned), frame (thick, solid, strong), and clothing size, indicating that a large frame was culturally acceptable and, perhaps, even desirable. (c) Children were considered overweight if seen as inactive or lazy or if they were being teased by peers. None had ever known a young child they considered obese. (d) Children were not considered overweight as long as they were active, playful, happy, and had good appetites. Two themes concerning *Etiology* (beliefs about what causes a child to be overweight) were: (a) belief that a child's size and growth pattern was fixed and predestined by nature, genetics, and heredity; and (b) belief that parents' behaviors and family environment also influenced a child's diet and activity patterns. In terms of *management* (4 themes), mothers described difficulties limiting or structuring their children's eating. (a) They reported that they were unable or did not wish to deny them food. (b) Some mothers used food as a reward for good behavior. (c) Other family members challenged mothers' control over children's diets. And, (d) mothers' own obesity affected their outlook on children's weight management.

- *Are the results valid?* Yes. Sampling reflects an effective strategy. That is, this example of a focus group study used a two-stage recruitment process. In the first stage, telephone calls to mothers of the 31 children identified by clinic records as being overweight resulted in 17 acceptances. And, because it was anticipated that some mothers would not arrive for the focus group, a second recruitment stage involved contacting 5 additional mothers whose children were identified as at increased risk for later obesity. Thus, of the total of 22 mothers who agreed to participate, 18 arrived for the 1-hour focus group session. Accuracy and validity were assured by the previously described procedures involving two of the authors' leadership in the focus groups, independent coding of transcripts by the six authors and an additional independent reviewer, and agreement on themes and most representative comments for presentation by consensus (credibility and dependability). Findings are linked to the data from which they were generated (confirmability) and are transferable, as best judged by a firsthand reading of the article.

- *Will the results help me in caring for my patients?* Findings suggest that growth charts will not be meaningful to mothers who do not share health providers' definitions of what it means to be "overweight." Therefore, it may be more effective to focus on areas of agreement (that children should follow healthy diets and be physically active) and to discuss mothers' management issues in that context rather than to approach issues by labeling children as overweight.

#3   Dixon-Woods, M., Findlay, M., Young, B., et al. (2001). Parents' accounts of obtaining a diagnosis of childhood cancer. *Lancet, 357,* 670–674.

Question: How do the time before and the process of obtaining the diagnosis of childhood cancer affect parents?

Design: Semi-structured interviews

Sample: 20 U. K. parents of children (ages 4-18 years) with a confirmed diagnosis of cancer or brain tumor.

Procedures: Purposeful sampling was explained to be an accepted method in qualitative research that does not aim for statistical representativeness. Interviews were open-ended, but a prompt guide was used to ensure that similar topics were discussed every time. All interviews were recorded and transcribed verbatim. Medical records also were analyzed. Data collection and analysis occurred concurrently. Emerging themes were refined, refocused or altered as new transcripts were analyzed; and sampling was continued to achieve theoretical saturation, i.e., when additional interviews added nothing to what was already known about the properties of categories and themes. A qualitative data analysis software program facilitated processing and analyzing textual material.

Appraisal:

● *What were the results of the study?* Parents noticed two types of *initial signs and symptoms*: (a) behavioral and affective cues indicating that something was wrong (e.g., not himself/herself, not wanting to play, quiet, nightmares, wetting self); and (b) "medical" signs and symptoms prompting help seeking (e.g., earache, fever, flu-like symptoms, weakness, vomiting). Most parents had a "wait and see" period in which they monitored symptoms and attempted to manage them with simple remedies. Unusual or frightening events (e.g., seizures, fainting, loss of coordination, or blood in urine that were judged to be abnormal) sometimes began to appear after innocent-type symptoms had been present for some time. After parents decided that their child's symptoms required further investigation, their accounts fell into two categories: *disputes and nondisputes* with ten families in each category. (a) Parents were satisfied when their child received prompt and appropriate investigation and referral. This tended to happen when a simple test, such as a blood test, could be done by the general practitioner. (b) Parents were not satisfied when they had had to insist that the doctor take action. Seven families experienced lengthy disputes, most often in cases that were harder to diagnose. Five families reported a long wait for their first appointment with a specialist, which caused considerable distress since their children deteriorated during this wait. Other families had difficulty convincing specialists of the seriousness of the situation and told stories of incompetence and delay. Some delays ended only if parents demanded action or when a medical crisis (e.g., kidney failure) happened. Two families were not referred to secondary care at all. *Parents' reactions to diagnosis* were affected by their experiences of obtaining the diagnosis. Some who had had to struggle to obtain a diagnosis felt vindicated or relieved by an identifiable condition for which something could be done. Those parents whose child was diagnosed within hours or days described feeling shock, numbness, and disbelief. And, some parents felt guilty and self-reproachful for not having more effectively advocated for their child.

● *Are the results valid?* Yes. This example of a qualitative interview study used purposeful sampling to enroll participants who met study criteria. "To avoid distressing parents or introducing bias by interviewing them when their child was in a critical condition, parents were approached only when a consultant said that the child was sufficiently stable" (p.671). Out of 21 families approached, 20 agreed to participate. A constant comparative approach supported trustworthiness (dependability and credibility) of findings. Interviews and transcripts were analyzed concurrently and emerging themes were refined, refocused, or altered as new interview transcripts were analyzed. Sampling continued until theoretical saturation was reached at the fourteenth interview. "Thereafter, every new statement could be fitted into existing themes without amendment – later interviews confirmed this analysis" (p. 671). Parents gave very detailed accounts; and verbatim quotes accompany the reported results (confirmability). Findings are plausible and believable; but further judgments of meaningfulness and transferability must be made independently by readers of this article.

● *Will the results help me in caring for my patients?* These interviews offer insights into parents' experiences, including disputes with physicians and delays in obtaining a diagnosis. It may make health providers more sensitive to the need for trusting parents' specific knowledge of their children and their usual health and behavioral pattern and more alert to training, communication, and systems issues that could be causes of errors and delays.

#4   Wise, B.V. (2002). In their own words: The lived experience of pediatric liver transplantation. *Qualitative Health Research, 12,* 74–90.

Question: What are children's perspectives on the period prior to liver transplantation, through surgery, and beyond; and what meanings do they give to this experience and to what they discover in their everyday lives after transplantation?

Design: van Manen's (1990) hermeneutic phenomenological approach

Sample: 9 children between the ages of 7 and 15 (5 girls and 4 boys representing school age and adolescent developmental periods) who were 3 to 9 years post–liver transplantation.

Procedures: Purposeful sampling was used. As an opening to in-depth conversations, children were asked to tell a story about the persons in two pictures they were asked to draw: one of themselves before transplant and another that reflected their current status. (An art therapist provided an initial interpretation of the drawings.) Taped interviews were transcribed and contextual fieldnotes were added to describe the setting, nonverbal behavior of the children/adolescents, and interruptions in the flow of conversations. Analysis occurred simultaneously with data collection. Techniques included use of reading and rereading, reflection and clarification, a dialectic process to identify themes, and reflective writing. A qualitative data analysis software program facilitated processing and analyzing of textual material.

Appraisal:

● *What were the results of the study?* Only one child followed directions and drew two pictures. The rest drew themselves that day, choosing colors identical to those in which they were dressed. Most stated they did not remember what they looked like before transplantation. One brought out family pictures of periods before and after transplant. (Many had received transplants as an infant with family pictures their only clue to their appearance and degree of illness.) Four major themes were described. The first theme, *"Searching for connections: Being the same and different,"* describes children's peer relationship experiences before and after transplant and their connecting to a donor. Children reported visible differences (e.g., appearance, energy level) that attracted the attention of others. All sought a "best friend" to help normalize their experiences at school and with other children. The experience of transplantation produced feelings of chaos and an understanding that their former lives were over. But peers tended not to understand the serious nature of their illness and misinterpreted long absences from school. Few children indicated an interest in learning about the donor. However, one participant met the donor family in a planned donor awareness event. And, two had living-related liver transplants using parental donors. The second theme, *"Being surrounded by sick people can be weird: Ordinary experiences,"* concerned what was perceived as ordinary and extraordinary about the hospital milieu. Though children could relate "scary" or "weird" aspects, the hospital was not new or unknown to them. Families and children attempted to fit the experience of transplantation into their ordinary lives by normalizing it (i.e., fitting medication regimes, clinic visits, or repeat hospitalizations around other school, work, and play events). Children sought routines and avoided calling attention to themselves. The third theme, *"It really hurted and I had to scream,"* involved the notion of pain, being hurt, or out of control with their lives. Three types of painful experiences were described: recurrent experiences (e.g., drawing blood), surgical pain, and procedural pain. Accounts were graphic and poignant. The fourth theme, *"I know my mom is upset, she worries too much,"* concerned parental responses. Children stated they did not like to tell their parents how they felt because it worries them. They felt they had a responsibility to protect their parents and to stay well. Maintaining normalcy was important to the children. And transforming their lives after transplantation involved maintaining a sense of self by connecting past realities with newly emerging realities at home, school, and with peers.

- *Are the results valid?* Yes. This is a good example of a study using van Manen's (1990) approach to hermeneutic phenomenology. Three criteria to evaluate the rigor of the research were discussed. Trustworthiness (dependability) of data to establish validity was ensured by the researcher stating preunderstandings, describing relationships with and steps taken to approach participants, and documenting data gathering and analysis decisions and processes. Credibility was assured by presenting the written text to participants and/or expert consultants for validation. Coherence of the evolving interpretation was assured by purposeful sampling to obtain accounts from children of different ages, genders and races and with varied complexities of illness experience and outcomes. Themes are illustrated by stories and quotes to show how findings fit the data from which they were generated (confirmability). These make results plausible, believable, and transferable as best judged by a first-hand reading of the article.

- *Will the results help me in caring for my patients?* Findings reveal how children with chronic and life-threatening disease strive for normalcy in their lives. Therefore, "it is imperative that interventions focus on normal development rather than on what is different about the child... [and] encourage independence" (p.88). Meeting psychosocial needs for support during every phase of transplantation (from time of diagnosis through resuming life as a transplant recipient) is emphasized through use of examples. "Dialoguing with children... listening to what

[they] have to say about what is important to them and encouraging them to be active participants in their care (p. 88)" is a central theme throughout.

#5   Farmer, T. J. (2002). The experience of major depression: Adolescents' perspectives. *Issues in Mental Health Nursing, 23,* 567–585.

Question: What are adolescents' perspectives on what it is like to be depressed?

Design: Colaizzi's (1978) descriptive phenomenological approach.

Sample: Purposive sample of 5 depressed adolescents from a Southwestern U.S. mental health facility (3 female and 2 male, ages 13 to17, and of Caucasian, Hispanic, or African American ethnicity).

Procedures: The data-eliciting statement – "Tell me as fully as you can what it is like for you to be depressed" – was given to participants a week in advance of in-depth audio taped interviews. Interviews ended when participants felt they had completed what they wished to say. Analysis involved extracting significant statements and restating them in more general terms, followed by formulation of meanings that attempted to capture underlying meanings. Meanings were grouped by themes and then into larger clusters and general categories. All findings were incorporated into a narrative description used as the basis for identifying the essential structure of the experience of depression for adolescents.

Appraisal:

- *What were the results of the study?* Adolescents focused on anger, fatigue, and interpersonal difficulties as characteristic of depression. Eight theme categories were identified: (a) dispirited weariness; (b) emotional homelessness: sense of aloneness; (c) emotional homelessness: no safety where expected; (d) unrelenting anger; (e) parental break-up: caught in the middle; (f) spectrum of escape from pain; (g) perspectives on friendship; and (h) gaining a sense of getting well. Pervasive, unrelenting, easily triggered, and rapidly escalating anger directed against self, parents, siblings, friends, and teachers was the most frequently discussed experience. Strong perceptions of aloneness, diminished sense of closeness, mourning losses, and weariness beyond physical fatigue led to loss of motivation to see friends, do school work, and invest in self. Decline of academic performance produced guilt and lowered self-esteem. Depressive symptoms increased with being both witness and victim of discord, divorce, abuse, and manipulation. Friends played a variable role in the experience, from being sources of support to sources of pain and rejection. Escape from the pain was sought through temporary measures or by suicidal thoughts and actions. Therapy began with the recognition of the need for help and was experienced as an up and down course. Part of the sense of getting well involved thinking of adequate descriptors of the experience, trying to understand reasons for becoming depressed, measuring symptomatic improvement, and recognizing that unresolved issues remain. Four of the five participants claimed to have had symptoms of depression for a year or more before receiving treatment.
- *Are the results valid?* Yes. This is an example of a study using Colaizzi's (1978) descriptive phenomenological approach. "Application of trustworthiness strategies [credibility and dependability]...to enhance scientific rigor included conducting lengthy, in-depth interviews; recording careful fieldnotes on interview details; checking transcripts against audiotapes for

accuracy; initial identification and then bracketing and subsequent reviewing of the investigator's beliefs about adolescent depression to increase validity of the emerging themes; careful documenting of data analysis steps to provide an audit trail; debriefings with faculty advisors; and sharing of findings with faculty members, practicing psychotherapists, and formerly depressed adolescents with subsequent refinement of results" (p. 572). Stories and quotes link findings to the data from which they were generated (confirmability). A sense of the meaningfulness and transferability of these findings is better obtained through a thoughtful reading of the article that attempts to put oneself in the place of the other.

- *Will the result help me in caring for my patients?* Findings underscore a need for those in contact with adolescents to be more aware of symptoms such as falling grades, fatigue and anger and to be mindful of responses to such things as friendship and family changes. Teen reports of suffering symptoms for a year or more prior to treatment are noteworthy. "Certainly the recognition of potential problems by a nurse, physician, teacher, or parent could have resulted in an illness of shorter duration and less discomfort" (p. 582).

#6   Machoian, L. (2001). Cutting voices: Self-injury in three adolescent girls. *Journal of Psychosocial Nursing, 39,* 22–29.

Question: What do adolescent girls know about why they inflict harm on themselves?

Design: Case study analysis using in-depth, semi-structured interviews.

Sample: Purposeful sample of 3 Caucasian girls between the ages of 12 to 17, from working class to upper middle class families, whose self-injury involved cutting. They were selected purposefully from among participants in a larger research project examining suicidal and self-injurious behavior in adolescents.

Procedures: Interviews were audio taped and transcribed. The Listener's Guide method of data analysis (Brown et al, 1988) was used. It involves multiple focused readings of the same text to listen for the presence of different themes and requires the reader to maintain a trail of evidence for interpretation by connecting interpretive statements to verbatim parts of the transcript using worksheets.

Appraisal:

- *What were the results of the study?* Three prominent themes that emerged were: (a) cutting gained a response when girls' speaking voices failed (i.e., cutting is noticed and taken seriously by others); (b) communicative cutting leads to affect regulation (i.e., cutting becomes a way to cope with psychological pain); and (c) adults listening is very important (i.e., girls described not being listened to and not receiving help for psychological distress until they inflicted harm on themselves). Each girl described a history of trauma and familial alcoholism that might explain this perceived lack of responsiveness. "A catch-22 for girls who cut is that, although their self-directed violence may have its onset in the service of self-preservation, it can lead them to be pejoratively labeled as manipulative in mental health settings, which may perpetrate further dismissal.... [Girls' awareness of this may] contribute to and exacerbate preexisting feelings of self-blame and self-loathing...[and] the pejorative label may increase risk, interfere with or lead to negativity with treatment providers, and may perpetuate a cycle of using violence" (p.27).

- *Are the results valid?* Yes. This is a good example of a qualitative case study analysis based on in-depth interviews. As noted, the three study participants were purposefully selected. And the voice-centered relational method used involved multiple readings of the data and maintaining a trail of evidence for interpretations (dependability). A structured analytic approach helped to assure accuracy and credibility of findings. "The first reading is for the general plot....The second reading is for the girl's first-person voice. And the third and fourth readings depend on the research question(s) and may be derived directly from the data. Hypothetically, there can be any number of readings" (p. 25). Sensitivity to what study participants had to say about their experiences (confirmability and transferability) of self-injury requires reflective first-hand engagement with the written text.

- *Will the results help me in caring for my patients?* Study conclusions emphasize the importance of listening, responding, and taking adolescents seriously. On the basis of evidence provided by these findings, adults are encouraged to understand the language and signals that convey distress even when they are "complex, dangerous, and seemingly dramatic" (p.28). And professionals in clinical settings are advised to avoid inflicting further pain by use of pejorative labeling of behaviors.

#7 Knobf, M. T. (2002). Carrying on: The experience of premature menopause in women with early stage breast cancer. *Nursing Research, 51*, 9–17.

Question: What substantive theory will describe and explain women's responses to chemotherapy induced premature menopause within the context of breast cancer?

Design: Grounded theory

Sample: 27 women with a primary breast cancer diagnosis who were premenopausal at the beginning of adjuvant chemotherapy and had documented menstrual irregularities or subjective menopausal symptoms following therapy.

Procedures: Collected data included participant interviews, informal discussions with specialty physicians and nurses, fieldnotes from national conferences and seminars, laywomen's writings, and memos (analytic notes). Based on analysis of data from the first ten purposively selected participants, theoretical sampling was used to maximize variation in the data, discover the range of data with confirming and disconfirming cases, and verify relationships among the data. Constant comparative method was used to simultaneously collect, code, and analyze data.

Appraisal:

- *What were the results of the study?* Vulnerability was identified as the basic social problem for women, as it relates to concerns about a cancer diagnosis, responses to chemotherapy side effects, alterations in self concept, threatened sense of control over body and health, uncertainty, unpredictability of symptoms, and unknown risks of future health problems related to early menopause. Carrying on was identified as the basic social psychological process (BSPP) that explains how women respond to vulnerability as they begin to assimilate early menopause into their recovery from breast cancer. Women did not move through the four stages of this process in a distinct linear fashion, but often moved back and forth between stages. The first stage of *Being Focused* represents the time during chemotherapy when getting through the treatment is the main priority. Women's responses at this time were *minimizing menopausal symptoms* and *isolating the meaning of menopause* in order to deal with it objectively and secondarily to their cancer experience. The second stage of *Facing Uncertainty* involved a transition from a crisis response to one of greater reflection. Uncertainty reflected difficulty in distinguishing what part of the experience was attributable to breast cancer or to menopause. This stage was characterized by *structured silence* (absence of dialogue about menopause with physicians and nurses), *relying on self* to define and interpret symptoms and hormonal changes, and *being prepared* for experiencing induced menopause (that ranged from not being prepared at all to some degree of preparation). The stage of *Becoming Menopausal* involved *exploring meaning* (perceived as a shock and a sadness, a nonnatural body experience which was not age appropriate, and feeling old) and *living with symptoms*. Women's acceptance of symptoms ranged from accepting, being resigned and tolerating them, to adjusting and taking action toward symptom relief. Responses were influenced by uncertainty of cause (chemotherapy, breast cancer, menopause), time since treatment, level of discomfort, and interference with daily activities. The final stage of *Balancing* involved use of three strategies aimed at protecting physical and psychological health. *Being wary* reflected a heightened awareness of risks associated with anything that affects the physical body. *Keeping healthy* involved taking actions toward symptom relief and lifestyle changes to minimize health risks (e.g., exercise and diet plans). *Struggling with the system of care* relates to women's awareness that physicians may be limited by the mindset of their specialty and unable to focus holistically on their needs for information and support.

- *Are the results valid*? Yes. The author of this example of grounded theory described the following research activities addressing criteria of credibility, transferability, dependability, and confirmability: using multiple data sources, sharing data with two nonparticipant women from the target population for common findings, consultation with methods experts and faculty, and developing an audit trail of memos and field notes. Diagrams and quotes demonstrate the connection between findings and the data from which they were generated. These help to draw the reader into the experience, as best judged by reading the article.

- *Will the results help me in caring for my patients*? Findings provide insights into the complexity of experiencing two major life events for women – breast cancer and menopause – simultaneously and the process of carrying on. There is evidence of a need for anticipatory guidance and understanding support. For example, women reported that "physicians generally did not describe the various patterns of menstrual irregularities and rarely discussed menopausal symptoms other than hot flashes. For women who were symptomatic, not being well prepared was associated with more emotional distress (Knobf, 1999), but even asymptomatic women would have liked being better prepared for the experience" (p. 13).

#8 **Sturge-Jacobs, M. (2002). The experience of living with fibromyalgia: Confronting an invisible disability.** *Research and Theory for Nursing Practice: An International Journal, 16,* 19–31.

Question: What is it like to live with fibromyalgia (FM)?

Design: Thematic analysis, using van Manen's (1990) phenomenological methodology.

Sample: 9 women diagnosed with a primary diagnosis of FM for at least one year (age range 20-57) who attended a 6-week outpatient education program at a tertiary care facility in Newfoundland, Canada.

Procedures: Purposeful sampling was used to select women who would be introspective and self reflective about their experiences as they told their stories.

Unstructured interviews to elicit definitive and broad statements about personal experiences were followed by telephone contact at 2-week and 4-week intervals to obtain further information or to clarify existing material. Analysis was a collaborative process, with each participant being asked for feedback on her transcribed interview and perceptions about identified themes.

Appraisal:

- *What were the results of the study?* The essence of living with FM was *confronting an invisible disability.* Eight themes were identified: (a) *Pain* – the constant presence was a prominent theme throughout. (b) *Fatigue* – the invisible foe and (c) *sleep* – the impossible dream further defined women's experience of overwhelming exhaustion. (d) *Thinking in a fog* described difficulties with problem solving, abstract thinking, and inability to make appropriate judgment calls or on the spot decisions. And, (e) *dealing with a flare-up* signified the unpredictability and fluctuating nature of the symptoms that were primary concerns. During flare-ups, a decrease in muscular strength and inability to walk without stumbling was evident. Others told stories of disorientation and frightening situations with inability to judge distance and space. (f) *Longing for a normal life* was a common desire. All participants spoke of the importance of "doing family things" and "keeping up a good front"; but these attempts at "normalizing" were often at great physical and emotional expense. (g) Women's stories reflected *the power of naming* – seeking a diagnosis where, more often than not, numerous visits and consultations with a variety of specialists added to confusion and chaos. The complexity of symptoms, coupled with poor understanding of the syndrome by many physicians, made it difficult to obtain an appropriate diagnosis. Finally, (h) *living within the boundaries* was vital to participants being in control of the condition, rather than the condition controlling them. However, this acceptance did not happen without a period of mourning losses. Well-meaning family and friends were not always understanding, thinking the mourning to be out of proportion, given that the condition was neither disfiguring nor life-threatening.

- *Are the results valid?* Yes. The processes of purposeful sampling and other procedures were described and sample size was adequate for this phenomenological study (dependability). As noted, participants provided feedback on their interview transcripts and also on emerging themes, ensuring accuracy and credibility. "Because of this activity, some participants suggested minor changes in naming a theme...hence, most titles of the themes came from the participants' own words. This collaborative process was necessary to ensure that interpretations were truly reflective of the participants' lived experiences [confirmability]"(p. 23). The result is an article that, on first-hand reading, provides insight on what persons with fibromyalgia experience that may be transferable and increase sensitivity to their suffering.

- *Will the results help me in caring for my patients?* Findings that enhance understanding of what living with FM is like may enable care providers to be more empathetic and supportive. Because FM is a poorly understood rheumatic condition and difficult to diagnosis, "some medical practitioners even question its existence... For years FM was thought to be the result of a psychological condition... It is now believed that depression and anxiety are the result of, not the cause of FM" (p. 20). Therefore, care providers need to acknowledge women's struggles respectfully and compassionately, seeking to empower them by "eliciting their own strengths to manage and control their lives" (p. 29). (See also Schaefer, 1995, for a feminist grounded theory of women living with fibromyalgia.)

#9 Hilton, E. L. (2002). The meaning of stroke in elderly women: A phenomenological investigation. *Journal of Gerontological Nursing, 28,* 19–26.

Question: What is the meaning of having and surviving a stroke within the daily life context of elderly noninstitutionalized women?

Design: van Manen's (1990) humanistic hermeneutic phenomenological approach to thematic analysis.

Sample: A purposive sample of 5 noninstitutionalized elderly women, ranging in age from 66 to 80, who were at least 65 years old when the stroke occurred, were at least 1 year poststroke, and who had sufficient recall and communication abilities to describe and discuss their experiences.

Procedures: Data collection involved open-ended questions; and participants were interviewed twice. Second interviews focused on fuller descriptions of transcribed and narrated experiences and validation of interpreted data. Redundancy ensured data saturation. Data analysis followed van Manen's method to identify thematic structures.

Appraisal:

- *What were the results of the study?* The overarching theme was that women believed they were in a state of transition with transformation as a result of the stroke. "An important facet of the central theme was the women's ability to survive this challenging and paradoxical process, and actively engage in transformation. They sought new roles, identified new strategies of coping, and reconciled with realities of stroke-imposed limitations" (p.23). Five subthemes were embedded within transformation: (a) deterioration and decline; (b) losses and helplessness; (c) regret; (d) uncertainty and anxiety about the future; and (e) resiliency. Six interwoven additional themes were: (a) dawning awareness of self as disabled – the nature of stroke; (b) life and suffering through inexorable losses; (c) quest for self, embodiment of disability; (d) adaptation to change; (e) existential reestablishment of self; and (f) reconciliation and reengagement.

- *Are the results valid?* Yes. This study is procedurally consistent with van Manen's approach to phenomenology (dependability), the steps of which are designed to ensure validity and credibility. These activities are described and involve: turning to the nature of the research question focused on the phenomenon (the lived experience); existential investigation, including searching for anything that may, on reflective imagination, yield something of its fundamental nature; using allusions and hidden meanings to consider data within context and to view experiences from primary sources; phenomenological writing and rewriting; maintaining a strong, pedagogical relationship to the phenomenon, involving constant engagement in readings and discussions about elderly women with stroke; and considering the research context of the lives of participants, in particular, effects of the research method on informants (several of whom said they had a clearer understanding of stroke processes as a result of their participation) (p. 22). Participants were interviewed twice; and redundancy ensured data saturation, negating the need for additional informants or data collection sessions (credibility). "Initial bracketing acknowledged and set aside specific investigator biases" (p. 22). Results present a multi-layered picture of the phenomenon from the perspective of elderly women stroke survivors enhanced by quotes and personal details (confirmability and transferability) best appreciated through a first-hand reading of the article.

- *Will the results help me in caring for my patients?* Awareness of meanings of individual stroke experiences may help healthcare providers understand more completely the kinds of support that elderly women need. "This information enables increased specificity in planning, rendering, and evaluating care" (p. 26). A humanistic approach based on insights from evidence supplied by this report may include: (a) facilitating transformation into disability by exploring their views of and plans for the future; (b) encouraging exploration of change through use of life review; (c) helping them discern and define priorities for recovery; (d) facilitating an awareness of their progress to instill hope; (e) actively listening as a form of validation and acknowledgment of the importance attributed to understanding women's experiences; (f) being sensitive to and facilitating recovery from dysfunctional grieving or mourning; and (g) demonstrating acceptance of women's coming to terms with an uncertain future (pp. 25-26).

#10 Wilde, M. H. (2002). Urine flowing: A phenomenological study of living with a urinary catheter. *Research in Nursing & Health, 25,* 14–24.

Question: What is it like to live with a long-term indwelling urinary catheter?

Design: Merleau-Ponty's phenomenology and van Manen's methodology.

Sample: A purposeful sample of 14 persons (9 women and 5 men, age span of 35-95 years) from urban, suburban, and rural settings with long-term (6 months to 18 years) indwelling urinary catheters. "The primary reason for wearing the catheter was urinary retention caused by disease conditions, including multiple sclerosis, cerebrovascular accident, enlarged prostate, and spinal cord injury (SCI)...Because younger people were expected to have different experiences, four people with SCI (ages 35-48) were recruited after interviews with the first ten participants revealed that no one in the sample was less than 56 years old" (p.16).

Procedures: Data collection involved audio taped interviews in participants' homes. Second interviews (n=7) early in the data collection period helped to clarify and expand emerging ideas. A computer software program supported data management. Data analysis was guided by Merleau-Ponty's phenomenology (1962, 1968), specifically related to a philosophy of embodiment. "Embodiment...is defined as how humans live in and know about the world through their bodies, especially through movement, perception, language, time, sexuality, and emotions" (Wilde, 1999) (p. 16). Because Merleau-Ponty's philosophy does not contain a specific research approach, van Manen's (1990, 1997) methodology Was used to guide "research activities". These included "turning to" and investigating the nature of the lived through hermeneutic (interpretive) phenomenological reflection, writing, and rewriting.

Appraisal:

- *What were the results of the study?* "Living with the forces of flowing water" was the dominant recurring metaphor that emerged from the analysis and interpretation of participants' descriptions of their experiences. "People talked about lacking control of urine flow, the sound and weight of urine in the bag, and sensations in their bladders attributed to changes in urine flow" (p. 19). The following themes were identified and discussed: (a) vulnerability: the force of flowing water; (b) embarrassment at lack of control: "Swish/Woosh;" (c) watchful attention to urine flow: "Running all the while;" (d) noise in the urine bag: "Slosh-Slosh;" (e) the metaphor of "the Spring" (from the embodied speech of a man who called his catheter the 'waterworks' and his bladder the 'spring'); and (f) embodied knowledge of urine flow: "paying attention" (i.e., skills people developed by "paying attention to what their bodies could teach them, especially about keeping their urine flowing freely (p. 21)" and avoiding painful blockages and complications related to catheter care).

- *Are the results valid?* Yes. This is a good example of a study that is guided by Merleau-Ponty's phenomenology and uses van Manen's methodology to advance procedurally. Validity, therefore, involves maintaining a strong connection to the philosophical foundation with its emphasis on embodiment while engaging in research activities structured to ensure an accurate and credible interpretation of the experience. Both the philosophy and methodological steps are described (dependability and credibility). The latter included: turning to the nature of the lived experience, investigation of the lived experience, and a dialectic, iterative process of hermeneutic phenomenological reflection and writing. Accuracy and clarification of data were accomplished through restatement to participants of what had been heard and recorded earlier. "By following how data were analyzed, readers can evaluate the reasonableness of procedures and therefore the trustworthiness of the findings" (p. 19). Findings are linked to the data from which they were generated (confirmability). Understanding of the meaningfulness and transferability of this report requires a first-hand reading.

- *Will the results help me in caring for my patients?* The purpose of this research was to understand what persons who wear long-term indwelling catheters experience as well as to discover their taken-for-granted knowledge about management of day-to-day issues and catheter maintenance so that nurses might provide more thoughtful and meaningful care. Nurses may tell persons with new urinary catheters "that they can expect to become aware of certain sensations and sounds associated with the catheter;... help [them] become prepared for dealing with urine flow issues when outside the home, [enabling them] to prevent urine accidents and remain active. Finally, because of the silence about catheters, nurses may need to begin discussions to draw out their patients' responses. Individuals with catheters may minimize embarrassing or frustrating experiences and even laugh about mishaps, but they would still benefit from empathic listening and support from their nurses" (p.22).

References

Anderson, D. G., & Imle, M. A. (2001). Families of origin of homeless and never-homeless women. *Western Journal of Nursing Research, 23,* 394–413.

Anderson, N. L. R. (1990). Pregnancy resolution decisions in juvenile detention. *Archives of Psychiatric Nursing, 4,* 325–331.

Anderson, N. L. R. (1994). Resolutions and risk-taking in juvenile detention. *Clinical Nursing Research, 3,* 297–315.

Anderson, N. L. R. (1996). Decisions about substance abuse among adolescents in juvenile detention. *IMAGE: Journal of Nursing Scholarship, 28,* 65–70.

Anderson, N. L. R. (1999). Perceptions about substance use among male adolescents in juvenile detention. *Western Journal of Nursing, 21,* 342–351.

Anderson, N. L. R., Nyamathi, A., McAvoy, J. A., Conde, F., & Casey, C. (2001). Perceptions about risk for HIV/AIDS among adolescents in juvenile detention. *Western Journal of Nursing Research, 23,* 336–359.

Aston, M. L. (2002). Learning to be a normal mother: Empowerment and pedagogy in post-partum classes. *Public Health Nursing, 19,* 284–293.

Benner, P. (1984). *From novice to expert.* Menlo Park, CA: Addison-Wesley.

Brown, L. M., Argyris, D., Antanucci, J., Bardige, B., Gilligan, C., Johnston, K., Miller, B., Os-borne, D., Tappan, M., Ward, J., Wiggins, O., & Wilcox, D. (1988). *A guide to reading narra-tives of conflict and choice for self and moral voice.* Cambridge, MA: Harvard Project on Women's Psychology and girls' development.

Butcher, H. K., Holkup, P. A., & Buckwalter, K. C. (2001). The experience of caring for a family member with Alzheimer's Disease. *Western Journal of Nursing Research, 23,* 33–55.

Chase-Ziolek, M., & Gruca, J. (2000). Clients' perceptions of distinctive aspects of nursing care received within a congregational setting. *Journal of Community Health Nursing, 17,* 171–183.

Chase-Ziolek, M., & Iris, M. (2002). Nurses' per-spectives on the distinctive aspects of providing nursing care in a congregational setting. *Journal of Community Health Nursing, 19,* 173–186.

Colaizzi, P. F. (1978). Psychological research as the phenomenologist views it. In R. S. Valle & M. King (Eds.), *Existential-phenomenological alternatives for philosophy* (pp. 48–71). New York: Oxford.

Dixon-Woods, M., Findlay, M., Young, B., Cox, H., & Heney, D. (2001). Parents' accounts of obtaining a diagnosis of childhood cancer. *The Lancet, 357,* 670–674.

Farmer, T. J. (2002). The experience of major de-pression: Adolescents' perspectives. *Issues in Mental Health Nursing, 23,* 567–585.

Hilton, E. L. (2002). The meaning of stroke in eld-erly women: A phenomenological investigation. *Journal of Gerontological Nursing, 28,* 19–26.

Hinds, P. S., Vogel, R. J., & Clark-Steffin, L. (1997). The possibilities and pitfalls of doing a secondary analysis of a qualitative data set. *Qualitative Health Research, 7,* 408–423.

Hurlock-Chorostecki, C. (2002). Management of pain during weaning from mechanical ventila-tion: The nature of nurse decision-making. *Canadian Journal of Nursing Research, 34,* 33–47.

Jain, A., Sherman, S. N., Chamberlin, L. A., Carter, Y., Powers, S. W., & Whitaker, R. C. (2001). Why don't low-income mothers worry about their preschoolers being overweight? *Pe-diatrics, 107,* 1138–1146.

Knobf, M. T. (1999). The influence of symptom distress and preparation on responses of women with early-stage breast cancer to induced menopause. *Psycho-Oncology, 8,* (6 suppl.), 88.

Knobf, M. T. (2002). Carrying on: The experience of premature menopause in women with early stage breast cancer. *Nursing Research, 51,* 9–17.

Lupton, D. (1997). Foucault and the medicalisa-tion critique. In A. Petersen & R. Bunton (Eds.), *Foucault, health and medicine* (pp. 94–110). London: Routledge.

Lupton, D., & Fenwick, J. (2001). 'They've for-gotten that I'm the mum': constructing and practising motherhood in special care nurseries. *Social Science & Medicine, 53,* 1011–1021.

Machoian, L. (2001). Cutting voices: Self-injury in three adolescent girls. *Journal of Psychosocial Nursing, 39,* 22–29.

McGrath, P. (2002). Qualitative findings on the ex-perience of end-of-life care for hematological malignancies. *American Journal of Hospice & Palliative Care, 19,* 103–111.

Merleau-Ponty, M. (1962). *Phenomenology of per-ception* (C. Smith, Trans.). New York: Rout-ledge Kegan Paul. (Original work published 1945.)

Merleau-Ponty, M. (1968). *The visible and the in-visible: Followed by working notes* (C. Lefort, Ed.; A. Lingis, Trans.). Evanston, IL: North-western University Press. (Original work pub-lished 1964.)

Merritt-Gray, M., & Wuest, J. (1995). Counteract-ing abuse and breaking free: The process of leaving revealed through women's voices. *Health Care for Women International, 16,* 399–412.

Norton, S. A., & Bowers, B. J. (2001). Working to-ward consensus: Providers' strategies to shift patients from curative to palliative treatment choices. *Research in Nursing & Health, 24,* 258–269.

Norton, S. A., & Talerico, K. A. (2000). Facilitat-ing end-of-life decision-making: Strategies for communicating and assessing. *Journal of Gerontological Nursing, 26,* 6–13.

Powers, B. A. (2003). *Ethics in long-term care: Issues affecting nursing home residents with dementia*. New York: Springer.

Rose, L., Mallinson, R. K., & Walton-Moss, B. (2002). A grounded theory of families responding to mental illness. *Western Journal of Nursing Research, 24,* 516–536.

Samuelsson, M., Radestad, I., & Segesten, K.. (2001). A waste of life: Fathers' experience of losing a child before birth. *BIRTH, 28,* 124–130.

Schaefer, K. M. (1995). Struggling to maintain balance: a study of women living with fibromyalgia. *Journal of Advanced Nursing, 21,* 95–102.

Spradley, J. P. (1979). *The ethnographic interview*. New York: Holt, Rinehart, & Winston.

Sturge-Jacobs, M. (2002). The experience of living with fibromyalgia: Confronting an invisible disability. *Research and Theory for Nursing Practice: An International Journal, 16,* 19–31.

Tuck, I., & Wallace, D. C. (2000). Exploring parish nursing from an ethnographic perspective. *Journal of Transcultural Nursing, 11,* 290–299.

van Kaam, A. (1966). *Existential foundations of psychology*. New York: Image.

Varcoe, C. (1996). Theorizing oppression: Implications for nursing research on violence against women. *Canadian Journal of Nursing Research, 28,* 61–78.

Varcoe, C. (2001). Abuse obscured: An ethnographic account of emergency nursing in relation to violence against women. *Canadian Journal of Nursing Research, 32,* 95–115.

Wallace, D. C., Tuck, I., Boland, C. S., & Witucki, J. M. (2002). Client perceptions of parish nursing. *Public Health Nursing, 19,* 128–135.

Wilde, M. H. (1999). Why embodiment now? *Advances in Nursing Science, 22*(2), 25–38.

Wilde, M. H. (2002). Urine flowing: A phenomenological study of living with a urinary catheter. *Research in Nursing & Health, 25,* 14–24.

Wise, B. V. (2002). In their own words: The lived experience of pediatric liver transplantation. *Qualitative Health Research, 12,* 74–90.

Wuest, J. (1995). Feminist grounded theory: An exploration of congruency and tensions between two methods of knowledge discovery in nursing. *Qualitative Health Research, 5,* 125–137.

Wuest, J., & Merritt-Gray, M. (1997). Participatory action research: Practical dilemmas and emancipatory possibilities. In J. Morse (Ed.), *Completing a qualitative research project: Details and dialogue* (pp. 283–306). Thousand Oaks, CA: Sage.

Wuest, J., & Merritt-Gray, M. (1999). Not going back: Sustaining the separation in the process of leaving abusive relationships. *Violence against women, 5,* 110–133.

Wuest, J., & Merritt-Gray (2001). Beyond survival: Reclaiming self after leaving an abusive male partner. *Canadian Journal of Nursing Research, 32,* 79–94.

Young, H. M., McCormick, W. M., & Vitaliano, P. P. (2002a). Attitudes toward community-based services among Japanese American families. *The Gerontologist, 42,* 814–825.

Young, H. M., McCormick, W. M., & Vitaliano, P. P. (2002b). Evolving values in community-based long-term care services for Japanese Americans. *Advances in Nursing Science, 25*(2), 40–56.

appendix B

527

Approved Consent Form
for a Study

appendix C

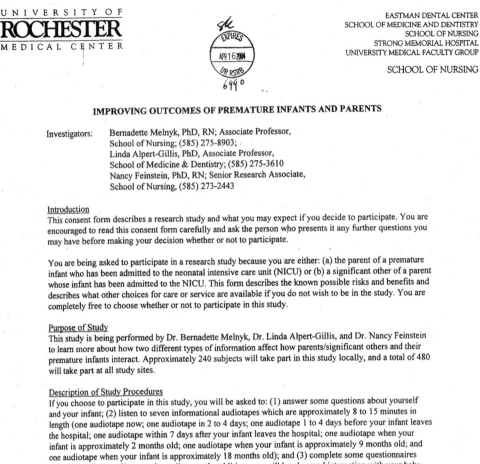

UNIVERSITY OF
ROCHESTER
MEDICAL CENTER

EASTMAN DENTAL CENTER
SCHOOL OF MEDICINE AND DENTISTRY
SCHOOL OF NURSING
STRONG MEMORIAL HOSPITAL
UNIVERSITY MEDICAL FACULTY GROUP

SCHOOL OF NURSING

EXPIRES
APR 16 2004
UR RSRB
699°

IMPROVING OUTCOMES OF PREMATURE INFANTS AND PARENTS

Investigators: Bernadette Melnyk, PhD, RN; Associate Professor,
School of Nursing; (585) 275-8903;
Linda Alpert-Gillis, PhD, Associate Professor,
School of Medicine & Dentistry; (585) 275-3610
Nancy Feinstein, PhD, RN; Senior Research Associate,
School of Nursing, (585) 273-2443

Introduction
This consent form describes a research study and what you may expect if you decide to participate. You are encouraged to read this consent form carefully and ask the person who presents it any further questions you may have before making your decision whether or not to participate.

You are being asked to participate in a research study because you are either: (a) the parent of a premature infant who has been admitted to the neonatal intensive care unit (NICU) or (b) a significant other of a parent whose infant has been admitted to the NICU. This form describes the known possible risks and benefits and describes what other choices for care or service are available if you do not wish to be in the study. You are completely free to choose whether or not to participate in this study.

Purpose of Study
This study is being performed by Dr. Bernadette Melnyk, Dr. Linda Alpert-Gillis, and Dr. Nancy Feinstein to learn more about how two different types of information affect how parents/significant others and their premature infants interact. Approximately 240 subjects will take part in this study locally, and a total of 480 will take part at all study sites.

Description of Study Procedures
If you choose to participate in this study, you will be asked to: (1) answer some questions about yourself and your infant; (2) listen to seven informational audiotapes which are approximately 8 to 15 minutes in length (one audiotape now; one audiotape in 2 to 4 days; one audiotape 1 to 4 days before your infant leaves the hospital; one audiotape within 7 days after your infant leaves the hospital; one audiotape when your infant is approximately 2 months old; one audiotape when your infant is approximately 9 months old; and one audiotape when your infant is approximately 18 months old); and (3) complete some questionnaires before and after you listen to the audiotapes. In addition, you will be observed interacting with your baby once while your baby is still in the NICU. Also, at some sessions you may be asked to do some activities with your baby. Two different types of information will be used. The type of information you listen to will be decided by chance, like flipping a coin. The time that it will take to complete the questionnaires at any one point will be no longer than 25 minutes. In addition, information will be collected from your infant's primary staff nurse and your infant's medical record (for example, diagnosis and days hospitalized).

You also will participate in eight home or office visits (one home visit that will take place 1 to 4 days before your baby leaves the hospital; one home visit within 7 days after your baby leaves the hospital; one home visit when your baby is approximately 2 months old; one home or office visit when your baby is approximately 6 months old; one home visit when your baby is approximately 9 months old; one home or office visit when your baby is approximately 12 months old; one home visit when your child is approximately 18 months old; and the final home or office visit when your child is approximately 24 months old). During all visits, you will answer questionnaires which will take about 25 minutes each time. In addition, as described above, you will listen to an informational audiotape during the first, second, third, fifth, and seventh home visits. During the fourth, sixth, and eighth home or office visits (when your baby is approximately 6, 12, and 24 months old), you will be observed interacting with your baby and your baby will have developmental testing done by a member of the research team. Each visit will take approximately 1 to 1 ½ hours.

Helen Wood Hall
601 Elmwood Avenue, Box SON
Rochester, New York 14642-8404

Page 1 of 3

Risks of Participation
It is not anticipated that participation in this study will present any risks to you or your infant.

Benefits of Participation
The benefit of participating in this study is that you may find the information and activities helpful to you and your infant.

Circumstance for Leaving the Study
You may be asked to leave the study if you do not complete the study activities or if the study sponsor decides to stop or cancel the study.

Payment
After completing the two sets of questionnaires in the hospital, you will receive $10.00. You also will receive $15.00 for each of the first 7 home visits and $25.00 for the eighth home visit. The total amount you will receive for participating in this study is $140.00.

Confidentiality of Records and HIPAA Authorization

While we will make every effort to keep information we learn about you private, this cannot be guaranteed. Other people may need to see the information. While they normally protect the privacy of the information, they may not be required to do so by law. Results of the research may be presented at meetings or in publications, but your name will not be used.

The federal Health Insurance Portability and Accountability Act (HIPAA) requires us to get your permission to use health information about you that we either create or use as part of the research. This permission is called an Authorization. We will use admission logs, your research record, related information from your medical records, results of laboratory tests, and both clinical and research observations made while you take part in the research.

We will use your health information to conduct the study, to monitor your health status, to determine research results, and possibly to develop new tests, procedures, and commercial products. Health information is used to report results of research to sponsors and federal regulators. It may be audited to make sure we are following regulations, policies and study plans. Strong Health policies let you see and copy this information after the study ends, but not until the study is completed. If you have never received a copy of the Strong Health HIPAA Notice, please ask the investigator for one.

To meet regulations or for reasons related to this research, the study investigator may share a copy of this consent form and records that identify you with the following people: the Department of Health and Human Services; the University of Rochester; data monitoring committees; and research study team members at Strong Memorial Hospital and at our other study site, Crouse Hospital.

If you decide to take part, your Authorization for this study will not expire unless you cancel (revoke) it. The information collected during your participation will be kept indefinitely. You can always cancel this Authorization by writing to the study investigator. If you cancel your Authorization, you will also be removed from the study. However, standard medical care and any other benefits to which you are otherwise entitled will not be affected. Canceling your Authorization only affects uses and sharing of information after the study investigator gets your written request. Information gathered before then may need to be used and given to others. For example, by Federal law, we must send study information to the FDA for drug and device studies it regulates. Information that may need to be reported to FDA cannot be removed from your research records.

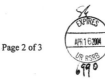

As stated in the section on Voluntary Participation below, you can also refuse to sign this consent/Authorization and not be part of the study. You can also tell us you want to leave the study at any time without canceling the Authorization. By signing this consent form, you give us permission to use and/or share your health information.

<u>Voluntary Participation</u>
Participation in this study is completely voluntary. You are free not to participate or to withdraw your consent at any time for whatever reason, without risking loss of present or future care you would otherwise expect your infant to receive. In the event that you do withdraw from this study, the information you have already provided will be kept in a confidential manner, unless you direct otherwise.

<u>Contact Persons</u>
For more information concerning this research, you should contact:

Dr. Bernadette Melnyk (585) 275-8903.

If you have any questions about your rights as a research subject, you may contact the Human Subjects Protection Specialist at the University of Rochester Research Subjects Review Board, Box 315, 601 Elmwood Avenue, Rochester, NY 14642-8315, Telephone: (585) 506-0005, for long-distance you may call toll-free, (877) 449-4441.

I have read the contents of this consent form, asked questions, and received answers concerning areas I did not understand. I give my consent to participate in this study by signing this form. I will receive a copy of this form for my records.

Study subject
(Parent/
Significant other): _____PRINT NAME

_____SIGNATURE

_____DATE

INVESTIGATOR- I have presented the consent form to the subject and answered questions completely.

_____SIGNATURE

_____DATE

Page 3 of 3

Rochester Consent
4/03

A Data and Safety Monitoring Plan for an Intervention Study

appendix D

Study: Improving Outcomes of LBW Premature Infants and Parents

Funded by the National Institutes of Health/National Institute of Nursing Research (R01#NR05077)

Principal Investigator (PI): Melnyk, Bernadette; Co-Investigators: Alpert-Gillis, Linda and Feinstein, Nancy Fischbeck

Data and Safety Monitoring Plan

The potential risk of this clinical trial is considered to be minimal because of the nature of the intervention. The study has no adverse events expected for participants based upon the pilot study. Since this grant application fits in the category of Clinical Trial (Phase II) study, we developed a plan for appropriate oversight and monitoring of the conduct of the clinical trial to ensure the safety of the participants and the validity and integrity of the data.

a) The PI had already obtained the policies of the University of Rochester IRB specifically regarding the adverse events associated with clinical trials. The PIs will adhere to those policies, and maintain a copy of the policies in the study file.

b) The PI will meet with the research assistants, and the co-investigators on a bi-weekly basis during the data collection phase, and identify any risks of adverse effects resulting from the data collection process and data review.

c) The PI, co-investigators and consultants will make decisions about necessary protocol and operational changes based on discussion and review of data and the data collection process. Any proposed changes in the consent form or research procedures resulting from the report will be prepared/identified by the PI and submitted with the report to the IRB for approval.

d) The following policies required by our IRB and NIH will be adhered to: (1) any adverse events that are serious and unexpected and are related (possibly or probably) to the study will be reported to the IRB and NIH within 15 calendar days; (2) adverse events that are both un-expected and related that are either life-threatening or result in death will be reported to IRB and NIH immediately; and (3) for adverse events that do not meet the criteria above will be documented in the summary report submitted to the IRB and NIH annually at the time of the study's continuing review. Because the proposed study has a low risk intervention, we do not anticipate any serious adverse effects described in the first two categories from a result of participating in this study.

e) The PI will ensure that the NIH (funding Institute and Center) is informed of actions, if any, taken by the IRB as a result of its continuing review, and recommendations that emanate from the monitoring activities.

f) The Rochester site will be responsible for reporting adverse events or unanticipated problems involving risks to subjects or others to the local IRB. If problems are considered related to the trial, the IRB at the Syracuse site will also be notified.

g) The PI will be responsible for the monitoring of this plan throughout the life of the study.

Case Example of an Evidence-Based Approach to Answer a Clinical Problem: Smoking Cessation and Women With Cardiovascular Disease

appendix E

Looking for Best Evidence: What If It Isn't There?

Case Example: Smoking Cessation and Women with Cardiovascular Disease

Rona F. Levin, Joanne K. Singleton, and Harriet R. Feldman

This example provides an inside look at how a team of researchers came together with a keen interest in developing an evidence-based approach to find answers to a common clinical problem, how to prevent cardiovascular disease in women between the ages of 40 to 65 years of age. We took a few turns to get to the point of clearly defining a focused clinical question. In so doing, we learned a number of valuable lessons that we share later in the chapter. The context for the clinical problem was the desire to address aspects of healthy aging that individuals could change.

The Background

National demographics on aging show that by 1994, one in eight or 33.2 million Americans were over the age of 65. Middle series projections by the U.S. Census Bureau expect that between now and 2050 the older adult population will reach 80 million, with the greatest period of growth projected between 2010 and 2030 as the baby boom generation enters older adulthood. Recognition and acceptance of these facts presents a call for a proactive approach across multiple sectors in America if this reality is to be addressed as a challenge rather than a problem. Although it is anticipated that the impact of the aging population will have tremendous affects on the future of the healthcare delivery system, it is also predicted that baby-boomers have the potential to redefine aging through their understanding of strategies for healthy aging and by participating in the prevention of disease and disabilities and the management of chronic illnesses. Healthcare professionals are especially positioned to help Americans to turn and focus on aging rather than continuing to turn away from it, by making available to the public the knowledge gleaned through practice and research.

Twenty years ago the focus of gerontology was on disease, disability, and perceived limitations based on chronological age. Now aging is understood to include biological, psychological, lifestyle, and social factors. New multidisciplinary strategies that address all factors encompassed in aging must be identified, developed, championed, and made available to meet the needs of older adults today and in the future. Meeting these needs traverses a variety of settings in which education and care are provided to older adults and baby boomers. Resources must be directed toward maintaining health and fitness in the absence or presence of chronic conditions. An expected outcome of this approach is redefining the concept of health at individual and societal levels to incorporate the ability of older adults to live productively, exercising self-reliance and autonomy to the maximum extent possible.

Focus on Healthy Aging

In 2000, the Institute for Healthy Aging at the Lienhard School of Nursing, Pace University (IHA) was established for the purposes of educating healthcare professionals, healthcare recipients, and the public on the realities of aging, and to conduct research and guide practice in this area. To address its mission the IHA focuses on providing information to individuals 40 years of age and older, as well as healthcare providers and allied professionals. Through evidence-based information, the IHA is a benchmark for reliable, truthful information and education on healthy aging.

Understanding healthy aging begins with the concept of health, defined by the American Nurses Association in 1980 as a "dynamic state of being in which the developmental and behavioral potential of an individual is realized to the fullest extent possible." Health is an active process that requires conscious intent. As defined in most dictionaries, aging is the process of existing over time. Healthy aging then, is the conscious intent and participation in the bio-psycho-social-spiritual care-of-self over time. According to Ken Dychtwald (1999), a noted gerontologist and visionary on aging:

> As informed as we've become about the factors that influence health, too many people continue to take too little responsibility for their own well-being. With maturity, the real challenge frequently shifts from knowing what to do, to doing what you know. (p. 131)

The expected increase in the aging population will have a tremendous impact on society in general and specifically on the healthcare delivery system. The size of the aging baby-boom population, however, also predicts the potential for this group to redefine the dynamics of aging, as long as the essential aspects of healthy aging are understood and intentionally acted on.

Key components of healthy aging include behavioral lifestyle choices, including diet, exercise, health habits, and exposure to toxic environmental sources (tobacco, UV radiation, pollution), which have potent effects on the body's aging process (National Institute of Aging [NIA], 2001). The mechanism of normal, healthy aging involves dynamic interactions between physiological, behavioral, and social factors (NIA, 2001b). Results of the past 40 years of research have been instrumental in defining the implications of normal aging of the body and mind and have emphasized the importance of health promotion, including diet and exercise, throughout life for health, longevity, and quality of life. Through this body of evidence, exercising the body and the mind, healthful eating, not smoking, and staying socially active have all been identified as critical to healthy aging.

The Clinical Problem

To carry out its mission the IHA planned a two-directional approach. In fall 2002, we held our first conference at which we presented the existing evidence that supports and directs recommendations for healthy aging in the areas of nutrition and exercise for the body and mind. At the same time, we developed a research agenda that focused on women, specifically women with cardiovascular disease, and we wanted to know what risk factors were modifiable and the best approaches for directing practice in this area. Our interest was grounded in the rapidly increasing incidence and significance of heart disease in women.

Smoking is a worldwide problem and a major risk factor for the development of cardiovascular and pulmonary disease and cancer (Sarna & Llington, 2002). During the past decade there has been an increased recognition of the incidence and effects of heart disease in women. More importantly, once diagnosed with cardiovascular disease, women have greater morbidity and mortality (Krummel, et al., 2001; Sparks & Frazier, 2002). Although smoking is a major risk factor for heart disease, it also is modifiable. Given the natural history of cardiovascular disease in women, smoking cessation interventions targeted for this population may be an important preventative strategy.

Part II: The Process

In chapters 1 and 2 of his second edition of *Evidence-Based Medicine* (2000), Sackett presents a step-by-step process for focusing clinical questions and finding the answers. We began our project by following these steps. Yet, the answers were not there, and we were burning to find them. This is our experience of how the process really worked, an honest recounting of successes and mistakes along the way. Table 1 provides a summary of the steps we took to try to answer our burning clinical question. We hope our experience will help you to avoid some pitfalls, making your experience as smooth and efficient as possible.

Initial Steps: Asking a Clinical Question and Looking for the Answer

The first step in our process was to formulate the clinical question. As an outgrowth of our desire to frame the IHA as an EBP institute, we decided initially to conduct a systematic review of research that would be relevant to healthy aging and the results of which we could disseminate at the next IHA-sponsored program. In particular, we were concerned with the lack of attention to women and cardiovascular disease (CVD), especially in relation to prevention of this major health problem. Since a major risk factor for development of CVD is smoking, we decided to see if we could find sufficient clinical trials that dealt with the comparative effectiveness of smoking cessation interventions for men versus women in order to conduct a meta-analysis. Our initial clinical question was: "For women with CVD, what is the best smoking cessation intervention?"

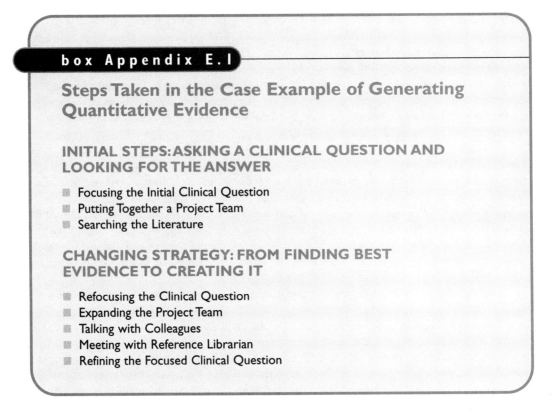

box Appendix E.1

Steps Taken in the Case Example of Generating Quantitative Evidence

INITIAL STEPS: ASKING A CLINICAL QUESTION AND LOOKING FOR THE ANSWER

- Focusing the Initial Clinical Question
- Putting Together a Project Team
- Searching the Literature

CHANGING STRATEGY: FROM FINDING BEST EVIDENCE TO CREATING IT

- Refocusing the Clinical Question
- Expanding the Project Team
- Talking with Colleagues
- Meeting with Reference Librarian
- Refining the Focused Clinical Question

The next step was to put together a project team. The first meeting about this project was between the co-directors of the IHA, Drs. Joanne Singleton and Marie Londrigan, and the visiting scholar in residence at the Lienhard School of Nursing (LSN), Dr. Rona Levin. This meeting focused on trying to determine how to go about using EBP as a framework to move the mission of the IHA forward. An outcome of the meeting was that we agreed that asking a focused clinical question related to the mission and synthesizing current best evidence would be a reasonable way to proceed. Our next step was to figure out what research expertise we already had on the team and then invite colleagues with the expertise we still needed to join us.

Drs. Singleton and Londrigan have clinical expertise as nurse practitioners as well as expertise in qualitative research methods; Dr. Levin's expertise is in quantitative methods. Dr. Harriet R. Feldman, the LSN dean, was asked to join the team since she and Dr. Levin had worked together on a meta-analysis in the 1980's. We also needed a statistician who knew meta-analytic techniques. Dr. Michael Barnes, a professor of Clinical Psychology at Hofstra University and a visiting scholar at the LSN who had presented classes on meta-analysis at our university in conjunction with Dr. Levin, agreed to join the team.

In addition, Dr. Singleton invited her colleagues from St. Vincent's Catholic Medical Centers of New York City, Dr. Steve Garner, Chief Medical Officer, and Dr. Subrahmanya Bhatt, Director of Cardiology for the Brooklyn Queens Division, both experts in cardiovascular disease, to join the research team.

We also needed graduate assistants (GA) to work with us on the project. The Center for Nursing Research, Clinical Practice and International Affairs (CNRCPIA) at the LSN provides such assistance to faculty engaged in scholarly projects. Given the work to be done in terms of literature retrieval and review and project management, we needed two assistants, one with a nursing background and a grasp of research concepts and methods, and one who could search data bases, take minutes of meetings, and maintain project files. The first student, Edward McMillan, was newly enrolled in our MS-Family Nurse Practitioner Program, having recently graduated from the Baccalaureate Completion Program for RNs. The second student, Ping Xu, was a student in the Computer Information Systems graduate program and also had a master's degree in Health Care Administration. We believed the team we put together that had the expertise to carry out the project and conduct a meta-analysis.

Our next step was to search the literature for existing evidence to answer the clinical question. Our first search yielded over 150 studies from seven databases. Table 2 provides the search terms we used and the databases that were searched. It may be used as a template for an evidence search.

An initial review of the retrieved studies indicated that of those accessed only approximately 25 were potentially relevant to the study problem. Of those studies that were deemed potentially relevant, there was a lack of gender specific research and an inability to tease out gender data from the information contained in the studies. Thus, the literature did not provide the data needed to conduct a meta-analysis to answer our clinical question.

Changing Strategy: From Finding Best Evidence to Creating It

Since we were not able to find sufficient research, specifically clinical trials to answer the initial clinical question, we had to refocus our question and revise our strategy for finding the answer. The first step was to integrate the literature related to our question in a formal, systematic way. To do this, the two primary investigators wrote a proposal for and received funding from Pace University's Scholarly Research Award competition. This proposal presented the major clinical question as: "In non-pregnant women, what is the comparative effectiveness of smoking cessation programs on smoking behavior?" Our initial literature review spawned questions about the effect of timing and duration of smoking cessation programs on smoking cessation behavior and the interactive effect of time and smoking cessation programs on smoking cessation behavior.

None of our questions were answered by the current literature. Therefore, it became quite obvious that we needed to conduct a clinical trial for that purpose. It was at this point that we realized the need for greater involvement from our clinical partners.

When it was determined that our project was reshaping itself into a clinical trial, Dr. Singleton discussed conducting a trial with Dr. Garner as study co-investigator. Dr. Garner identified that the Medical Center had a shared interest in understanding the role of patient characteristics in first-line evidence-based smoking cessation interventions. Not only was the medical center interested in gender differences, but as providers of healthcare to a highly diverse patient population, they also were interested in ethnic differences in smoking cessation. This synergy between the direction the research project was taking and the medical center's expressed interest in best practices for smoking cessation resulted in Dr. Garner, on behalf of the medical center, formalizing a clinical partnership. Through this clinical partnership, the Pace University LSN, and SVCMC began to identify and share resources in order to move the clinical trial project forward. Areas for additional expertise were identified and members added to the team of co-inves-

appendix table E.1. Initial search terms and databases

Search Terms

1. smoking cessation
2. smoking cessation & intervention
3. smoking cessation & intervention & clinical trials
4. smoking cessation & intervention & clinical trials
5. smoking cessation & interventions & women
6. smoking cessation & interventions & women & clinical trials
7. smoking cessation & interventions & women & clinical trials & cardiovascular disease
8. smoking cessation & intervention & transtheoretical model
9. smoking cessation & interventions & stages of change & cardiovascular disease

Databases searched	Smoking cessation & intervention	Smoking cessation & intervention & clinical trials	Smoking cessation & intervention & clinical trials & cardiovascular disease	Smoking cessation & women	Smoking cessation & intervention & women & clinical trials	Smoking cessation & intervention & women & clinical trials & cardiovascular disease
1. CINAHL						
2. Cochrane Library						
3. Dissertation Abstracts Online						
4. Medline						
5. PsycINFO						
6. Nursing journal						

tigators to include Dr. Harriet Enubuzor, Associate Program Director, Family Practice and Ms. Roseanne Russo, Administrative Coordinator, Oncology. Additionally, SVCMC agreed to have their director of pharmacy available for project support and Robert DiGregorio, PharmD, a colleague of Dr. Singleton's, joined the team as a co-investigator.

Beyond searching for evidence from databases, one of the most important strategies to use for finding information is networking with colleagues. During fall 2002, Dr. Bernadette Melnyk visited the Lienhard School of Nursing for 2 days as a visiting scholar. During this visit, she met with Drs. Singleton, Londrigan, and Levin about making the IHA an evidence-based unit. We also discussed the smoking cessation study we were planning to conduct. As a result of this interchange, we learned that a nursing faculty member at the University of Rochester School of Nursing was conducting research related to smoking cessation. Serendipitously, two members of our research team were planning to attend the evidence-based conference in Rochester in December 2002. Thus, at a dinner meeting one of the authors learned that there was much more literature available on our topic of interest than the initial search yielded. Therefore, we deemed it imperative to reconduct the search. We decided, however, that it would be more productive for the two primary investigators to be "hands on" with the search.

Upon returning from Rochester, Drs. Singleton and Levin set up a meeting with one of the Pace University reference librarians and included the GA who had done the initial literature review. During this session, we realized that our GA had several misunderstandings about our directions and also did not know about certain tools contained in databases, such as a thesaurus or controlled vocabulary. Because of the GA's lack of this knowledge, the initial search was inefficient and costly in terms of time and energy. As we realized after the discussion with our Rochester colleague, there was much more literature on our clinical question than was yielded by the initial search, including an updated set of guidelines for smoking cessation interventions published by the Agency for Health Care Research and Quality (AHRQ). Table 3 presents the template we constructed for the second database search. After reviewing the AHRQ guidelines, it became clear that we were on the right track from the beginning, which at this point gave us a needed "shot in the arm."

We needed to reformulate the clinical question to assure that we covered all the PICO components. One area in which there was insufficient evidence had to do with how gender and ethnicity might influence the effectiveness of first line smoking cessation interventions. And so the refined and final, focused clinical question to guide our research became: "In 40 to 65 year olds (P), what are the effects of gender (I) and ethnicity (C) on the efficacy of evidence-based smoking cessation interventions (O)?" A well-formulated question gave us a clearer, more focused direction, and then we were able to develop grant proposals to support the conduct of a clinical trial in the hope of answering this question.

Determining the Study Setting and Assessing Feasibility

We were lucky to have already put together a multidisciplinary team with members who were the head of clinical areas at a major medical center with multiple divisions and services. Thus we did not have to go through the complex task of finding a clinical agency in which to conduct a clinical trial. In fact our physician co-investigators brought staff from various related services to the table to help us determine the resources and support we needed for and the feasibility of proceeding with a complex clinical study. After these initial meetings and reviewing utilization statistics, we realized that several of the divisions within two New York boroughs provided care

appendix table E.2. **Template for second database search**

Pace University & SVCMC Research Partnership

Search terms	Number of citations	Number retrieved	Number used
CINAHL 1997-2002 Smoking cessation and (English) and (Journal article) and (clinical trial or doctoral dissertation or practice guidelines or research or "systematic review") Smoking Cessation and (English) and (Experimental studies or intervention trials) and (journal article) and (clinical trial or doctoral dissertation or practice guidelines or research or "systematic review" Smoking Cessation and (English) and (Experimental studies or intervention trials) and (journal article) and (clinical trial or doctoral dissertation or practice guidelines or research or "systematic review") and not (pregnant or pregnancy) Smoking cessation and qualitative studies and (English) and (journal article) Smoking cessation and qualitative studies and (English) and (journal article) or doctoral dissertation Smoking cessation and qualitative studies and (English) and (journal article) or doctoral dissertation and not (pregnant or pregnancy) Smoking cessation and qualitative studies and (English) and (journal article) or doctoral dissertation and not (pregnant or pregnancy) and not inpatients			
Dissertation Abstracts International: 1997-2002 Smoking cessation Smoking cessation and intervention Smoking cessation and intervention and clinical trial			

(continued)

to a relatively large and appropriate population of out-patients. In order to ensure a sufficient study sample, we also decided to include employees through the Medical Center's employee health service. These multidisciplinary meetings also helped us to delineate roles and responsibilities of project staff. For example, we needed to determine who would recruit study participants and whether or not these individuals needed to be hired as project personnel or whether

appendix table E.2. Template for Second Database Search *(continued)*

Search terms	Number of citations	Number retrieved	Number used
Medline: Date published: 1997-2002 Publication Type: Clinical Trial or Journal Article or Practice Guideline and Gender: Female and Age Related: Middle Age.			
Smoking cessation and intervention studies not (pregnant or pregnancy)			
Smoking cessation not inpatients not (pregnant or pregnancy)			
Smoking cessation and outpatients not (pregnant or pregnancy)			
Smoking cessation not (pregnant or pregnancy)			
Smoking cessation			
PsychINFO: 1997-2002 English			
Population Group: female + outpatient + and Age Groups: 40-64			
Smoking cessation not (pregnant or pregnancy)			
Smoking cessation			
Smoking cessation (journal article + dissertation abstract)			
Smoking cessation (clinical trial + journal article +dissertation abstract)			

Search terms	Number of completed reviews retreived	Number of abstracts of quality assessed reviews retreived	Number used
The Cochrane Library: 1997-2002			
Smoking cessation not (pregnant or pregnancy)			

individuals currently employed at the Medical Center could carry out this role. Other issues we had to grapple with were which first line smoking cessation interventions to administer, what type of control groups to use and how to keep study subjects from discussing the treatments they were getting with other participants, and how to ensure that participants were screened for health related exclusion criteria.

After at least 6 months of discussion, overcoming (at least conceptually) the challenges and issues involved in clinical research, putting a proposal together, and developing a budget, we realized what a complex, detailed, and expensive study we were developing. Because of this, particularly the cost of conducting a large-scale clinical trial, we realized we had to first conduct a pilot study. This is where we are as of this writing – on the brink of submitting a grant proposal to begin our pilot study.

Lessons Learned

As with all new experiences there are lessons to be learned that help us to do it better the next time around. We found several challenges throughout the process of forming the team in terms of expectations and how to "work smarter." For example, we engaged the services of graduate students without knowing well what their abilities and strengths were in relation to what we were aiming to do. We presumed incorrectly that they would have a more than a working knowledge of how to search databases related to our topic. We found out that our expectations were unfounded and that very clear instructions and monitoring were needed to guide the work of the GA. Also, periodic review of the findings of the GA would have revealed earlier on that the search terms were not sufficiently descriptive.

Another lesson had to do with organization of the team and our space to assure an efficient system that would be supportive of a collaborative project. For example, learning and applying Endnote* right from the beginning of the project would have placed all references into the proper style format, thereby saving time and energy. Also, having a central location where documents and files are kept, a computer and printer, and a designated work area would have facilitated meetings and access by all team members to information as needed.

We learned during the early part of the process and then at various points along the way that we needed to be clear on what the commitments of team members were to this project and what was realistic for them to accomplish to meet established timelines. An adjunct to this lesson is the challenge of staying focused on the project despite the many responsibilities each of us had for teaching, practice, professional organization work, and so on. In order to make progress according to our goals, we learned that we needed to use many forms of communication. Besides "in person" meetings, we conducted our business via conference call and e-mail. If someone could not be present for a particular meeting we were sure to ask for input either immediately before or immediately following the meeting. We also learned that expanding the team to assure adequate expertise and numbers would be essential to our success.

An important lesson, and perhaps a universal principle, is that putting together a clinical trial will take twice as long as you expect even with a research team that has all the expertise required, has access to a clinical setting, and is invested in the study. Finally, an investigator should always consider conducting a pilot study first when designing a large, complex, and expensive clinical trial.

Summary

In this example, we shared how we arrived at our initial clinical question and presented some of the particulars that needed to be addressed when we attempted to find the answer to that question. We learned that it is especially important to be open and flexible when you discover that the body of evidence thought to answer your question actually does not. We hope that our strategies of refocusing the clinical question and changing our project priorities to conduct a clinical trial may be of value to other clinicians and researchers pursuing an evidence-based approach to practice. In addition, significant consideration should be given to the types of expertise required for research team members, from principal investigator to graduate assistant. The principal investigator should determine how to assess needed expertise for the project; when and how much to orient and/or teach graduate assistants about data retrieval; and, find a place to call your own (space for the team to do its work). Also, it is important to determine the resources need to support a clinical trail, whether or not they are available, how much they will cost, and the feasibility of conducting the study within a reasonable budget and time frame. An important step in addressing these issues is to first carry out a pilot study. We hope that these writings will enable you to benefit in some small way from our experience.

References

American Nurses Association. (1980). *Nursing: A social policy statement.* Kansas City, MO: Author.

Dychtwald, K. (1999). *Age Power: How the 21st century will be ruled by the new old.* New York: Peguin Putnam.

Krummel, D. A., Koffman, D. M., Bronner, Y., Davis, J., Greenlunk, K., Tessaro, I., Upson, D. et al. (2001). Cardiovascular health interventions in women: What works? *Journal of Women's Health & Gender Based Medicine, 10,* 117–136.

Sackett, S. L., Strauss, S. E., Richardson, W. S., Rosenberg, W., & Haynes, R. B. (2000). *Evidence-based medicine. How to practice and teach EBM* (2nd ed.). Edinburgh: Churchill Livingstone.

Sarna, L., & Lillington, L. (2002). Tobacco: An emerging topic in nursing research. *Nursing Research, 51, 245–253.*

Sparks, E. A., &Frazier, L. Q. (2002, March-April). Heritable cardiovascular disease in women. *Journal of Obstetric, Gynecologic, and Neonatal Nursing, 217–228.*

National Institute of Aging (2001a). Strategic Plan for Fiscal Years 2001–2005. Retrieved January, 15, 2001, from http://www.nih.gov/nia/strat-plan/2001-2005/.

National Institute of Aging. (2001b). The Baltimore longitudinal study of aging. Retrieved: February 10, 2001, from http://www.nih.grc.nia.gov/branches/blsa/blsa.htm.

Case Example for an Ethnographic Study Resolving Ethical Issues of Daily Living

appendix F

Looking for Best Evidence: "A Rose by Any Other Name..."

Case Example for an Ethnographic Study Resolving Ethical Issues of Daily Living Affecting Nursing Home Residents With Dementia*

Bethel Ann Powers

> *Romeo and Juliet*
> Act II. Scene II. *Capulet's Orchard*
>
> *Jul.* 'Tis but thy name that is my enemy;
> What's Montague? it is nor hand, nor foot,
> Nor arm, nor face, nor any other part
> Belonging to a man. O be some other name!
> What's in a name? that which we call a rose
> By any other name would smell as sweet;
> So Romeo would were he not Romeo call'd

---

*This research was supported by a grant from the New York State Department of Health, Bureau of Long Term Care.

> Retain that dear perfection which he owes
> Without that title. Romeo, doff thy name,
> And for that name which is no part of thee
> Take all myself.
>
> *Rom.* I take thee at thy word:
> Call me but love, and I'll be new baptized;
> Henceforth I never will be Romeo.
>
> (Shakespeare, 1594/5, p.1627)

Perhaps for Shakespeare's Juliet "a rose by any other name would smell as sweet," meaning that a thing is what it is, no matter what it is called. However, this passage also suggests how the language people use to label things shapes their perceptions of reality. Thus, as data collection for an ethnographic study of everyday ethical issues affecting nursing home residents with dementia began, the language serving to frame the proposal produced some staff member uncertainty about what kinds of information might be applicable to this research focus. For example, individuals often are sensitized to the use of the term *ethics* in connection with reports of unethical or immoral behavior. Therefore, persons who associate ethics with criticism of wrongdoing that leads to judgments have a perspective on what constitutes an ethical issue that differs from that of persons who see ethical evaluation as an impartial synthesis of different views on a wider variety of concerns that leads to recommendations. *Ethical dilemmas* also may tend to call to mind dramatic examples of life and death issues. Examples that occur frequently in nursing homes involve ethical decision-making associated with honoring advance directives and discontinuing treatments, such as nutritional support, for dying persons. In contrast, there are many ordinary issues arising daily in the care of nursing home residents (e.g., residents' refusal of care or interpersonal difficulties with roommates) that may not immediately be identified as ethical issues, particularly if a problem or concern is labeled as something else (e.g., a behavior issue). This begins to explain how some ethical elements of resident care issues may be taken for granted or exist below the level of persons' conscious awareness when the issues themselves are thought of as unremarkable, manageable, usual, and expected occurrences in a given practice environment. Consequently, what counts as an ethical matter to persons depends a lot on how they use and tend to think about the term *ethics*. And, therefore, it was not surprising that staff wondered aloud about what might be considered as evidence of everyday ethical issues.

Principles of a Qualitative Study

Using this introduction as a point of departure, the story now will pick up on how the study was designed and executed in order to locate and present meaningful evidence that could be validated by nursing home staff (and readers of subsequent reports). It will be organized around the general principles described in Chapter 11, and will conclude with a discussion of the ethnographic reporting practices used to date to represent findings and communicate about practical applications of this field investigation.

Identify a Study Question

The primary study question was: What are commonly recurring ethical issues embedded in the daily life experiences of nursing home residents with dementia and the people who care for them?

Sub-questions included: How may similar cases differ in form and complexity? What may different cases have in common? What patterns exist in terms of nature and origination, communication about, and resolution of common forms of ethical dilemmas? What ethical perspectives are used to guide thinking about appropriate responses and interventions?

Review the Literature

In this study, literature was used in several ways. First, to introduce and frame the study problem, attention was drawn to the literature related to the ethics of long-term care and the concept of *everyday ethics* (Powers, 2000, 2001). Second, the researcher's previous knowledge of and contributions to extant literature on nursing home culture provided a backdrop for the study and a theoretical lens or perspective to guide the research toward issues to be examined and participant perspectives to be elicited. And third, relevant work related to dementia, long-term care, nursing home ethnography, and ethics was integrated into written reports at the end of the study as a basis for situating the research findings within those areas of the literature to which they pertain (Powers, 2003a).

Define the Theoretical Perspective

The theoretical lens or perspective, as noted above, was derived from the literature on nursing home culture that constitutes the genre known as nursing home ethnography, and also from long-term care literature focused on quality of life/care issues, social and environmental studies, and culture change in nursing homes. This background positioned the researcher to identify, observe and ask questions about, as well as to reflectively examine, specific challenges of providing dementia care within the cultural environment of the nursing home from the perspectives of residents, family, and nursing home staff members.

Select an Appropriate Research Design

Ethnography is the research method in which the researcher, a nurse and anthropologist, specializes. It was the design of choice for this study because of its purpose to provide an interpretation of particular kinds of human experiences in cultural context.

Formulate a Purpose Statement

The research objective was to critically examine ethical issues of daily living affecting nursing home residents with dementia and to construct a descriptive taxonomy inductively derived from ethnographic fieldwork data. The taxonomy (a type of conceptual framework) is an attempt to extend understanding of what may count as an ethical matter in the care of persons in nursing homes who have dementia. This evidence-based interpretation of field observation, interview, and cultural artifact data addresses some of the language/labeling issues mentioned above.

Establish the Significance of the Study

The significance of this study flowed from the above-described steps involving problem identification, review of the literature, definition of a theoretical perspective, formulation of the purpose statement and study questions, and selection of the overall design. However, though separately itemized, these activities actually occurred simultaneously.

A three-fold rationale was set forth. First, it was observed that the research findings would contribute to the generally underdeveloped literature on nursing home ethics. In addition, the emphasis on residents with dementia was noted to be important because extant gerontological studies of everyday ethics have not been specifically focused on these individuals, who constitute 60-80% of this special, vulnerable population. Second, products of the research analysis (guidelines for nursing home ethics committees and evidence-based hypothetical narratives designed for use as practice cases for committees or as staff in-service education offerings) were anticipated to be of practical use to individuals who care for nursing home residents with dementia. And third, an interpretive ethnographic approach was thought to be a good vehicle to ensure transferability, and hence applicability, of findings by drawing out the unifying strands of institutional cultural experiences in ways that could transcend differences across individual nursing home settings. That is, it would have the capacity to produce meaningful food for thought embedded in highly plausible scenarios with which persons across a variety of settings and circumstances would be able to identify.

Describe Research Procedures

This was a two-year study in the natural setting of a 147-bed, voluntary, not-for-profit nursing home. All residents with a diagnosis of dementia were eligible to participate. Since the unit of analysis was individual cases, purposeful sampling (i.e., deliberate, researcher-directed, and choosing from all residents with dementia) was used to identify a range of residents across a spectrum of situations. The desired sampling mix was both male and female residents at different stages of dementia on different units in the facility whose family members, along with nursing home staff, were good informants who could provide additional perspectives on residents' past history and current aspects of their daily life. As sampling and analysis of incoming data progressed, specific types of cases were sought that could provide new insights regarding particular emerging issues. Observations and interviews with participants, both formal and informal, were ongoing from time of enrollment in the study until cessation of data collection. Data collection ended at thirty cases, when it was determined that informational categories in the database were sufficiently saturated.

Ethical considerations included obtaining Institutional Review Board approval and following a process of informed consent that included signed consent of family and staff members and signed and witnessed assent of family members to approach residents for consent, to whatever degree they were able to provide it. Care was taken to respect personal autonomy, particularly with regard to showing awareness of different understanding and comfort levels of cognitively impaired individuals. Participants were assured of confidentiality in terms of record keeping and reporting. In addition, because of the need for broader participant observation activities on the part of the researcher in the setting, the nursing home community as a whole was made aware of the study. And names and identifiers of nonparticipants were not included in the researcher's recorded field observations.

Data collection included such examples of researcher participation as: (a) transporting residents and actively participating in organized activities; (b) assisting residents at mealtimes; (c) observing and helping nursing assistants perform resident care activities; (d) informal visiting and talking with residents; (e) attending staff development programs; (f) attending family council and family support meetings; and (g) continuing membership and participation on the ethics committee. Data from participant observation experiences were recorded in field notes. In-depth interviews involved taped conversations using an interview guide. Available documents collected to supplement recorded data included: (a) newsletters; (b) activity calendars; (c) daily care worksheets; (d) in-service education calendars and teaching tools; (e) annual reports; and (f) documents associated with the work of the ethics committee devoid of personal identifiers. The principal investigator conducted all data collection. Data were analyzed and organized continually and secured in computer files and locked storage areas.

Data analysis occurred simultaneously with data collection. Information was broken down, compared, and placed in categories during earlier stages. As data were reconstituted, analysis focused on similarities and differences of individual experiences and patterns related to resolution of common dilemmas. Paradigm cases (composite, fictionalized narratives) based on the analyzed research evidence were designed to exemplify everyday ethical issues. When staff members were given examples of these to read and comment upon, one nurse exclaimed, "Now I know what you were looking for. I know you explained it to me, but I couldn't understand it. I don't know why. It makes so much sense. These certainly are the kinds of things that we confront every day." Another said, "We deal with these issues all the time. We're so used to dealing with them I'm not sure we stop often enough to really think about them." These remarks illustrate the power of language categories (folk taxonomies) that influence how people conceptualize situations. In this instance, taken-for-granted ways of thinking about everyday occurrences with residents in this setting made it difficult for staff to recognize ordinary concerns as ethical issues (Powers, 2001).

Final levels of analysis involved creation of a classification scheme (the taxonomy) to organize and interpret findings. This involved (a) searching the data for the frames of reference study participants used to think about resident-focused issues and concerns and (b) creating an alternate model with four domains crosscut by dimensions of individual/social values and positive/negative moral rights(Powers 2000, 2001, 2003b). The evidence on which this model was based came from the findings in the data (combined information from observations, interviews, and review of cultural artifacts) and the inferences drawn from them.

Standards of quality and scientific rigor were addressed. Principle strategies validating data accuracy and confirmability included: (a) cross-examining evidence from different sources of information (sometimes called triangulation) as a means of justifying reported findings and interpretations; (b) asking participants to validate, clarify, and/or expand upon their own contributions to the data (member-checking); and (c) developing in-depth understanding of phenomena related to the study through prolonged time in the field.

Principle strategies addressing credibility and transferability involved: (a) using detailed, culturally grounded description to convey findings in ways designed to give readers a feeling for the setting and a sense of sharing experiences; (b) soliciting reviewers to assess the credibility of the interpretation and whether or not it resonated with persons other than the researcher (peer debriefing); and (c) obtaining expert consultation (external auditor concept) on the project's overall and specific use and application of ethics and ethical concepts.

Discuss Limitations

A delimitation of the study was that the scope of this in-depth field investigation was narrowly focused on observing and interviewing persons in one nursing home.

In contrast, some limitations of the study included that the research findings were theoretically/ analytically generalizable (transferable) to the extent that descriptions of the evidence and related insights are thought to be meaningful and applicable to similar cases in other nursing home situations. It also should be understood that the outcome reflects one interpretation of the data, which means that findings could be subject to other interpretations.

Reporting Practical Applications of the Research

A variety of texts may be produced from a single qualitative research study. These texts constitute unique representations of the data that serve particular purposes. Ethnographers also employ many different reporting styles to construct cultural portraits designed to reach certain audiences. To date, several styles and formats have been used to report practical applications of this research.

Ethnographic Analysis of Everyday Ethics in the Care of Nursing Home Residents with Dementia: A Taxonomy
(Powers, 2001)

This overview of the findings describes the research process and resultant taxonomy of everyday ethical issues for a primarily collegial audience in the discipline of nursing. It follows a conventional research journal format that conforms to the standard quantitative report style of: *introduction, literature, method, results,* and *discussion.* It highlights *cultural perspectives, concerns,* and *ethical perspectives* related to each of the taxonomy's four domains: (a) learning the limits of intervention; (b) tempering the culture of surveillance and restraint; (c) preserving individual integrity; and (d) defining community norms and values. It explains how the domains are oriented toward (a) individual and social values and (b) positive and negative moral rights. And, it calls attention to how language is used - as frames of reference or taxonomies – to shape people's views of reality, a tendency that can pose challenges to recognizing the ethical in the ordinary. In this regard, the report is similar in purpose to that of other qualitative studies whose aim is to increase understanding and raise awareness about a phenomenon of interest. Thus, the possibilities for practical application of this text rest on its ability to encourage readers' thoughtfulness about the moral basis of ordinary issues of daily living affecting quality of life for nursing home residents with dementia.

Everyday Ethics of Dementia Care in Nursing Homes: A Definition and Taxonomy
(Powers, 2000)

This overview of the findings follows a conventional journal report format as well. It describes the research process in less detail and presents a summarization of the domains of the taxonomy for an interdisciplinary audience interested in reading about dementia research. However, this summarization is provided for the purpose of suggesting that the taxonomy could be used to sensitize nursing home ethics committee members to issues that they might not otherwise have thought worthy of consideration. Raising awareness of the ethical in the ordinary by providing a new way to think about taken-for-granted everyday occurrences continues to be a major goal. But also included are some suggestions about what committees might do to expand their horizons. The practical application here is in the paper's focus on agenda setting/case finding problems sometimes experienced by ethics committees.

The Significance of Losing Things for Nursing Home Residents with Dementia and Their Families
(Powers, 2003b)

This paper is a report of a focused analysis of a subset of information in the data about a discrete topic - the meaning of personal possessions and issues related to their loss. It was written with readers in the field of gerontological nursing in mind.

      Persons with dementia often lose or misplace their belongings. Residents who take each other's belongings because they cannot distinguish them from their own further complicate possession loss in nursing homes. And, the possibility of deliberate theft when things go missing also cannot be discounted. Findings from analysis of this data subset are described as themes, supplemented by tables displaying a number of quotes by residents, family and staff members. One set of themes is related to the value of personal possessions — in terms of former life connections, self-expression, intrinsic value, and care related value (in the case of often-expensive devices such as eyeglasses, hearing aids and dentures). The other set of themes focuses on the experience of losing things — in terms of expressed concerns related to resident behaviors, challenges of providing care, and problems or worries about theft and security. Discussion of ethical considerations in cultural context addresses hypothetical questions such as: *Who can place a value on these things? Who is responsible when residents with dementia lose things or take items that belong to others? If a resident seems to have no interest in the objects that surround him/her, does it matter? Should we be doubtful about complaints of theft by residents with dementia who lose and misplace things? Should residents be denied the use of expensive devices that easily could be lost or destroyed?*

      Practice implications, expressed as *principles and strategies*, are discussed and summarized in a third table. Some of these are relevant to all nursing home residents. Others target issues that relate specifically to caring for residents with dementia. Thus, in contrast to the previous two reports, the practical applications in this paper are more narrowly problem-focused and action-oriented.

Nursing Home Ethics: Everyday Issues Affecting Residents with Dementia
(Powers, 2003a)

The monograph format of this text accomplished a number of things that journal articles cannot do. The major advantage was a greater amount of space to present the data in more detail and to describe the cultural contexts that make findings (evidence) more understandable and meaningful. Specifically, the book-length text made it possible to: (a) demonstrate the use of the taxonomy more thoroughly through examples; (b) present the 12 paradigm cases together in a dialogue-like format similar to conversations that might take place between staff or ethics committee members about pros and cons of various actions; and (c) include the guidelines for nursing home ethics committees in an appendix.

      The style, content, and organization of this research report also made it possible to reach out to a wider audience defined as: (a) persons who work or volunteer in nursing homes; (b) laypersons who wish to know more about dementia and long-term care, especially those who have kin or significant others with dementia who are living in nursing homes; and (c) educators and students in the field of gerontology. The writing tone is conversational because anthropologists often use this personal down-to-earth style when they want to convey more than factual information. In this way it often is possible to engage a wider audience because those who are new to the material will find it easy to become informed. And those who are more expert will be able to appreciate the information at a higher level – in this instance, one that enables them to reflect on how the interpretive rendition of the study participants' and researcher's shared experiences and insights may resonate with and/or contribute to what they already know. Expert professionals and educators also are in a good position to use the material in this text for educational purposes.

The design of a narrative structure to help readers understand, not issues alone, but also their complexity, involved: (a) the use of vignettes and quotes so that readers could vicariously get a feel for what being involved with an issue is like; (b) the use of a conversation-type ethical evaluation approach to simulate discussion about the issues presented in case examples; and (c) the use of a wide literature base to show where various explanations and interpretations of the data fit with what already is known about dementia, dementia and nursing home care, ethics, and ethical case analysis.

The organizational flow across chapters was closely tied to the research analysis that always began with how dementia shaped the experiences of residents and their families in the time leading up to decisions to live in a nursing home as well as what happened thereafter. Thus, the first two chapters on *Living with Dementia* and *The Nursing Home Experience* introduce the major focus of the book – *Ethics in Action* that describes a practical approach to ethical evaluation which is demonstrated by five abbreviated and twelve extensive case examples (fictionalized accounts based on the data) with titles, such as the following: *My Favorite Things; It Feels Just Like Jail; Timing is Everything;* and *Please, Just One More Bite.*

Finally, information within chapters is most often organized around actual quotes from the data that serve to signal transitions in ways that help sustain the personal nature of experiences that the researcher and readers are privileged to share with the experts – the participants in this study who live with dementia day in and day out. For example, the section headings within the first chapter on *Living with Dementia* lead the reader through family members' accounts of theirs and their loved ones' experiences in the following manner: *"It was such an unexpected thing"; "It came to the point where we needed a diagnosis"; "She fought me tooth and nail"; "It was traumatic for her and for us"; There was no way we could let her live alone"; "I don't think they watched her very well"; "We decided to move in with her"; "I wanted to make everything right, and you just can't"; "I felt like I'd be betraying him";* and *"It's brought us close together."* However, the information in the chapter is not only about personal experiences. Through a writing process called *interweaving*, participants' words and stories are used to draw attention to information that everybody should know about dementia and dementia-related issues in long-term care at the same time that they are used to ground this information in real-life human experiences.

In summary, reporting practical applications of this research on resolving ethical issues of daily living affecting nursing home residents with dementia has moved beyond the design of the now completed execution phase of the research – involving looking for best evidence - to the current dissemination phase - involving the design of how the evidence may best be represented. Representation in ethnographic work is about the many ways in which social reality can be conveyed to effectively communicate study findings and to address the specific interests of different audiences. It also is about teasing out and mining the richness of the data because no single report is likely to be able to do justice to it all. And it is, above all, about being true to one's data. That is, as long as the analysis and reanalysis of the evidence continues with each representation of its various aspects, the data are kept alive. And living data are essential for the creation of accurate, sensitive, respectful portrayals of the subject matter of human science research, such as that above, from which practical applications may be drawn.

*This research was supported by a grant from the New York State Department of Health, Bureau of Long Term Care.

references

Powers, BA (2000). Everyday ethics of dementia care in nursing homes: A definition and taxonomy. *American Journal of Alzheimer's Disease, 15*(3), 143–151.

Powers, BA (2001). Ethnographic analysis of everyday ethics in the care of nursing home residents with dementia: A taxonomy. *Nursing Research, 50*, 332–339.

Powers, BA (2003a). *Nursing home ethics: Everyday issues affecting residents with dementia.* New York: Springer.

Powers, BA (2003b). The significance of losing things for nursing home residents with dementia and their families. *Journal of Gerontological Nursing, 29*, 43–52.

Shakespeare, W. (1594/5). *Romeo and Juliet.* In Rowse, A.L.(Ed.), *The annotated Shakespeare: The comedies, histories, sonnets and other poems, tragedies, and romances complete* (pp.1610–1669). New York: Greenwich House, 1988.

Example of a Slide Show for a 20-Minute Paper Presentation

appendix G

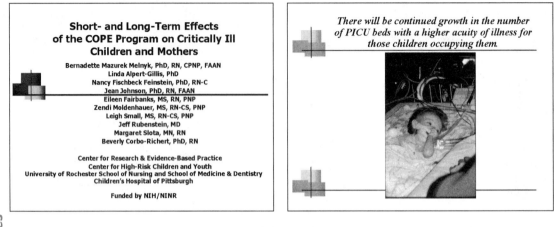

**Short- and Long-Term Effects
of the COPE Program on Critically Ill
Children and Mothers**

Bernadette Mazurek Melnyk, PhD, RN, CPNP, FAAN
Linda Alpert-Gillis, PhD
Nancy Fischbeck Feinstein, PhD, RN-C
Jean Johnson, PhD, RN, FAAN
Eileen Fairbanks, MS, RN, PNP
Zendi Moldenhauer, MS, RN-CS, PNP
Leigh Small, MS, RN-CS, PNP
Jeff Rubenstein, MD
Margaret Slota, MN, RN
Beverly Corbo-Richert, PhD, RN

Center for Research & Evidence-Based Practice
Center for High-Risk Children and Youth
University of Rochester School of Nursing and School of Medicine & Dentistry
Children's Hospital of Pittsburgh

Funded by NIH/NINR

*There will be continued growth in the number
of PICU beds with a higher acuity of illness for
those children occupying them.*

*Critically ill children are especially vulnerable to a
multitude of negative emotional and behavioral outcomes.*

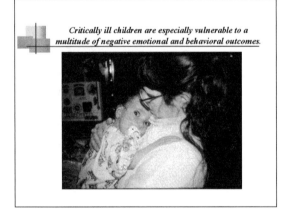

*Parents of critically ill children also are at risk for a host of
negative mental health outcomes, including PTSD.*

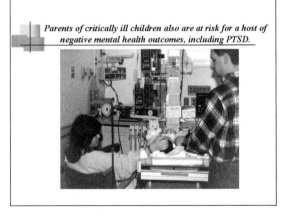

The Primary Aim of This Study

- To evaluate both the short- and long-term effects of the COPE (Creating Opportunities for Parent Empowerment) intervention program on the process and outcomes of mother and child coping with critical illness within the context of a full-scale randomized trial, as long as 12 months after hospitalization

The Theoretical Framework

- **Self-regulation theory (Leventhal & Johnson)**

- **Control theory (Carver & Scheier)**

- **The emotional contagion hypotheses (VanderVeer)**

Hypothesized Effects of the COPE Program on the Process and Outcomes of Maternal and Child Coping

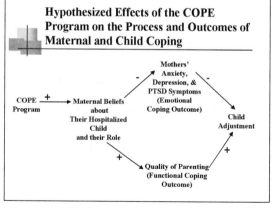

Methods

Study design: a randomized, controlled trial
Sites for the study:

- **Golisano Children's Hospital at the University of Rochester Medical Center**

- **Children's Hospital of Pittsburgh**

Randomization: Subjects were randomly assigned to either the COPE intervention or control intervention by 1-week blocks of time in order to decrease the probability of contamination.

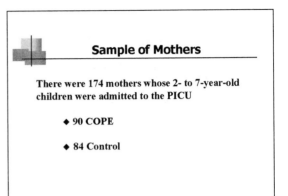

The Three Phases of the COPE and Control Intervention Programs

♦ Phase I: 6 to 16 hours after admission to the PICU

♦ Phase II: within 2 to 16 hours after transfer from the PICU to the general pediatric unit

♦ Phase III: within 2 to 3 days after discharge from the hospital

Sample of Mothers

There were 174 mothers whose 2- to 7-year-old children were admitted to the PICU

◆ 90 COPE

◆ 84 Control

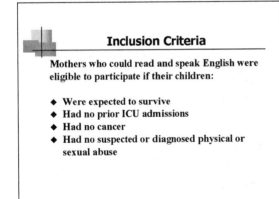

Inclusion Criteria

Mothers who could read and speak English were eligible to participate if their children:

◆ Were expected to survive
◆ Had no prior ICU admissions
◆ Had no cancer
◆ Had no suspected or diagnosed physical or sexual abuse

Exclusion Criteria

Mothers were excluded from data analysis if:

◆ Their children were readmitted to the PICU

◆ Their children were hospitalized in the PICU longer than 21 days

◆ They made a personal decision to withdraw from the study

The Sample

Of 212 eligible mothers, 38 (18%) refused to participate due to:

◆ Being too stressed or tired

◆ The desire to focus only on their children

Analysis of major demographic variables between those mothers who refused to participate and those who participated revealed no significant differences

The Final Sample

Of the 174 mothers enrolled, data from 11 mothers were excluded from the final data analysis because of:

◆ **Prior admission to the PICU**
◆ **A planned admission**
◆ **Readmission to the PICU**
◆ **Death after multiple readmissions to the PICU**

The final sample consisted of 163 mothers and their children

Demographics on the Sample of Mothers

Mean age = 31.2 years (SD = 6.3 years)
Mean number of other children at home = 1.7 (SD=1.4)
Racial/Ethnic Breakdown

◆ White = 116 (71.2%)
◆ African American = 33 (20.3%)
◆ Hispanic = 3 (1.8%)
◆ Native American = 2 (1.2%)
◆ Other = 9 (5.5%)

Demographics on the Sample of Children

Mean age = 50.2 months (SD = 18.9 months)

Gender
  ◆ Males = 99 (60.7%)
  ◆ Females = 64 (39.3%)

Major reasons for hospitalization
  ◆ **Respiratory problems (n = 71, 43.6%)**
  ◆ **Accidental trauma (n = 26, 16%)**
  ◆ **Neurological problems (n = 22, 13.5%)**
  ◆ **Infections (n = 18, 11%)**

Demographics on the Sample of Children

No prior hospitalizations, n = 93 (57%)

Mean pediatric risk of mortality score = 4.4 points (SD = 4.9 points)

Mean length of stay in the PICU = 63.9 hours (SD = 64.5 hours)

Mean length of hospital stay = 6.9 days (SD = 6.3 days)

The First Component of the COPE Program

Educational information that was audiotaped, which focused on:

◆ Creating a cognitive schema to increase parents' knowledge and understanding of the range of behaviors that young children typically display during and after hospitalization (guided by self-regulation theory)

◆ Removing barriers so that parents could participate in their child's care and facilitate their children's adaptation to hospitalization (guided by control theory)

The Second Component of the COPE Program

Behavioral workbook with activities for parents to perform with their children to enhance their adjustment:

◆ Therapeutic medical play

◆ Puppet play

◆ Jenny's Wish Book

From: *Jenny's Wish*

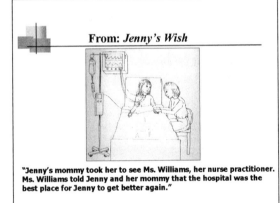

"Jenny's mommy took her to see Ms. Williams, her nurse practitioner. Ms. Williams told Jenny and her mommy that the hospital was the best place for Jenny to get better again."

The Control Intervention Program

♦ Control audiotaped information about the hospital's services and polices

♦ Control parent–child behavioral workbook with activities (coloring, reading a non-hospital–related story)

Dependent Variables and Measures of Emotional Coping

Variable	Measure	Cronbach Alphas
Mothers' state anxiety	State Anxiety Inventory (A-State) Spielberger et al., 1977	0.94 – 0.96
Mothers' mood state	Profile of Mood States (POMS) Lorr & McNair, 1989	0.92 – 0.96
Mothers' stress related to PICU	Parental Stressor Scale: PICU Miles & Carter, 1982	0.90 – 0.91

Dependent Variables and Measures of Functional Coping

Variable	Measure	Cronbach Alphas
Mothers' participation in care	Index of Parent Participation (IPP) Melnyk, 1994	0.85
	Visual analogue scales (VAS-EC, VAS-PC) Melnyk, 1994	N/A
Mothers' support during procedures	Index of Parental Support (IPS) Melnyk, 1994	0.81 – .85

Dependent Variables and Measures of Post-Hospital Adjustment

Variable	Measure	Cronbach alphas
Mothers' PTSD symptoms	Post-hospital Stress Index for Parents (PSI-P) Melnyk & Alpert – Gillis, 1997	0.83 – 0.88
Child adjustment	Behavioral Assessment Scale for Children (BASC) Reynolds & Kamphaus, 1992	0.92 – 0.95
	Post-hospital Stress Index for Children (PSI-C) Melnyk & Alpert – Gillis, 1997	0.78 – 0.85

appendices

Process Variable

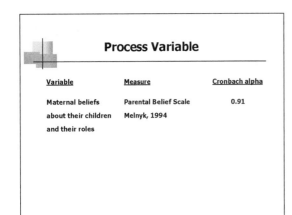

Variable	Measure	Cronbach alpha
Maternal beliefs about their children and their roles	Parental Belief Scale Melnyk, 1994	0.91

Manipulation Checks

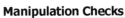

- ◆ Twelve multiple choice questions after each of the three interventions assessed processing of the educational information.
- ◆ Higher scores by the COPE mothers on the set of questions related to the COPE information and higher scores by the control mothers on the set of questions related to the control program documented processing of the appropriate information.

Statistical Analyses

- ◆ No distribution abnormalities were found.
- ◆ Subjects at each of the two sites were similar on most demographic and clinical variables, except for gender of the child, type of admission, use of restraints, and the father's level of education.
- ◆ Maternal trait anxiety correlated with multiple dependent variables.
- ◆ Study site and maternal trait anxiety were statistically controlled for in all data analyses.

Study Attrition by 1 Year Post-Discharge

- ◆ 50% in the COPE group (n = 44)
  67% in the control group (n = 51)
- ◆ There were no significant differences in demographic and baseline clinical variables as well as outcomes at 6 months post-discharge between the subjects who stayed in the study and those who dropped out of the study.
- ◆ Because of the smaller numbers at the 6- and 12-month post-discharge points that resulted in low observed power of our statistical tests, a decision was made to calculate effect sizes as part of the analytic strategy to avoid Type II errors.

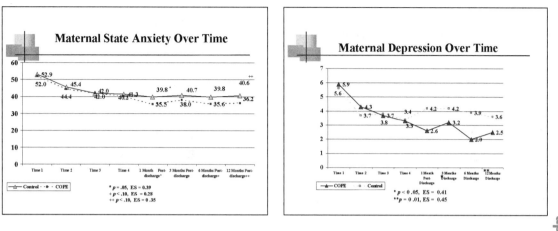

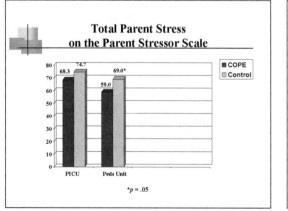

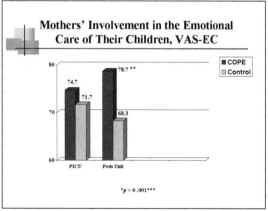

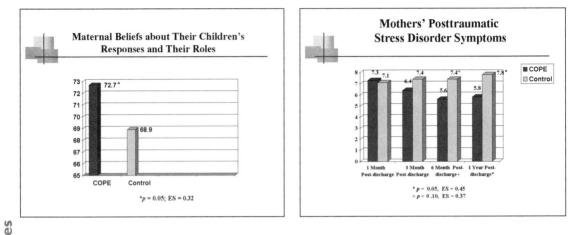

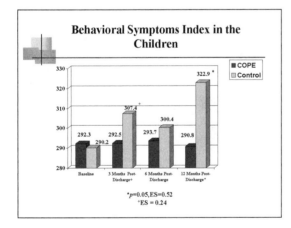

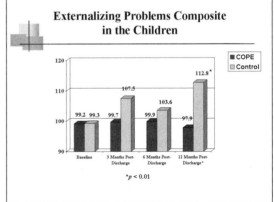

Clinically Significant Maladaptive Behaviors at the 12-Month Follow-up

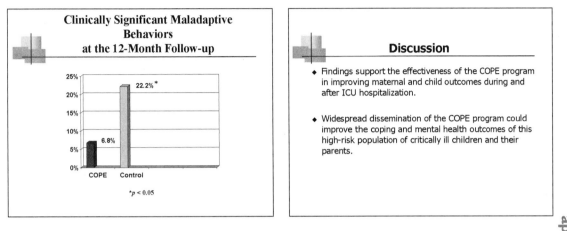

25% | 20% | 15% | 10% | 5% | 0%

22.2%*

6.8%

COPE   Control

*$p < 0.05$

Discussion

♦ Findings support the effectiveness of the COPE program in improving maternal and child outcomes during and after ICU hospitalization.

♦ Widespread dissemination of the COPE program could improve the coping and mental health outcomes of this high-risk population of critically ill children and their parents.

A Limitation of This Clinical Trial

♦ **The attrition rate.** However, there were no significant differences found on major demographic and baseline clinical variables as well as the 6-month outcomes between those mothers and children who remained in the study and those who did not.

The COPE Program should be routinely provided to critically ill children and their parents.

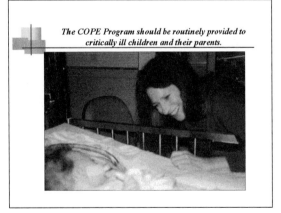

Example of a Health Policy Brief

appendix H

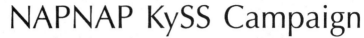

NAPNAP KySS Campaign

Keep your children/yourself Safe and Secure

20 Brace Road, Suite 200, Cherry Hill, NJ 08034-2634   Website: www.napnap.org
Voice: 856/857-9700   Fax: 856/857-1600   E-mail: info@napnap.org

National Study and Summit Urges the Need for Expanded Mental Health Services by Primary Care Providers

One in four (i.e., 13.7 million) U.S. children and teenagers has a mental health/psychosocial problem that affects their functioning at home or school. The incidence is believed to be underestimated due, in large part, to inadequate screening by primary care providers. Of children and teens affected by these problems, 70 percent do not receive any mental health services. There are only 6,300 child psychiatrists in the U.S. while need is estimated at 30,000 and there is a severe maldistribution. The costs associated with mental health problems are over 69 billion dollars per year. President George W. Bush's New Freedom Commission on Mental Health says that "the mental health system is failing Americans" and one of the major barriers to care is fragmentation and gaps in care for children."

As a result of mental health problems beginning to surpass the incidence of physical health problems in children and teens, the National Association of Pediatric Nurse Practitioners (NAPNAP) launched a new campaign called KySS (Keep your children/yourself Safe and Secure) in the spring of 2001. The goal of KySS is to prevent and reduce psychiatric problems in children and youth with one arm specifically geared to enhancing the knowledge and skills of primary care doctors and nurse practitioners to screen for and deliver early interventions to prevent more severe mental health problems. The campaign, which addresses several of the leading health indicators in Healthy People 2010 (e.g., mental health, tobacco and substance use, responsible sexual behavior, access to care, injury and violence, overweight and obesity, and physical activity), is now endorsed/supported by 23 national professional organizations, including the American Academy of Pediatrics, the American School Health Association, the National Association of Social Workers, the National Association of School Psychologists, the American Nurses Association, and the Association of Faculties of Pediatric Nurse Practitioners. The KySS Campaign is tackling the problem from an interdisciplinary perspective, across multiple health professions, which is the only way to assure that the right solutions are generated and implemented.

The first phase of the KySS Campaign was a national survey of over 1900 children/teens, parents, and pediatric primary care providers from 24 states. Findings from the KySS Survey, originally reported in the September/October, 2002 issue of *Journal of Pediatric Healthcare* indicated that the top five mental health worries of children/teens and their parents included: 1) how to cope with stressful things in their lives, 2) depression, 3) anxiety, 4) self-esteem, and 5) parent-child relationships. Twenty-five percent of the children/teens worried about how to cope with stressful things often to nearly always. Despite the high level of worries reported by the children/teens and their parents, only a small percentage reported talking to their doctors or nurse practitioners about their concerns.

Primary care providers answered only 64% of the mental health knowledge questions correctly on the KySS survey. Approximately 70 to 80 percent of the providers who completed the survey reported that they did not always consistently screen for various mental health problems in school-aged children and teenagers. About half of the providers felt that their professional education programs id not prepare them well to assess and intervene effectively with children and teens who have mental health/psychosocial morbidities. The majority of the providers stressed that what is needed to tackle these problems is better reimbursement in order to compensate them for their time if they were going to make screening and early intervention for these problems standard practice, better professional and continuing education training, and more effective evidence-based intervention programs that can be delivered in primary care settings.

As part of the KySS campaign, a national summit funded by HRSA/Maternal and Child Health Bureau was conducted on March 28 and March 29, 2003. The KySS Summit convened an unprecedented gathering of over 70 experts from 20 national health care organizations – a combination of specialties never before gathered – to plan initiatives and hammer out specific changes for health care providers to improve the mental health and safety of children and adolescents.

Former U.S. Surgeon General, Dr. David Satcher, was the featured speaker at the KySS Summit. During his talk, Dr. Satcher emphasized the importance of childhood as the foundation for the rest of adult health. He also emphasized that most mental health treatment can be provided by primary care providers if they are well trained in the assessment and early management of these problems.

Outcomes of the KySS Summit include plans for influencing health policy to: (1) increase funds for more health professional educational programs (both basic and professional continuing education programs) that enhance primary care providers' knowledge and screening, early and preventive intervention skills for the broad spectrum of mental health problems in children and teens, (2) increase funds for educational programs that prepare practitioners who are dually prepared in pediatrics and psychiatric mental health, which would improve access and decrease stigma for families with affected children, (3) expand reimbursement for early intervention/counseling services delivered by primary care providers, and (4) improve access to mental health services for all children.

Other outcomes of the KySS summit include plans for: (1) developing easy to use and efficient screening tools for the identification of mental health problems, (2) creating a core curriculum for professional educational programs to assist future clinicians in better detecting and treating psychosocial problems, (3) a national KySS continuing education institute and on-line courses that will train health care providers to deal with psychological problems in children and teens before they progress into dangerous behaviors and complex psychiatric mental health problems, (4) a KySS clearinghouse website for healthcare providers, parents and teens to learn more about these problems, (5) a major public health campaign to raise awareness of these problems and to decrease the ongoing stigma associated with them, (6) disseminating evidence-based effective interventions to primary care providers, and (7) developing and testing efficient mental health interventions for use in primary care.

The keys to decreasing the staggering human and financial costs of mental health problems in adulthood is increasing reimbursement for pediatric healthcare providers to deal with these problems in primary care settings, increasing funds for the training of health professionals to be competent in the delivery of these services, and decreasing stigma through major public health awareness campaigns. The detection of these problems and early mental health interventions with all children and teens in primary care will translate into healthier and more functional adults who can be productive in our society.

For more information about the KySS Campaign, please contact NAPNAP's national office or Bernadette Melnyk, PhD, RN, CPNP, NPP, FAAN, founder and director of the KySS campaign, at Bernadette_Melnyk@urmc.rochester.edu or 585-275-8903.

Example of a Press Release

appendix I

NAPNAP KySS Campaign

Keep your children/yourself Safe and Secure

20 Brace Road, Suite 200, Cherry Hill, NJ 08034-2634   Website: www.napnap.org
Voice: 856/857-9700   Fax: 856/857-1600   E-mail: info@napnap.org

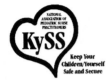

Sept. 10, 2002

FOR IMMEDIATE RELEASE

For further information, contact
Joe Casey at NAPNAP, or
Mark Liu
Mark_Liu@urmc.rochester.edu
(585) 275-1309

Before and After 9/11: Anxiety Plagues Children;

Parents and Healthcare Providers Need to Offer More Support

Children and teens in the United States who were surveyed after the September 11 attacks were significantly more worried about how to cope with stress than those surveyed before, while parents surveyed after 9-11 actually worried *less* about their children coping, according to surprising results of a national survey.

The 24-state survey, conducted in summer and fall 2001 by the National Association of Pediatric Nurse Practitioners (NAPNAP) in collaboration with the University of Rochester School of Nursing, also found a major gap between the perception of children and their parents as to how much the two groups talk to each other about children's anxiety, depression and stress, and a serious deficiency in discussion between children and their primary health care providers about their mental health problems. The findings appear in the Sept. 18 issue of the *Journal of Pediatric Health Care* and in the on-line version on Sept 11.

The gap between increased worries in children after Sept. 11 and parents' concerns about their children's worries was significant. Before 9/11, 21 percent of children and teens worried often, nearly always or always about coping with stressful things; after 9/11, 32 percent did. But among parents before 9/11, 39 percent worried often, nearly always or always about their children's ability to cope with stress, while after 9/11 only 26 percent did. One factor, hypothesizes Bernadette Melnyk, Ph.D., R.N. and primary investigator of the study, is that parents may have been more focused on how they could help the families directly affected by the tragedy – a common coping strategy.

Regardless of the reason, it points to a widening gap in parent-child communication and perception. Approximately 80 percent of parents said they talk to their children at least sometimes about anxiety, while only about 37 percent of their children said the same about talking with their parents. And 72 percent of parents said they talk at least sometimes with their children about depression, while only 36 percent of their children said the same.

"Parents think they're talking to their kids, but their kids don't think so or they're not hearing it," says Melnyk. "Many of the children and teens said they needed more information about mental health problems. It's an area where health care providers need to focus more of their attention."

The study bears this out. A large percentage of children and teens reported having mental health and psychosocial worries (25 percent worried often, nearly always or always about how to cope with stressful things, and 36 percent worried sometimes; 49 percent worried sometimes, often, nearly always or always about depression). Yet very few talked to their nurse practitioner or doctor about those worries. Eighty percent said they never talked about depression to their nurse practitioner or doctor.

Since mental health problems such as depression can be factors in risky behavior such as substance abuse and unsafe sex, Melnyk sees this lack of communication as a lost chance to help children.

"Pediatric health care providers should see office visits as windows of opportunity to draw out their patients' concerns and worries," Melnyk says. "The key is providing the right environment to get children, teens and parents to talk more about these mental health issues."

One promising solution comes from the survey itself. Simply from answering the survey questions about their worries and concerns,
- 48.5 percent of children and 50 percent of their parents reported better awareness of emotions and behaviors affecting children and teens
- 41 percent of the children and 52 percent of parents said that answering the survey will lead them to get more information about emotional and behavioral problems affecting children and teens
- 44 percent of the children and 63.5 percent of parents said that answering the survey will help them talk to their child/parent about these issues
- And 32.5 percent of children and 56 percent of parents said that answering the survey will help them talk to their nurse practitioner or doctor about these issues.

"Having this survey or similar ones for children, teens and their parents to complete while waiting to see their primary care providers could serve as a good way to screen for these problems," says Melnyk. "That could lead to earlier intervention with children and teens affected by mental health problems."

A total of 1224 children, teens and their parents completed the survey, part of the Keep your Children/yourself Safe and Secure (KYSS) campaign launched by Melnyk in July 2001 with the backing of the National Association of Pediatric Nurse Practitioners. With recent funding from the U.S. Department of Health and Human Services/Maternal-Child Health Bureau, the KySS campaign will convene a summit of experts in **March** to plan ways to help primary care providers intervene earlier with children who have mental health/psychosocial problems.

The University of Rochester School of Nursing is addressing these same issues with its new dual Pediatric Nurse Practitioner and Psychiatric Mental Health Nurse Practitioner Master's program – one of the first of its kind in the country.

Studies have shown that families tend to feel more comfortable seeking mental health treatment for children in primary care settings, making the nurse practitioner role a crucial one in detection and treatment.

"In this program, we want to provide a new, holistic model of primary care for children geared not just to their biological needs but also their psychological and social health care needs as well," says Melnyk.

###

Case Example of a Successful Media Dissemination Effort

appendix J

Case Example: When Rocking Chairs in Nursing Homes Make the News[1]

Nancy Watson

I'm the case study of what happens when the media strikes! I'm going to tell you what it was like to have your research or your story picked up by the public press. It all began when I was sitting in my office and the phone rang. It was a person from the public relations (PR) office at the university where I worked. He had heard I was presenting my research about our rocking chair study at a conference, and he wanted to know about it. He had a research abstract, but wanted me to explain it to him in laymen's terms.

The rocking chair study was directly aimed at improving the clinical problem that we examined in prior studies, the well-being of people with dementia in nursing homes. Our research team, led by the original Principal Investigator Dr. Thelma Wells, tried a simple intervention of using rocking to improve psychological well-being and improve balance.

What we found was that it worked. We were able to reduce anxiety/depression when the residents rocked long enough and also improved balance in

---

[1] 2001 Sigma Theta Tau International Research Dissemination Award

those who seemed to like it. This study spoke directly to a clinical need that came straight from practice and has gone back to practice. We have received hundreds of requests for intervention teaching materials. It is exciting when an intervention actually changes practice in a variety of settings.

The PR representative asked really hard and very specific questions, (e.g. "how many people improved;" "how much did they improve in numerical terms;" and "what does that mean for a patient"). These questions required rethinking and reframing, even recalculating numbers to recast the findings in a form that would be most easily understood by the average reader. The PR representative also asked why we thought rocking might be beneficial (i.e., what was the idea (theory) behind it, and what was the clinical hunch that led to it). All of this was a preparation for the actual interviews that followed.

The press release came next. This document translated our research into a form that would hopefully catch the public's imagination. But, before the press release went out, I had to check it very carefully to make sure it was accurate. It was a bit of a culture shock to see our technical research reframed in terms that the public would care about. But that reframing was *key* to why our story was so far reaching.

The first interview was with the Boston Globe Science Reporter. I was scared to death. It was on the Thursday before the Saturday conference at which we were to present our research. The interview lasted about 40 minutes, I think, though it seemed like forever. Though the interview was intense, our PR representative had primed me well. I had a sheet of paper in front of me with all the bits and pieces of things I might need to have at my fingertips (e.g., sample size, significant findings with the statistics). I also had the citations for key supportive studies and the references for the theoretical basis of the study right in front of me...and I was glad I had them. The reporter actually wanted to know the *exact* citations that this work was based upon and wrote them down. I'm certain the reporter must have looked them up as a way of being sure that we were "for real," and knew what we were talking about.

The reporter wanted to release the story before the "embargo" (i.e., an agreed upon time before which information about a study cannot be released) that was Saturday 12 noon when the study would be presented at the conference. The reporter really pushed, as he wanted to release the story for the Saturday morning paper, promising that he was sure he could get it on the front page of the Saturday edition. Our PR representative had told me to stand firm, so I did.

Low and behold, the story showed up on the front page of the Sunday edition. The Boston Globe headline was "Rock of Aged: Chairs' Sway May Soothe Ailing Elders." One important point is that they attributed the study to a nurse researcher. And this is no small point and not by accident. It was because I went to great pains to convince this reporter that this was important *to me*. I made it clear every time I talked to a reporter that I wanted them to be sure to mention that I was a nurse. I didn't care about being a PhD, but the nurse part was very important to me.

Even on Saturday, the press release started the phone ringing. On the day of the conference, in between sessions, I was on a pay phone calling reporters back who were interested in the story. In addition, on that same day, two of the local networks picked up the story, and it quickly went national. San Francisco, New York City, Seattle, Los Angeles, Philadelphia, Boston, Richmond, Columbus, and Tulsa, to name a few, aired the story.

I think part of the reason the story got so much television coverage was because we had the pictures of people using the rocking chairs, and this made the story visually interesting.

To use the pictures, we had to alert families, who had already given permission for the training video, that their loved one might be on television. This preparation was done ahead of time, when we first learned that this story might hit the press.

When the Boston Globe article hit on Sunday, things really heated up...and the phone was ringing off the hook. Our PR representative and I were tied at the hip! He could reach me anywhere; I had all his numbers and he had all my numbers, and he needed them.

The biggest thing that happened was that USA Today called on Sunday to do a story for the next morning. The reporter stated at 5pm on Sunday evening that she had to talk to me *immediately*. I called her right back and we did the interview over the phone. The next morning the story was on the front page of the Life Style Section of USA Today. I bought 10 copies (almost cleaned out the Seven-Eleven Store) and delivered copies to the nursing home that had been the study site. I left one for the Administrator and one for the Director of Nursing. I made sure to put one on the unit where we did the study.

The lesson to be learned here is that you have to act fast and be available to respond to the many reporters wanting to get the story out. USA Today was just ready to go to press when I called them back on Sunday. They were eager to get the story that the Boston Globe had scooped in their next day's edition. So being *reachable* and *ready* made the difference.

The next week was wild. Most notable were the radio reports and interviews on most of the major networks, including a long interview with the BBC that aired world-wide. These interviews included such questions as "how could people living the jungle fashion somewhat to rock — like a swing in a tree?" So I had to translate the principles of the rocking experience into terms that could be applied in a very foreign culture. This was a wonderful opportunity to reach a world-wide audience. I again told the reporter that it was really important to me that he mention that I was a nurse.

The next onslaught came from the wire services, wanting to pick up the story, including Reuters, Associated Press, UPI. As a result of the wire services running the story, newspaper articles popped up everywhere. We had alumni sending us articles from their local papers from across the country. This spin-off effect was very exciting. But there was also a feeling that the story was taking on a life of its own; and it *was*!

Next Time Magazine wanted to pick up the story and included a piece in their "GOOD NEWS" Health Report about three weeks later. It was attributed to the Eastern Nursing Research Society, thus, keeping the nursing connection. Websites were also picking up the story, including ABC, CBS, Associated Press, and NewsDay. These stories also involved interviews with freelance writers who would call and need to talk to us directly to get their *own* spin on the story. To be prepared, I needed to keep my notes out and ready for these calls too.

One of the most meaningful articles was the one in the Alzheimer's Association's "Advances" for families and caregivers. It was significant because it directly reached the people who needed it most, the people who love and care for persons with dementia, and that really meant a lot. This story lent real credibility to our work. Families and caregivers saw that nurses were important contributors to the effort to care for those persons with dementia.

That is how my story unfolded and some of what it is like to be caught up in the maelstrom of the public press. It was harrowing; it was very exciting; and it was rewarding. It was an opportunity to get the research to the people who could truly use it, and that made it worth it. My experience may not be typical, but I learned a lot from it. I hope that some of my experience may help you prepare for a similar experience with your work.

A science reporter for the university PR department calling on that April day enabled this to happen. He really walked me through it, and as a novice to this process, I really appreciated his sage advice. You may wonder how everything turned out and what happened as a result of our media attention. Our experience with the rocking chair study served to get the word out that nurses do research that matters. Nursing, having waited long and hard, had an opportunity to have the work nurses do be recognized!

But more than that, the initial coverage has continued to have a ripple effect. Recently, I did a live interview, via phone, with a news radio in London about the use of rocking chairs to relieve stress. For the last five years, I have had reporters call periodically wanting to know about whether or not rocking might be good for older people in general or if rockers in airports are a good idea. These questions stretch beyond our research, but that is fine. What I say is that our research was on people with dementia, but it is possible that it *could* have application for older persons, *BUT WE DON'T KNOW THAT FROM OUR* RESEARCH. Nevertheless, it is good to be asked and to be willing to help the reporter to be able to reference for their piece in a different context.

In addition to the continuing ripple effect with the media, we have gotten numerous phone calls from families, clinicians, and entrepreneurs. First, you would be surprised how many people (i.e., the entrepreneurs) have created rocking devices and contacted us wanting an endorsement. Our stand has always been that we cannot endorse specific products, only the idea that there *may* be value in rocking that is *self-propelled*. Our experience is somewhat typical in this respect, as press coverage may result in this type of response quite often, and you need to be ready for it. One variation on the calls from entrepreneurs has been the calls from the sales representatives from the company that manufactured the chair we used in the study. They have been interested in using our research to recommend that particular chair. However, we have taken the position that there are many chairs that meet the basic requirements that could be used safely for rocking, *not* just one brand. We have tried not to let our research be used for promotional purposes.

The families we have heard from have been our real joy. We have had phone calls from families with loved ones at home and in nursing homes, all wanting to know "what rocking chair we used" and if they should get one for their family member. These calls are our reward. They are our opportunity to make our research really matter. We have an opportunity to talk one-to-one with caregivers, and to explain to them how to go about it, and what to look for in a chair. As a part of our funding, we already had created a video to teach people how to select a chair, orient a person to the chair and teach them to rock. So, when families called we were ready with the video and clear written instructions to help them.

We also have had calls from nurses and other professionals, asking questions about using rocking chairs in their facilities. We have heard from nurses working in nursing homes, in psychiatric facilities, and in Veterans Administration (VA) hospitals. They have reported wonderful success with the rocking therapy, especially in calming people down when they are acutely upset. That is something that we observed anecdotally, but did not study directly.

Here is one testimonial that we just received this past August. It is from an Occupational Therapist (OT) working the VA system in California. She wrote, "Thank you very much for sending the video. Yesterday, I gave an inservice on Rocking Chair Therapy. It was such a huge success that three units — dementia, nursing home and hospice — would like to implement rocking chairs *ASAP*. I was able to get one [of the manufacture's chairs] for a trial use for one month. The manufacture's representative drove up from Southern California to deliver the chair to me the day before the inservice. I did a [slide] presentation, the chair was on display and I showed a two-minute clip of your video. Tomorrow, I am giving an inservice to the dementia nurses to implement the one rocking chair.

Today, my OT supervisor and I spent one hour with one of [our] more difficult dementia patient[s] and had him rock in the chair. At first, it wasn't working, but we gave him a teddy bear. Oh it was, incredible! He didn't want to leave the chair. He just kept on rocking. The patient has three children and maybe he thought he was rocking one of them. We're planning another rocking session with him tomorrow. I just want to thank you for all your great work on the rocking chair study and I want you to know that I know it is going to benefit the west coast VA sites in many positive ways. Again, thank you and I will keep you informed of our progress."

This is just one example of what we are still hearing. This truly is our reward. The media coverage has helped us get a clinical innovation out to the world in much shorter time than the usual 17 years that it usually takes to change clinical practice. It has communicated the "evidence" to those who can use it. The research article (Watson, Wells & Cox, 1998) is important to communicate the science to the professionals, but the public media is how this simple idea of rocking has been so widely disseminated, to all those it affects, professional and lay persons.

Based on our experience, the media is an important tool for nurses to use in communicating their research and in making our practice more evidence-based. I hope you will have the opportunity to use it to get your story out too.

References

Watson, N. W., Wells, T. J. & Cox, Christopher (1998). Rocking Chair Therapy For Dementia Patients: Its Effect on Psychosocial Well-Being and Balance, *American Journal of Alzheimer's Disease 13*,(6), 296–308.

glossary

A

Action research: A general term for a variety of approaches that aim to resolve social problems by improving existing conditions for oppressed groups or communities.

Adoption of research evidence: A process that occurs across five stages of innovation (i.e., knowledge, persuasion, decision, implementation, and confirmation).

Analytic notes: Notes researchers write to themselves to record their thoughts, questions, and ideas as a process of simultaneous data collection and data analysis unfolds.

Applicability of study findings: Whether or not the effects of the study are appropriate for a particular patient situation.

Attrition: When subjects are lost from or drop their participation in a study (see loss of subjects to follow up).

Axial coding: A process used in grounded theory to relate categories of information by using a coding paradigm with predetermined subcategories (Strauss & Corbin, 1990).

B

Background questions: Questions that need to be answered as a foundation for asking the searchable, answerable foreground question. They are questions that ask for general information about a clinical issue and they have two components: the starting place of the question (e.g., what, where, when, why, and how), and the outcome of interest (e.g., the clinical diagnosis).

583

Basic social process (BSP): The basis for theory generation—recurs frequently, links all the data together, and describes the pattern followed regardless of the variety of conditions under which the experience takes place and different ways in which persons go through it. There are two types of BSP, a basic social psychological process (BSPP) and a basic social structural process (BSSP).

Benchmarking: The process of looking outward to identify, understand, and adapt outstanding [best] practices and [high performance] to help improve performance.

Bias: Divergence of results from the true values or the process that leads to such divergence.

Biography: An approach that produces an in-depth report of a person's life. Life histories and oral histories also involve gathering of biographical information and recording of personal recollections of one or more individuals.

Biosketch: A 2 to 3 page document, similar to a resume or brief curriculum vitae, that captures an individual's educational and professional work experience, honors, prior research grants, and publications.

Blind review: A review process in which identification of the author/creator/researcher is removed and, likewise, the identity of the reviewers so that anonymity of both parties is assured.

Blocking: A strategy introduced into a study that entails deliberately including a potential extraneous intrinsic or confounding variable in a study's design in order to control its effects on the dependent or outcome variable.

Booster interventions: Interventions that are delivered after the initial intervention or treatment in a study for the purpose of enhancing the effects of the intervention.

Bracketing: Identifying and suspending previously acquired knowledge, beliefs, and opinions about a phenomenon.

C

Care delivery outcomes: The outcomes that are influenced by the delivery of clinical care.

Case-control study: A type of research that retrospectively compares characteristics of an individual who has a certain condition (e.g., hypertension) with one who does not (i.e., a matched control or similar person without hypertension); often conducted for the purpose of identifying variables that might predict the condition (e.g., stressful lifestyle, sodium intake).

Case reports: Reports that describe the history of a single patient, or a small group of patients, usually in the form of a story.

Case study: An intensive investigation of a case involving a person or small group of persons, an issue, or an event.

Categorical data: Data that is classified into categories (e.g., gender, hair color) instead of being numerically ordered.

Ceiling effects: Participant scores that cluster toward the high end of a measure.

Clinical forethought: All the anticipated actions and plans relevant to a particular patient's possible trends and trajectories that a clinician prepares for in caring for the patient.

Clinical grasp: Clinical inquiry in action. Includes problem identification and clinical judgment across time about the particular transitions of particular patient/family clinical situations. Four aspects of clinical grasp include making qualitative distinctions, engaging in detective work, recognizing changing relevance, and developing clinical knowledge about specific patient populations.

Clinical inquiry: A process in which clinicians gather data together using narrowly defined clinical parameters; it allows for an appraisal of the available choices of treatment for the purpose of finding the most appropriate choice of action.

Clinical practice guidelines: Systematically developed statements to assist clinicians and patients in making decisions about care; ideally the guidelines consist of a systematic review of the literature, in conjunction with consensus of a group of expert decision-makers, including administrators, policy-makers, clinicians, and consumers who consider the evidence and make recommendations.

Clinical significance: Study findings that will directly influence clinical practice, whether they are statistically significant or not.

Cochrane Central Register of Controlled Trials: A bibliography of controlled trials identified by contributors to the Cochrane Collaboration and others.

Cochrane Database of Methodology Reviews: Contains full text of systematic reviews of empirical methodological studies prepared by The Cochrane Empirical Methodological Studies Methods Group.

Cochrane Database of Systematic Reviews: Contains reviews that are highly structured and systematic with evidence included or excluded on the basis of explicit quality criteria, to minimize bias.

Cochrane Methodology Register: A bibliography of articles and books on the science of research synthesis.

Cohort study: A longitudinal study that begins with the gathering of two groups of patients (the cohorts), one that received the exposure (e.g., to a disease) and one that does not, and then following these groups over time (prospective) to measure the development of different outcomes (diseases).

Computer assisted qualitative data analysis: An area of technological innovation that, in qualitative research, has resulted in uses of word processing and software packages to support data management.

Confidence interval: A measure of the precision of the estimate. The 95% confidence interval (CI) is the range of values within which we can be 95% sure that the true value lies for the whole population of patients from whom the study patients were selected.

Confirmability: Demonstrated by providing substantiation that findings and interpretations are grounded in the data (i.e., links between researcher assertions and the data are clear and credible).

Confounding: Occurs when two factors are closely associated and the effects of one confuses or distorts the effects of the other factor on an outcome. The distorting factor is a confounding variable.

Confounding variables: Those factors that interfere with the relationship between the independent and dependent variables.

Constant comparison: A systematic approach to analysis that is a search for patterns in data as they are coded, sorted into categories, and examined in different contexts.

Construct validity: The degree to which an instrument measures the construct it is supposed to be measuring.

Contamination: The inadvertent and undesirable influence of an experimental intervention on another intervention.

Content analysis: In qualitative analysis, a term that refers to processes of breaking down narrative data (coding, comparing, contrasting and categorizing bits of information) and reconstituting them in some new form (e.g., description, interpretation, theory).

Content validity: The degree to which the items in an instrument are tapping the content they are supposed to measure.

Control group: A group of subjects who do not receive the experimental intervention or treatment.

Controlled vocabulary or thesaurus: A hierarchical arrangement of descriptive terms that serve as mapping agents for searches; often unique to each database.

Convenience sampling: Drawing readily available subjects to participate in a study.

Correlational descriptive study: A study that is conducted for the purpose of describing the relationship between two or more variables.

Correlational predictive study: A study that is conducted for the purpose of describing what variables predict a certain outcome.

Co-variate: A variable that is controlled for in statistical analyses (e.g., analysis of co-variance); the variable controlled is typically a confounding or extraneous variable that may influence the outcome.

Critical inquiry: Theoretical perspectives that are ideologically oriented toward critique of and emancipation from oppressive social arrangements or false ideas.

Critical theory: A blend of ideology (based on a critical theory of society) and a form of social analysis and critique that aims to liberate people from unrecognized myths and oppression in order to bring about enlightenment and radical social change.

Cronbach alpha: An estimate of internal consistency or homogeneity of an instrument that is comprised of several subparts or scales.

Cross-contamination: Diffusion of the treatment or intervention across study groups.

Cross-sectional study: A study designed to observe an outcome or variable at a single point in time, usually for the purpose of inferring trends over time.

Culture: Shared knowledge and behavior of people who interact within distinct social settings and subsystems.

D

Database of Abstracts of Reviews of Effects (DARE): Database that includes abstracts of systematic reviews that have been critically appraised by reviewers at the NHS Centre for Reviews and Dissemination at the University of York, England.

Data and safety monitoring plan: A detailed plan for how adverse effects will be assessed and managed.

Dependent or outcome variable: The variable or outcome that is influenced or caused by the independent variable.

Descriptive studies: Those studies that are conducted for the purpose of describing the characteristics of certain phenomena or selected variables.

Design: The overall plan for a study that includes strategies for controlling confounding variables, strategies for when the intervention will be delivered (in experimental studies) and how often and when the data will be collected.

Dialogical engagement: Thinking that is like a thoughtful dialogue or conversation.

Dimensional analysis: A method for generating grounded theory using an explanatory matrix (Schatzman, 1991).

Direct costs: Actual costs required to conduct a study (e.g., personnel, subject honoraria, instruments).

Discourse analysis: A general term for approaches to analyzing recorded talk and patterns of communication.

E

Educational prescription (EP): A written plan (usually self-initiated) for identifying and addressing EBP learning needs. The EP contains each step of the EBP process, but may have a primary focus on one or two steps, such as searching or critical appraisal.

Effect measures: Measures used to compare the differences in occurrences of outcomes between groups.

Effect size: The strength of the effect of an intervention.

Emergence: Glaser's (1992) term for conceptually driven ("discovery") versus procedurally driven ("forcing") theory development in his critique of Strauss and Corbin (1990).

Emic and etic: Contrasting "insider" views of informants (emic) and the researcher's "outsider" (etic) views.

Epistemologies: Ways of knowing and reasoning.

Essences: Internal meaning structures of a phenomenon grasped through the study of human lived experience.

Ethnographic studies: Studies of a social group's culture through time spent combining participant observation and in-depth interviews in the informants' natural setting.

Event rate: The rate at which a specific event occurs.

Evidence-based clinical practice guidelines: Specific practice recommendations that are based on a methodologically rigorous review of the best evidence on a specific topic.

Evidence-based decision making: The integration of best research evidence in making decisions about patient care, which should also include the clinician's expertise as well as patient preferences and values.

Evidence-based practice (EBP): A problem solving approach to practice that involves the conscientious use of current best evidence in making decisions about patient care; EBP incorporates a systematic search for and critical appraisal of the most relevant evidence to answer a clinical question along with one's own clinical expertise and patient values and preferences.

Evidence-based theories: A theory that has been tested and supported through the accumulation of evidence from several studies.

Evidence summaries: Syntheses of studies (see systematic reviews).

Evidence-user: Anyone who uses valid evidence to support or change practice; demonstrating skills in interpreting evidence, not generating evidence.

Exclusion criteria: Investigator-identified characteristics that are: (a) possessed by individuals that would exclude them from participating in a study; (b) specified to exclude studies from a body of evidence

Experiential learning: Experience requiring a turning around of preconceptions, expectations, sets, and routines or adding some new insights to a particular practical situation; a way of knowing that contributes to knowledge production; should influence the development of science.

Experimental design/experiment: A study whose purpose is to test the effects of an intervention or treatment on selected outcomes. This is the strongest design for testing cause and effect relationships.

External validity: Generalizability; the ability to generalize the findings from a study to the larger population from which the sample was drawn.

Extraneous variables: Those factors that interfere with the relationship between the independent and dependent variables.

F

Face validity: The degree to which an instrument appears to be measuring (i.e., tapping) the construct it is intended to measure.

Factorial design: An experimental design that has two or more interventions or treatments.

False positive: A condition where the test indicates that the person has the outcome of interest when, in fact, the person does not.

False negative: A condition where the test indicates that the person does not have the outcome of interest when, in fact, the person does.

Feminist epistemologies: A variety of views and practices inviting critical dialogue about women's experiences in historical, cultural, and socioeconomic perspectives.

Fieldnotes: Self-designed observational protocols for recording notes about field observations.

Field studies: Studies involving direct, first-hand observation and interviews in informants' natural settings.

Fieldwork: All research activities carried out in and in relation to the field (informants' natural settings).

Fixed effect model: Traditional assumption that the event rates are fixed in each of the control and treatment groups.

Floor effects: Participant scores that cluster toward the low end of a measure.

Focus groups: This type of group interview generates data on designated topics through discussion and interaction. Focus group research is a distinct type of study when used as the sole research strategy.

Foreground questions: Those questions that can be answered from scientific evidence about diagnosing, treating, or assisting patients with understanding their prognosis, focusing on specific knowledge.

Forest plot: (Colloquially called a "blobbogram") Diagrammatic representation of the results (i.e., the effects or point estimates) of trials (i.e., squares or "blobs") along with their confidence intervals (i.e., straight lines through the squares).

Funnel plot: The plotting of sample size against the effect size of studies included in a systematic review. The funnel should be inverted and symmetrical if a representative sample has been obtained.

G

Generalizability: The extent to which the findings from a study can be generalized or applied to the larger population (i.e. external validity).

Gold standard: An accepted and established reference standard or diagnostic test for a particular illness.

Grey literature: Refers to publications such as brochures and conference proceedings.

(Grounded) formal theory: A systematic explanation of an area of human /social experience derived through meta-analysis of substantive theory.

(Grounded) substantive theory: A systematic explanation of a situation-specific human experience/social phenomenon.

Grounded theory: Studies to generate theory about how people deal with life situations that is "grounded" in empirical data and describes the processes by which they move through experiences over time.

H

Harm: When risks outweigh benefits.

Health Technology Assessment Database: Database containing information on healthcare technology assessments.

Hermeneutics: Philosophy, theories, and practices of interpretation.

Hierarchy of evidence: A mechanism for determining which study designs have the most power to predict cause-and-effect. The highest level of evidence is systematic reviews of RCTs, and the lowest level of evidence is expert opinion and consensus statements.

History: The occurrence of some event or program unrelated to the intervention that might account for the change observed in the dependent variable.

Hits: Studies obtained from a search that contain the searched word.

Homogeneous study population/Homogeneity: When subjects in a study are similar on the characteristics that may affect the outcome variable(s).

Hyperlink: A connection to organized information that is housed in cyberspace and usually relevant to the site on which it was found.

Hypotheses: Predictions about the relationships between variables (e.g., adults who receive cognitive behavioral therapy will report less depression than those who receive relaxation therapy).

I

Incidence: New occurrences of the outcome or disorder within the at-risk population in a specified time frame.

Inclusion criteria: Essential characteristics specified by investigator that: (a) potential participants must possess in order to be considered for a study; (b) studies must meet to be included in a body of evidence.

Independent variable: The variable that is influencing the dependent variable or outcome; in experimental studies, it is the intervention or treatment.

Indirect costs: Costs that are not directly related to the actual conduct of a study, but are associated with the "overhead" in an organization, such as lights, telephones, office space.

Informatics: How data, information, knowledge, and wisdom are collected, stored, processed, communicated, and used to support the process of healthcare delivery to clients, providers, administrators, and organizations involved in healthcare delivery.

Integrative reviews: Systematic summaries of the accumulated state of knowledge about a concept, including highlights of important issues left unresolved.

Internal consistency reliability: The extent to which an instrument's subparts are measuring the same construct.

Internal validity: The extent to which it can be said that the independent variable (i.e., the intervention) causes a change in the dependent variable (i.e., outcome), and the results are not due to other factors or alternative explanations.

Interpretive ethnography: Loosely characterized, a movement within anthropology that generates many hybrid forms of ethnographic work as a result of crossing a variety of theoretical boundaries within social science.

Inter-rater reliability: The degree to which two individuals agree on what they observe.

Interval data: Data that has quantified intervals and equal distances between points, but without a meaningful zero point (e.g., temperature in degrees Fahrenheit); often referred to as continuous data.

Introspection: A process of recognizing and examining one's own inner state or feelings.

K

Key informant: A select informant/assistant with extensive or specialized knowledge of his/her own culture.

L

Level I evidence: Evidence that is generated from systematic reviews or meta-analyses of all relevant randomized controlled trials or evidence-based clinical practice guidelines based on systematic reviews of randomized controlled trials; the strongest level of evidence to guide clinical practice.

Level II evidence: Evidence generated from at least one well-designed randomized clinical trial (i.e., a true experiment).

Level III evidence: Evidence obtained from well-designed controlled trials without randomization.

Level IV evidence: Evidence from well-designed case-control and cohort studies.

Level V evidence: Evidence from systematic reviews of descriptive and qualitative studies.

Level VI evidence: Evidence from a single descriptive or qualitative study.

Level VII evidence: Evidence from the opinion of authorities and/or reports of expert committees.

Likelihood ratio: The likelihood that a given test result would be expected in patients with a disease compared to the likelihood that the same result would be expected in patients without that disease.

Lived experience: Everyday experience, not as it is conceptualized, but as it is lived (i.e., how it feels).

Loss of subjects to follow up: The proportion of people who started the study but do not complete the study, for whatever reason.

M

Macro level change: Change at a large-scale level (e.g., nation-wide systems or large institutions).

Magnitude of effect: Expressing the size of the relationship between two variables or difference between two groups on a given variable/outcome (i.e., the effect size).

Manipulation checks: Assessments verifying that subjects have actually processed the experimental information that they have received or followed through with prescribed intervention activities.

Maturation: Developmental change that occurs, even in the absence of the intervention.

Mean: A measure of central tendency, derived by summing all scores and dividing by the number of participants.

Mediating processes: The mechanisms through which an intervention produces the desired outcome(s).

Mediating variable: The variable or mechanism through which an intervention works to impact the outcome in a study.

Meta-analysis: A process of using quantitative methods to summarize the results from the multiple studies, obtained and critically reviewed using a rigorous process (to minimize bias) for identifying,

appraising, and synthesizing studies to answer a specific question and draw conclusions about the data gathered. The purpose of this process is to gain a summary statistic (i.e., a measure of a single effect) that represents the effect of the intervention across multiple studies.

Method: The theory of how a certain type of research should be carried out (i.e., strategy, approach, process/overall design, and logic of design). Researchers often subsume description of techniques under a discussion of method.

MeSH: MEDLINE®'s controlled vocabulary; Medical Subject Headings.

Micro level change: Change at a small-scale level (e.g., units within a local healthcare organization or small groups of individuals).

N

Narrative analysis: A term that refers to distinct styles of generating, interpreting, and representing data as stories that provide insights into life experiences.

National Guidelines Clearinghouse: A comprehensive database of up-to-date English language evidence-based clinical practice guidelines, developed in partnership with the American Medical Association, the American Association of Health Plans, and the Association for Healthcare Research and Quality.

Naturalistic research: Commitment to the study of phenomena in their naturally occurring settings (contexts).

News embargo: A restriction on the release of any media information about the findings from a study before they are published in a journal article.

NHS Economic Evaluation Database: A register of published economic evaluations of healthcare interventions.

Nominated/snowball sample: A sample obtained with the help of informants already enrolled in the study.

Nonexperimental study design: A study design in which data are collected but whose purpose is not to test the effects of an intervention or treatment on selected outcomes.

Nonhomogeneous sample: A sample comprised of individuals with dissimilar characteristics.

Null hypothesis: There is no relationship between or among study variables.

Number needed to harm (NNH): The number of clients, who, if they received an intervention, would result in one additional person being harmed (i.e., having a bad outcome) compared to the clients in the control arm of a study.

Number needed to treat (NNT): The number of people who would need to receive the experimental therapy to prevent one bad outcome or cause one additional good outcome.

O

Observation continuum: A range of social roles encompassed by participant–observation and ranging from complete observer to complete participant at the extremes.

Observer drift: A decrease in inter-rater reliability.

Occurrence rate: The rate at which an event occurs.

Odds ratio (OR): The odds of a case patient (i.e., someone in the intervention group) being exposed (a/b) divided by the odds of a control patient being exposed (c/d).

Opinion leaders: Individuals who are typically highly knowledgeable and well respected in a system; as such, they are often able to influence change.

Ordinal data: Variables that have ordered categories with intervals that cannot be quantified (e.g., mild, moderate, or severe anxiety).

Outcomes management: The use of process and outcomes data to coordinate and influence actions and processes of care that contribute to patient achievement of targeted behaviors or desired effects.

Outcomes measurement: A generic term used to describe the collection and reporting of information about an observed effect in relation to some care delivery process or health promotion action.

Outcomes research: The use of rigorous scientific methods to measure the effect of some intervention on some outcome(s).

P

Paradigm: A worldview or set of beliefs, assumptions, and values that guides all types of research by identifying where the researcher stands on issues related to the nature of reality (ontology), relationship of the researcher to the researched (epistemology), role of values (axiology), use of language (rhetoric), and process (methodology) (Creswell, 1998).

Participant-observation: Observation and participation in everyday activities in study informants' natural settings.

Participatory action research (PAR): A form of action research that is participatory in nature (i.e., researchers and participants collaborate in problem definition, choice of methods, data analysis, and use of findings); democratic in principle; and reformatory in impulse (i.e., has as its objective the empowerment of persons through the process of constructing and using their own knowledge as a form of consciousness raising with the potential for promoting social action).

Patient preferences: Values the patient holds, concerns the patient has regarding the clinical decision/treatment/situation, choices the patient has/prefers regarding the clinical decision/treatment/situation.

Peer reviewed: Project critiqued by a team of reviewers that has expertise in the subject.

Phenomenologic: Pertaining to the study of essences (i.e., meaning structures) intuited or grasped through descriptions of lived experience.

Phenomenological reduction: An intellectual process involving reflection, imagination, and intuition.

PICO format: A process in which clinical questions are phrased in a manner that yields the most relevant information; P = patient population; I = Intervention of interest; C = Comparison intervention or status; O = Outcome.

Power: The ability of a study design to detect existing relationships between or among variables.

Power analysis: Procedure used for determining the sample size needed for a study.

Prevalence: Refers to the persons in the at-risk population who have the outcome or disorder in a given "snapshot in time."

Principal investigator (PI): The lead person who is responsible and accountable for the scientific integrity of a study as well as the oversight of all elements in the conduct of that study.

Prognosis: The likelihood of a certain outcome.

Purposeful/theoretical sample: A sample intentionally selected in accordance with the needs of the study.

***p* value:** The statistical test of the assumption that there is no difference between an experimental intervention and a control. *p* value indicates the probability of an event given the assumption that there is no true difference. By convention, a *p* value of 0.05 is considered a statistically significant result.

Q

Qualitative data analysis: A variety of techniques that are used to move back and forth between data and ideas throughout the course of the research.

Qualitative data management: The act of designing systems to organize, catalogue, code, store, and retrieve data. System design influences, in turn, how the researcher approaches the task of analysis.

Qualitative description: Description that "entails a kind of interpretation that is low-inference (close to the 'facts'), or likely to result in easier consensus (about the 'facts') among researchers" (Sandelowski, 2000b, p. 335).

Qualitative evaluation: A general term covering a variety of approaches to evaluating programs, projects, policies, and so on using qualitative research techniques.

Qualitative studies: Research that involves the collection of data in nonnumeric form, such as personal interviews, usually with the intention of describing a phenomenon.

Quantitative research: The investigation of phenomena using manipulation of numeric data with statistical analysis. Can be descriptive, predictive, or causal.

Quantitative studies: Research that collects data in numeric form and emphasizes precise measurement of variables; often conducted in the form of rigorously controlled studies.

Quasi-experiments: A type of experimental design that tests the effects of an intervention or treatment but lacks one or more characteristics of a true experiment (e.g., random assignment; a control or comparison group).

R

Random error: Measurement error that occurs without a pattern, without purpose or intent.

Random sampling: Selecting subjects to participate in a study by using a random strategy (e.g., tossing a coin); in this method of selecting subjects, every subject has an equal chance of being selected.

Random assignment (also called randomization): The use of a strategy to randomly assign subjects to the experimental or control groups (e.g., tossing a coin).

Randomized block design: A type of control strategy used in an experimental design that places subjects in equally distributed study groups based on certain characteristics (e.g., age) so that each study group will be similar prior to introduction of the intervention or treatment.

Randomized controlled trial (RCT): A true experiment, (i.e., one that delivers an intervention or treatment), the strongest design to support cause and effect relationships, in which subjects are randomly assigned to control and experimental groups.

Ratio data: The highest level of data; data that has quantified intervals on an infinite scale in which there are equal distances between points and a meaningful zero point (e.g., ounces of water; height); often referred to as continuous data.

Reference population: Those individuals in the past, present, and future to whom the study results can be generalized.

Relative risk (RR): Measures the strength of association and is the risk of the outcome in the exposed group (Re) divided by the risk of the outcome in the unexposed group (Ru). RR is used in prospective studies such as RCTs and cohort studies.

Reliability: The consistency of an instrument in measuring the underlying construct.

Reliability coefficients: A measure of an instrument's reliability (e.g., often computed with a Cronbach alpha).

Reliability of study findings: Whether or not the effects of a study have sufficient influence on practice, clinically and statistically; that is the results can be counted on to make a difference when clinicians apply them to their practice.

Reliable measures : Those that consistently and accurately measure the construct of interest.

Representation: Part of the analytic process that raises the issue of providing a truthful portrayal of what the data represent (e.g.,

essence of an experience; cultural portrait) that will be meaningful to its intended audience.

Research design meeting: A planning meeting held for the purpose of designing a study and strategizing about potential funding as well as the roles of all investigators.

Research subjects review board (RSRB): Often referred to as an institutional review board (IRB); a group of individuals who review a study before it can be conducted to determine the benefits and risks of conducting the research to study participants.

Research utilization: The use of research knowledge, often based on a single study, in clinical practice.

Risk: The probability that a person (currently free from a disease) will develop a disease at some point.

Risk ratio: See relative risk.

Rules of evidence: Standard criteria for the evaluation of domains of evidence; these are applied to research evidence to assess its validity, the study findings, and its applicability to a patient/system situation.

S

Saturation: The point at which categories of data are full and data collection ceases to provide new information.

Saturation level: The level at which a searcher no longer finds any new references, but instead, is familiar and knowledgeable with the literature.

Semiotics: The theory and study of signs and symbols applied to the analysis of systems of patterned communication.

Semistructured interviews: Formal interviews that provide more interviewer control and question format structure but retain a conversational tone and allow informants to answer in their own ways.

Sensitivity: The probability of a diagnostic test finding disease among those who have the disease or the proportion of people with disease who have a positive test result (true positive).

SnNout: When a test has a high **Sen**sitivity, a **N**egative result rules **out** the diagnosis.

Sociolinguistics: The study of the use of speech in social life.

Solomon four group design: A type of experimental study design that uses a before-after design for the first two experimental groups and an after-only design for the second experimental and control groups so that it can separate the effects of pretesting the subjects on the outcome measure(s).

Specificity: The probability of a diagnostic test finding NO disease among those who do NOT have the disease or the proportion of people free of a disease who have a negative test (true negatives).

SpPin: When a test has a high **Sp**ecificity, a **P**ositive result rules **in** the diagnosis.

Standard error: An estimate due to sampling error of the deviation of the sample mean from the true population mean.

Statistical significance: That the results of statistical analysis of data are unlikely to have been caused by chance, at a predetermined level of probability.

Stratification: A strategy that divides the study population into two or more subpopulations and then samples separately from each.

Structured, open-ended interviews: Formal interviews with little flexibility in the way that questions are asked but with question formats that allow informants to respond on their own terms (e.g., "What does.... mean to you?" "How do you feel/think about...?").

Symbolic interaction: Theoretical perspective on how social reality is created by human interaction through ongoing, taken-for-granted processes of symbolic communication.

Systematic review: A summary of evidence, typically conducted by an expert or expert panel on a particular topic, that uses a rigorous process (to minimize bias) for identifying, appraising, and synthesizing studies to answer a specific clinical question and draw conclusions about the data gathered.

T

Techniques: Tools or procedures used to generate or analyze data (e.g., interviewing, observation, standardized tests and measures, constant comparison, document analysis, content analysis, statistical analysis). Techniques are method-neutral and may be used, as appropriate, in any research design—either qualitative or quantitative.

Test–retest reliability: A test of an instrument's stability over time assessed by repeated measurements over time.

Textword: A word that is not a part of the database's controlled vocabulary/thesaurus. Textwords are searched only in titles and abstracts. Sometimes called keywords.

Thematic analysis: Systematic description of recurring ideas or topics (themes) that represent different, yet related, aspects of a phenomenon.

Theoretical framework: The basis upon which a study is guided; its purpose is to provide a context for selecting the study's variables, including how they relate to one another as well as to guide the development of an intervention in experimental studies.

Theoretical generalizability: See transferability.

Theoretical sampling: Decision making, while concurrently collecting and analyzing data, about what further data and data sources are needed to develop the emerging theory.

Theoretical sensitivity: A conceptual process to accompany techniques for generating grounded theory (Glaser, 1978).

Theoretic interest: A desire to know or understand it better.

Thick description: Description that does more than describe human experiences by beginning to interpret what they mean, involving detailed reports of what people say and do, incorporating the textures and feelings of the physical and social worlds in which people move, with reference to that context (i.e., an interpretation of what their words and actions mean).

Transferability: Demonstrated by information that is sufficient for a research consumer to determine whether findings are meaningful to other people in similar situations (analytic or theoretical *vs.* statistical generalizability).

True experiment: A strongest type of experimental design for testing cause and effect relationships: true experiments possess three characteristics: (1) a treatment or intervention; (2) a control or comparison group; and (3) random assignment.

Type 1 error: Mistakenly rejecting the null hypothesis when it is actually true.

Type 2 error: Mistakenly accepting (not rejecting) the null hypothesis when it is false.

U

Unstructured, open-ended interviews: Informal conversations that allow informants the fullest range of possibilities to describe their experiences, thoughts, and feelings.

V

Validity of study findings: Whether or not the results of the study were obtained via sound scientific methods.

Valid measures: Those that measure the construct that they are intended to measure (e.g., an anxiety measure truly measures anxiety, not depression)

Volunteer sample: A sample obtained by solicitation or advertising for participants who meet study criteria.

Y

Yield: The number of hits obtained by a literature search; this can be per database and/or total yield; there can be several levels of yield (e.g., first yield and final yield, that is, only those studies that were kept for review).

All Cochrane definitions came from
http://www.update-software.com/cochrane/content.htm

index